I0066369

Animal Medicine for Veterinarians

Animal Medicine for Veterinarians

Edited by Andrea Santoro

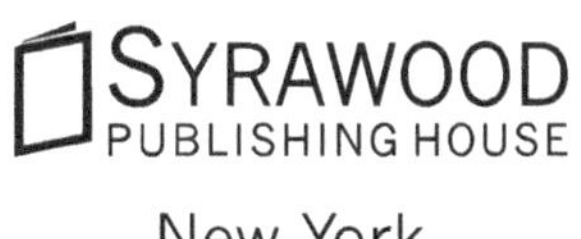

New York

Published by Syrawood Publishing House,
750 Third Avenue, 9th Floor,
New York, NY 10017, USA
www.syrawoodpublishinghouse.com

Animal Medicine for Veterinarians
Edited by Andrea Santoro

International Standard Book Number: 978-1-68286-441-8 (Hardback)

Cataloging-in-publication Data

Animal medicine for veterinarians / edited by Andrea Santoro.
p. cm.
Includes bibliographical references and index.
ISBN 978-1-68286-441-8
1. Veterinary medicine. 2. Veterinarians. 3. Veterinary medicine--Methodology. 4. Animals--Diseases. I. Santoro, Andrea.
SF745 .A55 2017
636.089--dc23

Printed in the United States of America.

TABLE OF CONTENTS

PREFACE

This book elucidates the concepts and innovative models around prospective developments with respect to animal medicine. It includes some of the vital pieces of work being conducted across the world, on various topics related to this subject. Animal medicine concerns itself with the treatment, diagnosis and prevention of diseases that affect animals. Various laboratory tests are conducted to diagnose diseases and treatment plans are formed accordingly. This book explores all the important aspects of animal medicine in the present day scenario. The various studies that are constantly contributing towards advancing technologies and evolution of this field are examined in detail in the book. It will help veterinarians by foregrounding their knowledge in this branch. It will serve as a valuable source of reference for graduate and post graduate students.

This book has been the outcome of endless efforts put in by authors and researchers on various issues and topics within the field. The book is a comprehensive collection of significant researches that are addressed in a variety of chapters. It will surely enhance the knowledge of the field among readers across the globe.

It gives us an immense pleasure to thank our researchers and authors for their efforts to submit their piece of writing before the deadlines. Finally in the end, I would like to thank my family and colleagues who have been a great source of inspiration and support.

Editor

PREFACE

Causes of Morbidity in Wild Raptor Populations Admitted at a Wildlife Rehabilitation Centre in Spain from 1995-2007

Rafael A. Molina-López[1,2], Jordi Casal[2,3], Laila Darwich[2,3]*

1 Centre de Fauna Salvatge de Torreferrussa, Catalan Wildlife-Service, Forestal Catalana, Spain, 2 Departament de Sanitat i Anatomia Animals, Faculty of Veterinary, Universitat Autònoma de Barcelona, Barcelona, Spain, 3 Centre de Recerca en Sanitat Animal, UAB-IRTA, Campus Universitat Autònoma de Barcelona, Barcelona, Spain

Abstract

Background: Morbidity studies complement the understanding of hazards to raptors by identifying natural or anthropogenic factors. Descriptive epidemiological studies of wildlife have become an important source of information about hazards to wildlife populations. On the other hand, data referenced to the overall wild population could provide a more accurate assessment of the potential impact of the morbidity/mortality causes in populations of wild birds.

Methodology/Principal Findings: The present study described the morbidity causes of hospitalized wild raptors and their incidence in the wild populations, through a long term retrospective study conducted at a wildlife rehabilitation centre of Catalonia (1995–2007). Importantly, Seasonal Cumulative Incidences (SCI) were calculated considering estimations of the wild population in the region and trend analyses were applied among the different years. A total of 7021 birds were analysed: 7 species of Strigiformes (n = 3521) and 23 of Falconiformes (n = 3500). The main causes of morbidity were trauma (49.5%), mostly in the Falconiformes, and orphaned/young birds (32.2%) mainly in the Strigiformes. During wintering periods, the largest morbidity incidence was observed in *Accipiter gentillis* due to gunshot wounds and in *Tyto alba* due to vehicle trauma. Within the breeding season, *Falco tinnunculus* (orphaned/young category) and *Bubo bubo* (electrocution and metabolic disorders) represented the most affected species. Cases due to orphaned/young, infectious/parasitic diseases, electrocution and unknown trauma tended to increase among years. By contrast, cases by undetermined cause, vehicle trauma and captivity decreased throughout the study period. Interestingly, gunshot injuries remained constant during the study period.

Conclusions/Significance: Frequencies of morbidity causes calculated as the proportion of each cause referred to the total number of admitted cases, allowed a qualitative assessment of hazards for the studied populations. However, cumulative incidences based on estimated wild raptor population provided a more accurate approach to the potential ecological impact of the morbidity causes in the wild populations.

Editor: Justin David Brown, University of Georgia, United States of America

Funding: The study has been supported by the Catalan Wildlife-Service and Forestal Catalana. The funders had no role in study design, data collection and analysis, decision to publish, or preparation of the manuscript.

Competing Interests: The authors have declared that no competing interests exist.

* E-mail: laila.darwich@uab

Introduction

Birds of prey are valuable sentinels of environmental changes because of their position at the top of the ecological food chain and because they are widespread across large geographical areas. In addition, they are particularly sensitive to ecological changes at a range of spatial scales [1,2] and, as such, some species of free-living birds of prey and owls have decreased in numbers and become threatened or even endangered around the world. In fact, in Europe, 36 species (64%) of the total 56 different raptor species have an unfavourable conservation status [3].

Morbidity studies complement the understanding of hazards to raptors by identifying natural or anthropogenic factors. Therefore, the analysis of morbidity and mortality reports of free-living raptors presented to rehabilitation centres has provided insight into the primary and secondary causes, as well as in the evaluation of the health status of wild populations [4,5]. However, there are few studies on morbidity in wild raptors of Spain, and these have focused on a limited number of species or specific causes [6–10]. In addition, global epidemiological studies of wild raptor diseases are also scarce, especially long term studies [11,12]. Finally, while the information reported by such studies is critical for the rehabilitation centres management, this information has been mainly based on the proportion of cases in the total number of admissions at the centre. Only rarely have the data been referenced to the overall wild population, that could provide a more accurate assessment of the potential impact of the morbidity/mortality causes in populations of wild birds.

The purpose of this study was to analyze the causes of morbidity in a large population of raptors admitted at one rehabilitation centre in Spain from 1995 to 2007 using specific epidemiological data (species, gender, age, season, and year) as well as the Seasonal

Cumulative Incidences (SCI) considering estimations of the wild population in the region for the different raptor species.

Results

Descriptive analyses

A total of 7553 admission reports were reviewed. Of those, 532 cases were excluded for not fulfilling the inclusion criteria. Thus, the final study population was 7021 individuals homogenously distributed in two orders: Order Strigiformes with 3521 animals corresponding to seven species of owls and Order Falconiformes with 3500 animals of 23 different diurnal raptor species. The majority of animals (89.5%, n = 6282) were alive when admitted. Within the species represented in the study, there were some important species catalogued as "in danger of extinction" (*Gypaetus barbatus*) and "vulnerable" (*Circus pygargus, Achila fasciata, Milvus milvus, Neophron percnopterus and Pandion haliaetus*) by the Spanish Catalogue of Menaced Species [13].

Most of the animals, 58.7% (n = 4119), were classified as undetermined gender, 22.5% (n = 1579) of raptors were sexed as female (F) and 18.8% (n = 1323) as males (M). Within the undetermined gender group, the majority of birds belonged to the Strigiformes order, representing 67% (2746/4119) of birds; the remaining 33% (1373/4119) of undetermined sex belonged to the Falconiformes order. Only three species -*Achila fasciata, Accipiter nisus* and *Otus scops*- showed significant differences between genders with ratios of 6F/15M ($\chi^2 = 105$, $P = 0.0001$), 329F/96M ($\chi^2 = 4.69$, $P = 0.03$) and 91F/61M ($\chi^2 = 12.58$, $P = 0.0004$), respectively.

The age distribution showed that 44% (3091/7021) of birds were within the first year calendar, 32.7% (2294/7021) > 1 year calendar and 23.4% (1636/7021) were of unknown age (Table 1). The dynamic of cases throughout the study period showed a homogenous entry of cases per year (ranging from 478 to 643 cases), with similar number of cases of raptors by order, gender and age among the different years (Fig. 1).

Distribution of primary causes of morbidity

The two most frequent causes of admission were trauma (49.5%; 95% CI: 48.3–50.7) and orphaned young birds (32.2%; 95% CI: 31.1–33.3). The other primary causes had frequencies below 10% (Table 2). Trauma was more frequently observed in Falconiformes. This order showed the highest risk of gunshot or electrocution. Risks of falling into traps, power lines or being predated were similar between both raptor orders and traumas with motor vehicles and fences were considerably higher in nocturnal raptors likely due to their habit of hunting along roads and their feature to be easily dazzled (Table 2). It is interesting to note that owls and *Falco tinnunculus* ($\chi^2 = 21.39$, $P < 0.0001$) represented the largest group of animals found inside buildings (Table 3), while most of *Accipiter gentillis* birds were captured inside chicken farms ($\chi^2 = 153.70$, $P < 0.0001$). Trichomoniasis was the most frequent cause of infectious/parasitic disease with positive cases in the following species: *Falco tinnunculus* (19 cases), *Strix aluco* (7), *Tyto alba* (5), *Accipiter gentillis* (5), *Falco peregrinus* (4), and *Accipiter nisus, Circus pygargus, Bubo bubo* and *Achila fasciata* with 1 case each, respectively (Table 2). Fatal intoxication was diagnosed in: *Gyps fulvus* for lead toxicity (1), *Tyto alba* for Bromodiolone (2), *Buteo buteo* (2) and *Circaeuts gallicus* (1) for carbofuran, and *Falco naumanni* for cipermetrine (1).

No differences between genders related to any of the analyzed causes were observed ($\chi^2 = 17.73$, $P > 0.05$). However, the first year calendar group had a higher risk of metabolic and nutritional diseases (OR = 3.7; 95%CI: 2.7–5.1), and infectious diseases (OR = 3.1; 95%CI: 1.95–4.85) compared to older birds. Conversely, the >1 year calendar group had a slightly higher risk of trauma with motor vehicles (OR = 1.36; 95%CI: 1.01–1.76) compared to the other age groups.

Seasonality of specific causes of morbidity

A significantly higher number of cases were detected during the breeding period ($\chi^2 = 1226.97$, $P < 0.001$), mainly due to orphaned young birds (Table 4). Metabolic or nutritional disease was significantly lower during the wintering season. Gunshot was concentrated during the autumn-winter hunting season (87.2%). Only 3.2% (22/689) of gunshot cases were recorded during the small game period at the end of August. The remaining 9.6% of cases (66/689) were detected out of hunting season. No statistically significant differences were observed among proportions of infectious/parasitic ($\chi^2 = 1.76$, $P > 0.05$), fortuity ($\chi^2 = 2.46$, $P > 0.05$) and electrocution ($\chi^2 = 5.88$, $P > 0.05$) casualties.

Seasonal cumulative incidence (SCI) of the overall causes of admission regarding the main raptor species (those with at least 100 cases) are summarized in Table 5. The highest number of incidences during the wintering period was observed in *Accipiter gentillis* mainly due to gunshot and *Tyto alba* due to vehicle trauma. Species such as *Falco tinnunculus* (mainly due to orphaned young) and *Bubo bubo* (due to electrocution and metabolic disorders) represented the highest affected populations during the breeding season (Table 5).

Inter-years distribution of specific causes of morbidity

The number of admissions increased throughout the study period and a significant increase of cases was observed among the twelve years of the study in orphaned young birds, infectious/parasitic diseases, electrocution and unknown trauma. By contrast, a decreasing tendency was observed in the number of admissions due to undetermined cause, trauma with vehicles and captivity (Fig. 2).

Discussion

Descriptive epidemiological studies of wildlife are an important source of information about natural and non-natural hazards to the wild animal population. In addition, studies of the causes of mortality and morbidity in wildlife have become an important source for ecosystem health monitoring [14,15]. However, there are still important limitations of the information available due to lack of randomization, overrepresentation of human induced casualties, the heterogeneity of analytical methods [7,16] and the low number of cases of free-living birds of prey reported [4,5,8,17,18]. Moreover, in most studies, disease frequency is estimated as a proportion of the cases of disease in the total number of admissions at the centres, lacking any information concerning the wild bird population and the particular risk for each species in the area of study.

The data presented in the current study were based on a large number of cases of very diverse wild raptor species, admitted to a wildlife rehabilitation centre during a long term period (12 years). Besides descriptive frequencies of morbidity cases admitted at the centre, the data included Seasonal Cumulative Incidences (SCI) based on the estimated wild raptor populations, for both wintering and breeding seasons. Thus, depending on the type of analyses performed, different information and conclusions can be obtained. Whereas, disease frequencies of morbidity entities (calculated as the proportion of each cause referred to the overall number of admitted cases) could allow a qualitative assessment of the hazards, the SCI (based on estimated wild raptor population) provides a more accurate approach to the potential ecological impact of the

Table 1. Frequency of admission in the rehabilitation centre and demographic data of raptors included in the study during the period 1995-2007.

Species descriptive: Common name (*scientific name*)	**Cases**	**Sex**		**Age (one year calendar)**		
Order Strigiformes	**Number**	**F/M***	**Unknown**	**<1 year**	**>1 year**	**Unknown**
Family Tytonidae						
Common barn owl (*Tyto alba*)	500	81/74	345	157	174	169
Family Strigidae						
Eurasian scops owl (*Otus scops*)	878	61/91	726	655	129	94
Eurasian eagle-owl (*Bubo bubo*)	198	54/62	82	28	110	60
Tawny owl (*Strix aluco*)	731	56/63	612	475	168	88
Little owl (*Athene noctua*)	1120	98/107	915	729	220	171
Northern long-eared owl (*Asio otus*)	82	18/7	57	19	25	38
Short-eared owl (*Asio flammeus*)	12	2/1	9	0	6	6
Order Falconiformes						
Family Pandionidae						
Osprey (*Pandion haliaetus*)	6	1/2	3	1	3	2
Family Accipitridae						
Western Honey-buzzard (*Pernis apivorus*)	61	12/8	41	19	22	20
Red kite (*Milvus milvus*)	7	1/6	17	1	4	2
Black kite (*Milvus migrans*)	24	1/1	5	6	7	11
Bearded vulture (*Gypaetus barbatus*)	2	0/2	0	0	2	0
Egyptian vulture (*Neophron percnopterus*)	2	0/0	2	1	1	0
Eurasian griffon (*Gyps fulvus*)	49	2/4	43	16	17	16
Short-toed Snake-eagle (*Circaetus gallicus*)	52	10/10	32	3	34	15
Western Marsh-harrier (*Circus aeruginosus*)	38	20/10	8	3	22	13
Hen harrier (*Circus cyaneus*)	14	6/4	4	0	11	3
Montagu's harrier (*Circus pygargus*)	13	3/8	2	8	5	0
Eurasian Sparrowhawk (*Accipiter nisus*)	466	329/96	41	103	227	136
Northern Goshawk (*Accipiter gentillis*)	231	108/84	39	93	106	32
Eurasian buzzard (*Buteo buteo*)	934	245/210	479	71	413	450
Golden eagle (*Aquila chrysaetos*)	7	3/3	1	1	5	1
Bonelli's eagle (*Aquila fasciata*)	31	6/15	10	6	16	9
Booted eagle (*Aquila pennata*)	30	5/10	15	4	17	9
Family Falconidae						
Lesser kestrel (*Falco naumanni*)	88	28/27	33	54	26	8
Common kestrel (*Falco tinnunculus*)	1295	382/361	552	591	451	253
Red-footed falco (*Falco vespertinus*)	2	1/1	0	0	2	0
Merlin (*Falco columbarius*)	7	3/3	1	0	4	3
Eurasian hobby (*Falco subbuteo*)	35	5/10	20	3	21	11
Peregrine falcon (*Falco peregrinus*)	106	38/43	25	44	46	16
Total	**7021**	**1579/1323**	**4119**	**3091**	**2294**	**1636**

*F/M, female/male ratio.

morbidity/mortality causes in the wild populations than the raw data.

Based on the present data it is evident that the anthropogenic origin was confirmed as the most frequent cause of hospitalization, comprising direct persecution (gunshot, poisoning, illegal captivity or traps) to involuntary human induced threats (collisions with vehicles, fences or electric lines and electrocution). Another clear finding was the high numbers of young orphaned cases admitted to the centre, which represented 32% of the total cases, and the fact that these cases increased throughout the study period. These values slightly differ from the ones reported by others [5,17]. One of the most significant characteristics of this region is the large diversity of bird populations, in part due to its location within the migratory routes, in part to the great variety of habitats. On the other hand, this region is highly populated, and species with nesting areas close to urban settlements and other buildings are the most likely to be found and brought to the wildlife rehabilitation centres. In fact, *Falco tinnunculus* and *Otus scops*, the species with higher SCI for the orphaned category, use man-made structures to nest and so are directly exposed to anthropogenic interaction.

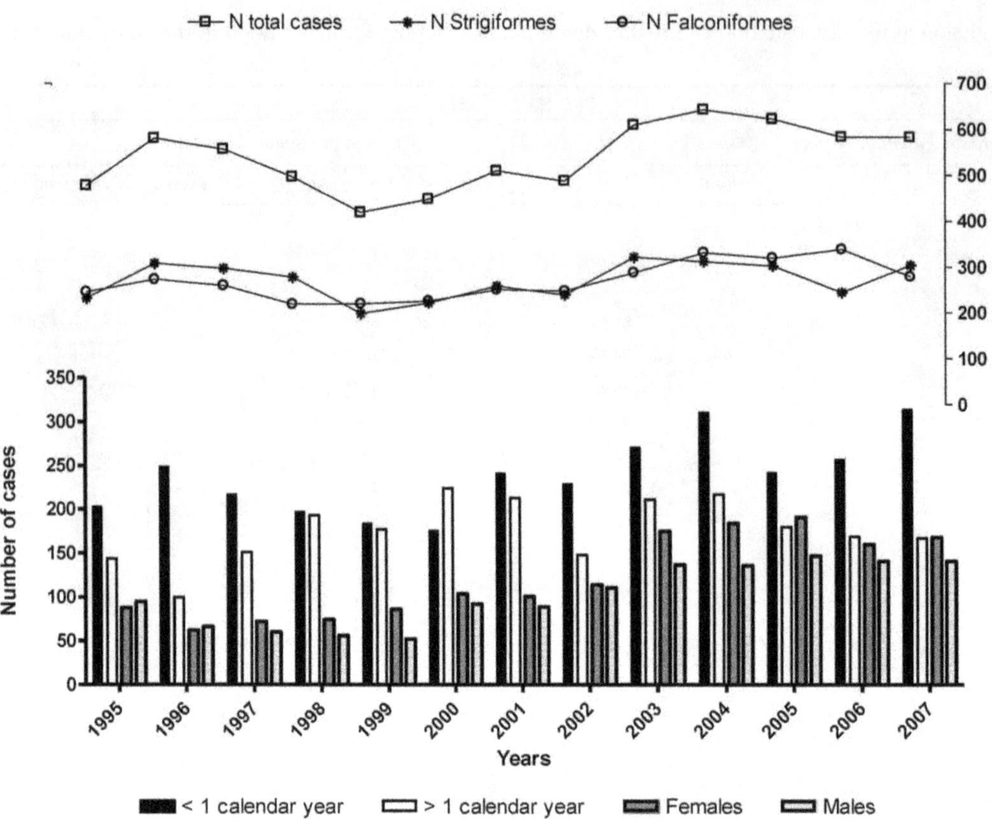

Figure 1. Admissions of birds of prey stratifying by raptor order, age and sex, yearly distributed along the period 1995-2007.

The analysis of data collected during the period of this study revealed that the number of animals with known information about age and gender increased in the later years of the study, indicating an improvement in data examination and collection by the centre. The high number of specimens with undetermined gender (67%), especially in birds belonging to the Strigiformes order, was mainly due to the high number of young or immature animals seen at the centre.

Trauma represented the main cause of admission (50% of cases, 60% when excluding orphaned bird category), with a prevalence similar to that described in other studies [4,5,8,17–19]. The main source of traumas was either anthropogenic origin or unknown. The unknown trauma have been reported in very different proportions in the published reports, ranging from 32% of cases in *Accipiter nisus* [19] to 84% of cases in *Falco peregrinus* [20] and could be due to the different classification of the cases in the different studies.

Within the trauma category, gunshot represented the most common cause of admission (10% of the total). Although considerably lower than the 36% reported by Martínez et al. (2001) [8] in the East of Spain, it is of relevance that almost 10% of the casualties have been recorded out of the hunting season, as indication of deliberate prosecution. Even though birds of prey are legally protected species under Spanish law, shooting is still a major concern, especially in endangered species such as *Achila fasciata, Pandion haliaetus and Circus pygargus*. Interestingly, *Accipiter gentillis* and *Falco peregrinus* showed the highest SCI for gunshot. Both species have traditionally been considered as competing with small game hunters, and those values are again indication of deliberate shooting [21].

On the other hand, collision trauma with vehicle (8%) was the second highest cause of trauma, although in a lower proportion than previously reported in other studies [5,17,18]. This difference might be due to the high diversity of species analysed in the present study. Basically, the highest incidence of collision has been observed in owls -basically in *Athene noctua*, *Tyto alba* and *Strix aluco*- during the breeding and post-breeding period, which agrees with the results by Frías (1999) [22]. When we analyzed the SCI during the winter season, the highest risk was for *Tyto alba*, reinforcing the major vulnerability of this species for collision trauma [23]. In the Falconiformes order, *Buteo buteo* was the most affected species. This high risk could be related to its scavenging behaviour in the vicinity of roads. Moreover, we have also observed a winter peak of admissions in *Buteo buteo* and *Tyto alba*, possibly related to higher densities of these migratory species at this time of the year.

Another important cause of trauma was electrocution representing approximately 6% of the cases which is higher than studies in other areas [5,17,18]. The species distribution obtained in our study coincides with data published previously in Catalonia [24,25]. *Bubo bubo* was the most affected owl with the highest SCI value, highlighting the potential impact of electrocutions in their wild population [9]. For diurnal raptors, the highest SCI was for *Accipiter gentillis* during winter and *Buteo buteo* in the breeding season. Both species have similar anatomical features that make them highly vulnerable to electrocution. On the other hand, we found a higher percentage of electrocutions in *Falco tinnunculus* compared to a previous report in Spain [26]. Despite the small size of this falcon, the perching behaviour of this species is a well-known risk factor that could explain the present results.

Captivity of birds of prey, especially Falconiformes, is still an important cause of admission in Spain [8]. However, the frequency was clearly lower than the 18% reported by Martínez et al. (2001) [8]. Noteworthy, the most commonly captive species was Falco *tinnunculus* -mostly related with illegal trade of birds and

Table 2. Frequency of primary causes of admission and statistical comparison between Strigiformes and Falconiformes orders.

	Overall Prevalence		Strigiformes (N = 3521)		Falconiformes (N = 3500)		Odds Ratio (OR)	
Primary Causes	**Total number**	**Percentage (95% CI)**	**Total number (%)**	**Percentage**	**Total number (%)**	**Percentage**	**OR (CI 95%)**	**p-value**
Trauma:	3476	49.5 (48.3–50.7)	1182 (33.6)	100	2294(65.5)	100	0.3 (0.2–0.3)	<0.0001
Unknown	1817	25.9 (24.8–26.9)	694 (19.7)	58.7	1123 (32.1)	49	1.4 (1.2–1.7)	<0.0001
Gunshot	689	9.8 (9.1–10.5)	48 (1.4)	4.1	641 (18.3)	27.9	0.1 (0.08–0.1)	<0.0001
Vehicles	571	8.1 (7.5–8.7)	322 (9.1)	27.2	249 (7.1)	10.9	3.0 (2.5–3.6)	<0.0001
Electrocution	281	4.0 (3.5–4.5)	60 (1.7)	5.1	221 (6.3)	6.3	0.5 (0.3–0.6)	<0.0001
Buildings	58	0.8 (0.6–1)	28 (0.8)	2.4	30 (0.9)	1.3	1.8 (1.1–3.1)	<0.010
Traps	19	0.3 (0.2–0.4)	5 (0.1)	0.4	14 (0.4)	0.6	0.7 (0.2–1.9)	ns
Fences	24	0.3 (0.2–0.5)	21 (0.6)	1.8	3 (0.1)	0.2	13.8 (4.1–46.4)	<0.0001
Power lines	11	0.2 (0.1–0.3)	2 (0.1)	0.2	9 (0.3)	0.4	0.4 (0.1–1.9)	ns
Predation	6	0.1 (0.05–0.2)	2 (0.1)	0.2	4 (0.1)	0.2	0.9 (0.1–5.3)	ns
Orphaned young	2260	32.2 (31.1–33.29)	1768 (50.2)	100	492 (14.1)	100	6.1 (5.4–6.9)	<0.0001
Fortuity:	398	5.7 (5.1–6.2)	249 (7.1)	100	149 (4.3)	100	1.7 (1.3–2.1)	<0.0001
Buildings	289	4.1 (3.6–4.6)	191	76.7	98	65.8	1.7 (1.1–2.6)	0.0179
Others[a]	65	0.9 (0.7–0.2)	37	14.9	28	18.8	0.7 (0.4–1.3)	ns
Water ponds	44	0.6 (0.4–0.8)	21	8.4	23	15.4	0.5 (0.2–0.9)	0.0311
Undetermined	379	5.4 (4.8–5.9)	161 (4.6)	100	218 (6.2)	100	0.7 (0.5–0.8)	<0.005
Metabolic/nutritional:	235	3.3 (2.9–3.8)	76 (2.2)	100	159 (4.5)	100	0.4 (0.3–0.6)	<0.0001
Emaciation	151	2.1 (1.8–2.5)	52	68.4	99	62.3	1.3 (0.7–2.3)	ns
Others[b]	48	0.6 (0.5–0.9)	16	21.1	32	20.1	1.4 (0.7–2.6)	ns
MBD	36	0.5 (0.3–0.7)	8	10.5	28	17.6	0.5 (0.2–1.2)	ns
Captivity	158	2.3 (1.9–2.6)	47 (1.3)	100	111 (3.2)	100	0.2 (0.1–0.2)	<0.0001
Infectious/parasitic:	108	1.5 (1.2–1.8)	34(1)	100	74(2.1)	100	0.4 (0.2–0.6)	<0.0001
Others[c]	55	0.7 (0,5–1)	21	61.8	34	45.9	1.9 (0.8–4.3)	ns
Trichomoniosis	44	0.6 (0,4–0.8)	13	38.2	31	41.9	0.8 (0.3–1.9)	ns
Toxicoses	7	0.1 (na)	4 (0.1)	100	3 (0.1)	100	1.3 (0.3–5.9)	ns

CI: confidence interval. ns: no statistical significance (p>0.05). na: not applicable. MBD, metabolic bone diseases. Others:
a, manure heaps, bad weather;
b, rest of diagnoses grouped by organic systems such as musculoskeletal, digestive, nervous, integument, and ocular diseases;
c, mycobacteriosis, helminthiasis, mites, abscess.

falconry- followed by *Athene noctua* and *Otus scops*. Both owl species were probably captured when young birds and kept as pets in captivity. Finally, the proportion of undetermined causes showed similar values to other retrospective surveys [11,18,20], indicating that the lack of obtaining a specific diagnosis in birds of prey is around 10% of the total admissions.

Data from rehabilitation centres based on live birds is useful for detecting primary infectious or parasitic diseases. Digestive tract disease caused by *Trichomonas gallinae* was the most frequent disease observed in both diurnal raptors and owls, in agreement with Wendell et al. (2002) [5].

Trichomoniasis was diagnosed by both direct examination and cytology (Diff-Quick stained) of scraping of oral or upper digestive tract lesions. Since we have focused our study in primary causes of admissions, the role of underlying infectious or parasitic diseases has been underestimated, because of no complete microbiological and parasitological analyses were done routinely in all cases due to financial constraints, autolysis or the statement of a primary diagnosis. Finally, intoxication was anecdotally included in our study due to financial limitations in the diagnosis.

Analysis of the principal causes of morbidity throughout the twelve years of study showed a decrease in the undetermined cause category that could be an indication of an improvement in the quality of the diagnostic protocols and staff experience. Similarly, the increase of hospitalized cases by electrocution and the decrease of casualties by captivity could be explained by increased efficiency of the wildlife police services. As suggested above, the increase of cases in the young orphaned category could be related to both the human demographic traits of Catalonia and a better knowledge by the inhabitants about the role of wildlife rehabilitation centres. On the other hand, the increased cases by unknown trauma could be due to a greater participation of people taking care of injured animals, but also suggest the difficulty in the trauma classification. Another interesting finding was that gunshot fatalities have become stable over the years, pointing out the enormous deficiencies in the police investigative process and the necessity of stronger legal action from the relevant authorities.

In conclusion, the long term epidemiological research conducted at the wildlife rehabilitation center determined the main environmental and anthropogenic causes of morbidity in wild raptor populations of Catalonia. In addition, the weight of different epidemiological markers such as the seasonal cumulative incidence can provide more accurate statistics about the dynamics of wild raptor populations in the studied area.

Table 3. Number of cases and frequency distribution by primary causes of admission and species.

	TRAUMA: Number of cases (%)									OTHERS: Number of cases (%)							
Species	**Unknown**	**Gunshot**	**Vehicles**	**Electrocuted**	**Building**	**Fences**	**Traps**	**Power Lines**	**Predation**	**Orphaned young**	**Fortuity**	**Undetermined**	**Metabolic diseases**	**Captivity**	**Infectious diseases**	**Toxicity**	**Total**
Accipiter gentillis	65 (28)	77 (33)	4 (2)	12 (5)	1 (0)	0	1 (0)	0	1 (0)	11 (5)	25 (11)	16 (7)	5 (2)	8 (4)	5 (2)	0	**231**
Accipiter nisus	224 (48)	122 (26)	26 (6)	1 (0)	20 (4)	2 (0)	1 (0)	1 (0)	0	12 (3)	11 (2)	27 (6)	7 (1)	5 (1)	7 (2)	0	**466**
Aquila chrysaetos	3 (43)	0	0	1 (14)	0	0	0	0	0	0	0	3 (43)	0	0	0	0	**7**
Asio flameus	6 (50)	6 (50)	0	0	0	0	0	0	0	0	0	0	0	0	0	0	**12**
Asio otus	37 (45)	7 (8)	9 (11)	1 (1)	0	2 (2)	0	0	0	13 (16)	5 (6)	4 (5)	4 (5)	0	0	0	**82**
Athene noctua	255 (23)	16 (1)	105 (9)	4 (0)	6 (1)	5 (0)	3 (0)	0	0	585 (52)	59 (5)	43 (4)	16 (1)	18 (2)	5 (1)	0	**1120**
Bubo bubo	49 (25)	8 (4)	16 (8)	48 (24)	0	10 (5)	0	2 (1)	0	13 (7)	20 (10)	12 (6)	14 (7)	3 (2)	3 (2)	0	**198**
Buteo buteo	279 (30)	272 (29)	138 (15)	79 (8)	0	0	1 (0)	3 (0)	1 (0)	16 (2)	26 (3)	62 (7)	32 (3)	13 (1)	11 (1)	1 (0)	**934**
Circaetus gallicus	18 (35)	2 (4)	3 (6)	15 (29)	0	1 (2)	0	2 (4)	0	1 (2)	1 (2)	5 (10)	2 (4)	0	1 (2)	1 (2)	**52**
Circus aeruginosus	17 (45)	6 (16)	0	0	0	0	0	0	0	0	4 (10)	6 (16)	4 (11)	0	1 (3)	0	**38**
Circus cyaneus	6 (43)	6 (43)	0	0	0	0	0	0	0	1 (7)	0	1 (7)	0	0	0	0	**14**
Circus pygargus	7 (54)	1 (8)	0	0	0	0	0	0	0	0	0	1 (8)	1 (8)	0	3 (23)	0	**13**
Falco columbarius	4 (57)	2 (29)	0	0	0	0	0	0	0	0	1 (14)	0	0	0	0	0	**7**
Falco naumanni	21 (24)	0	4 (4)	0	0	0	0	0	2 (2)	22 (25)	2 (2)	14 (16)	9 (10)	12 (14)	1 (1)	1 (1)	**88**
Falco peregrinus	30 (28)	28 (26)	6 (6)	9 (8)	0	0	0	1 (1)	0	7 (7)	2 (2)	8 (7)	5 (5)	4 (4)	6 (6)	0	**106**
Falco subbuteo	15 (43)	6 (17)	2 (6)	1 (3)	0	0	0	0	0	0	2 (6)	2 (6)	2 (6)	2 (6)	3 (9)	0	**35**
Falco tinnunculus	373 (29)	89 (7)	54 (4)	87 (7)	6 (1)	0	11 (1)	0	0	415 (32)	63 (5)	54 (4)	45 (3)	66 (5)	32 (3)	0	**1295**
Falco vespertinus	0	0	0	0	1 (50)	0	0	0	0	0	0	1 (50)	0	0	0	0	**2**
Gypaetus barbatus	2 (100)	0	0	0	0	0	0	0	0	0	0	0	0	0	0	0	**2**
Gyps fulvus	6 (12)	3 (6)	2 (4)	0	0	0	0	0	0	2 (4)	0	2 (4)	33 (67)	0	1 (2)	0	**49**
Hieraetus fasciatus	7 (23)	4 (13)	0	5 (16)	0	0	0	1 (3)	0	0	2 (7)	8 (26)	2 (6)	0	2 (7)	0	**31**
Hieraetus pennatus	8 (27)	12 (40)	1 (3)	5 (17)	0	0	0	0	0	2 (7)	0	0	1 (3)	1 (3)	0	0	**30**
Milvus migrans	9 (37)	0	5 (21)	1 (4)	0	0	0	1 (4)	0	1 (4)	4 (17)	1 (4)	1 (4)	0	1 (4)	0	**24**
Milvus milvus	1 (14)	1 (14)	0	3 (43)	0	0	0	0	0	1 (14)	0	1 (14)	0	0	0	0	**7**
Neophron percnopterus	1 (50)	0	0	0	0	0	0	0	0	0	0	1 (50)	0	0	0	0	**2**
Otus scops	127 (14)	0	37 (4)	0	8 (1)	1 (0)	0	0	1 (0)	586 (67)	55 (6)	28 (3)	11 (1)	17 (2)	7 (1)	0	**878**
Pandion haliaetus	0	1 (17)	0	1 (17)	0	0	0	0	0	0	1 (17)	2 (33)	1 (17)	0	0	0	**6**
Pernis apivorus	27 (44)	9 (15)	4 (7)	1 (2)	2 (3)	0	0	0	0	1 (2)	5 (8)	3 (5)	9 (15)	0	0	0	**61**
Strix aluco	88 (12)	2 (0)	76 (10)	2 (0)	3 (0)	2 (0)	0	0	1 (0)	441 (60)	61 (8)	30 (4)	12 (2)	4 (1)	9 (1)	0	**731**
Tyto alba	132 (26)	9 (2)	79 (16)	5 (1)	11 (2)	1 (0)	2 (1)	0	0	130 (26)	49 (10)	44 (9)	19 (4)	5 (1)	10 (2)	4 (1)	**500**
Total	**1817**	**689**	**571**	**281**	**58**	**24**	**19**	**11**	**6**	**2260**	**398**	**379**	**235**	**158**	**108**	**7**	**7021**

Table 4. Intra-year distribution of primary causes of admission at the wildlife center according to seasonal periods (cases registered from 1995 to 2007).

Cause category	Breeding		Post-nuptial migration		Wintering		Total
	n	%	n	%	n	%	n
Orphaned young	1994	53.7	224	14.9	42	2.3	2260
Unknown trauma	672	18.1	503	33.5	642	35.5	1817
Gunshot	41	1.1	171	11.4	477	26.4	689
Motor vehicles	215	5.8	140	9.3	216	11.9	571
Fortuity	212	5.7	95	6.3	91	5.0	398
Undetermined	168	4.5	95	6.3	116	6.4	379
Electrocution	132	3.6	60	4.0	89	4.9	281
Metabolic/nutritional	102	2.7	103	6.9	30	1.7	235
Illegal	64	1.7	43	2.9	51	2.8	158
Infectious	60	1.6	26	1.7	22	1.2	108
Others (<100 cases)							
Trauma with building	23	0.6	20	1.3	15	0.8	58
Fences	8	0.2	6	0.4	10	0.6	24
Trap	9	0.2	6	0.4	4	0.2	19
Power lines	3	0.1	5	0.3	3	0.2	11
Intoxication	5	0.1	2	0.1	0	0.0	7
Predation	4	0.1	1	0.1	1	0.1	6
Total	**3712**	**100**	**1500**	**100**	**1809**	**100**	**7021**

Materials and Methods

Study design and animals

A retrospective study was performed using the original medical records of birds of prey admitted at the Wildlife Rehabilitation Centre of Torreferrussa from 1995 to 2007. The centre receives animals from all of Catalonia (North-East Spain, 3°19′-0°9′ E and 42°51′-40°31 N), mainly from the South and Central areas. More than thirty species of diurnal raptors and eight different owl species have been observed in this area, most of which are breeding species [27].

The centre directly depends on the governmental Catalan Wildlife-Service. Thus, protocols, amendments and other resources were done according to the guidelines approved by the government of Catalonia.

Definition of variables

Species, gender, age, date and primary cause of admission were included in the data analyses. Sex was determined when possible by inspection in dimorphic species [28] or by gonadal examination at necropsy. Age was categorized as "first year calendar" and ">1 year calendar" according to Martínez et al. (2001) [8]. The year was divided into three seasons: breeding (from March to July), post-nuptial migration (August to October) and wintering (November to February).

Our general classification of primary morbidity causes was adapted from different studies [4,5,29] as follows: trauma, infectious/parasitic disease, metabolic/nutritional disease, toxicosis, orphaned young birds, and unknown/undetermined. Two more categories of causes were added: captivity and fortuity. The captivity category included wild birds maintained illegally in captivity for more than 6 months and the fortuity category included all animals with no associated medical primary cause (birds found inside buildings, farms, water ponds, entangled in plants or manure heaps). The orphaned young category integrated chicks and fledging raptors (Table 2). To assign these categories we used different information obtained from different sources: (a) the physical examination performed by the veterinarian at the admission instance; (b) the anamnesis of people that recovered the bird; (c) the medical reports or case history; and when possible (d) from complementary diagnostic tools, as now radiography (basically to corroborate gunshots), blood chemistry and haematology, cytology and toxicology. Post-mortem diagnoses were done when birds arrived dead to the centre, when they had to be euthanized for bad prognoses or died due to the primary cause.

The trauma category was subdivided into: collision, electrocution, gunshot, trap, predation, and unknown trauma (for those cases with clinical signs of trauma but without clear information about the circumstances of the accident). Collision traumas were further subdivided into impacts with motor vehicles, buildings, power lines, fences, and others. The diagnosis of electrocution was based on the information recorded in the anamnesis and the clinical signs (presence of electric burns mainly affecting feathers, skin and soft tissues).

The metabolic and nutritional disorder category comprised birds with low body condition or weakness, suffering from metabolic bone diseases (MBD) and the rest of diagnoses were grouped by organic systems (Table 2). The infectious disease category was applied when a pathogenic microorganism was confirmed by microbiological, parasitological or histopathological diagnosis.

Statistical analysis

Descriptive statistics, normality test and inferential analyses were done at 95% of confidence with SPSS Advanced Models ™ 15.0 (SPSS Inc. 233 South Wacker Drive, 11th Floor Chicago, IL

Table 5. Seasonal incidence rate values of the different raptors species admitted during the 12 years of the study.

	Number of total cases[a]		Estimated[b] population number		Overall causes[c]		Orphaned young[c]	Unknown trauma[c]		Gunshot[c]	Motor vehicles[c]		Fortuity[c]		Undetermined[c]		Electrocution[c]		Metabolic/ nutritional[c]		Infectious/ Parasitic[c]	
Raptor species*	W	B	W	B[d]	W	B	B	W	B	W	W	B	W	B	W	B	W	B	W	B	W	B
Accipiter gentillis	99	54	1438	750	5.74	0.73	0.15	1.39	0.20	2.78	0.12	0.01	0.64	0.08	0.46	0.05	0.17	0.08	0.00	0.03	0.06	0.01
Accipiter nisus	254	66	22954	1500	0.92	0.28	0.04	0.44	0.14	0.30	0.04	0.03	0.02	0.00	0.06	0.03	0.00	0.00	0.01	0.00	0.01	0.00
Athene noctua	112	844	5449	11669	1.71	0.67	0.65	0.81	0.11	0.18	0.24	0.04	0.11	0.03	0.06	0.03	0.02	0.00	0.03	0.01	0.02	0.00
Bubo bubo	56	95	1055	631	4.43	1.79	0.43	1.34	0.30	0.40	0.40	0.13	0.32	0.19	0.16	0.11	1.50	0.45	0.00	0.23	0.08	0.02
Buteo buteo	652	180	25710	1404	2.11	1.53	0.24	0.62	0.48	0.73	0.36	0.17	0.05	0.08	0.13	0.17	0.13	0.18	0.05	0.08	0.01	0.03
Falco peregrinus	37	36	1028	249	3.00	1.38	0.29	1.05	0.34	1.13	0.16	0.08	0.00	0.04	0.24	0.08	0.32	0.15	0.00	0.08	0.08	0.19
Falco tinnunculus	239	787	32003	3794	0.62	1.88	1.35	0.27	0.41	0.13	0.04	0.06	0.03	0.09	0.03	0.06	0.03	0.13	0.01	0.08	0.01	0.05
Otus scops	18	651	166	6515	9.06	0.93	0.98	2.01	0.12	0.00	0.50	0.03	0.50	0.06	0.00	0.03	0.00	0.00	0.00	0.01	0.00	0.01
Strix aluco	98	560	5981	13618	1.37	0.38	0.42	0.40	0.02	0.03	0.22	0.03	0.29	0.02	0.14	0.01	0.00	0.00	0.01	0.00	0.00	0.01
Tyto alba	124	240	1240	2765	8.34	0.76	0.52	3.16	0.13	0.34	2.22	0.08	0.74	0.07	0.94	0.04	0.07	0.01	0.07	0.02	0.13	0.02

[a]Total number of admissions at the center during the period of the study.
[b]Estimation of resident population (individuals) of the region during the wintering and breeding seasons according to the Catalan wintering bird Atlas 2009 and the Catalan breeding bird Atlas 1999-2002. Post-nuptial migration population is highly fluctuant and is not considered.
[c]Seasonal cumulative incidence (SCI) cases per 1000 animal/year = [(total season cases[a]/estimated season population[b])* 1000]/12.
[d]Number of individuals. Estimated population at the breeding season was calculated from the number of pairs multiplied by the number of chicks.
*Only species with at least up to 100 cases are represented in the table.
W = Wintering period; B = Breeding period.

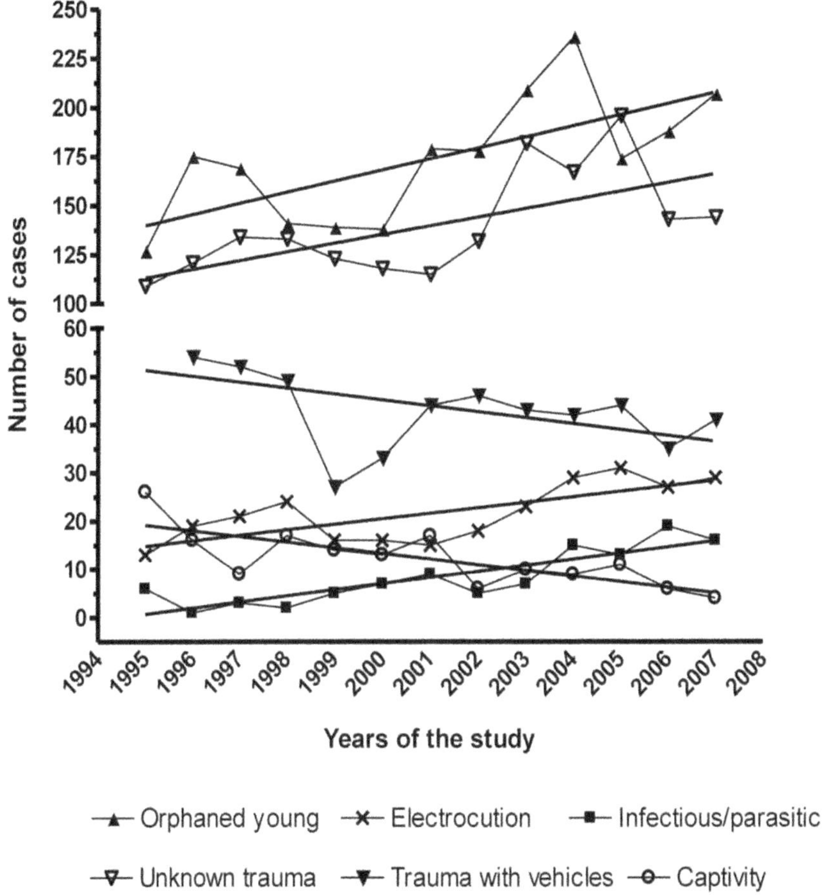

Figure 2. Different causes of admissions during the period 1995–2007 (number of cases). Only causes with significant statistical tendency are represented.

60606-6412). Chi-square (χ^2) or Fisher exact tests were used for comparison between proportions. Odds ratio measure of association was employed for disease comparisons. Seasonal cumulative incidences (SCI) were calculated for the wintering and breeding seasons, and were defined as the number of cases per season divided by the estimated population at that season. Results were expressed per 1000 animal and year. Reference populations of the region were obtained from published data [27,30]. Breeding and wintering estimated populations were considered as stable during the seasons and over the period of study. Trend analyses were applied for specific causes with a minimum of 100 cases in order to detect differences among years.

Acknowledgments

We are grateful to Paul Cairns, Sonia Almeria, Eugenia de la Torre and Santi Mañosa (Universitat de Barcelona) for the technical advice and review of the manuscript. We thank all the staff of the Torreferrussa Rehabilitation Centre (Berta Balcells, Gregori Conill, Ana Ledesma, Joan Mayne, Conxi Millán, Elena Obón, Laura Olid, and Albert Petit) for devoted care of patients. We also thank Chema López (Direcció General del Medi Natural) and Sergi Herrando (ICO) for the information about wild avian population in Catalonia.

Author Contributions

Conceived and designed the experiments: RM-L JC LD. Performed the experiments: RM-L. Analyzed the data: RM-L. Contributed reagents/materials/analysis tools: RM-L JC LD. Wrote the paper: RM-L JC LD.

References

1. Kovács A, Mammen UCC, Wernham CV (2008) European Monitoring for Raptors and Owls: State of the Art and Future Needs. Ambio 37: 408–412.
2. Sergio F, Newton I, Marchesi L, Pedrini P (2006) Ecologically justified charisma: preservation of top predators delivers biodiversity conservation. J Appl Ecol 43: 1049–1055.
3. Burfield IJ (2008) The Conservation Status and Trends of Raptors and Owls in Europe. Ambio 37: 401–407.
4. Morishita TY, Fullerton AT, Lownestine L, Gardner IA, Brooks DL (1998) Morbidity and mortality of free-living raptorial birds of Northern California: a retrospective study, 1983-1994. J Avian Med Surg 12: 78–90.
5. Wendell MD, Sleeman JM, Kratz G (2002) Retrospective study of morbidity and mortality of raptors admitted to Colorado state university veterinary teaching hospital during 1995 to 1998. J Wildl Dis 38: 101–106.
6. Hernández M (1988) Road mortality of the little owl (*Athene noctua*) in Spain. J Raptor Res 22: 81–84.
7. Real J, Grande JM, Mañosa S, Sánchez-Zapata JA (2001) Causes of death in different areas for Bonelli's eagle *Hieraetus fasciatus* in Spain. Bird Study 48: 221–228.
8. Martínez JA, Izquierdo A, Zuberogoitia I (2001) Causes of admisión of raptors in rescue centres of the East of Spain and proximate causes of mortality. Biota 2: 163–169.
9. Martínez JA, Martínez JE, Mañosa S, Zuberogoitia I, Calvo F (2006) How to manage human-induced mortality in the Eagle Owl *Bubo bubo*. Bird Conserv Int 16: 265–278.
10. González LM, Margalida A, Mañosa S, Sánchez R, Oria J, et al. (2007) Causes and spatio-temporal variations of non-natural mortality in the Vulnerable Spanish imperial Eagle *Aquila adalberti* during a recovery period. Oryx 41: 1–8.

11. Newton I, Wyllie I, Dale L (1999) Trend in the number and mortality patterns of sparrohawks (*Accipiter nisus*) and kestrels (*Falco tinnunculus*) in Britain, as revealed by carcass analyses. J Zool 148: 139–147.
12. Rodríguez B, Rodríguez A, Siverio F, Siverio M (2010) Causes of raptor admissions to a wildlife rehabilitation Center in Tenerife (Canary Islands). J Raptor Res 44: 30–39.
13. Dirección General para la Biodiversidad. Ministerio de Medio Ambiente (2006) Catálogo Nacional de Especies Amenazadas (1990-2006). Madrid: Listado de taxones por categorías de amenaza. 29 p.
14. Brown JD, Sleeman JD (2002) Morbidity and mortality of reptiles admitted to the Wildlife Center of Virginia, 1991 to 2000. J Wildl Dis 38: 699–705.
15. Sleeman JM (2008) Use of Wildlife Rehabilitation Centers as monitors of ecosystem health. In: Fowler ME, Miller RE, eds. Zoo and Wild Animal Medicine. pp 97–104.
16. Newton I (2002) Diseases in wild (free-living) raptors. In: Cooper JE, ed. Birds of prey Health and disease. pp 217–234.
17. Deem SL, Terrell SP, Forrester DJ (1998) A retrospective study of morbidity and mortality of raptors in Florida: 1988-1994. J Zoo Wildl Med 29: 160–164.
18. Komnenou AT, Georgopoulou I, Savvas I, Dessiris A (2005) A retrospective study of presentation, treatment, and outcome of free-ranging raptors in Greece (1997-2000). J Zoo Wildl Med 36: 222–228.
19. Kelly A (2006) Admissions, diagnoses, and outcomes for Eurasian sparrowhawks (Accipiter nisus) brought to a wildlife rehabilitation center in England. J Raptor Res 40: 231–235.
20. Harris MC, Sleeman JM (2007) Morbidity and mortality of bald eagles (Haliaeetus leucocephalus) and peregrine falcons (Falco peregrinus) admitted to the Wildlife Center of Virginia, 1993-2003. J Zoo Wildl Med 38: 62–66.
21. Mañosa S (2002) The conflict between game bird hunting and raptors in Europe. Unpublished report to REGHAB Project European Commission, Available from http://www.uclm.es/irec/Reghab/informes_3.htm.
22. Frías O (1999) Seasonal dynamics of avian traffic casualties on Central Spain: age and number of individuals and species richness and diversity. Ardeola 46: 23–30.
23. Martínez JA, Zuberogoitia I (2004) Habitat preferences and causes of population decline for barn owls *Tyto alba*: a multi-scale approach. Ardeola 51: 303–317.
24. Mañosa S (2001) Strategies to identify dangerous electricity pylons for birds. Biodiversity Conserv 10: 1997–2012.
25. Tintó A, Real J, Mañosa S (2010) Predicting and correcting the electrocution of birds in mediterranean areas. J Wildl Manage 74: 1852–1862.
26. Guzmán J, Castaño JP (1998) Raptor mortality by electrocution in power lines in eastern Sierra Morena and Campo de Montiel (Spain). Ardeola 15: 161–169.
27. Estrada J, Pedrocchi V, Brotons L, Herrando S, eds (2004) Catalan breeding bird Atlas 1999-2002. Institut Català d' Ornitologia (ICO). In: Lynx Editions.
28. Baker K (1993) Identification Guide to European Non-Passerines. BTO Guides. British Trust for Ornithology.
29. Samour JH (2004) Causes of morbidity and mortality in Falcons in Saudi Arabia. J Avian Med Surg 18: 229–241.
30. Herrando S, Brotons L, Estrada J, Guallar S, Anton M (2011) Atles dels ocells de Catalunya a l'hivern 2006-2009. In: Lynx Editions In Press.

2

EU-Approved Rapid Tests for Bovine Spongiform Encephalopathy Detect Atypical Forms: A Study for Their Sensitivities

Daniela Meloni[1], Aart Davidse[2], Jan P. M. Langeveld[2], Katia Varello[1], Cristina Casalone[1], Cristiano Corona[1], Anne Balkema-Buschmann[3], Martin H. Groschup[3], Francesco Ingravalle[1], Elena Bozzetta[1]*

1 Centro di Referenza Nazionale per le Encefalopatie Animali, Istituto Zooprofilattico Sperimentale del Piemonte, Liguria e Valle d'Aosta, Turin, Italy, **2** Central Veterinary Institute of Wageningen UR, Lelystad, The Netherlands, **3** Friedrich-Loeffler Institut, Federal Research Institute for Animal Health, Insel Riems, Germany

Abstract

Since 2004 it become clear that atypical *bovine spongiform encephalopthies* (BSEs) exist in cattle. Whenever their detection has relied on active surveillance plans implemented in Europe since 2001 by rapid tests, the overall and inter-laboratory performance of these diagnostic systems in the detection of the atypical strains has not been studied thoroughly to date. To fill this gap, the present study reports on the analytical sensitivity of the EU-approved rapid tests for atypical L- and H-type and classical BSE in parallel. Each test was challenged with two dilution series, one created from a positive pool of the three BSE forms according to the EURL standard method of homogenate preparation (50% w/v) and the other as per the test kit manufacturer's instructions. Multilevel logistic models and simple logistic models with the rapid test as the only covariate were fitted for each BSE form analyzed as directed by the test manufacturer's dilution protocol. The same schemes, but excluding the BSE type, were then applied to compare test performance under the manufacturer's versus the water protocol. The *IDEXX HerdChek ® BSE-scrapie short protocol* test showed the highest sensitivity for all BSE forms. The *IDEXX® HerdChek BSE-scrapie ultra short protocol*, the *Prionics® - Check WESTERN* and the *AJ Roboscreen® BetaPrion* tests showed similar sensitivities, followed by the *Roche® PrionScreen*, the *Bio-Rad® TeSeE™ SAP* and the *Prionics® - Check PrioSTRIP* in descending order of analytical sensitivity. Despite these differences, the limit of detection of all seven rapid tests against the different classes of material set within a 2 $\log_{10}$ range of the best-performing test, thus meeting the European Food Safety Authority requirement for BSE surveillance purposes. These findings indicate that not many atypical cases would have been missed surveillance since 2001 which is important for further epidemiological interpretations of the sporadic character of atypical forms.

Editor: Corinne Ida Lasmezas, The Scripps Research Institute Scripps Florida, United States of America

Funding: The authors have no funding or support to report.

Competing Interests: The authors have declared that no competing interests exist.

* E-mail: elena.bozzetta@izsto.it

Introduction

Transmissible spongiform encephalopathies (TSEs) or prion diseases include a group of progressive, neurodegenerative as yet untreatable disorders affecting several mammalian species, including Creutzfeldt-Jakob disease (CJD) in humans, bovine spongiform encephalopathy (BSE) in cattle and scrapie in small ruminants. TSEs are characterized by the concentration of an anomalous isoform (PrP^{Res}) of the natural prion protein (PrP^c) in the central nervous system (CNS) and peripheral tissues. PrP^{res} differs from PrP^c in its aggregated state and partial protease resistance. These characteristics are exploited by the majority of the methods currently used for TSE diagnosis. The protease resistant disease related PrP entity, varies in its extent of degradation by proteinase K (PK) which is influenced by the strain-dependent conformational variations of the secondary and tertiary structure of PrP^{res}. In different TSE strains, the pathological prion protein displays disease-specific features such as different cleavage sites after proteolytic treatment, glycosylation profile, and deposition patterns, which make strain identification possible [1].

The existence of different BSE strains was discovered in 2004. The classical form (C-BSE) coexists with the atypical H-type BSE (H-BSE) originally described in France [2] and the L-type BSE (L-BSE), also known as bovine amyloidotic spongiform encephalopathy (BASE), an unusual form of BSE first identified in Italy [3]. Their diagnostic differentiation is based mainly on the molecular features of the PrP^{res} identified by Western blot analysis. After PK digestion, PrP^{res} shows a triplet of non-, mono-, and diglycoforms, which, while expressing their quantitative ratio and migration positions, peculiarly typify the original BSE strain [4]. H- and L-BSE have a higher or a lower discernible molecular mass of unglycosylated PrP^{res}, respectively, at Western blot analysis; in addition, L- BSE has smaller proportion of diglycosylated PrP^{res} with levels between 40–55% than C-BSE where values range between 60–80%. Subsequently, occurrence of the two atypical forms to several European countries, Japan and North America has been reported. The origin of different BSE forms is still cryptic.

C-BSE, which was isolated during the epizootic disease, was postulated to have occurred after the recycling of a scrapie agent insufficiently deactivated in destructor plants [5,6]. However, this has been questioned after the detection of atypical BSE forms that seem to occur spontaneously in older cattle [7] and that, under certain circumstances, are able to change their biochemical properties into those of classical BSE. The accidental use of bovine material derived from an animal that had succumbed to a spontaneous form of BSE in the feed and food production may therefore also have been the origin of the BSE crisis. Such hypothesis seems to be also compatible with the peculiar distribution by year of birth of cattle affected by atypical BSEs, in comparison to bovines affected by C-type BSE observed in France [8]. Moreover, it has been shown in several transmission experiments to primates [9,10] and in human and bovine PrP transgenic mice [11,12] that L-type BSE seems to have a higher zoonotic potential than C-type BSE. The use of rapid tests that are able to reliably detect such cases is therefore crucial in the frame of the protection of the consumer from an accidental exposure to the BSE agent.

Until 1999 EU surveillance systems for bovine spongiform encephalopathy (BSE) were primarily passive, *i.e.* relying on the examination of diseased adult cattle showing clinical signs reported to the veterinary authorities, in compliance with the Decision 98/272/EC which modifies Decision 94/474/EC [13]. Brains were examined by histopathology and immunhistochemistry for PrP^{res} identification. Rapid molecular diagnostic assays became officially available in the late 1990s. With the enforcement of Regulation (EC) No. 999/2001 [14] the use of rapid tests became mandatory: a large number of countries subsequently detected the first BSE cases.

To provide dependable tools for an active surveillance system, in 1999 the European Commission (EC) carried out the first scientific evaluation of four new rapid *post mortem* BSE tests to assess their diagnostic accuracy and analytical sensitivity on brain tissue from clinically affected bovines [15]. Subsequent EU validation exercises enhanced the estimating parameters, including test robustness on autolyzed samples and testing of negative field samples to address the test specificity and to simulate routine activity [16,17,18].

To date, the EC has assessed 19 rapid tests in the frame of three "successive" evaluations and approved 9 for survey purposes [19].

In 2009 the Community Reference Laboratory (EURL) for TSEs assessed the analytical sensitivity of all the currently approved TSE rapid tests to determine their continued suitability for active surveillance plans [20]. The analytical sensitivity study was then evaluated by the European Food Safety Authority (EFSA) [21,22] on the basis of current EFSA requirements for the evaluation of TSE rapid *post mortem* tests [23].

In that context, the lowest limit of detection (LOD) of rapid tests approved for the diagnosis of TSEs in bovines was assessed. The pre-prepared positive and negative dilution series (EURL protocol) were compared with the manufacturer's dilution series. The rapid tests with a LOD poorer than 2 $\log_{10}$ as compared to the best-performing assay could not be recommended for use in the frame of BSE monitoring in cattle and TSE in small ruminants within the EU.

At same time, the BIOHAZ Panel recommended that a similar study should have been conducted with regard to the other TSE strains. Furthermore, because experimental transmission of atypical BSE prions suggests that they might be more insidious than classical BSE [24], the assessment of approved rapid-test performance on detecting atypical BSE strains remains a priority.

The aim of this study was to compare the analytical sensitivity of all presently EU-approved rapid *post mortem* tests for the detection of atypical BSE forms in bovines by assessing their lower LOD against atypical L- and H-type BSE. The outcome will be of interest for the interpretation of epidemiological surveillance data of all three BSE types.

Materials and Methods

Study Design

Consistent with the methodology of the EFSA analytical sensitivity study, the strategy of the Italian TSE National Reference Laboratory (NRL) was to compare the performance of all approved rapid tests against the same sample pools. Thus, the test results could be directly compared and their performance ranked according to their respective LOD.

Each test was challenged with decreasing amounts of confirmed BSE-positive material in a consistent background of negative material prepared following two protocols: the one using the EURL standard method of homogenate preparation (50% w/v protocol) [23] and the other as directed by the test kit manufacturer's instructions. This was done to permit comparison between the two preparation protocols.

The study design was set up to account for several confounders (e.g., the operator, the day of the test, plates, etc.). Factors were controlled by minimizing variability (e.g., all tests were performed by only two operators) and fitting multilevel logistic models in which the confounders were set as random or fixed effects [25,26,27].

The first step was a basic descriptive analysis. The second involved only the manufacturer's protocol, and a multilevel logistic model was fitted for each BSE type in order to compare test kit performance. The date of testing execution constituted the first level of the models (level 1); replicated crossover and nesting of the plates were the second level (level 2). The intraclass correlation coefficient (ICC) of the replicates obtained from these models allowed us to verify that their residual variance was due only to the replicates [25,26,27]. In this case, when the number of positive replicates was monotone decreasing in the dilutions, we could neglect the fixed effect of the dilution and focus instead on the effect of the different test kits. In the third step, simple logistic models [28,29] were fitted with the specific test kit as the only covariate.

Finally, the test results obtained under the two preparation protocols were compared. As mentioned, we fitted the multilevel logistic models not referring to each BSE type but instead to each test kit. Seven simple logistic models [28,29] one for each test, were then fitted: the interaction between BSE type and protocol was the only covariate in the model.

Tissue Background

Briefly, atypical L-BSE tissue was obtained from two Italian field cases. The atypical H-BSE tissue pool was provided to the Italian NRL by the Friedrich-Loeffler-Institut (FLI) (Germany) and originated from German calves experimentally inoculated intracranially [24]. Two C-BSE pools were included in the study, one strongly reacting at confirmatory Western blot, the second weakly. This was done in order to have reference data on known matrices for the comparison of unexplored results with atypical BSE. The strong C-BSE type tissue included a pool of five Dutch regularly slaughtered field cases (collected and tested in the frame of statutory BSE surveillance plane) provided by Central Veterinary Institute of Wageningen UR (CVI). The weak C-BSE tissue was a mixture of two Italian natural cases. All positive tissues originated from brain stem area and were confirmed by discriminatory Western blot analysis [4]. The negative tissue was created from 30 bovine brainstems randomly selected from Italian slaughtered surveillance samples which had tested negative at the *IDEXX® HerdCheck BSE-scrapie ultra short protocol* test [30] and confirmatory Western blot.

All details pertaining to sample origin were recorded.

Preparation of Diagnostic Test Material

To ensure that the samples would be homogeneous, they were prepared using the Veterinary Laboratory Agency (VLA) standard methods for TSE QA sample production (Veterinary Laboratory Agency, Standard Operating Procedure, "Instruction for the homogenisation and dilution of brainstem for preparation of QA Samples" – personal communication).

Accordingly, four CNS tissue pools (L, H, C strong, and C weak) were prepared from L-BSE-positive, H-BSE-positive, C-BSE strong and C-BSE weak positive tissues, respectively. The 100% CNS tissues were trimmed, pooled, mildly minced with scalpels, and then treated with a low-speed hand-held homogenizing unit for 30 s. A negative pool was prepared as described above. Each BSE-positive macerate pool was diluted in pre-homogenized negative tissue to obtain 2 base logarithm dilutions series down to 1:1024. As the 1:1024 dilution of the C-BSE strong pool tested positive at the *IDEXX® HerdCheck BSE-scrapie short protocol*, further 1:2048 and 1:4096 dilutions of the same tissue were investigated, with negative results.

To set up the dilution series, one half of the BSE-positive pools was prepared under the EURL homogenization protocol in *nuclease*-free water (50% w/v) using a low-speed hand-held homogenizing unit for a total of 90 s in three successive treatments. Each dilution underwent a final homogenization cycle to ensure the preparation was mixed thoroughly. All the homogenates were aliquoted into test-specific pre-labelled grinding tubes as directed by the manufacturer's instructions and stored at −20°C.

The other half of the BSE-positive and negative starting tissue pools was distributed in the manufacturer's tissue-disruption supports for the different test kits and then immediately submitted to the specific protocols as per the manufacturer's instructions.

Each dilution was tested in triplicate by each rapid test. The test panel consisted of 150 aliquots, with 30 samples per pool, for each dilution protocol.

Testing Exercise

The tests included in the study were those approved according to Regulation (EC) No. 999/2001 amended by Regulation 162/2009. Enfer Scientific [31] declined to participate in the study. The *Prionics® - Check LIA BSE Antigen Test Kit* [32] had been withdrawn from the market at the time the study was conducted.

A unique batch of each rapid test specifically provided for this study by the manufacturers largely before the relative expiring date was used for all the analyses. One rapid test was performed per day and all the dilution series were tested in triplicate. One out of three positive results interpreted according to the test specifications was selected as the criterion for judging the overall result as positive. For the evaluation of the *Prionics® - Check WESTERN* [33], the samples were considered positive if they exhibited a signal with a three-band pattern. A more diffuse pattern of PrP^{res} with the top band clearly visible, as reported by the manufacturer, was considered positive as well.

The laboratory test exercise was completed within 15 days from the starting point of generating and freezing the aliquots.

Results

The analyses of the different BSE samples – C-type strong, C-type weak, H-type and L-type – under both the EURL protocol or the manufacturers' protocol indicated that in principle, all tests were able to detect the different types of BSE though at different sensitivity (Table 1).

The ability of the rapid tests to identify positive replicates clearly differed between the tests when increasing dilutions were compared within the manufacturers' protocol and under the EURL 50% w/v protocol. Under the manufacturer's dilution protocol, the sensitivity of the *IDEXX® HerdCheck BSE-scrapie short protocol* test for all BSE types was higher than that of the other rapid tests. The sensitivity of the *IDEXX® HerdCheck BSE-scrapie ultra short protocol*, Prionics® - *Check WESTERN*, and *AJ Roboscreen® BetaPrion* [34] was similar, followed in decreasing order by the *Roche® PrionScreen* [35] *Bio-Rad® TeSeE™ SAP* [36] and *Prionics® - Check PrioSTRIP* [37], the last two of which displayed the lowest analytical sensitivity, notably for L-BSE.

The multilevel models fitted in the second step of the statistical analysis confirmed that the residual variance was almost entirely due to the replicates. For all BSE types, the ICC of the replicates was higher than 0.99. Therefore, apart from a few exceptions, it was assumed that the three replicates for each dilution would have the same result, whereupon a simplified logistic model was adopted. The *IDEXX® HerdCheck BSE-scrapie short protocol* was taken as the reference test, as it provided the highest analytical sensitivity for all BSE forms.

The logistic models showed that a loss of sensitivity up to two dilutions lower than the best-performing test was not statistically significant. Testing with the C-BSE strong pool showed that only the *IDEXX® HerdCheck BSE-scrapie ultra short protocol* test compared favourably with the *IDEXX® HerdCheck BSE-scrapie short protocol* test; while the sensitivity of the *AJ Roboscreen® BetaPrion*, *IDEXX® HerdCheck BSE-scrapie ultra short protocol*, *Prionics® - Check WESTERN* for detecting the other BSE types was not statistically different from that of the reference test.

To further discriminate between the quality of performance of the different test systems, logistic models were applied on the data obtained. On the basis of the odds ratio (OR) magnitude, each test can be ranked using the *IDEXX® HerdCheck BSE-scrapie short protocol* as reference test and it can be concluded that a higher OR is related to higher sensitivity. Ranking obtained under the manufacturer's protocol did not differ from that obtained under the water protocol (Figure 1).

Comparison of test performance under the two dilution protocols based on the descriptive analysis (Table 1) showed that all seven tests had a higher analytical sensitivity for the BSE-positive samples prepared under the manufacturer's protocol than those prepared as *per* the water protocol for all BSE types, except for H-BSE, toward which the tests performed generally better with the 50% w/v homogenates.

The same scheme to compare the tests under the manufacturers' protocol was then applied to compare their performance under the water protocol. A simple logistic model was fitted for each test. All seven rapid tests performed better under the manufacturers' dilution protocol than under the 50% w/v protocol (Figure 2), as already suggested by the descriptive analysis, however, upon the least approach, this result appeared to be statistically significant only for the *AJ Roboscreen® BetaPrion* and the *Bio-Rad® TeSeE™ SAP* kits.

Assessment of test specificity was not within the scope of this study; nevertheless, appropriate BSE-negative tissue amounts tested on each test platform displayed negative results.

Table 1. Detection limits obtained by the different rapid tests for the different BSE forms. The number of positives out of three replicates is also reported.

Test	Weak C – BSE		Strong C – BSE		L – BSE		H – BSE		Number of false positive/number of negative samples tested
	Manufacturer prepared dilutions	50% w/v	Manufacturer prepared dilutions	50% w/v	Manufacturer prepared dilutions	50% w/v	Manufacturer prepared dilutions	50% w/v	
IDEXX® HerdCheck BSE-scrapie Short	1:64	1:16	1:1024	1:512	1:512	1:512	1:256	1:512	0/30
	3/3	3/3	2/3	3/3	3/3	2/3	3/3	2/3	
IDEXX® HerdCheck BSE-scrapie Ultra Short	1:32	1:16	1:512	1:512	1:256	1:128	1:128	1:64	0/30
	3/3	3/3	3/3	3/3	3/3	3/3	1/3	3/3	
Bio-Rad ® TeSeE TM SAP	1:2	-	1:64	1:4	1:16	1:4	1:32	1:32	0/30
	3/3	0/3	3/3	3/3	3/3	3/3	2/3	3/3	
Prionics®-Check Western	1:32	1:16	1:128	1:64	1:256	1:32	1:128	1:128	0/30
	1/3	3/3	3/3	2/3	1/3	3/3	3/3	1/3	
Prionics®-Check PrioSTRIP	1:4	1:2	1:32	1:16	1:16	1:16	1:16	1:16	0/30
	1/3	1/3	2/3	2/3	3/3	3/3	3/3	3/3	
AJ Roboscreen® BetaPrion	1:32	1:16	1:128	1:64	1:512	1:128	1:128	1:32	0/30
	2/3	3/3	2/3	2/3	2/3	3/3	3/3	3/3	
Roche PrionScreen®	1:8	1:2	1:64	1:16	1:16	1:16	1:32	1:64	0/30
	3/3	3/3	2/3	3/3	3/3	1/3	3/3	2/3	

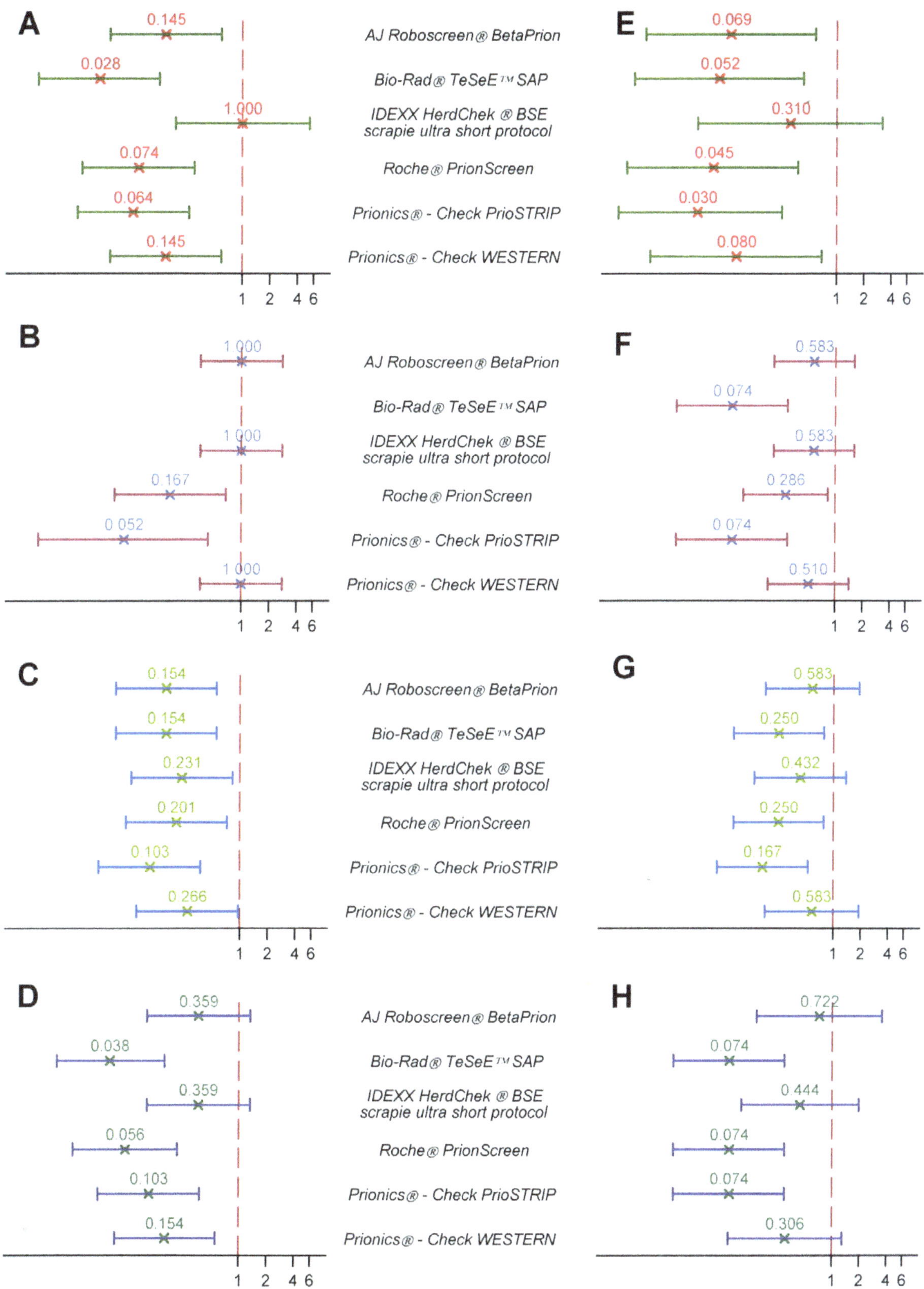

Figure 1. Test performance compared to the *IDEXX® HerdCheck BSE-scrapie short protocol.* The vertical axis reports the different rapid tests challenged. The horizontal axis reflects the odds ratio magnitude using *IDEXX® HerdCheck* BSE-scrapie short protocol as reference test. Panels A, B, C, D (left column) report the results obtained under the w/v protocol; panels E, F, G, H (right column) display the results under the manufacturers' instructions. BSE forms studied: panels A, E: strong C-type; panels B, F: weak C-type; panels C, G: H-type; panels D, H: L-type. All the weak C type water dilutions series tested negative with Bio-Rad® TeSeE™ SAP (notably, the optical densities were for all the three replicates of the 1:2 dilution just under the cut-off value), thereby, the odd ratio could not be calculated (Subfigure B).

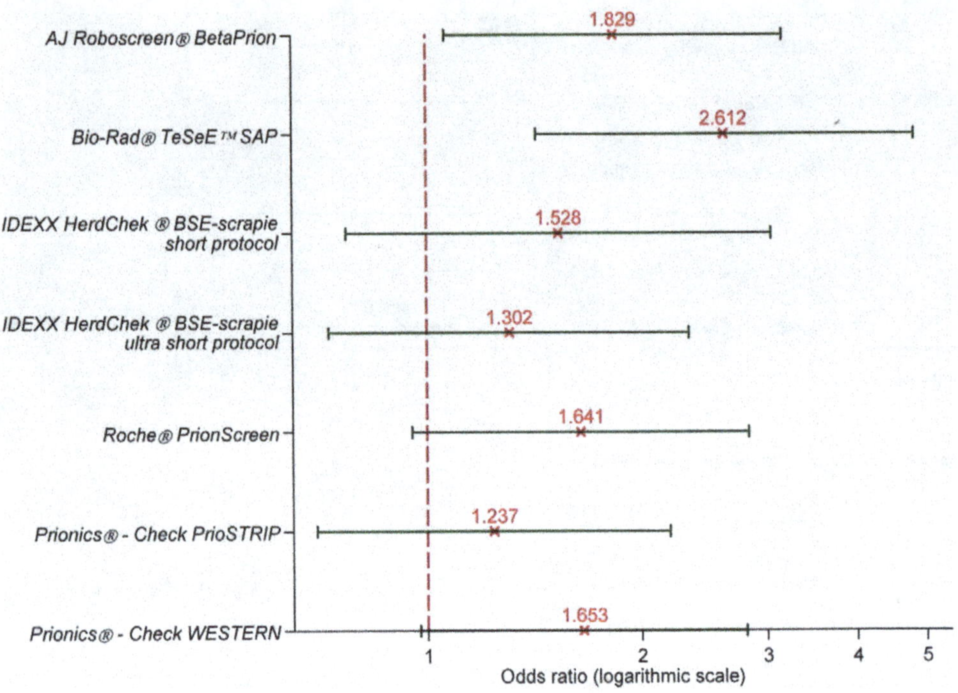

Figure 2. Comparison of test performance under the manufacturer's dilution protocol *versus* the 50% w/v protocol. The vertical axis reports the different rapid tests challenged. The horizontal axis reflects the odds ratio magnitude.

Discussion

In this study we have evaluated the analytical sensitivity of approved rapid tests for the current known atypical BSEs detection. It is to be noted that Seuberlich et al. [38] raised the possibility that a new prion disease not previously encountered and distinct from the known types of BSEs exists. Nevertheless, the information is really limited and the puzzle of the different observations has still to be assembled, considering that the results described remind the features of poorly digested normal PrP (known as the physiologically C2 fragment of PrP [39,40]).

Referring to the tissues origin, is to be remarked that the investigated H-BSE tissues originated from intracranially challenged cattle, whereas the three other forms derived from field cases. Nevertheless, recent studies showed that biochemical and histopathological features of experimental H-type BSE animals were identical to that found with field H-type [12,24,41].

According to our results, all tests were able to detect both H- and L-BSE types at a 1:16 dilution prepared as directed by the manufacturer's instructions, with the same performance as for classical BSE.

The LOD varied across the tests. The *IDEXX® HerdCheck BSE-scrapie short protocol* showed the highest analytical sensitivity, as previously reported in a EURL study on classical BSE [21]. The performance of the *AJ Roboscreen® BetaPrion*, *IDEXX® HerdCheck BSE-scrapie ultra short protocol*, and *Prionics® - Check WESTERN* compared favourably with one another at our statistical analysis. The *Prionics® - Check PrioSTRIP*, *Bio-Rad® TeSeE™ SAP* and *Roche® PrionScreen tests* showed the lowest sensitivities for all the BSE types analyzed. These results were confirmed also using other explorative statistical approaches (e.g., Poisson models for number of positive replicates, receiver operating characteristic [ROC] curves) which we had initially applied (results not reported).

The analytical sensitivity of the tests was investigated in accordance with the requirements set by the relevant evaluation protocols established by the European Commission, the SSC and EFSA, using serial dilutions of sample replicates.

Test differences between the last positive dilutions of weak and strong C-BSE samples varies among the different systems from two to four factors (2 base logarithm) for buffer dilutions and from two to five factors for water dilutions. In this context, the different tests showed parallel results between the dilutions prepared following the two protocols. The dynamic range of each rapid test or rather the concentration range of PrP^{res} that results in a change in response is a specific peculiarity of each diagnostic system.

The rate of conversion of substrate to coloured product should be proportional to the amount of PrP^{res} within the well, but there are many limits to this depending on the analyte itself, that tends to aggregate rapidly in solution, and on the combination of methods and materials used within the test kits other than on the equipments.

A gradual stratification of the signal represents a *surplus* value for TSE rapid assays.

In our study, the *Bio-Rad® TeSeE™ SAP* test could surprisingly detect only the 1:2 dilution when challenged with positive C BSE weak samples. A loss of analytical sensitivity for this test was observed also during the active surveillance activity carried out from 2004 to 2008 by the Italian Reference Center for TSEs applying *Bio-Rad® TeSeE™* test. In that context, a National batch testing was performed on every new batch prior to commercialization to provide reassurance that BSE rapid test kits were fit for the survey purpose. As a consequence, distribution of some kit batches was precluded because of the lack of signal showed on positive reference samples. Further to the unexpected poor performance of *Bio-Rad® TeSeE™* within this study even after test repetition, the same *Bio-Rad®* homogenate sample set, according to previous studies in which its suitability for the *IDEXX* test was shown, was challenged with the last test revealing signals miming the ones reported *for IDEXX* test (data not shown).

The question of whether the specific kit batch affected the test performance is of concern, but it is noteworthy that all producers were asked to provide a kit for this evaluation. Thereby, our results represent a picture of the kits available on the market.

The seven simple logistic models showed a meaningful difference between the dilution protocols only for the *AJ Roboscreen® BetaPrion* and *Bio-Rad® TeSeE^{TM} SAP*. The lower bounds of the 95% confidence intervals for the *Roche® PrionScreen* and *Prionics® - Check WESTERN* tests approached 1 (0.9528 and 0.9755, respectively); for the remaining tests, there was no statistical evidence of a higher test sensitivity between the manufacturer's dilution protocol and the 50% w/v protocol (Figure 2).

Whenever in order to evaluate the field performances of BSE rapid *post mortem* tests the manufacturers' protocol represents the term of reference, the relevance of water dilution-based results relies on the specific Annex X of Regulation (EC) 999/2001 requirements. NRLs for TSE periodically have to verify national diagnostic standards and methods by means of comparative trials. The objectives are to monitor national rapid test activity and to demonstrate to the EC that the rapid surveillance system is effective. EURL itself annually verifies the interlaboratory agreement of the rapid systems used by the NRLs.

As previously reported in the EURL study [20], the analytical sensitivity values obtained under the 50% w/v protocol were from one to three dilutions inferior to those obtained under the specific homogenization protocol. For all the tests except one, the discrepancies between the two modes of dilutions were similar whatever the sample tested. Particularly with the Bio-Rad test the strong positive C -BSE sample was four factors lower when the water protocol was applied. Anyway, this is congruent with the EFSA 2009 results [21], where the discrepancy set at three logarithms. This difference needs to be taken into account when organizing ring trials, during which a less sensitive test could be penalized.

To rule out a possible decrement of the signal related to the storage of the water aliquots, and because of the scarcity of atypical BSE material, the laboratory test exercise was completed within a 15-day period. This precautionary approach was taken as no data exist on the stability of atypical BSE homogenates, whereas differences in stability have been observed for atypical *versus* classical scrapie [21,42,43,44]. Further, as it is indeed known that the results of some tests can lapse while approaching the expiring date of kit batches, the kits provided for the evaluation were expected to expire from three to six months after the date of testing. Table S1 lists the kit batches used, the expiring dates and the days of testing.

With regard to the homogeneity of serial dilutions, as PrP^{res} is amyloidogenic, the fibrils tend to aggregate in solution [45], thus potentially hindering a real homogeneity of dilution series. In our study, the ICC of the replicates was higher than 0.99. This ensured that, whenever the amounts of BSE tissues available were extremely limited, the material tested was homogeneous.

When considering the working principle of rapid tests, summarized in the Text S1, all approved tests include a PK digestion step to unmask cryptic epitopes, except for the *IDEXX HerdChek® BSE-scrapie EIA*, which relies on conformational detection technology using a specific aggregate specific capture ligand on a dextran polymer (Seprion ligand technology, Microsens Biotechnologies, London, UK) [46]. The severe effects of proteinase K (PK) in digesting atypical PrP^{res} are well known. Depending on the PK concentration, signal loss after atypical BSE-related PrP^{res} PK digestion varies from less than 20% for the C-type isolates to more than 50% for both L- and H-type BSE tissues [4]. This could be the reason for the higher sensitivity of the IDEXX test in detecting atypical BSEs compared to the others. However, the type of detergent used in homogenates and the type of TSE strain used do affect the extent of PrP^{res} degradation, and this remains a matter of further study [47].

With regard to the interpretation of results, five of the rapid tests in this study are based on semi-quantitative ELISA methods that produce a qualitative result relative to a cut-off value. To minimize subjectivity, the study's *Prionics® - Check PrioSTRIP* results were interpreted with the use of the computerized *PrioSCAN®* software, although visual interpretation by two independent readers was also validated. The *Prionics® - Check Western* is both a qualitative and quantitative test, as it distinguishes PrP^{res} in non-, mono-, and diglycoforms while expressing their respective quantitative ratio and migration positions. The diagnostic criteria for positive results are based on the exhibition of a three-band signal, the top one corresponding to a protein with an approximate molecular weight of 30 kD. Signal intensity decreases from top to bottom, but the higher band should be clearly visible immediately under the PK band. Significant blot images of atypical BSE dilution series obtained on in the frame of this study are presented in the Figure S1. In addition, extremely weak samples, notably for atypical BSE strains, can vary in their conventional blot pattern that fit positive criteria. Glycoform separation on the *Sodium Dodecyl Sulphate PolyAcrylamide* gel by electrophoresis causes the PrP^{res} signal to thin out along the migration line rather than concentrate in a narrow area, as occurs with ELISA and immunochromatographic methods. This means that if the relative non-, mono-, and diglycoform immunoreactivity ratios of L-BSE are taken as corresponding roughly to 39%, 35%, and 26% [48], the blot signal characterizing the last tissue ratio meeting the non-negative criteria generates from only 39% of the total prion protein on the migration line. Despite this, the *Prionics® - Check Western* was found to be among the more sensitive systems, indicating that the interpretation of a specific PrP^{res} marker by an expert reader can increase the test's sensitivity.

In conclusion, despite the evidence of clear differences in relative analytical sensitivity, the LOD of all seven rapid tests included in this study, against all the classes of material used, was within a 2 $\log_{10}$ range of the best-performing test, thus meeting EFSA criteria for rapid tests for BSE monitoring.

No certain conclusions on the field of diagnostic performance of these rapid-test kits can be drawn from our results on their analytical sensitivity, as the two parameters are not directly linked, anyway samples from animals exhibiting subclinical signs [24], could be expected to behave similarly to extremely diluted CNS tissues used in analytical sensitivity studies.

The outcome of this study endorses the current epidemiological follow up and interpretation of all three BSE forms prevalence [49,50] and means that for epidemiological studies the data obtained in the different countries and regions of EU can be considered equally, as plausibly, most stronger atypical cases have been detected by the different rapid tests.

Acknowledgments

We would like to thank Maria Mazza, Danilo Pitardi and Antonio Longo (Istituto Zooprofilattico Sperimentale del Piemonte Liguria e Valle d'Aosta, Torino, Italy) for their helpful contribution, the AHVLA group for the advises towards the design of this study.

Author Contributions

Conceived and designed the experiments: DM JPML EB KV C. Casalone C. Corona FI. Performed the experiments: DM KV AD. Analyzed the data: DM JPML EB FI. Contributed reagents/materials/analysis tools: AD C. Casalone C. Corona ABB MHG. Wrote the paper: DM EB JPML ABB MHG FI.

References

1. Bessen RA, Marsh RF (1994) Distinct PrP properties suggest the molecular basis of strain variation in transmissible mink encephalopathy. J Virol 68:7859–7868.
2. Biacabe AG, Laplanche JL, Ryder S, Baron T (2004) Distinct molecular phenotypes in bovine prion diseases. EMBO Rep 5: 110–115.
3. Casalone C, Zanusso G, Acutis P, Ferrari S, Capucci L, et al. (2004) Identification of a second bovine amyloidotic spongiform encephalopathy: molecular similarities with sporadic Creutzfeldt-Jakob disease. Proc Natl Acad Sci U S A 101: 3065–3070.
4. Jacobs JG, Langeveld JPM, Biacabe AG, Acutis PL, Polak MP, et al. (2007) Molecular discrimination of atypical bovine spongiform encephalopathy strains from a geographical region spanning a wide area in Europe. J Clin Microbiol 45(6): 182–1829.
5. Wilesmith JW, Wells GA, Cranwell MP, Ryan JB (1988) Bovine spongiform encephalopathy: epidemiological studies. Vet Rec 123: 638–644.
6. Baron T, Biacabe AG (2006) Origin of bovine spongiform encephalopathy. Lancet 367: 297–298; author reply 298–299.
7. Brown P, Mc Shane LM, Zanusso G, Detwile L (2006) On the question of sporadic or atypical bovine spongiform encephalopathy and Creutzfeldt-Jakob disease. Emerging Infectious Diseases 12:1816–21.
8. Biacabe AG, Morignat E, Vulin J, Calavas D, Baron TGM (2008) Atypical bovine spongiform encephalopathies, France, 2001–2007. Emerging Infectious Diseases 14: 298–300.
9. Comoy EE, Casalone C, Lescoutra-Etchegaray N, Zanusso G, Freire S, et al. (2008) Atypical BSE (BASE) transmitted from asymptomatic aging cattle to a primate. PLoS One 20;3(8):e3017.
10. Ono F, Tase N, Kurosawa A, Hiyaoka A, Ohyama A, et al. (2011) Atypical L-type bovine spongiform encephalopathy (L-BSE) transmission to cynomolgus macaques, a non-human primate. Jpn J Infect Dis 64(1):81–4.
11. Kong Q, Zheng M, Casalone C, Qing L, Huang S, et al. (2008) Evaluation of the human transmission risk of an atypical bovine spongiform encephalopathy prion strain. J Virol 82: 3697–3701.
12. Buschmann A, Gretzschel A, Biacabe AG, Schiebel K, Corona C, et al. (2006) Atypical BSE in Germany–proof of transmissibility and biochemical characterization. Vet Microbiol 117(2–4):103–16.
13. (1998) European Commission Decision 98/272/CE which is related to epidemiological surveillance of spongiform encephalopathies and which modifies Decision 94/474/CE. Official Journal of the European Union L 122 p. 59.
14. (1999b) European Commission Regulation (EC) No. 999/2001 of the European Parliament and of the Council of 22 May 2001 laying down rules for the prevention, control and eradication of certain transmissible spongiform encephalopathies. Official Journal of the European Union L 147 pp 1–40.
15. Moynagh J, Schimmel H, Kramer GN (1999) The evaluation of tests for the diagnosis of transmissible spongiform encephalopathy in bovines. Nature 400: 105–105.
16. (2003) Opinion of the Scientific Steering Committee on the field trial evaluation of the evaluation of two new rapid BSE post mortem tests. Available: http://ec.europa.eu/food/fs/sc/ssc/out316_en.pdf.
17. Wolfang P, Pavel V (2004) The field trial of seven new rapid post mortem tests for the diagnosis of bovine spongiform encephalopathy in bovines. Available: http://irmm.jrc.ec.europa.eu/activities/TSE_testing/Documents/globalreportphaseii.pdf.
18. (2005) Scientific Report of the European Food Safety Authority on the evaluation of two rapid post mortem BSE tests. EFSA Journal 48: 1–10.
19. (2010) European Commission Regulation (EC) No 956/2010 of the European Parliament and of the Council amending Annex X to Regulation (EC) No. 999/2001 of the European Parliament and of the Council as regards the list of rapid tests. Official Journal of the European Union L 279 pp 10–12.
20. Webster K, Flowers M, Cassar C, Bayliss D (2009) Determination of analytical sensitivity (detection limit) for currently approved TSE rapid tests. Available: http://www.efsa.europa.eu/de/scdocs/doc/1436.pdf
21. (2009) Scientific Opinion of the European Food Safety Authority on the analytical sensitivity of approved TSE rapid tests. EFSA Journal 7(12):1436.
22. (2010) Scientific Opinion of the European Food Safety Authority on the analytical sensitivity of approved TSE rapid tests - new data for assessment of two rapid tests. EFSA Journal 8: 1591.
23. (2007) Scientific Opinion of the European Food Safety Authority on a protocol for the evaluation of new rapid BSE post mortem tests. The EFSA Journal 508, 1–20.
24. Balkema-Buschmann A, Ziegler U, Mc Intyre L, Keller M, Hoffmann C, et al. (2011) Experimental challenge of cattle with German atypical bovine spongiform encephalopathy (BSE) isolates. Journal of Toxicology and Environmental Health, Part A, 74: 2, 103–109.
25. Armstrong BK, White E, Saracci R (2001) In: Principle of exposure measurement in epidemiology. Oxford: Oxford University Press. 351 p.
26. Rabe-Hesketh S, Skrondal A (2008) In:Multilevel and longitudinal modelling using Stata. College Station, Texas: S. Stata Press. 562 p.
27. Szklo M, Nieto FJ (2006) Quality assurance and control. In: Epidemiology: beyond the basics. Sudbury, Massachusetts: Jones and Bartlett Publishers. 297–350 pp.
28. Altman DG (1991) In: Practical Statistics for Medical Research. London: Chapman & Hall/CRC. 611 p.
29. Fleiss JL, Levin B, Paik MC (2003) In: Statistical Methods for Rates and Proportions. New York: John Wiley & Sons. 760 p.
30. IDEXX® HerdCheck Bovine Spongiform Encephalopathy Antigen Test Kit, EIA. IDEXX Laboratories, Westbrook, ME, USA.
31. Enfer Scientific®, Newhall, Naas, County Kildare, Ireland.
32. Prionics® - Check LIA BSE Antigen Test Kit, Prionics AG, Schlieren-Zurich, Switzerland.
33. Prionics® - Check WESTERN Prionics AG, Schlieren-Zurich, Switzerland
34. BetaPrion® BSE EIA Test Kit, AJ Roboscreen, Leipzig, Germany.
35. PrionScreen® Test, Roche Diagnostics, Mannheim, Germany.
36. TeSeE™ Purification-Detection SAP Test Kit, Bio-Rad Laboratories, Marnes-La-Coquette, France.
37. Prionics® - Check PrioSTRIP, Prionics AG, Schlieren-Zurich, Switzerland.
38. Seuberlich T, Gsponer M, Drögemüller C, Polak PM, McCutcheon S, et al. (2012) Novel prion protein in BSE-affected cattle. Switzerland Emerging Infectious Diseases 18:1, 158–159.
39. Pirisinu L, Di Bari M, Marcon S, Vaccari G, D'Agostino C, et al. (2010) A new method for the characterization of strain-specific conformational stability of protease-sensitive and protease-resistant PrP^{Sc}. PLoS ONE 5(9): e12723.
40. Kittelberger R (2012) Novel prion protein in BSE-affected cattle, Switzerland. Emerg Infect Dis 18:890–2. doi: 10.3201/eid1805.111824.
41. Dobly A, Langeveld JPM, van Keulen L, Rodeghiero C, Durand S, et al. (2010) No H- and L-type cases in Belgium in cattle diagnosed with bovine spongiform encephalopathy (1999–2008) aging seven years and older. BMC Veterinary Research 6:26.
42. Everest SJ, Thorne L, Barnicle DA, Edwards JC, Elliott H, et al. (2006) Atypical prion protein in sheep brain collected during the British scrapie-surveillance programme. J Gen Virol 87, 471–477.
43. Gretzschel A, Buschmann A, Langeveld JPM, Groschup M (2006) Immunological characterization of abnormal prion protein from atypical scrapie cases in sheep using a panel of monoclonal antibodies. J Gen Virol 87, 3715–3722.
44. Klingeborn M, Wik L, Simonsson M, Renstrom LH, Ottinger T, et al. (2006) Characterization of proteinase K-resistant N- and C-terminally truncated PrP in Nor98 atypical scrapie. J Gen Virol 87, 1751–1760.
45. Caughey B, Baron GS, Chesebro B, Jeffrey M (2009) Getting a grip on prions oligomers, amyloids, and pathological membrane interactions. Annual Review of Biochemistry 78: 177–204.
46. Grassi J, Maillet S, Simon S, Morel N (2008) Progress and limits of TSE diagnostic tools. Vet Res 39: 33.
47. Breyer J, Wemheuer WM, Wrede A, Graham C, Benestad SL, et al. (2012) Detergents modify proteinase K resistance of PrP^{res} in different transmissible spongiform encephalopathies (TSEs). Vet. Microbiol. Doi:10.1016/j.vetmic.2011.12.008.
48. Dudas S, Yang J, Graham C, Czub M, McAllister TA, et al. 2010 Molecular, biochemical and genetic characteristics of BSE in Canada. PLoS ONE 5(5): e10638.
49. Langeveld JPM, Erkens JHF, Rammel I, Jacobs JG, Davidse A, et al. (2011) Four independent molecular prion protein parameters for discriminating new cases of C, L, and H bovine spongiform encephalopathy in cattle. Journal of Clinical Microbiology 49:8, 3026–3028.
50. Polak MP, Zmudzinski JF (2012) Distribution of a pathological form of prion protein in the brainstem and cerebellum in classical and atypical cases of bovine spongiform encephalopathy. The Veterinary Journal 191, 128–130.

3

Molecular Relatedness of Methicillin-Resistant *S. aureus* Isolates from Staff, Environment and Pets at University Veterinary Hospital in Malaysia

Erkihun Aklilu[1,2]*, Zunita Zakaria[1], Latiffah Hassan[1], Chen Hui Cheng[1]

1 Faculty of Veterinary Medicine Universiti Putra Malaysia, Serdang, Malaysia, **2** Faculty of Veterinary Medicine, Universiti Malaysia Kelantan, Pengkalan Chepa, Kota Bharu, Malaysia

Abstract

Methicillin-resistant *Staphylococcus aureus* (MRSA) has emerged as a problem in veterinary medicine and is no longer considered as a mere nosocomial pathogen. We studied the occurrence of MRSA in veterinary personnel, cats and dogs and the environmental premises in University Veterinary Hospital (UVH). We found the prevalence of MRSA as follows: UVH 2/28 (7.1%) staff, 8/100 (8%) of the pets [5/50 (10%) of the dogs and 3/50 (6%) of the cats)], and 9/28 (4.5%) of the environmental samples. Antibiotic sensitivity tests (AST) show multi-resistance characteristics of the MRSA and the minimum inhibitory concentration (MIC) values for the isolates ranged from 1.5 µg to >256 µg/ml. Molecular typing by using multi-locus sequence typing (MLST), staphylococcal protein A typing (*spa* typing) and pulsed-field gel electrophoresis (PFGE) was conducted and the results from MLST indicated that an isolate from a veterinary personnel (PG21), typed as ST1241 belonged to the same clonal complex (CC) as the two isolates from two dogs (DG16 and DG20), both being typed as ST59. The PFGE results revealed that the two isolates from two veterinary personnel, PG21 and PG16 belonged to closely related MRSA strains with isolates from dog (DG36) and from environmental surface (EV100) respectively. The fact that PFGE revealed close similarity between isolates from humans, a dog and environmental surfaces indicates the possibility for either of them to be the source of MRSA and the potential routes and risks of spread.

Editor: Tara C. Smith, University of Iowa, United States of America

Funding: This research was supported by the Ministry of Science Technology and Innovation MOSTI ScienceFund. The funders had no role in study design, data collection and analysis, decision to publish, or preparation of the manuscript.

Competing Interests: The authors have declared that no competing interests exist.

* E-mail: erkihun@umk.edu.my

Introduction

Reports of MRSA in the community beyond the hospital environment suggest the increasing prevalence of MRSA in humans [1]. In the past few years, there have been increasing reports of MRSA in companion animals [2,3] and veterinary professionals [4,5,6] which has made MRSA as a potential emerging problem in veterinary medicine [5] and human hospital environments [7].

Studies have shown that transmission of MRSA can occur from human to animal and vice versa and direct exposure to MRSA-positive animals may lead to transmission to humans [7,8,9]. The environmental contamination by MRSA has been implicated as sources of infections in human [10] and veterinary hospitals [11]. MRSA strains have been found to survive for long periods on many different surfaces in the hospital environment and in private homes [12,13].

Molecular typing methods have been used to track the sources and transmissions of pathogenic bacteria, thereby helping the establishment of national and global epidemiological data of pathogens like MRSA [3,14,15,16,17,18]. Among the molecular typing methods, PFGE has been considered as a highly discriminatory method and as the 'gold standard' for MRSA outbreak investigations [14]. The advantages of using PFGE for molecular typing are attributed to full typability of isolates, good reproducibility of results within centers and recognizable stability of genomic pattern relatedness over years and high discriminatory power [19]. PFGE has been used as a tool for monitoring and tracking the transmission and spread of MRSA between human and animals [3,5,15,20,21]. In addition, sequence-based typing methods such as MLST and *spa* typing have been used to study the evolution and epidemiology of MRSA [22,23].

In Malaysia, MRSA have been reported at 44.1% detection rate in teaching and referral hospital in Kuala Lumpur [24]. However, little is known about the molecular characteristics and MRSA prevalence in the veterinary settings. The current study described the isolation of MRSA in a local veterinary setting and the genetic relatedness of isolates from veterinary personnel, cats and dogs, and environmental surfaces.

Materials and Methods

Ethics Statement

Approval for the study was acquired from the university ethics committees for research involving humans and animals (University Committee for Medical Research Ethics and Committee for Ethics for Using Animals in Research). All human subjects involved here were breifed and signed a consent form. The data were also analysed anonymously.

Sampling

Sampling was conducted in such a way that the staff members are sampled over a one week period, while sampling from pets and environment was done over six months time period. All samplings were done once and there was no replicate sampling. A total of 28 staff, 100 pets (50 cats and 50 dogs) presented to UVH, and 200 environmental surfaces at UVH, Faculty of Veterinary Medicine, Universiti Putra Malaysia (UPM) were sampled between November 2007 and May 2008. The UVH staff members provided informed consent for voluntary participation in the study. Both nasal and oral swabs were collected from each staff member. From pets, nasal and peri-anal swabs were collected by using separate sterile swabs. Environmental sampling was done on selected surfaces of approximately 25 cm^2 areas at small animal hospital (waiting areas, chairs, reception desk, floors, examination table, markers, water taps, door handles), small animal ward (examination tables, cages), surgical and radiology wards. Sterile swabs were rinsed with sterile normal saline solution to wipe the selected surfaces for sampling. All samples were placed in Amies transport medium (Amies, Italy) and were kept at 4°C until processed.

Isolation and Phenotypic Characterization

Swab samples were enriched in Tryptone Soya Broth (Oxoid, UK) containing 6.5% NaCl at 37°C for 24 hours prior to culturing [25]. Enriched growths were cultured onto blood agar with 7% horse blood and incubated aerobically at 37°C for 18–24 h. Gram-staining, catalase and coagulase tests were used to identify *S. aureus*. Further confirmations of *S. aureus* isolates were done by culturing on mannitol salt agar (MSA, Oxoid, UK) and by latex agglutination test using Staphytect Plus® (Oxoid, UK). Oxacillin-resistant screening agar base (ORSAB, Oxoid, UK) supplemented with ORSAB selective supplement consisting of 1 mg oxacillin and 25,000 IU polymyxin B incorporated into 500 mL of the agar solution was used for selective growth of MRSA. The plates were aerobically incubated at 37°C for 24–48 h and colony morphologies were used to confirm the growth of presumptive MRSAs.

Antibiotic Sensitivity Test and MIC Determination

Antibiotic resistance profile for each MRSA isolate was determined by disc diffusion methods according to CLSI standards [34] (2006). Amikacin (AK30), Amoxicillin (AML25), Methicillin (MET10), Oxacillin (OX1), Cefoxitin (FOX30), Streptomycin (S10), Vancomycin (VA30), Minocycline (MH30), Rifampicin (RD15), Doxycycline Hydrochloride (DO30), Amoxycillin-Clavulanic acid (AMC30), Gentamicin (CN10), Impenem (IPM 10), Tetracycline (TE10), Erythromycin (E15) were the antimicrobials used. Isolates with intermediate and full resistance to vancomycin were further tested by vancomycin Etest.

The Oxacillin MIC for each isolate was determined by using Oxacillin Etest (AB Biodisc, Solana, Sweden) strips according the manufacturer's recommendations. A pure isolate of MRSA from overnight growth on blood agar was emulsified in normal saline (0.85% NaCl) to achieve a turbidity equivalent of 0.5–1.0 McFarland standard. Isolates with MIC ≥4 μg/mL were considered oxacillin resistant [26].

Detection of *mec*A, MLST and *spa* Typing

Staphylococcus aureus specific gene (*nuc*A) and methicillin-resistance gene (*mec*A) were amplified as described earlier [27]. Two human isolates, three pet isolates and two environmental isolates were typed by MLST and *spa* typing. Multilocus sequence typing was conducted as previously described [18]. The single-locus DNA repeat region of the Staphylococcus protein A gene (*spa*) was sequenced as described previously [28].

Pulsed-Field Gel Electrophoresis (PFGE)

Pulsed-Field Gel Electrophoresis of *Sma*I (Sigma) digested chromosomal DNA was conducted according to the Harmony protocols [29]. Briefly, bacterial colonies from overnight growth were incorporated into agarose plugs. The PFGE was done by using contour-clamped homogeneous electric field (CHEF) (Bio-Rad, Hercules, California) and was ran in two blocks with a total run time of 23 h; the first block switch time was 5 to 15 s for 10 h, and the second-block switch time was 15 to 60 s for 13 h. The voltage for the run was 6 V/cm or 200 V. The included angle was 120° and the ramping factor was linear. Gels were stained and analysed visually and using Bionumerics® software package Version 3.0 (Applied Math, Sint-Martens, Belgium), using the Dice coefficient and represented by unweighted pair group method using the arithmetic averages (UPGMA) clustering method with 1% band position tolerance and 0.5% optimization settings. A similarity cut-off of 80% [30] and criterion of a difference of ≤6 bands [31] were both used to define a cluster.

Results

Prevalence

About 7.1% of the UVH staff (2/28), 8% (8/100) of the pets [5/50 (10%) of the dogs and 3/50 (6%) of the cats)], and 4.5% (9/28) of the environmental samples were found to be MRSA positive based on selective growth on ORSAB.

Antibiotic Resistance and MIC

All but two environmental isolates were resistant to Oxacillin. The two isolates show intermediate resistance to OX1, however, 4 μg/mL Oxacillin MIC values were recorded for both. The oxacillin MIC values for the isolates ranged from 4 μg/mL to ≥256 μg/mL with an isolate from a cat and two environmental isolates showing the highest MIC values. The two human isolates showed multi-resistance including intermediate resistance against vancomycin. An environmental isolate, EV017 has shown resistance to vancomycin while other two isolates, EV080 and EV100 from the same source were intermediately resistant to the same antibiotic. Moreover, these two isolates had the highest MIC value ≥256 μg/mL (Table 1). However, these three isolates were typed as vancomycin susceptible with MIC values of 0.5 μg/mL for EV080 and EV100 and 1.5 μg/mL for EV017 by Etest.

Detection of *mec*A, MLST and *spa* Typing

Among the 19 culture positive isolates, 17 (89.5%) were *mec*A-positive, whereas the remaining two isolates from the environment (10.5%) were *mec*A negative. The *mec*A-negative isolates were considered as borderline Oxacillin resistant based on combination of phenotypic features such as selective growth on ORSAB, AST and MIC values. The seven isolates analyzed by MLST were grouped into three clonal complexes (CCs) and two singletons. A human isolate (PG21), typed as ST1241 belonged to the same clonal complex CC59 as the two isolates from dogs (DG16 and DG20), both being typed as ST59. While all the same isolates typed by MLST were assigned to unique *spa* types which shared no similarity in their repeat patterns (Table 1).

PFGE

Fingerprinting by PFGE grouped the isolates into 11 PFGE profiles. Close similarities were seen in isolates from dogs, cats and environmental surfaces. Three of the five isolates from dogs, two of

Table 1. Phenotypic and genotypic characteristics of MRSA Isolated from veterinary personnel, pets and environmental surfaces.

Isolate Source and ID			Antibiotic Resistance Profile															Oxacillin MIC (μg/mL)	*nucA*	*mecA*	*spa* type/ Repeat Pattern	MLST
			AK30	**AML25**	**MET10**	**OX1**	**FOX30**	**S10**	**VA30**	**MH30**	**RD15**	**DO30**	**AMC30**	**CN10**	**IPM10**	**TE10**	**E15**					
UVH Staff	Nose	PG16	R	R	R	R	R	R	I	R	R	S	R	R	R	R	R	16	(+)	(+)	t2636 UJGAGJ	ST5
	Nose	PG21	S	S	R	R	S	R	I	R	R	S	S	S	S	R	R	8	(+)	(+)	UJGEGEEJJ	ST1241
Dogs	Nose	DG13	R	R	R	R	R	I	S	S	S	S	S	S	S	S	S	12	(+)	(+)	–	–
	Nose	DG16	R	R	R	R	R	R	S	S	S	S	R	S	S	S	R	16	(+)	(+)	t3590 ZAMDMOB	ST59
	Nose	DG20	S	R	R	R	S	S	S	S	S	S	S	S	S	S	S	8	(+)	(+)	t267 UJGFMBBBPB	ST59
	Nose	DG36	R	R	R	R	R	R	S	S	S	S	R	S	S	R	R	16	(+)	(+)	–	–
	Nose	DG49	R	R	R	R	R	R	S	S	S	S	R	S	S	R	R	12	(+)	(+)	–	–
Cats	Nose	CT04	R	R	R	R	R	R	S	R	R	R	R	R	S	R	R	≥256	(+)	(+)	t346 UJGBGGJAGJ	ST55
	Nose	CT27	R	R	R	R	R	S	S	S	S	S	S	I	S	S	S	32	(+)	(+)	–	–
	Nose	CT33	I	R	R	R	S	S	S	S	S	S	R	S	S	S	S	32	(+)	(+)	–	–
Environmental Surfaces	Waiting area	EV007	R	S	R	R	R	S	I	R	R	R	R	R	R	R	R	24	(+)	(+)	–	–
	Reception desk	EV017	R	R	R	R	R	S	R	R	R	R	R	R	I	R	R	≥256	(+)	(+)	–	–
	SAW table	EV035	R	R	R	R	R	R	I	R	I	R	R	R	I	R	S	12	(+)	(+)	–	–
	SAW cage	EV039	R	R	R	R	S	I	S	R	S	S	R	I	S	R	S	8	(+)	(+)	–	–
	Radiology room	EV041	R	R	R	R	R	R	S	R	R	R	R	R	S	R	S	8	(+)	(+)	–	–
	Surgical ward	EV080	R	R	R	R	R	R	I	S	R	R	R	R	R	R	S	≥256	(+)	(+)	UKGEMBKBGK	ST658
	Surgical ward	EV100	R	R	R	R	R	R	I	R	R	R	R	S	S	R	S	≥256	(+)	(+)	UJGEGE3KELO	ST1156
	SA examination room (table)	EV122	S	R	R	I	S	S	S	S	S	S	R	S	S	R	S	4	(+)	(−)	–	–
	SA examination room (floor)	EV157	R	R	R	I	S	R	S	S	S	R	R	S	S	S	S	4	(+)	(−)	–	–

SA: Small Animal; SAW: Small Animal Ward; R, Resistant; I, Intermediate Resistance; S, Susceptible.

the three isolates from cats and four of the nine environmental isolates were designated as genetically related based on their PFGE profiles. An isolate from dog (DG36) and a human isolate (PG21) from veterinary personel shared more than 90% similarity in their PFGE profile and hence were grouped as having genetic similarity. Likewise, an isolate from veterinary personnel (PG16) had 83.3% PFGE profile similarity with an isolate from environmental surface (EV100) indicating the close similarity between the two (Fig. 1).

Discussion

There has been increase in the number of reports of the isolation of MRSA from veterinarians and companion animals [3,21,32,33]. This underscores that MRSA is an emerging problem in veterinary medicine. The current study isolated MRSA from veterinary personnel, pets, and environmental surfaces in small animal hospital. A similar study in the UK found that the epidemic MRSA strain (EMRSA-15) occur in staff, patients and environmental sites in the referral small animal hospital [21]. While concurrent colonization with MRSA has been identified in humans and animals, MRSA can be transmitted between humans and animals many times within a household or veterinary clinic [34].

In a recent study conducted in Japanreported that being in contact with an identified animal MRSA case and being an employee of a veterinary hospital are the two independent factors associated with MRSA carriage [35]. They also suggested that animal patients spread MRSA infection among human individuals in veterinary hospitals. Recent evidence indicates that the environment in veterinary hospitals may be a potential source of MRSA [36]. It has been implicated that a clone of MRSA may have spread from a veterinarian to a dog patient by direct contact or through the medium of contaminated environments [35]. Our findings are supported by another study that reported MRSA at 12% (19/157) of the veterinary hospital environments sampled [36]. According to a recent report [37], humans were found to represent the most important source of MRSA for dogs in both community and veterinary hospital settings. The environment was found to be secondary to humans in terms of importance and other dogs less still [37]. A contaminated environment has also been reported as a potential source of MRSA in human and animal hospitals. It was stated that MRSA contaminated environment can be a source of contamination to the gloves of

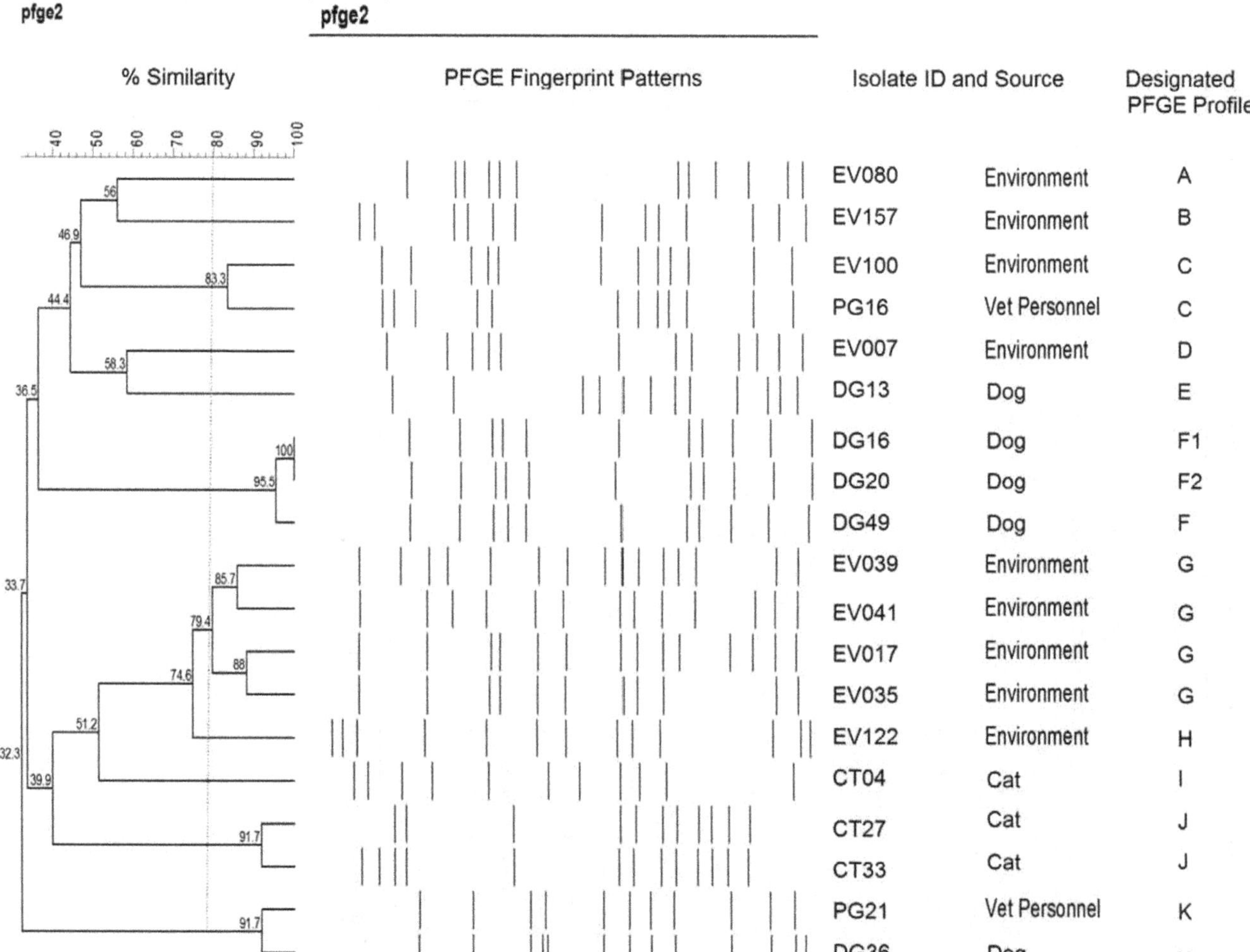

Figure 1. Dendrogram showing PFGE analyzed MRSA isolates from veterinary personnel, cats, dogs, and environmental surfaces at UPM. Data was analyzed using BioNumerics® (Applied Math, Sint-Martens, Belgium) Version 3.0. Dendrogram were derived from the unweighted pair group method using arithmetic averages (UPGMA) and based on Dice coefficient at band optimization of 0.5% and 1% band position tolerance.

healthcare workers and hence the pathogen gets transmitted to patients. A study conducted in Canadareported a widespread contamination of the veterinary hospital, which suggested the environment as an important source of MRSA infection [11]. MRSA contamination in veterinary hospitals has been reported in previous studies [21,37]. Though there is no evidence showing the direct transmission of MRSA from the environment to patients [38], the environment may serve as a source of MRSA exposure for animal health workers.

The PFGE pattern revealed that an isolate from a dog is closely related to an isolate from veterinary personnel in the present study. Likewise, an isolate from environmental surface was found to be closely related to a human isolate from other veterinary personnel. In a study conducted in Germany, an isolate from a cat was reported to be indistinguishable from the PFGE pattern of the human epidemic strain Barnim [39]. Furthermore, two studies conducted in UK [14] and Ireland [20] have respectively demonstrated that MRSA isolates in dogs and cats were indistinguishable or closely related to their attending personnel on PFGE. A similar finding has reported the genetic relatedness between MRSA isolates from human and environmental surfaces in veterinary teaching hospitals in UK [21]. In addition, MLST results in this study showed that a human isolate belonged to the same clonal complex (CC59) with two isolates from dogs, indicating the similar genetic background among the isolates. The fact that human isolates were closely related to isolates from a dog and environmental surfaces indicates the potential for either of the sources to serve as reservoirs for the other. This further implies the possibility of spread of the MRSA clones to an epidemic level, which in turn enables the strains to circulate and prevail in the small animal hospital premises and veterinary personnel. Furthermore, it is possible for veterinary staff to redistribute the strains into the community. A study has documented MRSA transmission between humans and dogs as they found the same MRSA strain in three staff members of small animal and equine hospital and three dogs, all being identical to the predominant human epidemic strain EMRSA-15 [40]. Other studies have also reported the similarity or close similarity of MRSA isolated from humans and companion animals [14,20,39,41].

Since *S. aureus* is resistant to desiccation and can survive longer in the environment [42,43], it is possible that a contaminated environment can serve as a source of colonization or infection with the bacteria. The environment has been indicated as potential source of MRSA in veterinary hospitals [36,37]. The significant contribution of environment in maintenance and propagation of MRSA was the possibility in the current study. However, further detailed studies are needed to affirm the importance of environment in MRSA transmission and its potential to serve as a source of infection in veterinary settings for animals and humans as well. In connection with this, the role of veterinary personnel as a possible vehicle for MRSA introduction into animal hospitals needs to be studied further and addressed to develop a sound MRSA control and prevention strategy. Though this study had limitations in ruling out the source of MRSA isolates in any of the sources, we believe that it paves the way for a more comprehensive study to be conducted in Malaysia.

Acknowledgments

The authors would like to thank the laboratory technicians and assistants at Bacteriology laboratory and staff at UVH, Faculty of Veterinary Medicine, Universiti Putra Malaysia for their kind cooperation over the course of this study. We also like to thank Ministry of Science, Technology and Innovation (MOSTI) for funding the research project.

Author Contributions

Conceived and designed the experiments: EA ZZ. Performed the experiments: EA. Analyzed the data: EA ZZ LH. Contributed reagents/ materials/analysis tools: ZZ. Wrote the paper: EA. Arranged and facilitated sample collection: CHC.

References

1. Hawkey PM (2008) Molecular epidemiology of clinically significant antibiotic resistance genes. Brit J Pharma 153: 406–413.
2. Jones RD, Kania SA, Rohrbach BW, Frank LA, Bermis DA (2007) Prevalence of oxacillin-and multidrug-resistant staphylococci in clinical samples from dogs: 1,772 samples (2001–2005). J Am Vet Med Assoc 230: 221–227.
3. van Duijkeren E, Wolfhagen MJHM, Box AT, Wannet WJ, Fluit AC (2004) Human-to-dog transmission of methicillin-resistant *Staphylococcus aureus*. Emerg Infect Dis 10: 2235–2237.
4. Anderson MEC, Lefebvre SL, Weese JS (2008) Evaluation of prevalence and risk factors for methicillin-resistant *Staphylococcus aureus* colonization in veterinary personnel attending an international equine veterinary conference. Vet Microbiol 129: 410–417.
5. Hanselman BA, Kruth SA, Rousseau J, Low DE, Willey BM, et al. (2006) Methicillin-resistant *Staphylococcus aureus* colonization in veterinary personnel. Emerg Infect Dis 12: 1933–1938.
6. Wulf MA, van Nes A, Eikelenboom-Boskamp J, de Vries W, Melchers C, et al. (2006) Methicillin-resistant *Staphylococcus aureus* in Veterinary Doctors and Students, the Netherlands. Emerg Infect Dis 12: 1939–1941.
7. Weese JS, van Duijkeren (2010) Methicillin-resistant Staphylococcus aureus and Staphylococcus pseudintermedius in veterinary medicine. Vet Microbiol 140: 418–429.
8. Stein RA (2009) Methicillin-resistant *Staphylococcus aureus*- the new Zoonosis. Int J Infect Dis 13: 299–301.
9. Moodley A, Nightingale EC, Stegger M, Nielsen SS, Skov RL, et al. (2008) High risk for nasal carriage of methicillin-resistant *Staphylococcus aureus* among Danish veterinary practitioners. Scand J Work Environ Health 34: 151–157.
10. Boyce JM, Potter-Bynoe G, Chenevert C, King T (1997) Environmental contamination due to methicillin-resistant *Staphylococcus aureus:* possible infection control implications. Infect Control Hosp Epidemiol 18: 622–627.
11. Weese JS, Goth K, Ethier M, Boehnke K (2004) Isolation of methicillin-resistant *Staphylococcus aureus* from the environment in a veterinary teaching hospital. J Vet Int Med 18: 468–470.
12. de Boer HE, van Elzelingen-Dekker CM, van Rheenen-Verberg CM, Spanjaard L (2006) Use of gaseous ozone for eradication of methicillin-resistant Staphylococcus aureus from the home environment of a colonized hospital employee. Infect Control Hosp Epidemiol 27: 1120–1122.
13. Neely AN, Maley M P (2000) Survival of enterococci and staphylococci on hospital fabrics and plastic. J Clin Microbiol 38: 724–726.
14. Moodley A, Stegger M. Bagcigil AF, Baptiste KE, Loeffler A, et al. (2006) *spa* typing of methicillin-resistant *Staphylococcus aureus* isolated from domestic animals and veterinary staff in the UK and Ireland. J Antimicrob Chemother 58: 1118–1123.
15. Weese JS, Archambault M, Willey BM, Dick H, Hearn P, et al. (2005) Methicillin-resistant *Staphylococcus aureus* in horses and horse personnel, 2000–2002. Emerg Infect Dis 11: 430–435.
16. McDougal LK, Steward CD, Killgore GE, Chaitram JM, McAllister SK, et al. (2003) Pulsed-Field Gel Electrophoresis Typing of Oxacillin-Resistant *Staphylococcus aureus* Isolates from the United States: Establishing a National Database. J Clin Microbiol 41: 5113–5120.
17. Straden A, Frei R, Windmer AF (2003) Molecular typing of methicillin- resistant *Staphylococcus aureus*: can PCR replace pulsed-field gel electrophoresis? J Clin Microbiol 41: 3181–3186.
18. Enright MC, Day NP, Davies CE, Peacock SJ, Spratt BG (2000) Multilocus sequence typing for characterization of methicillin-resistant and methicillin-susceptible clones of *Staphylococcus aureus*. J Clin Microbiol 38: 1008–1015.
19. Deplano A, Witte W, Van Leeuwen WJ, Brun Y, Struelens MJ (2000) of epidemic methicillin-resistant *Staphylococcus aureus* in and neighboring countries. Clin Microbiol Infect 6: 239–245.
20. O'Mahony R, Abbott Y, Leonard FC, MarkeyBK, Quinn PJ, et al. (2005) Methicillin-resistant *Staphylococcus aureus* (MRSA) isolated from animals and veterinary personnel in Ireland. Vet Microbiol 109: 285–296.
21. Loeffler A, Boag AK, Sung J, Lindsay JA, Guardabassi L, et al. (2005) Prevalence of methicillin-resistant *Staphylococcus aureus* among staff and pets in a small animal referral hospital in the UK. J Antimicrob Chemother 56: 692–697.
22. Nulens E, Stobberingh EE, van Dessel H, Sebastian S, van Tiel FH, et al. (1999) Molecular Characterization of *Staphylococcus aureus* Bloodstream Isolates Collected in a Dutch University Hospital between1999 and 2006. J Clin Microbiol 46: 2438–441.

23. Feil EJ, Enright MC (2004) Analyses of clonality and the evolution of bacterial pathogens. Curr Opin Microbiol 7: 308–313.
24. Ghaznavi-Rad E, Mariana NS, Zamberi S, Liew YK, Mohammad NA, et al. (2010) Predominance and Emergence of Clones of Hospital-Acquired Methicillin-Resistant *Staphylococcus aureus* in Malaysia. J Microbiol 48: 867–872.
25. Safdar N, Narans L, Gordon B, Maki DG (2003) Comparison of culture screening methods for detection of nasal carriage of methicillin-resistant *Staphylococcus aureus*: a prospective study comparing 32 methods. J Clin Microbiol 41: 3163–3166.
26. CLSI (2006) Performance Standards for Antimicrobial Disk Susceptibility Supplement, Clinical and Laboratory Standards Institute/National Committee for Clinical Laboratory Standards, Wayne, PA, USA. Document M100–S16.
27. Louie L, Goodfellow J, Mathieu P, Glatt A, Louie M, et al. (2002) Rapid detection of methicillin-resistant staphylococci from blood culture bottles by using a multiplex PCR assay. J Clin Microbiol 40: 2786–2790.
28. Harmsen D, Claus H, Witte W, Rothganger J, Turnwald D, et al. (2003) Typing of methicillin-resistant *Staphylococcus aureus* in a university hospital setting using novel software for *spa* repeat determination and database management. J Clin Microbiol 41: 5442–5448.
29. Murchan S, Kaufmann ME, Deplano A, de Ryck R, Struelens M, et al. (2003) Harmonization of pulsed-field gel electrophoresis protocols for epidemiological typing of strains of methicillin-resistant *Staphylococcus aureus*: a single approach developed by consensus in 10 European laboratories and its application for tracing the spread of related strains. J. Clin. Microbiol. 41: 1574–1585.
30. Struelens MJ, Deplano A, Godard C, Maes N, Serruys E (1992) Epidemiologic typing and delineation of genetic relatedness of methicillinresistant *Staphylococcus aureus* by macrorestriction analysis of genomic DNA by using pulsed-field gel electrophoresis. J Clin Microbiol 30: 2599–2605.
31. Tenover FC, Arbeit RD, Goering RV, Mickelsen PA, Murray BE, et al. (1995) Interpreting chromosomal DNA restriction patterns produced by pulsed-field gel electrophoresis: criteria for bacterial strain typing. J Clin Microbiol 33: 2233–2239.
32. Boost MV, O'Donoghue MM, Siu KHG (2007) Characterization of methicillin-resistant *Staphylococcus aureus* isolates from dogs and their owners. Clin Microbiol Infect 13: 731–733.
33. Rich M, Roberts L (2004) Methicillin-resistant Staphylococcus aureus isolates from companion animals. Vet Rec 154: 310.
34. Weese JS, Dick H, Willey BM, McGeer A, Kreiswirth BN, et al. (2006) Suspected transmission of methicillin-resistant *Staphylococcus aureus* between domestic pets and humans in veterinary clinics and in the household. Vet Microbiol 115: 148–155.
35. Ishihara K, Shimokubo N, Sakagami A, Ueno H, Muramatsu Y, et al. (2010) Occurrence and Molecular Characteristics of Methicillin-Resistant *Staphylococcus aureus* and Methicillin-Resistant *Staphylococcus pseudintermedius* in an Academic Veterinary Hospital. Appl Env Micorbiol 15: 5165–5174.
36. Hoet AE, Johnson A Nava-Hoet RC, Bateman S, Hillier A, et al. (2011) Environmental Methicillin-Resistant Staphylococcus aureus in a Veterinary Teaching Hospital During a Non-outbreak Period. Vector Borne Zoonotic Dis 11: 609–615.
37. Heller J, Kelly L, Reid SW, Mellor DJ (2010) Qualitative Risk Assessment of the Acquisition of Meticillin-Resistant Staphylococcus aureus in Pet Dogs. Risk Analysis 30: 458–472.
38. Hardy KJ, Oppenheim BA, Gossain S, Gao F, Hawkey PM (2006) A study of the relationship between environmental contamination with methicillin-resistant *Staphylococcus aureus* (MRSA) and patients' acquisition of MRSA. Infect Control Hosp Epidemiol 27: 127–132.
39. Walther B, Wieler LH, Friedrich AW, Hanssen AM, Kohn B, et al. (2008) Methicillin-resistant *Staphylococcus aureus* (MRSA) isolated from small and exotic animals at a university hospital during routine microbiological examinations. Vet Microbiol 127: 171–178.
40. Baptiste KE, Williams K, Williams NJ, Wattret A, Clegg PD, et al. (2005) Methicillin-resistant staphylococci in companion animals. Emerg Infect Dis 11: 1942–1944.
41. Vitale CB, Gross TL Weese JS (2006) Methicillin-resistant *Staphylococcus aureus* in cat and owner. Emerg Infect Dis 12: 1998–2000.
42. Dietze B, Rath A, Wendt C, Martiny H (2001) Survival of MRSA on sterile goods packaging. J Hosp Infect 49: 255–261.
43. Jawad A, Heritage J, Snelling M, Gascoyne-Binzi DM, Hawkey PM (1996) Influence of relative humidity and suspending menstrua on survival of *Acinetobacter* spp. on dry surfaces. J Clin Microbiol 34: 2881–2887.

4

A Vicious Cycle: A Cross-Sectional Study of Canine Tail-Chasing and Human Responses to It, Using a Free Video-Sharing Website

Charlotte C. Burn*

Veterinary Clinical Sciences, The Royal Veterinary College, North Mymms, Hertfordshire, United Kingdom

Abstract

Tail-chasing is widely celebrated as normal canine behaviour in cultural references. However, all previous scientific studies of tail-chasing or 'spinning' have comprised small clinical populations of dogs with neurological, compulsive or other pathological conditions; most were ultimately euthanased. Thus, there is great disparity between scientific and public information on tail-chasing. I gathered data on the first large ($n = 400$), non-clinical tail-chasing population, made possible through a vast, free, online video repository, YouTube^{TM}. The demographics of this online population are described and discussed. Approximately one third of tail-chasing dogs showed clinical signs, including habitual (daily or 'all the time') or perseverative (difficult to distract) performance of the behaviour. These signs were observed across diverse breeds. Clinical signs appeared virtually unrecognised by the video owners and commenting viewers; laughter was recorded in 55% of videos, encouragement in 43%, and the commonest viewer descriptors were that the behaviour was 'funny' (46%) or 'cute' (42%). Habitual tail-chasers had 6.5+/−2.3 times the odds of being described as 'Stupid' than other dogs, and perseverative dogs were 6.8+/−2.1 times more frequently described as 'Funny' than distractible ones were. Compared with breed- and age-matched control videos, tail-chasing videos were significantly more often indoors and with a computer/television screen switched on. These findings highlight that tail-chasing is sometimes pathological, but can remain untreated, or even be encouraged, because of an assumption that it is 'normal' dog behaviour. The enormous viewing figures that YouTube^{TM} attracts (mean+/−s.e. = 863+/−197 viewings per tail-chasing video) suggest that this perception will be further reinforced, without effective intervention.

Editor: Petter Holme, Umeå University, Sweden

Funding: The current study was carried out while the author was supported by a Wellcome Trust 'Value in People' Award (www.wellcome.ac.uk). The funders had no role in study design, data collection and analysis, decision to publish, or preparation of the manuscript.

Competing Interests: The authors have declared that no competing interests exist.

* E-mail: cburn@rvc.ac.uk

Introduction

Tail-chasing in dogs is widely celebrated in cultural references, such as its depiction in the cheerful, repetitive phrases of Chopin's Minute Waltz [1], and as performed by Sirius Black's *animagus* dog, Padfoot, in the Harry Potter series, when it is accompanied by a 'joyful bark' [2]. However, scientific literature exclusively refers to tail-chasing – or 'spinning', when the behaviour is not necessarily focussed towards the tail – in clinical contexts, because it can indicate welfare problems of varying severity, e.g. [3,4,5]. The most common reported diagnosis is canine compulsive disorder [6,7], but other conditions, such as dermatitis or anal sacculitis [8], are also reported. Even in otherwise healthy dogs, the behaviour could indicate externally triggered welfare problems including lack of stimulation ('boredom'), insufficient exercise, or various stressful situations [4,7,9]. Nevertheless, tail-chasing can simply comprise play or exercise in many dogs, and these 'normal' tail-chasers have never yet been included in scientific publications, partly because the sporadic nature of the behaviour makes it difficult to study.

Clinical texts, e.g. [3,4,10,11], often propose that compulsive tail-chasing develops from repeated exposure to triggering events or situations, but the behaviour gradually becomes dissociated from the original trigger, occurring ever more frequently in increasingly diverse contexts. In other words, the behaviour might develop through a vicious cycle. Like many stereotypic behaviours, tail-chasing can sometimes be temporarily eliminated by the opioid blocker, naloxone [12]. Attempted treatments for compulsive tail-chasing include behavioural therapy alongside drugs, including the tricyclic antidepressant, clomipramine, the selective serotonin reuptake inhibitor, fluoxetine [6,9], and the NMDA receptor blocker, memantine [7]. Tail-amputation has no reported success, and the problem can be so intractable, and distressing for the owners, that dogs are euthanased [7,12]. Indeed, all 32 dogs in Blackshaw et al.'s [12] study – the largest study to date – were euthanased due to the persistence of their condition.

Several breeds are prone to compulsive tail-chasing, including Bull Terriers [12], German Shepherds [6] and Anatolian sheepdogs [9]. However, the sample sizes of clinical studies to date have been too small to rule out high propensities in other breeds too, such as Jack Russells and West Highland White Terriers [12]. Breed differences could arise from environmental (e.g. opportunities to exercise) and/or genetic factors. If the latter, the behaviour could have been artificially selected for, even indirectly if tail-chasing is linked with a desirable characteristic, as with many inherited defects [13].

Despite the general renown of the behaviour and its potential severity in clinical cases, little is known about tail-chasing in home contexts or when no clinical causes have been diagnosed. Yet, a search for "dog chasing tail" on the most popular video-sharing website [14], YouTube™, returned almost 3500 hits in 2010. These videos provide a new opportunity for a hitherto untapped insight into tail-chasing in non-clinical contexts, and will include many 'normal' dogs (those with no relevant clinical diagnosis). For the first time, a large sample size is rapidly available and economically feasible. Furthermore, the videos reveal environments and contexts in which tail-chasing occurs, often together with audible and written responses of human observers (Figure 1).

Despite the increasing accessibility of broadband and video cameras/phones to a wide demographic, the dogs and humans on YouTube™ will not represent *all* dogs and humans; indeed truly representative sampling eludes most population studies. Dogs that tail-chase very rarely are likely to be under-represented, as videographers would have to catch the behaviour at exactly the right place and time. Conversely, dogs with clinical diagnoses may also be under-represented if owners are embarrassed (but not if they wish to raise awareness). Thus, the tail-chasing dogs on YouTube™ should approximately represent the centre of the normal distribution of dogs that chase their tails at some point in their lives. As with other survey methods, the use of video-sharing websites requires similar caution in generalizing conclusions beyond the sample population, because the populations are usually non-random and self-selecting to some extent. However, data from video-sharing websites reflects directly observed behaviour (rather than relying on respondents' descriptions), and data are unprompted by the researcher, so they are less likely to be biased towards the study purposes.

To date, video-sharing websites, such as YouTube™, have been studied regarding their potential for disseminating information to the public, in contexts including tobacco use [15], immunization [16] and sunbed use [17]. More recently, the actual video content has begun to be explored epidemiologically, providing insight into an asphyxiation 'game' in teenagers (using 65 video clips) [18], and into dietary messages given by adults to children playing with toy kitchens (115 clips) [19]. The current study goes further, using a larger sample size, plus a control group to examine the characteristics of and responses to tail-chasing in domestic dogs.

My aims were to describe (i) canine breed/morphological and (ii) behavioural characteristics, and the (iii) animal welfare implications and (iv) broad environmental contexts, associated with tail-chasing; and also (v) to describe human responses to it on YouTube™. I made no clinical diagnoses from the videos, but could broadly infer certain animal welfare implications from visible injuries and characteristics commonly associated with perseverative abnormal behaviours, including both frequent performance and persistence in the face of distraction.

Methods

Description of tail-chasing videos

I identified tail-chasing videos using the search term "dog chasing tail" on YouTube, which returned 3340 hits in November 2009. The videos were continually but gradually shuffled by YouTube's

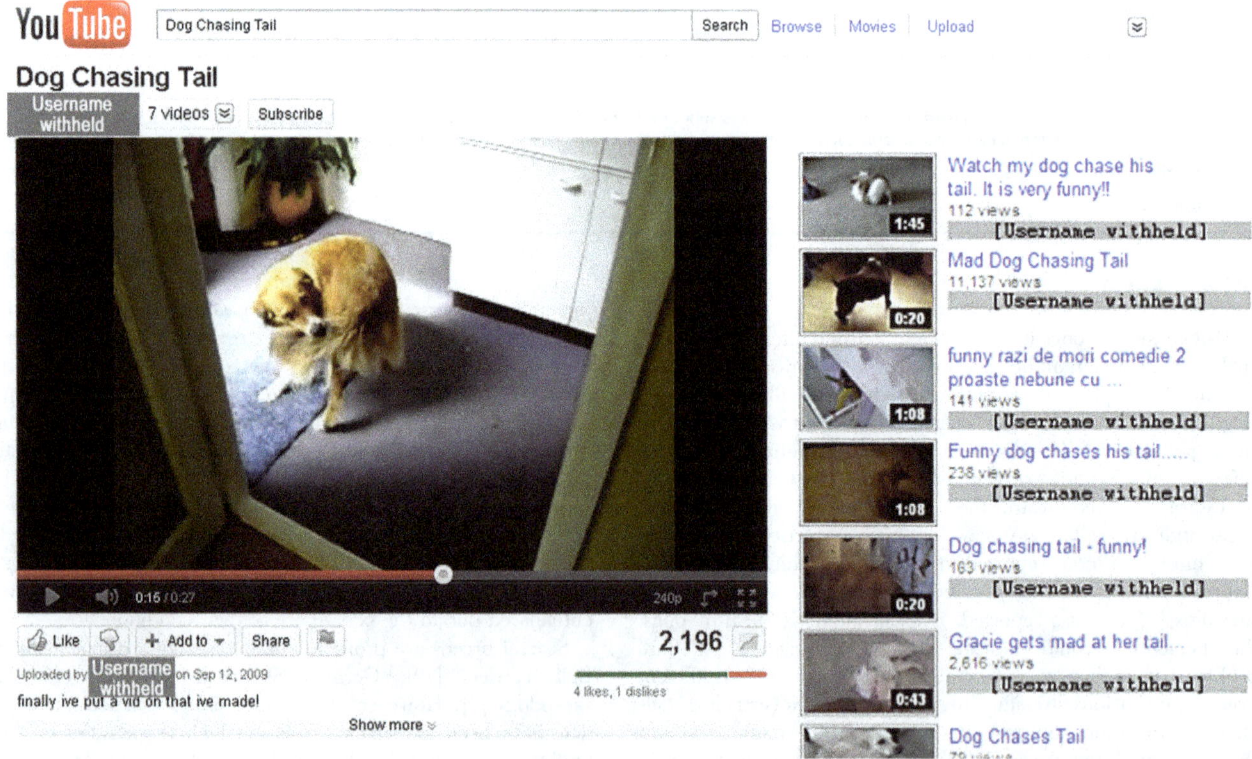

Figure 1. Screenshot of a video of a Golden Retriever chasing its tail on YouTube™. The sidebar on the right also offers views links to related videos, showing a thumbnail of the video content, the video title, and the number of times the video has been viewed. The usernames are withheld here for privacy reasons, but on YouTube™ they are hyperlinked to the uploaders' homepages, which usually contain information about their age, sex, country, and their other videos.

confidential search algorithms. Between Nov 2009 and August 2010, I collected data from the first 400 videos of the returned hits, subject to the following exclusion criteria: only one video was used per 'uploader' (person who uploaded a video to their YouTube™ account); and very dark or pixelated videos, or those not showing a domestic dog tail-chasing or spinning were discarded; photographic collages, professional videos, and advertisements were excluded, and in video collages, only the first continuous shot was used. It is worth noting that in some cases, the uploader may neither have owned the dog, nor have taken the footage themselves.

The following details were recorded from the videos (further details in Table S1):

- Clip ID and URL
- the reported sex, age and nationality of the uploader
- dog breed, sex and age
- dog tail morphology
- relevant human and dog behaviour observed in the video (summarized in Table 1)
- environmental context (indoors or outdoors; television switched on, off or unknown)
- relevant descriptive comments by the uploader and viewers (summarised in Table 2).

I structurally defined all the behaviours scored according to an ethogram (Table S1 and S2), and systematically categorized human comments after data collection using defined criteria (Table 2).

Comparisons of tail morphology and environmental context in breed-matched controls

I compared tail-chasing videos against 400 breed-matched control (non-tail-chasing) videos, to investigate associations between tail-chasing and tail morphology, such as whether docked tails were more or less frequently seen in tail-chasing versus control videos. The control videos were also used to identify whether dogs were more frequently indoors, and whether a television, computer, radio or music was switched on when tail-chasing. Breed- and age-matching was important because these factors affect the likelihood that dogs are taken outdoors and that their tails are docked. My control search terms were "[dog breed name]"+"dog" or "puppy" as appropriate to match each tail-chasing video. The first control video not yet scored for that breed was used in each case. Exclusion criteria were as before, but additionally, videos were excluded if the tail could not be clearly seen; if the control video included tail-chasing or spinning; or if the video seemed to involve animal cruelty, for ethical reasons (e.g. dog fights). The ensuing control videos included diverse footage: for example, dogs playing, vocalising, performing 'tricks', eating, dreaming, exercising, exploring novel stimuli, or interacting with other dogs, other pets, or humans.

Observer reliability

A subset of the variables described in Table S2 & S3, encompassing the more subjective aspects of dog and human behaviour, were checked for inter- and intra-observer reliability using 10% of the tail-chasing videos. Kappa observer reliability statistics are meaningless in overly homogenous samples [20–22], so Hoehler [21] suggests that investigators should 'concentrate on obtaining populations with trait prevalence near 50% rather than searching for statistical methods to rescue inefficient experiments." The 40 videos were therefore selected (using my ratings as the primary observer) to optimize the prevalence index for as many variables as possible, avoiding overly homogenous samples and allowing even rare scores to be tested [20,21]. For example, only 46 videos had comments revealing the dog's tail-chasing frequency as well as having a potentially distracting event occurring during the video, so 35 of these videos were included in the reliability sample (representing habitual, periodic and rare tail-chasing, in both perseverative (difficult to distract) and non-perseverative dogs). This meant that for key variables, such as tail-chasing frequency, distractibility, or play behaviour, the prevalence index was <0.4 [20], so no variable was too rare to test.

The order in which videos were re-watched was randomized. The other observer (OHB; see Acknowledgements) was an experienced observer of animal behaviour, and was blind to the hypotheses being tested. He received five practice videos for which he could see my original scores, and he was given a detailed description of the scoring criteria for each variable (Table S2), but he received no other training.

Intra- and inter-observer agreement was tested using Fleiss' Kappa statistics for binary variables, and Kendall's W for ordinal variables (Minitab 15). Thresholds for clinical acceptability were defined as Moderate (κ or $W \geq 0.4$), Substantial (≥ 0.6), or Excellent (≥ 0.8) according to convention, e.g. [22]. Only scores for panting behaviour failed to attain at least Moderate reliability, so results for that variable are not reported. The observer reliability scores are shown in Table S3.

Statistical methods

Within the 400 tail-chasing videos, I tested associations between specific tail-chasing behaviours and their predictors (other behaviours, dog characteristics, and human responses) using generalized linear mixed models (glmmPQL and glmmML in R). I included breed as a random factor in every model to control for non-independence of similar dogs, and compared breed groups (defined according to both the UK Kennel Club and genetic groupings found by Parker et al. [23]) either as random or as fixed factors in alternative models. Breed was nested within breed group. Video-length was always included, because certain events (e.g. play behaviour or potential distractions) will have been more likely to be observed in longer videos. For analyses of clinically relevant predictors, dogs with objects attached to their tails were excluded, because their tail-chasing was not necessarily ever a self-initiated behaviour.

I also used generalized linear mixed models, as before, to compare tail-chasing and control videos. In these analyses, tail morphology, the in- or outdoor location, and television/computer/radio activity were used as predictors.

I selected models using Akaike information criteria, and identified (and thus avoided) multicollinearity using inflated standard error terms. The α-level for statistical significance was set at $P \leq 0.05$ in this exploratory study [24]; the number of independent tests for each dependent variable ranged from six to 16, depending on the hypotheses relating to that variable. Of the total 76 tests carried out, just under four (5%) of the seemingly significant results can therefore be expected to be Type I errors, but follow up studies will be required to reveal which results can and cannot be replicated. No correction for multiple testing has been done here, because the risk of Type II errors, failing to report potentially significant results, is considered more serious in exploratory studies than that of Type I errors [24].

Results

Uploader and video characteristics

Of the 400 uploaders of the tail-chasing videos, 69.0% were from the USA, 13.8% from the UK, 5.8% from Canada, and

Table 1. Brief description of behavioural data collected from YouTube, and associations between them.

Behavioural characteristic	Description	Proportion of videos showing the characteristic (excluding videos with missing values)	Significant associations (↑ =positive association; ↓ =negative association	Odds ratio +/− S.E.; DF; P-value
Tail-chasing frequency as indicated by uploader comments*	'Habitual' (e.g. daily, "all the time", "a lot", "spends hours" tail-chasing, the dog is "obsessed"); 'Periodic' (e.g. "from time to time", "regularly", "[the dog] usually tail-chases when…"); or 'Rare' (e.g. "[the dog] rarely does this", I "managed to catch" the dog tail-chasing)	Habitual: 26/86 (30.2%); Periodic: 49/86 (57.0%); Rare: 11/86 (12.8%)	↑ Difficult to distract	8.06+/−2.50; 9; 0.049
"	"	"	↑ 'Stupid' in uploader comments	6.52+/−2.33; 23; 0.037
Difficult to distract	The dog did not stop chasing for more than 5 s despite a potential distraction (e.g. the owner commanded the dog to do something other than tail-chase, a sudden noise, or the dog collided with something hard enough to impede its progress)	76/198 (38.4%)	↓ Play	0.16+/−1.70; 102; 0.001
"	"	"	↓ Encouragement	0.28+/−1.40; 102; 0.000
"	"	"	↑ 'Funny' in public comments	6.82+/−2.09; 24; 0.016
"	"	"	Also see Habitual tail-chasing frequency	-
Vocalisations heard during or within 5 s of tail-chasing	Barking	54/366 (14.8%)	↓ Television and computer use	0.30+/−1.51; 201; 0.004
"	"	"	↑ Tail wagging	2.30+/−1.45; 201; 0.026
"	Growling	75/353 (21.2%)	↑ Hunter Group (Parker et al., 2007)	2.66+/−1.63; 83; 0.050
"	"	"	↑ Age (i.e. adults)	2.30+/−1.40; 206; 0.013
"	Whining	4/354 (1.1%)	(too rare to test)	-
Collision	Dog collided with an object during or up to 30 s after tail-chasing	101/393 (25.7%)	↓ Play	0.37+/−1.53; 262; 0.019
"	"	"	↑ Laughter	2.12+/−1.32; 230; 0.007
Play behaviour	Within 5 s of a chasing bout, the dog exhibits a play bow (characteristic posture with the forelegs extended on the ground), object play (manipulation of a toy or other available object), social play (with human or conspecific), or locomotor play (e.g., bounding, rolling)	66/389 (17.0%)	↑ Tail wagging	3.89+/−1.40; 259; 0.000
"	"	"	↓ Age	0.24+/−1.39; 259; 0.000
"	"	"	↑ Outside	3.26+/−1.63; 260; 0.016
"	"	"	↓ Funny	0.04+/−3.60; 68; 0.023
"	"	"	Also see Difficult to distract, and Collisions	-
Tail wagging	Dog rhythmically moves its tail laterally at least twice in each direction within 5 s of a chasing bout, rather than it remaining inanimate or moving irregularly	135/393 (25.7%)	↑ Age	2.77+/−1.36; 207; 0.001
"	"	"	↑ Television and computer use	2.15+/−1.33; 237; 0.008
"	"	"	↑ Mastiff-terriers	2.67+/−1.63; 84; 0.046
"	"	"	Also see Play Behaviour and Barking	-
Mouths tail	Dog is clearly seen to bite, lick or hold the tail or hindquarters/hind leg in its mouth for at least 1 s	248/392 (63.3%)	↑ Laughter	1.78+/−1.27; 235; 0.018
"	"	"	↑ 'Stupid' in uploader comments	4.16+/−1.67; 154; 0.006

When videos had no sound-track or the soundtrack was replaced by music, missing values were recorded for data reliant on sound; similarly missing values were recorded for videos without relevant comments or where the behaviour could not be clearly seen. The proportion of tail-chasing videos (excluding those with missing values) showing each characteristic is displayed, along with any significant associations with relevant predictors, for which the odds ratios, degrees of freedom, and P-values are displayed. *This odds ratio was calculated from a model using 'Habitual' vs other frequencies as a binary variable.

Table 2. Human encouragement and responses to tail-chasing in dogs on YouTube™.

Human response to tail-chasing (*n* = number of valid videos)	Proportion of videos (excluding videos with missing values)	Examples or synonyms (where relevant)
Human behaviour	-	-
Laughter	199/362 (55.0%)	Female: 66.4%; male 18.6%; both sexes: 15.0%
Verbal encouragement	119/362 (32.9%)	"Get your tail!", "Get it!"
'Growling' at dog	6/321 (1.9%)	
Physical manipulation	74/371 (19.9%)	Placing the tail in the mouth, pulling or pinching the tail, waving the tail near the dog's face, pushing the hindquarters
Tail attachment	14/371 (3.8%)	Attaching hair bands, dog toys or treats, a bottle, a section of plastic piping, or string to the tail
Verbal praise	12/362 (3.3%)	"Good dog", "Good girl/boy", and other variants
Physical praise	2/371 (0.6%)	Patting or stroking the dog, or feeding it a treat, after a chasing bout
Uploader description	-	-
'Funny'	149/253 (58.9%)	"Funny", "haha", "lol" (laugh out loud), "hilarious", "comedy", "humour", "XD" (a laughing emoticon), "lmao" (laugh my ass off)
'Crazy'	65/250 (26.0%)	"Crazy", "mad" (but not "gets mad" or "mad at" as these indicate perceived anger), "insane", "mental", "maniac", "nuts", "psycho", "nutcase"
'Cute'	47/250 (18.8%)	"Cute", "cutie", "sweet", "aww", "adorable"
'Stupid'	38/251 (15.1%)	"Stupid", "retard/retarded", "nerd", "dumb", "duh/doh", "dumbass", "dopey", "idiot", "moron"
'Silly'	28/250 (11.2%)	"Silly", "Goofy"
'Fun'	19/250 (7.6%)	"Fun", "amusing", "entertainment"
'Play'	12/250 (4.8%)	"Play", "playing", "game", "playful"
'Dizzy'	11/250 (4.4%)	"Dizzy"
'Weird'	10/250 (4.0%)	"Weird"
'Tricks'	8/249 (3.2%)	Tail-chasing is the dog's "party trick"
'Awesome'	8/250 (3.2%)	"Awesome", "cool", "amazing", "wow"
'Bored'	5/250 (2.0%)	"Bored"
'Hyper'	4/250 (1.6%)	"Hyper", "hyperactive", "energetic"
Other	N/A	Angry, classic, clever, confused, crack up, curious, dirty, enjoy, freak, frenzy, frustrated, inner battle, itchy, loser, nerd, nice, obsessed (x 2), possessed, serious problems, smart, spaz, tipsy, torture, wild, wrong, "I love that my dog actually chases her tail"
Explanations given	N/A	[The dog…] "loves/likes to tail-chase" (x6), "hates his tail", is "entertaining herself", is "having fun", is "either bored or has high cholesterol", "enjoys the dizziness", does it "out of dominance", "puts on a little show", "needs prozac", "chases on command" (x2), is "still a puppy", "hasn't figured [his tail] is connected to him", is showing "typical dog behaviour", is playing "his favourite game"
Viewer comments	-	-
'Funny'	64/138 (46.0%)	As for 'Uploader description', plus "hilarious"
'Cute'	58/138 (41.7%)	As for 'Uploader description'
'Awesome'	16/138 (11.5%)	As for 'Uploader description', plus "impressive"
'Stupid'	11/138 (7.9%)	As for 'Uploader description', plus "daft", "not that smart"
'Crazy'	4/138 (3.6%)	As for 'Uploader description', plus "bonkers"
Other	N/A	"Great" (x2), "excellent", "nice" (x3), "priceless", "entertaining", "weird", "gay", "fun" (x2), "cruel", "animal abuse", "I wonder why they do that", "My dog does/did that too" (x7), "My dog bites his tail to the point of bleeding", "My dog spins/chases faster than yours" (x4), "Dog chasing tail never gets old", "I want your dog", "I've never seen a dog do that", "I feel bad for him", "repetitive behaviours need to be checked by a vet", "I love it when dogs and cats do that"

Table 2. Cont.

Human response to tail-chasing (*n*= number of valid videos)	Proportion of videos (excluding videos with missing values)	Examples or synonyms (where relevant)
Explanations given	N/A	[The dog...] has "high cholesterol" (x2), has "canine compulsive disorder", is in "pain/discomfort", has "Schizophrenia", needs "the doggie chiropractor", is "happy", needs "toys", "doesn't know [the tail] is part of their body yet", has an "itchy tail", has "worms", is "hyper", is "bored", is "showing off", has "a flea stuck in his tail"

The percentages of videos are arranged in order of magnitude for each general category. The words that were accepted as valid synonyms for comment categories were shown. These were accepted only if they were consistent within the context of the whole comment, e.g. a comment was not included in the counts for 'funny' if the comment actually stated that the video was 'not funny', even though the keyword was present in the comment.

9.8% from 19 other countries. There was no significant sex bias in uploaders: 30% were female, 24% male and 46% undeclared (Binomial test of 119 females of the 215 declared: $P = 0.133$). The mean (s.e.) reported age of uploaders was 27.5+/−0.44, ranging between 11 and 68 years.

The mean tail-chasing video length was 59.8+/−2.8 s. Each video had a mean of 863+/−197 viewings by May 2011 (maximum = 58,613), giving a cumulative viewing figure of 313,225 for the 400 videos included here.

Tail-chasing characteristics and their associations

Associations between dog behaviour characteristics and context (excluding dogs with objects attached to their tails) are shown in Table 1. Of the 86 tail-chasing videos that had comments describing the frequency of tail-chasing, about 30% of dogs were stated as chasing their tails habitually (e.g. daily or 'all the time', rather than 'periodically' or 'rarely' (Table 1; Table S1), which is a clinical criterion for classifying tail-chasing as compulsive [7,25]).

Approximately 38% of dogs appeared difficult to distract, or 'perseverative' during tail-chasing. Perseverative dogs were more likely to tail-chase habitually and to collide with objects when tail-chasing, and they were less likely to show play behaviours than were other tail-chasing dogs (Table 1). Hair-loss from the tail or hind-quarters was seen in 1.25% of the tail-chasing dogs and there were no comments that suggested uploaders or viewers considered this as an indication of the tail-chasing being a potential clinical problem.

Play behaviours (defined in Table 1) were interspersed with tail-chasing bouts in 17% of videos, and were more likely to be seen in puppies than older dogs. When indoors, tail-chasing was less likely to include play behaviour than when outdoors, and with a screen switched on, tail-chasing dogs were less likely to bark but more likely to wag their tails (Table 1).

Problematic tail-chasing (as indicated by the percentage of all tail-chasing videos that appeared perseverative or habitual per breed group) was distributed widely across diverse Kennel Club breed groups (Table 3). The highest proportion of perseverative tail-chasing was observed in toy breeds (56% of videos), followed by crossbreeds (43%) and terriers and working dogs (42% of both), but around one quarter of videos of gundogs, hounds, and utility breeds also showed evidence for perseveration. Few breed groups contained enough videos to enable assessment of tail-chasing frequency, but of those with at least 10 such clips, the highest proportion of habitual tail-chasing was observed in crossbreeds (52%) and terriers (38%). The five dogs with visible hair-loss or injury to the tail or hindquarters comprised two German Shepherds, one Labrador-Staffordshire Bull Terrier cross, one Labrador and one Parsons Jack Russell Terrier.

Human responses and descriptions of tail-chasing videos

While 69.3% of tail-chasing videos were categorized as 'Pets and Animals', 18.8% were categorized as 'Comedy' and 6.3% as 'Entertainment'.

Human responses to tail-chasing are shown in Table 2. In 55% of videos, laughter could be heard, and this was significantly more likely to be female (in 81.6% of 114 clips with only one sex laughing; Binomial test: $P<0.001$). Laughter was positively associated with encouragement of the dog (Odds +/− S.E. = 2.83+/−1.28; DF = 234; $P<0.001$), but there were no significant associations with tail-chasing frequency or perseveration. Verbal or physical encouragement or praise was noted in 43% of videos, including attaching objects to the tail in almost 4% of videos (Table 2). Uploaders described 59% of tail-chasing videos as 'Funny', 26% as 'Crazy', 19% as 'Cute' and 15% as 'Stupid'. Similarly, 46% of videos with comments from viewers were described as 'Funny' by the viewers, and 42% as 'Cute'.

Viewers were 6.8 times more likely to describe perseverative dogs as 'Funny' (defined in Table 2) compared with more easily distracted dogs. Uploaders described dogs that tail-chased habitually as 'Stupid' (defined in Table 2) 6.5 times more often than other dogs. Examples of uploader comments describing habitual chasing are as follows: "*Ya it's funny she does this all the time:)*"; "*... my puppy does this ALL THE TIME. I've never seen a dog chase its tail so much. Maybe he enjoys the dizzyness??*"; "*This is just 1/100th of the allotted time [my dog] spends chasing his tail every day*"; "*This is him on a normal day. Chasing His Tail, Then eats his food, Watches a little TV, Chase's his tail some more then eat...*"; and (audible, rather than written) "*It's amazing how long he'll do that for... he never stops... it's your favourite game; you take it everywhere with you*".

In nine videos (2.3%), at least one comment offered clinical explanations for the behaviour or suggested that the dog should be checked by a veterinarian (three comments by uploaders, and seven videos had at least one such comment by viewers). However, none of the descriptions indicated that uploaders had posted their video on YouTube^{TM} specifically to raise awareness of clinical aspects of tail-chasing.

Comparisons of environmental context and tail morphology against breed-matched controls

Videos showing tail-chasing were approximately 6.5 times less likely to be outdoors than were breed- and age-matched control videos (8.8% of tail-chasing videos were outdoors versus 38.8% of controls; Odds +/− S.E = 0.15+/−1.25; DF = 317; $P<0.001$); and when indoors, tail-chasing videos were over three times more likely to show a television or computer switched on than were controls (32.1% of indoor tail-chasing videos showed one switched

Table 3. Perseverative and habitual tail-chasing described by Kennel Club group.

Kennel Club Breed group	Total tail-chasing videos (*n*)	Perseveration				Tail-chasing frequency				
		Distractible (*n*)	Perseverative (*n*)	Percentage perseverative	Breeds exhibiting perseveration	Rare (*n*)	Periodic (*n*)	Habitual (*n*)	Percentage habitual	Breeds exhibiting habitual tail-chasing
Gundog	56	22	8	26.7	Goldendoodle, Golden Retriever, Labrador	2	9	3	21.4	Labrador, Springer Spaniel
Hound	21	9	3	25.0	Beagle, Dachshund	1	1	0	0.0	N/A
Pastoral	28	5	0	0.0	N/A	1	5	1	14.3	Shetland Sheepdog
Terrier	86	28	20	41.7	American Staffordshire Bull Terrier, Jack Russell Terrier, Patterdale Terrier, Pitbull, Staffordshire Bull Terrier, Yorkshire Terrier	3	7	6	37.5	American Staffordshire Bull Terrier, Jack Russell Terrier, Patterdale Terrier, Pitbull Terrier, Staffordshire Bull Terrier
Toy	56	11	14	56.0	Chihuahua, Havenese, Papillon, Pekingese, Pug	3	10	2	13.3	Chihuahua, Shih Tzu
Utility	29	10	3	23.1	Lhasa Apso, Shih Tzu	0	4	2	33.3	Lhasa Apso
Working dog	24	7	5	41.7	Bernese Mountain Dog, Boxer	1	2	0	0.0	N/A
Crossbreeds	100	30	23	43.4	N/A	0	11	12	52.2	N/A

Breeds are grouped according to the Kennel Club, which takes into account the breed history and general usage. They can also be grouped both genetically, as described by Parker et al. (2007), but those data are not shown here because not all recognised breeds have been genetically characterised according to that system to date. Representative breeds that showed perseverative or habitual tail-chasing are listed for each breed group; these were identified from uploader descriptions, or if no breed was stated, the breed was estimated from the appearance of the dog. Only those videos that included a potentially distracting event ($n = 198$) are included in the figures for perseveration, and only those with comments describing the tail-chasing frequency ($n = 86$) are included in the habitual chasing calculations.

on versus 9.1% of controls; Odds +/− S.E. = 3.35+/−1.34; DF = 106; $P<0.001$).

Control and tail-chasing videos showed no significant differences in tail morphology, such as length, docking, or hair-type (initial analyses had suggested that tails were longer in tail-chasing than control videos [26], but this relationship proved not to be robust when other significant variables were included in the final statistical models).

Discussion

Descriptions of tail-chasing characteristics, context and human responses to it

The results here reveal new clinically relevant information that has been difficult to discover previously. Approximately one third of the dogs with complete data tail-chased habitually or appeared perseverative, and were significantly more likely than other tail-chasers to be described as 'Stupid' or 'Funny', respectively. Comments suggesting clinical explanations for habitual, perseverative tail-chasing were only seen on 2.3% of videos, so it seems that public awareness must indeed be very low. Regardless of clinical signs, about one quarter (25.1%) of tail-chasing videos were classified as Comedy or Entertainment, laughter was recorded in over half (55%) of videos, and encouragement in 43%; and almost half of viewer comments described the videos as 'funny' or 'cute'. The vast and ever growing numbers of viewings that these and similar videos receive on YouTube™ will likely reinforce these perceptions, normalising tail-chasing behaviour yet further [18].

The findings therefore indicate a gulf between public perception and indicators of poor welfare in tail-chasing dogs. This implies that many pathological tail-chasers may go untreated, and the behaviour is widely assumed to be normal and amusing regardless of its persistence. These results are perhaps not surprising considering that some owners also incorrectly perceive the – arguably less ambiguous – separation-related behaviours in their dogs (barking, whining, howling, scratching the door, destructive behaviour and inappropriate elimination) to indicate neutral or even positive welfare [27]. Similarly, owners can describe frequent signs of breathing difficulties in their brachycephalic (short-muzzle) dogs, but most later report that this not a 'breathing problem', being normal for the breed [28]. It appears that, although dogs seem readily to understand aspects of human behaviour [29,30], humans do not necessarily interpret all important aspects of canine behaviour accurately.

Results in Table 3 show that problematic tail-chasing as a proportion of all the tail-chasing videos per breed group was prevalent in Bull Terrier breeds, consistent with clinical literature [4,9,12], but it was also widely distributed across other breed groups, including Toy and other groups little represented in studies to date. The prevalences here should not be taken as absolute values, because some breeds may be owned by a more technologically active demographic than others, and might thus be over represented on YouTube™. Also, if owners of breeds known to tail-chase compulsively are more aware of the clinical implications of this behaviour than other owners, they may be reluctant to post videos of it (e.g. being embarrassed or saddened by it), so those breeds could be under-represented. Nevertheless, the results indicate the degrees to which tail-chasing videos show problematic signs in the different breed groups and suggest that it would be worthwhile investigating whether there are hitherto unrecognized clinical implications of tail-chasing across diverse breeds. Possibly behavioural anomalies in small or toy dogs may be less likely to be referred for veterinary attention than in larger, heavier breeds, whose behaviour may be more disruptive and obviously problematic to the owners. A previous survey indicated that owners of smaller dogs may also be less attentive to their dogs' behaviour and training in general [31].

In 17% of videos play behaviours were interspersed with tail-chasing; playing was less likely in perseverative dogs, but more likely in puppies than adult dogs. This is consistent with tail-chasing sometimes forming part of play, especially in puppies [4]. In these cases, as long as dogs infrequently chase their tails, owners need not necessarily be concerned about their dog's tail-chasing because play is often (but not always) an indicator of positive welfare [32]. A caveat is that even play can be a response to stress, lack of exercise or under-stimulation (a 'do-it-yourself enrichment', c.f. [33]), so owners should assess the context of the behaviour in case the trigger could be a negative one.

Encouragement of tail-chasing was recorded in 43% of videos, and laughter, which could also inadvertently be reinforcing for dogs, was heard in 55% of videos. The true prevalence of encouragement and laughter, will depend on how frequently people manipulate the dog for the film (e.g. attaching objects to the tail), play up to the camera, or deliberately remain quiet or offscreen during filming. Some encouragement seen on YouTu-be™ may have directly distressed the dogs: in almost 2% of videos, humans 'growled' at dogs, and almost 20% of people physically manipulated the tail (Table 2), often appearing to pull or pinch it with considerable force. In any case, whether reinforcement is through negative or positive means, it should be minimized to prevent tail-chasing from becoming compulsive. Equally, frequent tail-chasing must not be punished or prevented without addressing its cause, as this can increase stress and poor welfare in the affected dog, e.g. [34].

Comparisons of environmental context and tail morphology in breed-matched controls

Compared with breed- and age-matched controls, tail-chasing videos were approximately 6.5 times less likely to be outdoors, and – when indoors – televisions or computers (but not radios or music players) were more frequently switched on. The breed- and age-matching was intended to control for some breeds being kept indoors to a greater extent than others. However, the environmental differences could still be Type I errors (falsely significant) if, for example, tail-chasing were one of the few canine behaviours that people tend to record indoors while watching television, rather than it being performed more in that situation *per se*. Some control videos were by nature likely to be filmed outdoors, such as dogs exercising or interacting with other dogs, but others showed more typically indoor activities, such as eating, dreaming, or interacting with other pets, so further research will be necessary to confirm the environmental contexts of tail-chasing.

Nevertheless, the observed environmental differences are consistent with tail-chasing being triggered by a lack of exercise, under-stimulation, and/or insufficient attention from humans [4,7,9,11]. If so, the behaviour might indeed predominantly occur when dogs are indoors while humans are engaged in the sedate, non-interactive pastimes of television and computer use. Lack of exercise, stimulation and attention as triggers for tail-chasing have apparently not yet been tested empirically. If tail-chasing genuinely is associated with insufficient exercise, this would also be consistent with tail-chasing dogs having raised cholesterol levels, as found by Yalcin et al. [25].

The usual treatment for compulsive tail-chasing is drug therapy combined with behavioural therapy, such as increased owner attention and walks; the drugs may treat the clinical signs but behavioural change addresses the cause of the problem. However, owner compliance with behavioural recommendations is often poor, e.g. [7], and in general many dogs are walked very seldom (e.g. fewer than half of Australian owners surveyed walked their dogs at all [35], and 70% of dogs with acral lick dermatitis were never walked [36]). The finding that tail-chasing on YouTube™ appears to occur predominantly indoors with screens switched on might therefore reinforce the importance of exercise and stimulation for dogs.

Tail morphology and docking showed no significant differences between tail-chasing and control videos. A previous small-scale study [37] found neuromas in the docked tails of dogs showing 'tail-directed behaviour', so neuromas should be considered as a potential cause of tail-chasing in docked dogs, but no such association was found here (indeed the non-significant trend was in the opposite direction). A study focussing on breeds with frequently docked tails will be necessary to investigate whether a significant association exists.

Conclusions

In summary, YouTube™ has offered the first large, study population of dogs chasing their tails in non-clinical contexts. Approximately one third of the dogs showed signs of clinical relevance, but this was rarely recognised openly by uploaders or viewers; indeed, dogs showing problematic tail-chasing were more likely than other dogs to be described as 'Stupid' or 'Funny'. In 43% of videos tail-chasing was actively encouraged, which could risk reinforcing the behaviour excessively, and in some cases it included rough handling or goading the dog. The study also reveals that diverse dog breeds chase their tails on YouTube™, and that this seems predominantly to occur indoors when televisions or computers are switched on.

Future research could record more detail about the clinical signs: for example, details of tail-mouthing behaviour could indicate tail or hindquarter discomfort, and persistently chasing in one direction could help diagnose compulsivity [12]. It will also be necessary to determine what really triggers tail-chasing, to obtain meaningful prevalences of pathological and non-pathological tail-chasing, and to identify the most reliable indicators of whether the behaviour is of welfare concern. in the meantime, awareness of the clinical implications of frequent tail-chasing should be increased in the public domain if the associated canine welfare problems are to be addressed.

Supporting Information

Table S1 Condensed descriptions of all the data collected concerning YouTube™ videos of dogs chasing their tails. * indicates that the data were also collected for breed-matched control videos.

Table S2 The detailed description of criteria for scoring the presence or absence of particular characteristics in YouTube™ videos of dogs chasing their tails. This includes a subset of the behavioural ethogram used to score the dog behaviour throughout the study. This summary was sent to the animal behaviour expert (OHB) who scored the 40 videos to allow inter-observer reliability to be tested.

Table S3 Intra- and inter-observer reliability for selected variables describing dogs chasing their tails on YouTube™. For each variable, the raw percentage agreement (%), the prevalence index (P.I.) and the κ value (for categorical variables) or W value (for ordinal variables) is shown. * indicates that the κ value fell below the clinically acceptable threshold of 0.4 (e.g. Sim & Wright, 2005), so the variable should be discarded from further analysis. ¥ indicates that the variable is ordinal, rather than categorical.

Acknowledgments

Many thanks to Dr Oliver H. Burman for watching and behaviour-scoring the videos to allow testing for inter-observer reliability. Thanks also to Drs Holger Volk, Oliver H. Burman, Alex A. S. Weir, Prof. Alan Wilson and the anonymous referees for their constructive comments on the manuscript. I would like to acknowledge Verity J. Browning, who carried out her Bioveterinary Sciences Final Honours project on part of this subject under my supervision at the Royal Veterinary College, which effectively acted as a pilot for this study. The RVC has approved this manuscript (ID number: P/VCS/000147/) for publication.

Author Contributions

Conceived and designed the experiments: CCB. Performed the experiments: CCB. Analyzed the data: CCB. Contributed reagents/materials/analysis tools: CCB. Wrote the paper: CCB.

References

1. Small A (1994) World's Greatest Classic Themes. Harlow: Alfred Publishing Company.
2. Rowling JK (2003) Chapter 10. Harry Potter and the Order of the Phoenix. London: Bloomsbury Publishing PLC. 165 p.
3. Bowen J, Heath S (2005) Behaviour Problems in Small Animals: Practical Advice for the Veterinary Team. Philadelphia: Saunders Ltd. 288 p.
4. Hartigan PJ (2000) Compulsive tail chasing in the dog: A mini-review. Ir Vet J 53: 261–264.
5. Moon-Fanelli AA, Dodman NH (1998) Description and development of compulsive tail chasing in terriers and response to clomipramine treatment. J Am Vet Med Assoc 212: 1252–1257.
6. Irimajiri M, Luescher AU, Douglass G, Robertson-Plouch C, Zimmermann A, et al. (2009) Randomized, controlled clinical trial of the efficacy of fluoxetine for treatment of compulsive disorders in dogs. J Am Vet Med Assoc 235: 705–709.
7. Schneider BM, Dodman NH, Maranda L (2009) Use of memantine in treatment of canine compulsive disorders. J Vet Behav Clin Appl Res 4: 118–126.
8. Halnan CRE (1976) The diagnosis of anal sacculitis in the dog. J Small Anim Pract 17: 527–535.
9. Yalcin E (2010) Comparison of clomipramine and fluoxetine treatment of dogs with tail chasing. Tierärztliche Praxis Kleintiere 2010: 295–299.
10. Luescher AU (2004) Diagnosis and management of compulsive disorders in dogs and cats. Clin Tech Small Anim Pract 19: 233–239.
11. Lindsay SR (2001) Excessive Behavior. In: Lindsay SR, ed. Handbook of Applied Dog Behavior and Training, Volume 2: Etiology and Assessment of Behavior Problems Iowa State University Press. pp 131–159.
12. Blackshaw JK, Sutton RH, Boyhan MA (1994) Tail chasing or circling behavior in dogs. Canine Pract 19: 7–11.
13. Summers JF, Diesel G, Asher L, McGreevy PD, Collins LM (2010) Inherited defects in pedigree dogs. Part 2: Disorders that are not related to breed standards. Vet J 183: 39–45.
14. Cheng X, Dale C, Liu J (2007) Understanding the characteristics of internet short video sharing: YouTube as a case study. arXiv: 07073670v1.
15. Freeman B, Chapman S (2007) Is "YouTube" telling or selling you something? Tobacco content on the YouTube video-sharing website. Tob Control 16: 207–210.
16. Keelan J, Pavri-Garcia V, Tomlinson G, Wilson K (2007) YouTube as a source of information on immunization: a content analysis. J Am Med Assoc 298: 2482–2484.
17. Hossler EW, Conroy MP (2008) YouTube as a source of information on tanning bed use. Arch Dermatol 144: 1395–1396.
18. Linkletter M, Gordon K, Dooley J (2010) The choking game and YouTube: a dangerous combination. Clin Pediatr (Phila) 49: 274–279.
19. Lynch M (2010) Playing with food. A novel approach to understanding nutritional behaviour development. Appetite 54: 591–594.
20. Burn CC, Weir AAS (2011) Using prevalence indices to aid interpretation and comparison of agreement ratings between two or more observers. Vet J 188: 166–170.
21. Hoehler FK (2000) Bias and prevalence effects on kappa viewed in terms of sensitivity and specificity. J Clin Epidemiol 53: 499–503.
22. Sim J, Wright CC (2005) The kappa statistic in reliability studies: use, interpretation, and sample size requirements. Phys Ther 85: 257–268.
23. Parker HG, Kukekova AV, Akey DT, Goldstein O, Kirkness EF, et al. (2007) Breed relationships facilitate fine-mapping studies: A 7.8-kb deletion cosegregates with Collie eye anomaly across multiple dog breeds. Genome Res 17: 1562–1571.
24. Bender R, Lange S (2001) Adjusting for multiple testing–when and how? J Clin Epidemiol 54: 343–349.
25. Yalcin E, Ilcol YO, Batmaz H (2009) Serum lipid concentrations in dogs with tail chasing. J Small Anim Pract 50: 133–135.
26. Burn CC, Browning VJ. Dog tail-chasing behaviour & human responses to it: Preliminary insights from YouTube™ [poster presentation]. In: Lidfors L, Blokhuis H, Keeling L, eds. 2010; Uppsala Wageningen Academic Publishers, 165.
27. Mendl M, Brooks J, Basse C, Burman O, Paul E, et al. (2010) Dogs showing separation-related behaviour exhibit a 'pessimistic' cognitive bias. Curr Biol 20: R839–R840.
28. Packer RMA, Hendricks A, Axe JL, Burn CC (2011) Preliminary indications of a lack of owner recognition of clinical signs related to a conformational inherited disorder - a potential constraint to improving breeding practices in pedigree dogs. In: Kirkwood JK, Hubrecht R, Wickens S, eds. UFAW International Animal Welfare Symposium. Portsmouth: Universities Federation for Animal Welfare.
29. Miklosi A, Topal J, Csanyi V (2004) Comparative social cognition: what can dogs teach us? Anim Behav 67: 995–1004.
30. Riedel J, Schumann K, Kaminski J, Call J, Tomasello M (2008) The early ontogeny of human-dog communication. Anim Behav 75: 1003–1014.
31. Arhant C, Bubna-Littitz H, Bartels A, Futschik A, Troxler J (2010) Behaviour of smaller and larger dogs: Effects of training methods, inconsistency of owner behaviour and level of engagement in activities with the dog. Appl Anim Behav Sci 123: 131–142.
32. Held SDE, Špinka M (2011) Animal play and animal welfare. Anim Behav 81: 891–899.
33. Mason GJ, Latham NR (2004) Can't stop, won't stop: is stereotypy a reliable animal welfare indicator? Anim Welf 13: 57–69.
34. Mason GJ, Clubb R, Latham N, Vickery S (2007) Why and how should we use environmental enrichment to tackle stereotypic behaviour? Appl Anim Behav Sci 102: 163–188.
35. Bauman AE, Russell SJ, Furber SE, Dobson AJ (2001) The epidemiology of dog walking: an unmet need for human and canine health. Med J Aust 175: 632–634.
36. Pereira JT, Larsson CE, Ramos D (2010) Environmental, individual and triggering aspects of dogs presenting with psychogenic acral lick dermatitis. J Vet Behav Clin Appl Res 5: 165–165.
37. Gross TL, Carr SH (1990) Amputation neuroma of docked tails in dogs. Vet Path Online 27: 61–62.

Reproductive Capability Is Associated with Lifespan and Cause of Death in Companion Dogs

Jessica M. Hoffman[1], Kate E. Creevy[2]*, Daniel E.L. Promislow[1]*

1 Department of Genetics, University of Georgia, Athens, Georgia, United States of America, 2 Department of Small Animal Medicine and Surgery, College of Veterinary Medicine, University of Georgia, Athens, Georgia, United States of America

Abstract

Reproduction is a risky affair; a lifespan cost of maintaining reproductive capability, and of reproduction itself, has been demonstrated in a wide range of animal species. However, little is understood about the mechanisms underlying this relationship. Most cost-of-reproduction studies simply ask how reproduction influences age at death, but are blind to the subjects' actual causes of death. Lifespan is a composite variable of myriad causes of death and it has not been clear whether the consequences of reproduction or of reproductive capability influence all causes of death equally. To address this gap in understanding, we compared causes of death among over 40,000 sterilized and reproductively intact domestic dogs, *Canis lupus familiaris*. We found that sterilization was strongly associated with an increase in lifespan, and while it decreased risk of death from some causes, such as infectious disease, it actually increased risk of death from others, such as cancer. These findings suggest that to understand how reproduction affects lifespan, a shift in research focus is needed. Beyond the impact of reproduction on *when* individuals die, we must investigate its impact on *why* individuals die, and subsequently must identify the mechanisms by which these causes of death are influenced by the physiology associated with reproductive capability. Such an approach may also clarify the effects of reproduction on lifespan in people.

Editor: Samuli Helle, University of Turku, Finland

Funding: This work was partially supported by National Institutes of Health training grant T32GM007103. No additional external funding was received for this study. The funders had no role in study design, data collection and analysis, decision to publish, or preparation of the manuscript.

Competing Interests: The authors have declared that no competing interests exist.

* E-mail: creevy@uga.edu (KEC); promislow@uga.edu (DELP)

Introduction

Models for life history evolution assume that investment in reproduction comes at the cost of survival. Numerous studies in nematodes, fruit flies and mice have found that reproduction often–but not always–shortens lifespan [1,2,3,4], and scientists disagree over whether reproduction in humans increases, decreases, or has no effect on lifespan (e.g., [5,6,7], but see [8]). We submit that these inconsistent results are due to the fact that these studies examine the effect of reproduction on *when* individuals die, but not on *why* they die. Surprisingly, there currently are no comprehensive studies on the specific causes of mortality associated with reproductive capability or sterilization status. While invertebrate species such as *Caenorhabditis elegans* and *Drosophila melanogaster* serve as powerful model systems for genetic and molecular investigations, we know little about actual causes of mortality in these species. Studies on worms and flies are unlikely to explain whether reproduction itself and the physiology associated with reproductive capability affect all causes of mortality, or only certain ones. To address this question, we need a model system that is not only well characterized genetically, but is equally well characterized medically, so that we can investigate the underlying disease states that lead to mortality.

The domestic dog exhibits dramatic breed-associated phenotypic variation not only in morphology and behavior [9], but also in causes of death [10]. Additionally, elective surgical sterilization by ovariohysterectomy ("spay") or orchiectomy ("castration" or "neuter") is commonly performed at a young age in pet dogs in North America for the management and behavioral benefits it confers [11]. By electing whether or not to sterilize their dogs, dog owners have inadvertently carried out a large-scale epidemiologic experiment on the consequences of effectively eliminating reproductive capability. Previous studies in dogs have examined the effects of sterilization status on a variety of specific diseases. For example, sterilized dogs generally show an increase in rates of specific cancers [12,13,14,15] with the exception of mammary cancer, which is relatively rare in sterilized dogs [16]. However, in all but one of these studies [15], the relationship between sterilization and disease-specific risk of death is confounded with age. If elective sterilization increases life expectancy, then sterilized dogs might have a higher occurrence of diseases that occur late in life (such as cancer) simply because sterilized dogs live longer.

Here we determined the effects of sterilization not only on longevity, but also on the pathophysiological causes of death, controlling for the confounding effects of age. We examined causes of death in over 40,000 domestic dogs that died in veterinary teaching hospitals from 1984 to 2004. By comparing causes of death in dogs that had undergone elective surgical sterilization and those that had not, we were able to measure the lifespan cost of maintaining reproductive capability, and to determine the categories of disease associated with this cost.

Materials and Methods

Data Collection

The Veterinary Medical Data Base (VMDB, http://www.vmdb.org) contains abstracted medical records of animals presented to North American veterinary teaching hospitals since 1964. Each animal's record includes species, sex, sterilization status, age class, weight class, breed, and diagnoses made during the visit. We obtained the VMDB records for all dogs whose hospital visits resulted in death between the years 1984–2004, including all diagnoses recorded at the time of death. Dogs under one year of age or with unknown sterilization status were removed from analyses. Records of dogs meeting these criteria (Full Cohort, FC) were used to determine lifespan, and for assessment of all diagnoses present at the time of death.

For each dog, a single diagnosis was identified as the cause of death and categorized into one of nine pathophysiologic processes (PP; congenital, degenerative, infectious, immune-mediated, metabolic, neoplastic, toxic, traumatic and vascular) as previously described [10]. Some diagnoses contained insufficient information to allow PP categorization and these records were excluded from cause of death analysis. Congenital causes of death were also removed from subsequent analysis because they would have been present before the time that sterilization was or was not elected. Records remaining after these exclusions (Cause of Death Cohort, CODC) were used for cause of death analysis.

Lifespan

In the VMDB, dogs are classified into nine age bins (bins evaluated: bin 4:1–2 years; bin 5:2–4 years; bin 6:4–7 years; bin 7:7–10 years; bin 8:10–15 years; and bin 9:15 years and older). Age at death was assigned as the midpoint of each bin for all dogs in that bin, and for bin 9, the age assigned was 17.5 years. All analyses were performed using the software program R [17]. To determine the effect of sterilization on survival, we applied log-rank tests and generated Kaplan Meier plots using the R package "survival" [18] for FC dogs in the dataset, analyzing males and females separately.

Cause of Death

If sterilized dogs live longer and if the frequency of a particular cause of death increases with age, then it might appear that sterilization causes an increase in a particular cause of death, when it simply changes the age-distribution of death. To correct for this potential confound, we analyzed causes of death in the CODC dogs stratified by age using a Cochran-Mantel-Haenzel (CMH) test [19], which provides a stratified chi-squared test with one degree of freedom. Pooled odds ratios and 95% confidence intervals were calculated with intact dogs as the reference. We also evaluated differences between sterilized and intact dogs for each PP categorical cause of death within each age bin using a chi-squared test.

Different causes of death in dogs are more prevalent at different ages, so we ran a cumulative incidence model to determine the effects of age on the risk of a specific cause of death and to identify differences in these age-related effects between sterilized and intact dogs. We implemented a cumulative incidence model based on competing risks data using the "cmprsk" package in R [20].

Using the FC dogs, discretely defined infectious and neoplastic diagnoses that were present in more than 1% of the population at the time of death, regardless of cause of death, were also analyzed. To test for effects of sterilization within each diagnosis controlling for age, we used the CMH test described above.

Previous studies have shown that breeds differ both by rates and by causes of mortality [10]. To ensure that patterns observed in the CMH test were not confounded by differences among breeds, we carried out two additional analyses. First, we performed a logistic regression for each PP categorical cause of death using age and sterilization status as fixed effects and breed as a random effect using the "MASS" package in R [21]. Second, for each PP in which a pattern of sterilization-associated differences in frequency was detected, CMH tests were also run separately for each of the 24 most frequently encountered breeds within the dataset (mixed breed dogs were considered a single group). This allowed us to determine if sterilization had varying effects among breeds. Dog breed sizes were classified by the average of adult male and female body weights reported in breed standards, or compiled from veterinary and public resources for those breeds whose standard does not include a weight. We used the size categories small (up to 10 kg), medium (10.1–25 kg), large (25.1–40 kg), and giant (>40 kg).

Results

Full Cohort

The initial dataset contained 80,958 records of dog death. When juvenile dogs and those with unknown sterilization status were removed there were 70,574 FC dogs, representing 185 breeds. The average number of diagnoses recorded per dog was 2.9 (range 1–32). Overall, 30,770 (43.6%) dogs were intact and 39,804 (56.4%) dogs were sterilized at the time of death. The mean age of death for intact dogs was 7.9 years versus 9.4 years for sterilized dogs.

Cause of Death Cohort

We were able to identify the PP category for the specific cause of death in 41,045 dogs, and we removed 906 dogs whose cause of death was congenital (occurring primarily in the earliest of the age bins that we analyzed here). This enabled the inclusion of 40,139 dogs in the CODC for analysis of the relationship between sterilization and cause of death.

Lifespan

We found that sterilization significantly affected survival in both males ($\chi_1^2=446$, $P<10^{-6}$) and females ($\chi_1^2=1372$, $P<10^{-6}$) (Figure 1A). Sterilization increased life expectancy by 13.8% in males and 26.3% in females among the FC dogs.

Cause of Death

We found a striking effect of sterilization on cause of death (Figure 1B). Sterilized dogs were dramatically less likely to die of infectious disease ($\chi_1^2=184.4$, $P<10^{-6}$), trauma ($\chi_1^2=268.7$, $P<10^{-6}$), vascular disease ($\chi_1^2=8.25$, $P=0.004$), and degenerative disease ($\chi_1^2=7.7$, $P=0.006$). In contrast, sterilized dogs died more commonly from neoplasia ($\chi_1^2=300.4$, $P<10^{-6}$) and immune-mediated disease ($\chi_1^2=167.2$, $P<10^{-6}$). We saw effects of sterilization both on common causes of death, as well as on more rare causes (e.g., vascular disease). We also found that even within specific age bins, there were visible differences in causes of death for sterilized and intact dogs (Figure S1).

We expected that the consequences of sterilization would differ significantly between the sexes, as the endocrinological consequences of sterilization should differ between males and females. Surprisingly, both the direction and magnitude of the effect of sterilization on cause of death was markedly similar in males and females (Table 1). Results from the logistic regression, controlling

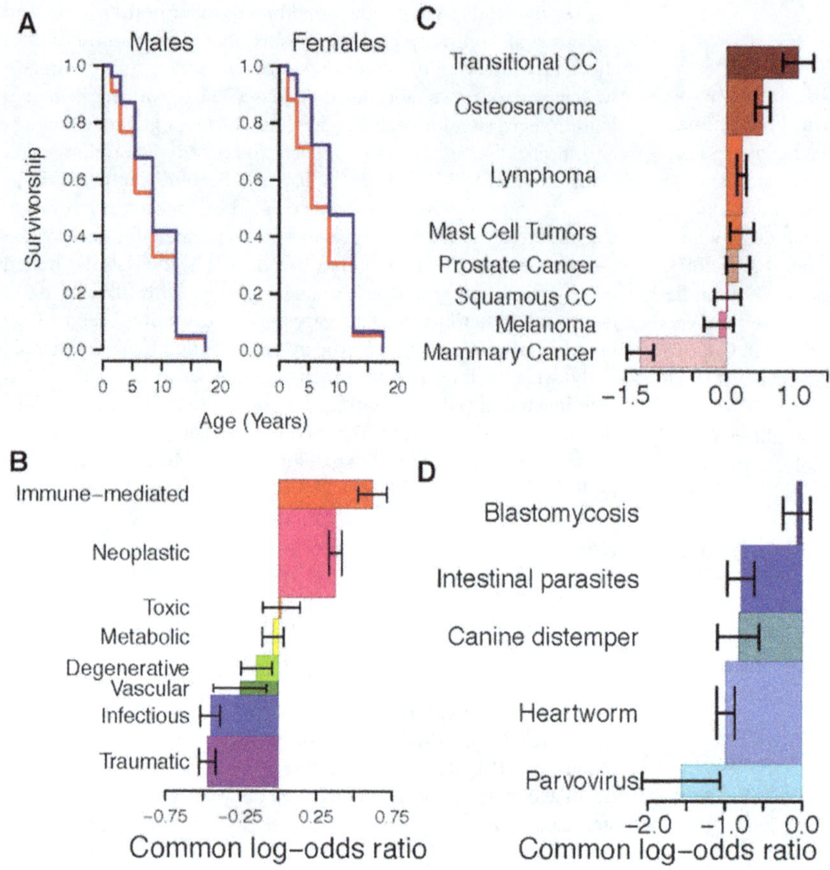

Figure 1. Effect of sterilization on longevity and diagnoses. (A) Kaplan-Meier plots of longevity for males (left) and females (right). Blue lines indicate sterilized dogs and red lines indicate intact dogs. (B) Common log-odds ratios with 95% confidence intervals (CI) for pathophysiological processes (PP). Height of each bar indicates the relative frequency of each PP among all deaths. (C) Effects of sterilization on specific neoplastic diagnoses, showing common log odds ratios and 95% CI. Height of each bar indicates fraction of individuals with this diagnosis at the time of death. Transitional CC - transitional cell carcinoma; Squamous CC - squamous cell carcinoma. All cancers significant at $P<0.01$ except prostate cancer, squamous cell carcinoma and melanoma ($P>0.05$). (D) As in Figure 1C, but for specific infectious disease diagnoses. All infectious diseases significant at $P<0.01$ except blastomycosis ($P>0.4$).

for the effects of breed as well as age, mirrored the initial findings (Table S1).

Because causes of death vary with age, we ran a cumulative incidence analysis to determine if the pathophysiological risks of death associated with sterilization status differ among age-classes (Figure S2). Most differences in causes of death between sterilized and intact dogs (intact dogs at greater risk for infectious and traumatic causes of death, sterilized dogs at greater risk for neoplastic and immune-mediated causes of death) remain significantly different under a cumulative incidence model using competing risk data (Table S2). However, while our CMH tests show that degenerative causes of death are significantly more frequent in intact dogs, the cumulative incidence model fails to find a significant difference between intact and sterilized dogs for this PP category.

Diagnoses at the Time of Death

Given the prevalence of neoplasia and infectious disease in these dogs and the relevance of those diseases to humans, within these categories we further examined specific diagnoses that were present in more than 1% of the FC dog population in a specific age class at the time of death, regardless of cause of death. Eight cancers met these criteria, five of which are among the top ten human cancer diagnoses in the US, according to the SEER Database [22]. Seven of the eight analyzed had higher or unchanged frequency in sterilized dogs; only mammary cancer showed a significantly lower prevalence (Figure 1C). Of five infectious diseases we considered, four had significantly lower frequencies in sterilized dogs (Figure 1D).

Within-breed Cause of Death

Finally, for the four PP causes of death most affected by sterilization status, the patterns that we observed were recapitulated within individual breeds (Figure 2). Since small-breed dogs are known to have longer lifespans than large-breed dogs [23,24], we divided the 24 most frequently observed breeds into four size classes (small, medium, large and giant). Despite the longer lifespans seen in small compared to large dogs, the effect of sterilization was relatively consistent among size classes (ANOVA, $P>0.11$ for all processes). Notably, even though death due to neoplasia is relatively rare in the smallest size classes [10], sterilization still increased the risk of neoplasia within these breeds.

Discussion

Despite a rich literature on the relationship between reproduction and lifespan [1,2,25], surprisingly little is understood about

Table 1. Risk of death by pathophysiologic process (PP) for sterilized dogs.

Sterilized males					
Process	**Odds-ratio**	**Lower**	**Upper**	**Chi-sq value**	**P-value**
Traumatic	−0.46	−0.54	−0.37	122.92	<2.2e−16
Infectious	−0.46	−0.56	−0.37	89.48	<2.2e−16
Vascular	−0.35	−0.61	−0.08	6.24	0.01
Degenerative	−0.15	−0.29	0.00	3.75	0.05
Metabolic	−0.09	−0.19	0.01	3.11	0.08
Toxic	0.04	−0.14	0.22	0.17	0.68
Neoplastic	0.43	0.37	0.49	194.26	<2.2e−16
Immune-Mediated	0.51	0.37	0.65	52.22	<2.2e−16
Sterilized females					
Process	**Odds-ratio**	**Lower 95% CI**	**Upper 95% CI**	**Chi-sq value**	**P-value**
Traumatic	−0.44	−0.53	−0.35	101.61	<2.2e−16
Infectious	−0.49	−0.59	−0.39	101.74	<2.2e−16
Vascular	−0.31	−0.56	−0.06	5.61	0.02
Degenerative	−0.20	−0.35	−0.04	6.10	0.01
Metabolic	0.00	−0.11	0.11	0.00	0.99
Toxic	−0.10	−0.28	0.08	1.15	0.28
Neoplastic	0.42	0.35	0.49	152.27	<2.2e−16
Immune-Mediated	0.54	0.39	0.68	56.32	<2.2e−16

Odds ratios for each of the eight PP are shown. Data for sterilized males (top) and sterilized females (bottom) are shown separately, and intact dogs of the same sex served as the reference population for each group.

the mechanisms by which investment in reproduction affects cause of death. Our analysis of causes of death associated with reproductive capability suggests that further and more detailed studies of reproduction and mortality in companion dogs could shed considerable light on this problem. Companion dogs are an established medical model for humans because the two species experience many of the same spontaneously-occurring diseases, participate in analogous high-caliber medical and surgical care, respond similarly to therapy, and share a daily environment [10,26,27,28,29]. No other species is similarly able to mirror the human experience of the impacts of environment, lifestyle choices, and medical care on health. Furthermore, in North America 50–75% of pet dogs are electively surgically sterilized, as recommended by the American and Canadian Veterinary Medical Associations, the American Society for the Prevention of Cruelty to Animals, and the Humane Society of the United States. The existence of large numbers of reproductively intact and electively sterilized companion dogs provides an unparalleled opportunity to evaluate outcome differences between the groups.

In our study on companion dogs, we identified many underlying causes of death that shape the composite trait of lifespan. In our study overall, lifespan was greater in the sterilized dogs compared with the reproductively intact dogs. While intact reproductive capability was associated with decreased lifespan in dogs, some causes of death were less frequent in intact dogs. Interestingly, we observed the largest–and opposite–effects in two of the most common causes of death among dogs within our dataset: neoplasia and infectious disease. It is not within the scope of our study to determine the causes of these associations. While the absence of gonadal hormones is an obvious physiological outcome of surgical sterilization, downstream consequences of the absence of gonadal hormones, including altered feedback on pituitary or adrenal hormonal axes, or changes in patterns of growth, development, or behavior may also be significant factors.

Sterilization increased the risk of death due to neoplasia, but did not increase risk for all specific kinds of cancer. Female dogs sterilized before sexual maturity are unlikely to develop mammary cancer because of the decrease in cumulative estrogen exposure associated with the absence of the estrus cycle [30]. However, it is not clear why the frequency of some cancers outside the reproductive system, including lymphoma and osteosarcoma, is influenced by sterilization, while the frequency of others, such as melanoma and squamous cell carcinoma, is not. The increased risk of death due to cancer observed in sterilized dogs could be due to the fact that in both sexes, dogs sterilized before the onset of puberty grow taller than their intact counterparts [31] as a result of reduced estrogen signaling [32]. Recent studies in humans suggest that growth is a risk factor for a number of different cancers [33].

Conversely, sterilized dogs had a decreased risk of death due to infection, and avoidance of infection may partly explain their longer lifespans. The relationship between sterilization and infectious disease could arise due to increased levels of progesterone and testosterone [34] in intact dogs, both of which can be immunosuppressive [35,36]. Studies in humans, mice and rats reveal patterns of infectious disease morbidity and mortality associated with testosterone and estrogen exposure. However, these patterns vary with host species, type of pathogen, and chronicity of infection [37]. Additionally, sterilization and disease risk might both be correlated with specific canine behaviors. Given the opportunity, intact male dogs are more likely than sterilized

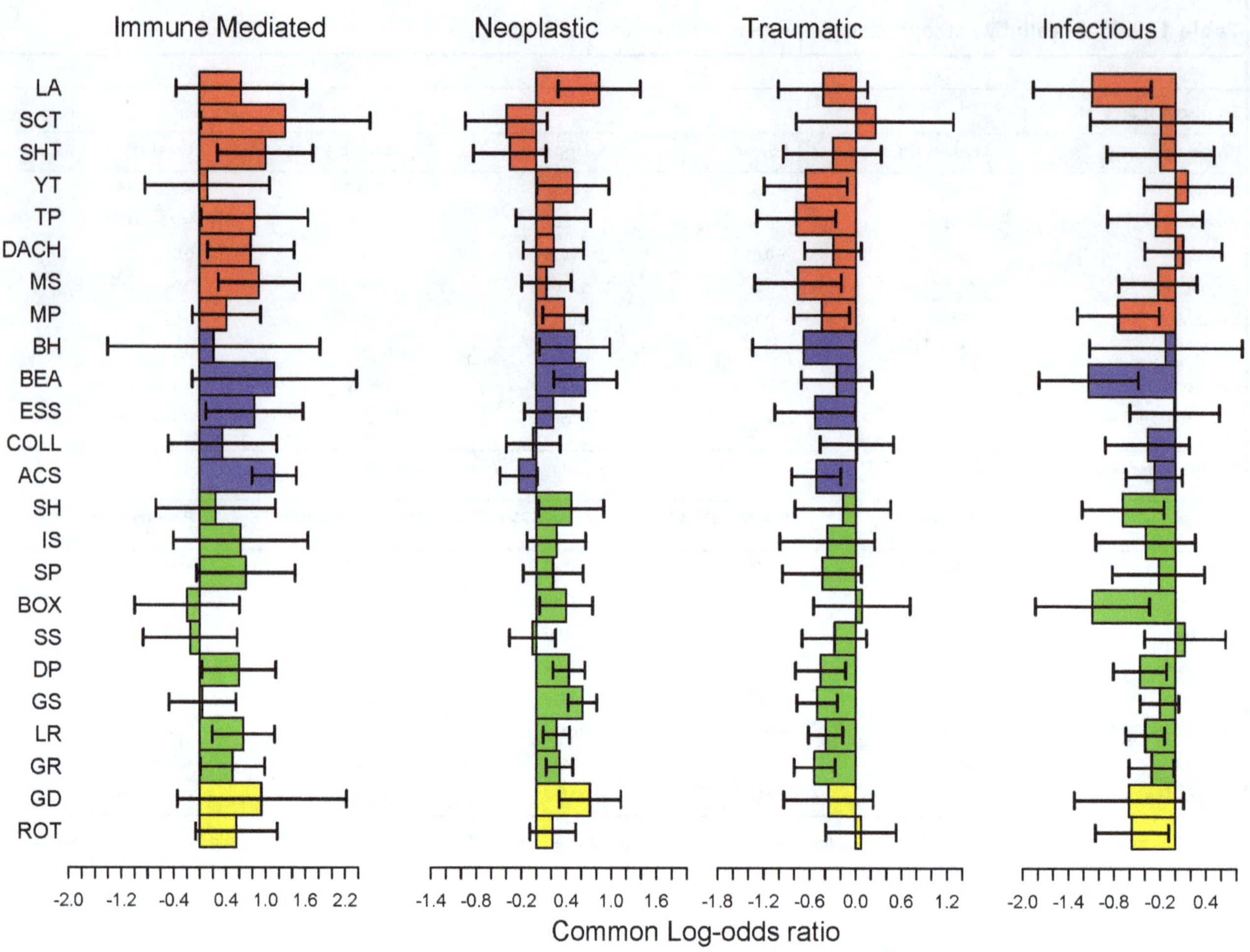

Figure 2. Breed specific causes of mortality. Effects of sterilization on the 24 pure breeds that appear most frequently in our dataset (minimum sample size = 319, median sample size = 517). Bars indicate 95% CI. Colors of odds ratio bars indicate size of the breed (red-small [up to 10 kg], blue-medium [10.1–25 kg], green-large [25.1–40 kg], yellow-giant [>40 kg]). Breed abbreviations are shown (LA: Lhasa Apso, SCT: Scottish Terrier, SHT: Shih Tzu, YT: Yorkshire Terrier, TP: Toy Poodle, DACH: Dachshund, MS: Miniature Schnauzer, MP: Miniature Poodle, BH: Basset Hound, BEA: Beagle, ESS: English Springer Spaniel, COLL: Collie, ACS: American Cocker Spaniel, SH: Siberian Husky, IS: Irish Setter, SP: Standard Poodle, BOX: Boxer, SS: Shetland Sheepdog, DP: Doberman Pinscher, GS: German Shepherd, LR: Labrador Retriever, GR: Golden Retriever, GD: Great Dane, ROT: Rottweiler).

dogs to roam, and to fight with other dogs, and intact female dogs show more dominance aggression than spayed females [38,39]. These behaviors might increase the risks of both infectious and traumatic causes of death among intact dogs.

Limited previous studies on the effects of gonadectomy in humans have found some results consistent with ours. Studies in two different populations have shown that eunuchs live longer than their intact male counterparts [40,41]. Interestingly, Hamilton and Gordon [40] found that the largest factor influencing the survival difference was the high rate of death due to infections among the intact men. However, the study failed to find differences between the two groups in death due to cancer or trauma, both categories in which sterilization was associated with a large effect in our dataset.

Retrospective studies such as this are not without potential weaknesses. For example, elective surgical sterilization and subsequent veterinary care are potentially associated with socio-economic status. Owners who cannot afford the cost of sterilization might also lack the resources to provide medical care for diseases that later occur, which might result in sterilized dogs who have access to better medical care appearing to live longer. This issue is unlikely to exert a significant impact on our results, however, as all dogs within our dataset were seen at referral institutions, where costs of care are high. Since dogs in our study were owned by people who could afford the cost of referral from their local veterinary practices to specialty hospitals when their pets became ill, it is unlikely that financial resources were a limiting factor in preventive health management choices such as sterilization [42].

A second potential bias is introduced by the fact that our dataset does not provide the age at which each dog was sterilized, the number of times that intact dogs reproduced, or whether sterilized dogs reproduced prior to sterilization. We cannot extrapolate this information from prior work because while most North American veterinary practitioners currently recommend sterilization at 6–9 months of age for pet dogs, and specifically before the first heat cycle in females [11], there is no large study which reports the actual age at which most dogs are sterilized. If the proportion of dogs becoming sterilized were constant within each age bin, then sterilized dogs could appear to live longer simply because the sterilized group steadily expands with increasing age. Previous research has shown that using gonadectomy as a time-dependent variable can give different estimates of the effect of sterilization on longevity than using sterilization status as a straight yes/no response, and that right-censored lifespans from retrospective studies underestimate population lifespan [43,44]. However, it was not our objective to define the precise life expectancy for any category of dog, merely the difference between two groups that varied only by sterilization status. Both sterilized and intact dogs were subject to the same limitation (i.e., enrollment at the time of death), and the impact on the groups is expected to be proportionate. Furthermore, when causes of death are compared between reproductively intact and sterilized dogs within age bins, the differential effects of sterilization persist. Thus, even in the youngest dogs, when the consequences of sterilization would have manifested over a shorter period of time, an impact is apparent (Figure S1). Regarding parity, we cannot state that all individuals within the sterilized group were nulliparous, nor that all individuals within the intact group had reproduced. Thus, it is likely that there is some crossover between groups with respect to actual reproductive experience. The effect of this crossover, however, would be to minimize any differences identified between groups; thus, the ability to identify a marked difference in lifespan and cause of death risk in the face of imperfect separation of lifetime reproductive experience substantiates the significance of the effect. We also note that parallel patterns of pathophysiologic process morbidity were evident within all age groups, suggesting that these effects are robust to variation arising from differences in parity within and between groups. Nonetheless, future studies would obviously benefit from data on parity in individual dogs.

Finally, as previously mentioned, the link between sterilization and the observed outcomes cannot currently be known. A direct cause-and-effect relationship between reproduction and cause of death is possible, but the actual relationship is likely more complex. In mammals, removal of gonadal hormones has been shown to alter hematological and coagulation parameters, the pituitary-adrenal axis, satiety, neurotransmitters, thymic tissue, and behavior [11,45,46,47,48,49,50]. Any or all of these factors could mediate the differential causes of death observed between the reproductively intact and sterilized dogs of this report. Documentation of these outcome differences now creates the exciting opportunity to investigate the possible causal mechanisms in dogs and other species.

Although a retrospective, epidemiological study such as this cannot prove causality, our results suggest that close scrutiny of specific causes of death, rather than lifespan alone, will greatly improve our understanding of the cumulative impact of reproductive capability on mortality. Our results strongly demonstrate the need to determine the physiologic consequences of sterilization that influence causes of death and lifespan. Shifting the focus from when death occurs to why death occurs could also help to explain contradictory findings from human studies [e.g., 8].

Supporting Information

Figure S1 Differences in cause of death for sterilized and intact dogs. Pathophysiological plots by age for sterilized (blue circles) and intact (red triangles) dogs. Error bars indicate +/ −1 SE. Black asterisks above each age bin indicate significant difference between sterilized and intact dogs for that age bin using a Chi-squared test. P value <0.05.

Figure S2 Competing risks plot for the four most significantly different causes of death between sterilized and intact dogs. Solid lines represent intact dogs, and dashed lines represent sterilized dogs. Each color represents a different cause of death: orange-neoplastic, red-traumatic, black-infectious, blue-immune-mediated.

Table S1 Mixed-effect model of the effects of sterilization on cause of death. Shown are the results for sterilization under each cause of death. The model includes sterilization and age as fixed effects and breed as a random effect.

Table S2 Competing risks analysis for each cause of death. Results indicate significant differences in risk for sterilized and intact dogs, with d.f. = 1 in each case.

Acknowledgments

The authors thank Bayer Animal Health for providing the APPA National Pet Owners Survey, used as reference material for this report. The Veterinary Medical Data Base (VMDB) does not make any implicit or implied opinion on the subject of the paper or study. The manuscript benefited from critical comments by Karen Cornell, Dave Hall, Sue Healy, Leslie Kean, Allen Moore, Simon Platt, and Crystal Weyman.

Author Contributions

Conceived and designed the experiments: JMH KEC DELP. Performed the experiments: JMH KEC DELP. Analyzed the data: JMH KEC DELP. Contributed reagents/materials/analysis tools: JMH KEC. Wrote the paper: JMH KEC DELP.

References

1. Flatt T (2011) Survival costs of reproduction in *Drosophila*. Experimental gerontology 46: 369–375.
2. Partridge L, Gems D, Withers DJ (2005) Sex and death: what is the connection? Cell 120: 461–472.
3. Chapman T, Liddle LF, Kalb JM, Wolfner MF, Partridge L (1995) Cost of mating in *Drosophila melanogaster* is mediated by male accessory gland products. Nature 373: 241–244.
4. Partridge L, Harvey P (1985) Costs of reproduction. Nature 316: 20.
5. Penn DJ, Smith KR (2007) Differential fitness costs of reproduction between the sexes. Proceedings of the National Academy of Sciences of the United States of America 104: 553–558.
6. Gagnon A, Smith KR, Tremblay M, Vezina H, Pare PP, et al. (2009) Is there a trade-off between fertility and longevity? A comparative study of women from three large historical databases accounting for mortality selection. American Journal of Human Biology 21: 533–540.
7. Helle S, Lummaa V, Jokela J (2002) Sons reduced maternal longevity in preindustrial humans. Science 296: 1085–1085.
8. Hurt LS, Ronsmans C, Thomas SL (2006) The effect of number of births on women's mortality: Systematic review of the evidence for women who have completed their childbearing. Population Studies-a Journal of Demography 60: 55–71.
9. Boyko AR, Quignon P, Li L, Schoenebeck JJ, Degenhardt JD, et al. (2010) A simple genetic architecture underlies morphological variation in dogs. PLoS biology 8: e1000451.
10. Fleming JM, Creevy KE, Promislow DEL (2011) Mortality in North American dogs from 1984 to 2004: An investigation into age-, size-, and breed-related causes of death. Journal of Veterinary Internal Medicine 25: 187–198.
11. Kustritz MV (2007) Determining the optimal age for gonadectomy of dogs and cats. J Am Vet Med Assoc 231: 1665–1675.
12. Bryan JN, Keeler MR, Henry CJ, Bryan ME, Hahn AW, et al. (2007) A population study of neutering status as a risk factor for canine prostate cancer. Prostate 67: 1174–1181.
13. Cooley DM, Beranek BC, Schlittler DL, Glickman NW, Glickman LT, et al. (2002) Endogenous gonadal hormone exposure and bone sarcoma risk. Cancer Epidemiology Biomarkers & Prevention 11: 1434–1440.
14. Ru G, Terracini B, Glickman LT (1998) Host related risk factors for canine osteosarcoma. Veterinary Journal 156: 31–39.

15. White CR, Hohenhaus AE, Kelsey J, Procter-Gray E (2011) Cutaneous MCTs: associations with spay/neuter status, breed, body size, and phylogenetic cluster. Journal of the American Animal Hospital Association 47: 210–216.
16. Sorenmo KU, Shofer FS, Goldschmidt MH (2000) Effect of spaying and timing of spaying on survival of dogs with mammary carcinoma. Journal of Veterinary Internal Medicine 14: 266–270.
17. R Development Core Team (2009) R: A language and environment for statistical computing. R Foundation for Statistical Computing.
18. Therneau T (2012) A package for survival analysis in S. R package version 2.36–14 ed.
19. Cochran WG (1954) Some methods for strengthening the common tests. Biometrics 10: 417–451.
20. Fine JP, Gray RJ (1999) A proportional hazards model for the subdistribution of a competing risk. Journal of the American Statistical Association 94: 496–509.
21. Venables W, Ripley B (1997) Modern applied statistics with S-plus Journal of Educational and Behavioral Statistics 22: 244–245.
22. Surveillance, Epidemiology, and End Results (SEER) Program. Available: www.seer.cancer.gov. SEER*Stat Database: Populations- Total U.S. (1969–2009). National Cancer Insitute. DCCPS. Surveillance Resrach Program. Surveillance Systems Branch. Released April 2011.
23. Greer KA, Canterberry SC, Murphy KE (2007) Statistical analysis regarding the effects of height and weight on life span of the domestic dog. Research in Veterinary Science 82: 208–214.
24. Li Y, Deeb B, Pendergrass W, Wolf N (1996) Cellular proliferative capacity and life span in small and large dogs. Journals of Gerontology, Series A: Biological Sciences and Medical Sciences 51: B403–B408.
25. Reznick D (1985) Costs of reproduction: an evaluation of the empirical evidence. Oikos 44: 257–267.
26. Breen M (2009) Update on genomics in veterinary oncology. Topics in Companion Animal Medicine 24: 113–121.
27. Fernandez-Varon E, Villamayor L (2007) Granulocyte and granulocyte macrophage colony-stimulating factors as therapy in human and veterinary medicine. Veterinary Journal 174: 33–41.
28. Reif JS, Dunn K, Ogilvie GK, Harris CK (1992) Passive smoking and canine lung-cancer risk. American Journal of Epidemiology 135: 234–239.
29. Withrow SJ, Wilkins RM (2010) Cross talk from pets to people: translational osteosarcoma treatments. Ilar Journal 51: 208–213.
30. Schneider R, Dorn CR, Taylor DON (1969) Factors influencing canine mammary cancer development and postsurgical survival. Journal of the National Cancer Institute 43: 1249–1261.
31. Salmeri KR, Bloomberg MS, Scruggs SL, Shille V (1991) Gonadectomy in immature dogs - effects on skeletal, physical and behavioral-development. Journal of the American Veterinary Medical Association 198: 1193–1203.
32. Grumbach MM (2000) Estrogen, bone, growth and sex: A sea change in conventional wisdom. Journal of Pediatric Endocrinology and Metabolism 13: 1439–1455.
33. Green J, Cairns BJ, Casabonne D, Wright FL, Reeves G, et al. (2011) Height and cancer incidence in the Million Women Study: prospective cohort, and meta-analysis of prospective studies of height and total cancer risk. Lancet Oncology 12: 785–794.
34. Frank LA, Rohrbach BW, Bailey EM, West JR, Oliver JW (2003) Steroid hormone concentration profiles in healthy intact and neutered dogs before and after cosyntropin administration. Domestic Animal Endocrinology 24: 43–57.
35. Klein SL (2004) Hormonal and immunological mechanisms mediating sex differences in parasite infection. Parasite Immunology 26: 247–264.
36. Folstad I, Karter AJ (1992) Parasites, bright males, and the immunocompetence handicap. American Naturalist 139: 603–622.
37. McClelland EE, Smith JM (2011) Gender specific differences in the immune response to infection. Arch Immunol Ther Exp 59: 203–213.
38. Hopkins SG, Schubert TA, Hart BL (1976) Castration of adult male dogs: effects on roaming, aggression, urine marking, and mounting. Journal of the American Veterinary Medical Association 168: 1108–1110.
39. Neilson JC, Eckstein RA, Hart BL (1997) Effects of castration on problem behaviors in male dogs with reference to age and duration of behavior. Journal of the American Veterinary Medical Association 211: 180–182.
40. Hamilton JB, Mestler GE (1969) Mortality and survival. Comparison of eunuchs with intact men and women in a mentally retarded population. Journals of Gerontology 24: 395–411.
41. Min KJ, Lee CK, Park HN (2012) The lifespan of Korean eunuchs. Current Biology 22: R792–R793.
42. Bartlett PC, Van Buren JW, Neterer M, Zhou C (2010) Disease surveillance and referral bias in the veterinary medical database. Preventive Veterinary Medicine 94: 264–271.
43. van Hagen MAE, Ducro BJ, van den Broek J, Knol BW (2005) Life expectancy in a birth cohort of Boxers followed up from weaning to 10 years of age. American Journal of Veterinary Research 66: 1646–1650.
44. Urfer SR (2008) Right censored data ('cohort bias') in veterinary life span studies. Veterinary Record 163: 457–458.
45. Bernichtein S, Petretto E, Jamieson S, Goel A, Aitman TJ, et al. (2008) Adrenal gland tumorigenesis after gonadectomy in mice is a complex genetic trait driven by epistatic loci. Endocrinology 149: 651–661.
46. Fettman MJ, Stanton CA, Banks LL, Hamar DW, Johnson DE, et al. (1997) Effects of neutering on bodyweight, metabolic rate and glucose tolerance of domestic cats. Research in Veterinary Science 62: 131–136.
47. Hince M, Sakkal S, Vlahos K, Dudakov J, Boyd R, et al. (2008) The role of sex steroids and gonadectomy in the control of thymic involution. Cellular Immunology 252: 122–138.
48. Nemeth N, Kiss F, Hever T, Brath E, Sajtos E, et al. (2012) Hemorheological consequences of hind limb ischemia-reperfusion differ in normal and gonadectomized male and female rats. Clinical Hemorheology and Microcirculation 50: 197–211.
49. Pinilla L, Seoane LM, Gonzalez L, Carro E, Aguilar E, et al. (1999) Regulation of serum leptin levels by gonadal function in rats. European Journal of Endocrinology 140: 468–473.
50. Tamas A, Lubics A, Lengvari I, Reglodi D (2006) Effects of age, gender, and gonadectomy on neurochemistry and behavior in animal models of Parkinson's disease. Endocrine 29: 275–287.

6

Centronuclear Myopathy in Labrador Retrievers: A Recent Founder Mutation in the *PTPLA* Gene Has Rapidly Disseminated Worldwide

Marie Maurer[1,2], Jérôme Mary[1,2,3], Laurent Guillaud[1,2], Marilyn Fender[4], Manuel Pelé[1,2], Thomas Bilzer[5], Natasha Olby[6], Jacques Penderis[7], G. Diane Shelton[8], Jean-Jacques Panthier[1,2,9], Jean-Laurent Thibaud[10], Inès Barthélémy[10], Geneviève Aubin-Houzelstein[1,2], Stéphane Blot[10], Christophe Hitte[11], Laurent Tiret[1,2]*

1 CNM Project, Université Paris-Est Créteil, Ecole Nationale Vétérinaire d'Alfort, Maisons-Alfort, France, **2** UMR955 de Génétique Fonctionnelle et Médicale, Institut National de la Recherche Agronomique, Maisons-Alfort, France, **3** Antagene, La Tour de Salvagny, France, **4** CNM Project, Pickett, Wisconsin, United States of America, **5** Institut für Neuropathologie, Heinrich-Heine-Universität, Düsseldorf, Germany, **6** College of Veterinary Medicine, Neurology Faculty, North Carolina State University, Raleigh, North Carolina, United States of America, **7** College of Medical, Veterinary and Life Science, School of Veterinary Medicine, University of Glasgow, Glasgow, United Kingdom, **8** Department of Pathology, University of California San Diego, La Jolla, California, United States of America, **9** Mouse Functional Genetics URA2578, Centre National de la Recherche Scientifique, Institut Pasteur, Paris, France, **10** Unité Propre de Recherche de Neurobiologie, Université Paris-Est Créteil, Ecole Nationale Vétérinaire d'Alfort, Maisons-Alfort, France, **11** UMR6290, Centre National de la Recherche Scientifique, Institut de Génétique et Développement de Rennes, Université de Rennes1, Rennes, France

Abstract

Centronuclear myopathies (CNM) are inherited congenital disorders characterized by an excessive number of internalized nuclei. In humans, CNM results from ~70 mutations in three major genes from the myotubularin, dynamin and amphiphysin families. Analysis of animal models with altered expression of these genes revealed common defects in all forms of CNM, paving the way for unified pathogenic and therapeutic mechanisms. Despite these efforts, some CNM cases remain genetically unresolved. We previously identified an autosomal recessive form of CNM in French Labrador retrievers from an experimental pedigree, and showed that a loss-of-function mutation in the protein tyrosine phosphatase-like A (*PTPLA*) gene segregated with CNM. Around the world, client-owned Labrador retrievers with a similar clinical presentation and histopathological changes in muscle biopsies have been described. We hypothesized that these Labradors share the same $PTPLA^{cnm}$ mutation. Genotyping of an international panel of 7,426 Labradors led to the identification of $PTPLA^{cnm}$ carriers in 13 countries. Haplotype analysis demonstrated that the $PTPLA^{cnm}$ allele resulted from a single and recent mutational event that may have rapidly disseminated through the extensive use of popular sires. *PTPLA*-deficient Labradors will help define the integrated role of *PTPLA* in the existing CNM gene network. They will be valuable complementary large animal models to test innovative therapies in CNM.

Editor: Reiner Albert Veitia, Institut Jacques Monod, France

Funding: This work was funded by the CNM Project (www.labradorcnm.com), the French Association against Myopathies (AFM), a FP6 EuroTransBio Grant from the European Commission (Biomarks), the American Kennel Club-Canine Health Foundation and the Centre National de la Recherche Scientifique (CNRS). The funders had no role in study design, data collection and analysis, decision to publish, or preparation of the manuscript.

Competing Interests: The authors have declared their affiliation to Antagene which employed JM, a PhD student in the UMR955 laboratory. Through a national scheme named CIFRE, dedicated to upgrading innovative capabilities of SME through hiring highly-educated employees, Antagene received subsidies from the French Ministry of Research. Antagene neither influenced our scientific strategy nor provided us with research or travel grants.

* E-mail: ltiret@vet-alfort.fr

These authors contributed equally to this work.

Introduction

In humans, myotubular/centronuclear myopathies, often referred to as CNM, are congenital inherited myopathies characterized by generalized muscle weakness associated with respiratory insufficiency, external ophthalmoplegia and normal function of the central and peripheral nervous system. Muscle biopsies show a type 1 fiber predominance and excessive numbers of fibers with internalized or centralized nuclei [1,2]. Clinical presentations in patients are very heterogeneous and in most instances, correlate with mutations in distinct genes. The very severe X-linked form (XLMTM, OMIM 310400) affects neonates and carries a poor prognosis. This form is due to mutations in the myotubularin gene (*MTM1*; www.hgmd.cf.ac.uk and [3]). Milder late-onset childhood or adult-onset autosomal dominant forms (ADCNM, OMIM 160150) are mainly due to mutations in the dynamin 2 gene (*DNM2*) or, in one reported case, in the ryanodine receptor gene (*RYR1*) [4,5]. Intermediate autosomal recessive forms (ARCNM, OMIM 255200) are due to mutations in the BIN1/amphiphysin 2 (*BIN1*), myotubularin-related 14 (*MTMR14*) [6,7] or *RYR1* genes [8,9]. Despite these major advances in the identification of CNM-causing genes in humans, 30% of sporadic or familial cases remain genetically unresolved, underlying the existence of additional causative genes in the CNM functional network.

Years ago, an autosomal recessive congenital canine CNM was described in Labradors from an experimental pedigree developed in France from two probands [10,11]. By linkage analysis, the locus was mapped to canine chromosome 2, and an associated mutation was identified in a gene annotated as the protein tyrosine phosphatase-like A (*PTPLA*) gene. In affected dogs, the homozygous genotype resulting from the insertion of a SINE within exon 2 of *PTPLA* correlated with a complex panel of splicing defects in skeletal muscles, eventually leading to a 99% decrease in the amount of wild-type *PTPLA* transcripts [12], compatible with a loss-of-function mutation. For decades, phenotypically similar myopathies have been reported in client-owned Labradors living in the USA, the United Kingdom, Australia, Canada and Europe [13,14,15,16,17], and have been named type II fiber deficiency [13], autosomal recessive muscular dystrophy [18] or hereditary myopathy of Labrador retrievers (HMLR) [19,20]. Here we demonstrate that regardless of the country of origin, every client-owned Labrador retriever diagnosed with any of these phenotypically similar myopathies carried the same *PTPLA* loss-of-function allele first identified in our experimental pedigree. Further, our findings provide evidence that this allele originated from a leading founder that sustained rapid dissemination worldwide. Finally, we show that the variable expression of disease severity in affected dogs does not rely on genetic polymorphisms within the inserted SINE sequence.

Results

Selection of an international panel of CNM/ Phenotypically similar Labrador retrievers

To perform a global genetic analysis on CNM/Phenotypically similar dogs, further referred to as CNM Labradors, we set up an initial confirmation panel of DNA from 32 client-owned Labradors living in the USA, Germany, the UK, France and Denmark, which had been initially diagnosed with type 2 fiber deficiency, autosomal recessive muscular dystrophy, HMLR or CNM (Table 1, Table 2 and Table S1). Two Labradors with a diagnosis of myasthenia gravis or primary neuropathy were included as controls. Although records were incomplete in some cases, clinical signs in affected dogs included gait abnormalities, generalized weakness, fatigability, absence of patellar reflexes, and generalized muscle atrophy prominently affecting limb, cervical and temporal muscles. Structural remodeling of skeletal muscles included atrophic (≤25 μm of diameter) and anguloid-round fibers, fiber size variation, endomysial and perimysial fibrosis, predominance of type I fibers and internalization or centralization of nuclei in some fibers (Figure 1 and Table S1).

Table 2. Numbers by genotype of Labradors diagnosed with HMLR or phenotypically similar myopathy.

	+/+	+/*cnm*	*cnm*/*cnm*	Total
US	0	1	14	15
Germany	4	0	7	11
UK	1	0	2	3
France	0	0	2	2
Denmark	0	0	1	1
Total	**5**	**1**	**26**	**32**

Countries of origin of dogs are listed. With the exception of two German Labradors used as controls, all Labradors were genotyped because they had initially been diagnosed with HMLR or phenotypically similar myopathies (Table S1).

A unique mutation in CNM Labradors

It was previously shown that Labradors from a French experimental pedigree segregating CNM carry two copies of the *PTPLA* g.9459-9460ins238 mutation (Figure 2A; [12]). First, to determine whether client-owned CNM Labradors from the USA carry the same recessive disease-causing mutation, one affected female proband from the initial confirmation panel (US-3), an unaffected sister, parents, and a great-grandfather were genotyped by PCR, as described [12]. DNA from the healthy sister yielded a unique product of 610 bp, which is the size of the wild-type *PTPLA* allele. In contrast, DNA from the female proband yielded a unique product of ~850 bp, a size corresponding to the CNM-causing allele. The two healthy parents and great-grandfather were heterozygotes (Figure 2B).

Second, genotypes of the 32 dogs from the initial confirmation panel were analyzed (Figure 2C and full list of results in Table S1). We confirmed that the two control dogs were homozygous for the wild-type allele (DE-3 and DE-5), and identified that 77% of dogs (23/30) were homozygous for the *PTPLA* mutation. One was heterozygous and six were homozygous for the wild-type allele. The heterozygous USA dog (US-11) expressed none of the early histopathological signs of CNM, but a type 1 predominance that has never been observed in heterozygous dogs from the experimental pedigree. An idiopathic etiology was favored for this dog. Wild-type dogs were from the UK and Germany and corresponded to orphan cases for which precise clinical or histopathological records were missing.

A genetic test was thus proposed to owners for diagnostic or breeding purposes (www.labradorcnm.com). In the last 7 years, we received and genotyped samples from 7,426 Labradors living in 18 countries (Figure 3 and Table 3). In this unique comprehensive

Table 1. Number of genotyped dogs used in this study.

	+/+	+/*cnm*	*cnm*/*cnm*	Total
Dogs tested for the mutation *(whole panel)*	6 173	1 173	80	7 426
Dogs with clinical or histopathological reports *(initial confirmation panel)*	5	1	26	32
Dogs included in the haplotype analysis	39	-	32	71
Dogs sequenced (SINE insertion)	-	-	12	12

The whole panel includes all dogs for which samples were received for testing purposes. The initial confirmation panel includes dogs with an early diagnosis of HLMR or phenotypically similar myopathies (Table S1).

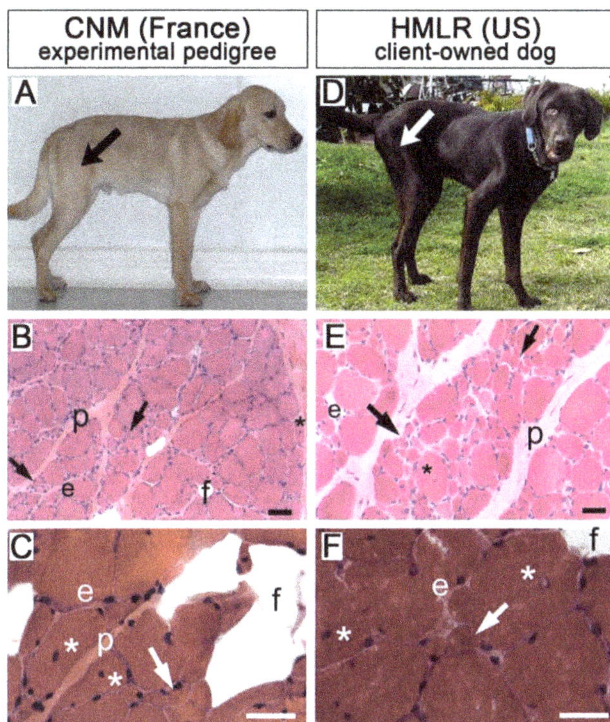

Figure 1. Client-owned US Labradors share similar morphological and histopathological features with French CNM dogs from the experimental pedigree. French CNM (A–C) and US HMLR (D–F) affected dogs have atrophic skeletal muscles, the most affected being those of pelvic limbs (e.g. *biceps femoris* muscle, arrows in A,D). B,C,E,F are Hematoxylin-Eosin-stained transverse sections of the *biceps femoris* muscle from 6-month-old (B, FR-4; E, US-18) or 10-year-old (C,F) affected Labradors. Early signs include groups of atrophic fibers, surrounded by endomysial (e) and perimysial (p) fibrosis. In older dogs, increased internalized or centralized nuclei (asterisks) and fatty infiltration (f) are observed. Scale bar = 50 µm.

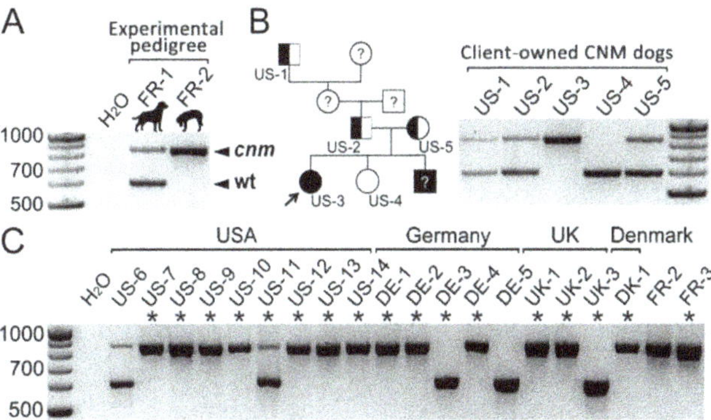

Figure 2. *PTPLA* mutation in the initial confirmation panel of CNM dogs. (A) Wild-type (wt = 610 bp) and $PTPLA^{cnm}$ (*cnm* = wt+238 bp) alleles in a healthy carrier (FR-1) and an affected (FR-2) Labrador from the French experimental pedigree. (B) Segregation of the $PTPLA^{cnm}$ allele in a four-generation pedigree of a client-owned US proband female (arrow). (C) Genotypes of client-owned Labradors from several countries, diagnosed with CNM-related myopathies (asterisks; Table S1). US-6 is a champion known to have produced CNM pups; DE-5 is a control affected by a neuropathy and FR-2 was reloaded for size comparison.

panel of client-owned dogs, we identified 80 dogs from six countries that were homozygous for the mutated *PTPLA* allele. Sixty-eight were young dogs that had already displayed clinical signs of CNM and twelve were asymptomatic one-month-old pups at the time of testing; a few weeks after testing, all pups displayed clinical signs consistent with CNM. On the contrary, none of the 1,172 heterozygous dogs living in 13 different countries displayed clinical signs of CNM, confirming the strict autosomal recessive mode of inheritance of CNM in Labradors. Affected and healthy carriers included both males and females with the three recognized yellow, black and chocolate coat colors (Table S2 and Table S3).

Reports of clinical signs in the 80 CNM genotyped dogs or of histopathological features in affected dogs from the initial confirmation panel suggested a spectrum in severity of the disease (Table S1). In the *SILV/PMEL* gene, the length of the oligo(dA)-rich tail of an inserted SINE was shown to influence the merle phenotype penetrance in dogs [21]. Thus, we visually checked the size of the $PTPLA^{cnm}$ allele amplified from DNAs of the 1,172 healthy carriers from the whole panel and the 80 affected dogs (representative panel in Figure S1). No fragment length polymorphisms were observed. The $PTPLA^{cnm}$ allele was further sequenced in 12 CNM dogs from the initial confirmation panel and no base pair polymorphisms were identified within SINE sequences (Figure S2).

In light of the finding that all affected Labradors share a unique well-conserved mutation causing muscle defects analogous to those seen in human forms of CNM, we propose that the mutated allele, initially named $PTPLA^{alf}$ [12], becomes $PTPLA^{cnm}$.

Founder effect for the $PTPLA^{cnm}$ allele

A unique origin for the $PTPLA^{cnm}$ allele was suggested by pedigree analyses showing that some affected Labradors from Germany and France had UK champions in their background (Table S1), where the prevalence of CNM is one of the highest (Table 3). To confirm that all occurrences of the disease were due to a single ancestral mutation, we constructed a series of haplotypes with SNPs from a 9-Mb region surrounding the *PTPLA* locus (Table S4 and Table S5) for each of 39 homozygous $PTPLA^{+/+}$ healthy Labradors and 32 $PTPLA^{cnm/cnm}$ affected Labradors.

A thorough analysis of genotyping data revealed that 100% of affected Labradors (n = 32) shared two copies of a common short haplotype of 489.4 kb, extending from SNP 21763 to SNP 22253 (Figure 4, Figure S3). The A-T-G short haplotype is highly predictive of the disease condition in the $PTPLA^{cnm/cnm}$ affected dogs ($P = 3.87\times10^{-21}$), and was identified at a carrier frequency of 12.8% (10/78 haplotypes) in healthy control dogs. Further analyses indicated that a second long haplotype of 3.8 Mb and covering 10 SNPs from SNP 20687 to SNP 24518 (G-G-A-T-A-T-G-C-A-A), remained highly associated with the disease ($P = 2.59\times10^{-19}$). The frequency of this longer haplotype segment in affected dogs was 77,4% (48/62 haplotypes) and was not found in healthy dogs (0/78 haplotypes).

A hierarchical clustering analysis using genotypes obtained for these 10 SNPs confirmed that at k = 8, all affected dogs segregated in a single highly predictive haplogroup, regardless of their geographic origin (Figure 5). Closer examination of this long haplotype segment revealed that CNM dogs finely stratified into distinct sub-groups, each diverging from the CNM haplotype by loss of homozygosity at one or two SNPs (Figure S3). Using the mutation-rate of 3.0×10^{-8} mutations/nucleotide/generation reported in humans [22], we calculated that 17.5 generations would separate today's Labradors from the original $PTPLA^{cnm}$ founder.

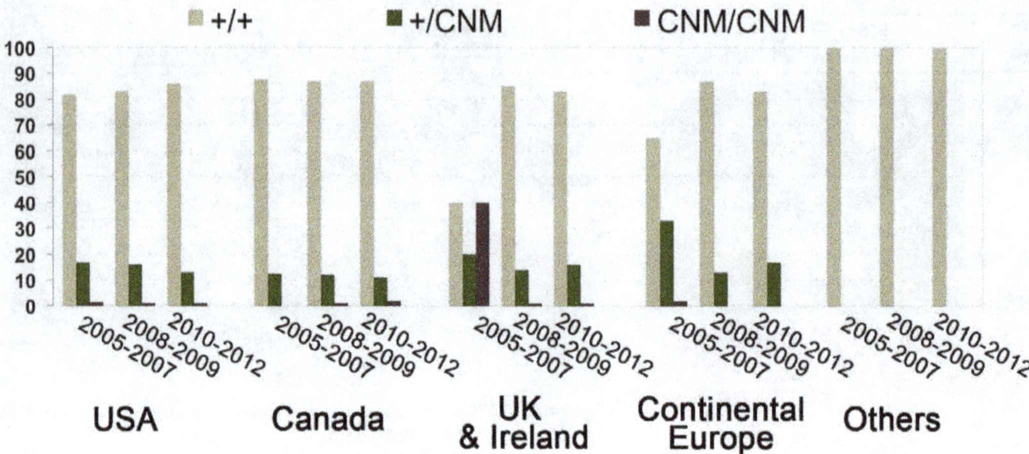

Figure 3. Percentage of wild-type homozygous (+/+), healthy carriers (+/*cnm*) and CNM affected (*cnm*/*cnm*) Labradors tested for medical or breeding purposes. The total number of dogs for each period is indicated above histograms. Additional dog samples from Australia (n = 15), New-Zealand (n = 2), Puerto Rico (n = 1) and Argentina (n = 1) were tested; they were all homozygous for the wild-type allele (+/+).

Assuming a generation time of 2.5–3 years in dogs, we estimate that the *PTPLA^cnm^* mutation arose ~50 years ago. Healthy Labradors were later subdivided into seven haplogroups, reflecting the genetic heterogeneity of the Labrador breed, the most popular in the world.

Discussion

*PTPLA^cnm^*, a prevalent and fully penetrant mutation with variable expressivity

This report shows that the *PTPLA^cnm^* allele, initially identified in a French experimental pedigree, is the worldwide fully penetrant allele causing CNM in client-owned Labradors. On the basis of the results obtained in the past 24 months, we estimate that one dog in seven is a CNM carrier (245/1,757 = 13,9%), with the highest percentages found in the UK (19%), the USA (13%) and Canada (11,5%). A high percentage of carriers in the UK (22%) has also been independently reported [23]. To date, the autosomal recessive CNM is the most prevalent hereditary myopathy segregating in Labradors.

Variable phenotypic expression of *PTPLA^cnm^* was revealed by differences in pups' gain of weight, age of first clinical signs or extent of muscle atrophy and remodeling. A first hypothesis relied on a variable *PTPLA* function resulting from a SINE-dependent modulation of the splicing machinery. For example, Merle ($SILV^{M}$) is a coat color mutation that is inherited in an autosomal, incompletely dominant fashion, with rare $SILV^{M/+}$ dogs not exhibiting the merle phenotype. These phenotypic reversions are due to a ~30 bp shortening of the oligo(dA)-rich tail of the SINE responsible for the $SILV^{M}$ mutation [21]. In CNM dogs, this mechanism can be excluded because no polymorphisms were detected in the inserted SINE. The variable phenotypic expression may thus depend upon undetected functional polymorphisms yet to be identified in *PTPLA*, its functionally redundant paralogs, or additional genetic modifiers.

Identifying the origin of the *PTPLA^cnm^* allele

The Labrador breed is characterized by a 785-kb linkage disequilibrium, the shortest in dogs [24]. The simplest explanation

Table 3. Numbers by genotype of Labradors tested for medical or breeding purposes.

	2005–2007			2008–2009			2010–2012			
	+/+	+/*cnm*	*cnm*/*cnm*	+/+	+/*cnm*	*cnm*/*cnm*	+/+	+/*cnm*	*cnm*/*cnm*	Total
US	1 954	400	32	1 575	302	19	1 195	186	9	5 672
– carriers		*16,8%*			*15,9%*			*13,4%*		
Canada	155	22	0	103	14	1	104	13	2	414
– carriers		*12,4%*			*11,9%*			*10,9%*		
UK & Ireland	10	5	10	253	41	2	141	28	1	491
– carriers		*20%*			*13,9%*			*16,5%*		
Continental Europe	140	71	4	324	50	0	201	40	0	830
– carriers		*33%*			*13,4%*			*16,6%*		
Others	5	0	0	7	0	0	7	0	0	19
Total	2 264	498	46	2 262	407	22	1 648	267	12	7 426

Dogs are grouped by geographical origin and period of testing. The percentage of healthy carriers (+/*cnm*), suggestive of the *PTPLA^cnm^* allele segregation in Labrador lines, is provided.

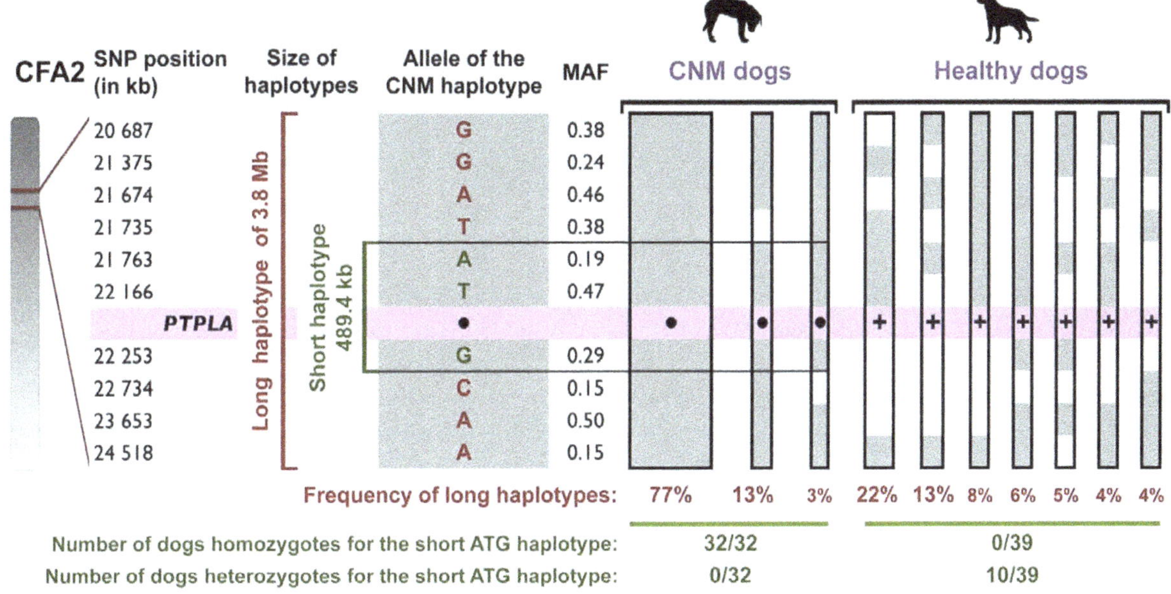

Figure 4. A 3.8-Mb haplotype is highly associated with CNM. The acrocentric region of the *PTPLA* locus within canine chromosome 2 (CFA2) is depicted. Positions of genotyped SNPs are indicated. The short and long haplotypes associated with CNM are shown in green and red, respectively. For each SNP, the allele detected in the CNM associated haplotype is indicated and represented as a grey box. The alternative allele is represented as a white box. For each SNP, the minor allele frequency (MAF) in the healthy population of Labradors is given. The $PTPLA^{cnm}$ allele is represented by a black dot (●) and the wild-type $PTPLA^{+}$ allele by a "+". Frequencies of long 3.8-Mb haplotypes in each population of CNM or healthy dogs are given below each haplotype. For haplotypes with frequencies >10%, width of haplotypes is proportional to its frequency. Haplotypes with frequencies below 3% have been omitted and are detailed in Figure S3.

for the presence of a long 3.8 Mb haplotype segment shared by CNM affected dogs, is that the ancestral $PTPLA^{cnm}$ allele arose recently, about 50 years ago, but sufficiently long ago for the accumulation of *de novo* mutations. The large size of the CNM haplotype and the high percentage of carriers favor a rapid expansion of the haplotype among Labradors, suggesting that the mutation appeared within the pedigree of a very famous stud. Accordingly, several National Stake winners of the 1950s and the 1970s are dominant in pedigrees of contemporaneous champion dogs [25], and the first clinical description has been reported in 1976 [13]. Absence of the associated haplotype in the tested healthy population highly suggests that this champion emerged from a marginal line of Labradors, or resulted from introduction of genetic diversity from other breeds.

CNM Labradors, a model in comparative pathophysiology and therapeutics

A global therapeutic strategy for this heterogeneous group of CNM may be economically relevant and to reach this goal, it is essential to understand how the different CNM-causing genes, including *PTPLA*, interact to build a functional muscle and to maintain its homeostasis. A collection of animal models with loss- or gain-of-function mutations in CNM-causing genes has been developed. They have been instrumental in identifying common defects in membrane organization, trafficking or remodeling (reviewed in [26,27]), mimicking structural aberrations observed in muscle biopsies from *BIN1*, *MTM1*, and *DNM2*-CNM patients [28,29]. In humans and CNM animal models, altered triad junctional complexes have been observed, suggesting deficient intracellular Ca^{2+} homeostasis and impaired excitation-contraction coupling [28,30,31,32,33]. A plausible mechanism is that DNM2 at the Z-disk would play a role in the transverse orientation of T-tubules through its interaction with BIN1, localized at the T-tubule [34]; the concomitant recruitment of DNM2 and BIN1, two phosphoinositide-binding proteins, would be tightly regulated by the phospahtidylinositol (PtdIns) 3-phosphatase activity of MTM1 and MTMR14 [7,35]. Once established, excitation-contraction complexes would be maintained and functionally regulated by CNM genes. Indeed deregulation of the Ca^{2+} handling in adult CNM muscles have been attributed to increased PtdIns(3,5)*P2* levels on the activity of the RYR1 Ca^{2+} sarcoplasmic channel [32], or to a PtdIns-independent consequence of MTM1 deficiency on mitochondrial positioning and homeostasis [29]. Abnormal membrane traffic at the neuromuscular junction has also been shown in MTM patients [36] and mice models [37]. Finally, it has been shown that deficiency of MTMR14 alone, or in combination with MTM1, promotes autophagy initiation through increased levels of PtdIns3*P*, thereby suggesting that the CNM pathomechanism is complex and may combine regulation of intracellular Ca^{2+} homeostasis, neuromuscular junction efficiency and autophagy.

PTPLA is a 3-hydroxyacyl-CoA dehydratase (HACD), which is an endoplasmic reticulum resident enzyme that catalyzes the third reaction of elongation of very long chain fatty acids (VLCFA) [38,39]. Saturated and monounsaturated VLCFA are components of sphingolipids, a large family of lipids that are enriched in lipid rafts and display crucial structural and signaling roles [40]. Directly or following their inclusion into sphingolipids and phosphoinositides, VLCFA may participate in muscle homeostasis by targeting phosphoinositides to specific cellular compartments or by regulating their levels. Indeed deficiency in the yeast *PTPLA* ortholog (*Phs1*) decreases the amount of VLCFA and corresponding sphingolipids and indirectly reduces the level of some phosphoinositides [38,41]. A complementary role of VLCFA may be to promote the clustering of neuromuscular junction components and signaling complexes in lipid rafts. In-depth

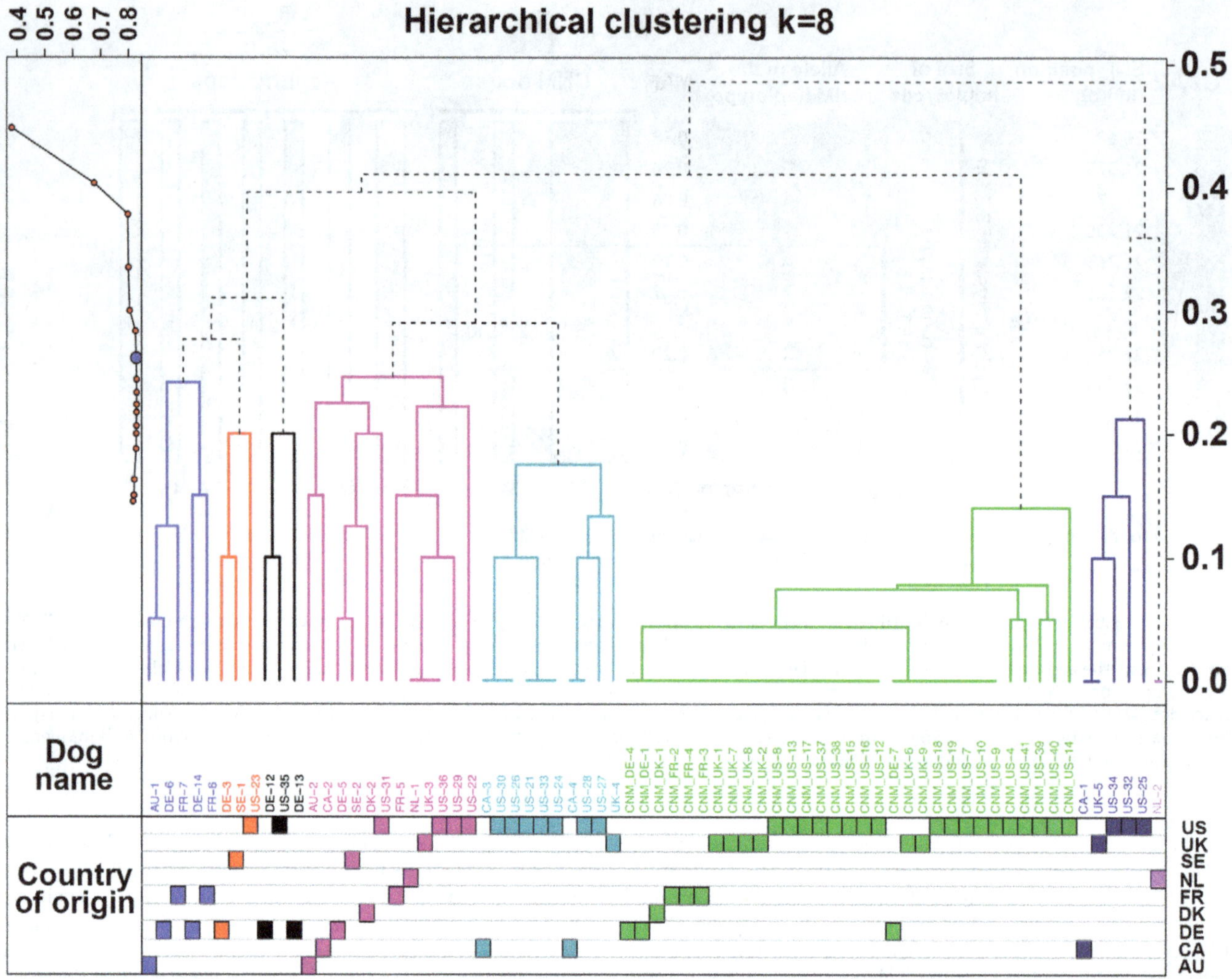

Figure 5. Hierarchical clustering from the 81 dogs at k = 8. The analysis was based on genotypes obtained for ten loci (SNP 20687 to SNP 24518). Hubert Gamma values are indicated for k≥2 on the top left panel. The scale on the right axis represents the genetics distances calculated by PLINK software. In the dendogram, each vertical line represents a dog and colors reflect the eight clusters obtained by the analysis. Grey dash lines indicate common ancestors inferred from the analysis. Below the dendogram, dogs are named by their unique identifier. The "CNM_" prefix was added to the name of affected Labradors.

analysis of PTPLA-deficient animals will help precisely understand the role of VLCFA in the functional network of other CNM genes. Ultimately, CNM Labradors will be a relevant large animal model for inclusion in pre-clinical trials of innovative drugs and gene or cell therapies.

Materials and Methods

Dogs Included in the Study

A total of 7,426 Labrador retrievers from 19 countries were included in the study (whole panel, Table 1). A subgroup of the whole panel was named the "international confirmation panel". It was composed of 32 dogs from the US, Germany, UK, Denmark and France for which clinical, histopathological or genetic reports were provided (Table 2, Table S1). Haplotype analyses were conducted on a representative group of 71 healthy (wild-type, +/+) or affected (CNM, *cnm/cnm*) Labradors from 9 countries. Each dog was assigned a unique identifier made of a 2-letter code for its country of origin, followed by an incremental number (e.g. UK-3).

Ethics statement

All but one dog, FR-2, were examined with the consent of their owners. Blood and biopsies were obtained as part of routine clinical procedures for diagnostic purposes. Cheek cells were collected by owners or veterinarians using non-invasive swabs. As the data were from client-owned dogs undergoing normal veterinary exams, there was no "animal experiment" according to the legal definitions in France, Germany, Denmark, the US and the UK. All local regulations related to clinical procedures were observed.

FR-2 was a founder dog of our experimental pedigree, and materials from FR-2 used in this study were frozen samples obtained in the 1990s by one of the co-authors (SB). At the time FR-2 was sampled, there was no animal welfare committee at the Ecole nationale vétérinaire d'Alfort; however, SB was accredited by the Veterinary Division of the French Ministry of Agriculture to perform research on animals.

DNA Extraction and SINE Sequence Analysis

Genomic DNA was extracted either from blood using a proteinase K digestion followed by a classical phenol/chloroform purification or from cheek swabs using the ChargeSwitch© gDNA buccal cell kit following manufacturer's instructions (Invitrogen).

SINE amplification by PCR was carried out as previously described [12], using the following primers: 5′-CCTCGAAGAAGGGTCAGTGTAA-3′ and 5′-CCAGCCACAATCACAGAAGTAG-3′. This produced 610-bp and 848-bp amplicons from the wild-type and mutated alleles, respectively. For a representative panel of 12 differentially affected dogs (bold numbers, Table S1), the mutated amplicon encompassing the SINE was purified and sequenced (GATC, Germany). Passed sequences were aligned using the Multalin version 5.4.1 software (multalin.toulouse.inra.fr).

SNPs Selection and Genotyping

These experimental steps were performed as previously described [42]. The list of the 15 selected SNPs with their positions is provided in Table S4. Primer sequences and optimal melting temperatures are detailed in Table S5.

Haplotype Analysis and Clustering

Haplotype phases were inferred using the program fastPHASE version 1.4.0. Haplotype frequencies and associations were calculated using the statistical software package PLINK (http://pngu.mgh.harvard.edu/purcell/plink) (v1.07). Clustering analyses were performed using PLINK to compute the IBS distance matrice, and hierarchical clustering using the R function Hclust (http://cran.r-project.org/). Both PLINK and HCLUST use distance matrix to perform clustering. For HCLUST, we used a method that merged clusters based on a point biserial correlation with the Hubert Gamma statistics, that measures the correlation between groupings and distances.

Supporting Information

Figure S1 Size conservation of the SINE insertion in 25 unrelated affected Labradors. Dogs were from the US (US; n = 20), the UK (UK; n = 3), Denmark (n = 1) and Canada (n = 1). In every tested dog, a unique band of the expected size is observed after the specific amplification of the SINE flanked by priming regions from exon 2.

Figure S2 Identity of SINE sequences amplified from 12 affected Labradors. Dogs (bolded in Table S1) were from the US (n = 7), Germany (n = 2), UK (n = 1), Denmark (n = 1) and France (n = 1; FR-2 is a founder dog of our experimental pedigree). The SINE sequence is shown in red, inserted within exon 2 of the *PTPLA* gene, which partial sequence is shown in green. The two 13-bp repeat sequences flanking the SINE are included in light-grey boxes.

Figure S3 Haplotypes of 71 Labradors in a 9-Mb region around the *PTPLA* locus. SNP positions (in kbp) from the centromeric to the telomeric end of the chromosome are listed on the left of charts. Dogs, identified by the two-letter code of their country followed by a unique incremental number for each country, are listed on the top of charts. For each dog, the two haplotypes are represented using a color code. The $PTPLA^{cnm}$ allele is represented by a black dot (•) and the wild-type $PTPLA^{+}$ allele by a "+".

Table S1 Summarized clinical signs, histopathological features and assigned genotypes of Labradors from the international confirmation panel. Dogs were sorted by their country of origin and individually identified by the two-letter code of their country followed by a unique incremental number for each country. The 12 dogs for which SINE sequences have been assessed are bolded and shaded in grey. When available, the age at which biopsies were obtained is indicated. The initial diagnosis made by co-authors, who are qualified veterinarians (NO, JP, SB) or pathologists (GDS, TB), is reminded. When available, informative data excerpted from their pedigree are provided. In the last column, the assigned genotype at the *PTPLA* locus is given. Abbreviations: AF, Atrophic fibers; ARF, Anguloid-Round fibers; FatI, Fatty infiltration; FSV, Fiber size variation; GA, Gait abnormalities; InternN, Internalized nuclei; HypoT, hypotrophy; NF, Necrotic myofibers; NonInf, Non inflammatory; NR, Nemaline rods; no PR, no patellar reflex; type 1P, type 1 fiber predominance; WK, Weakness.

Table S2 Numbers by genotype and sex of Labradors tested for medical or breeding purposes. The period of testing was 2005–2012.

Table S3 Numbers by genotype and coat colors of Labradors tested for medical or breeding purposes. The period of testing was 2005–2012.

Table S4 Positional information for the 15 polymorphic SNPs from CFA2 used in the haplotype analysis. Their names and position, from the centromere of CFA2, are indicated in the two first columns. The first group from BICF2P407690 to BICF2P583542 encompasses the ~4.2 Mb centromeric region of *PTPLA*. The second group from BICF2P642478 to BICF2S23249211 encompasses the ~4.8 Mb telomeric region of *PTPLA*.

Table S5 Experimental conditions to amplify the 15 polymorphic SNPs from CFA2 used in the haplotype analysis. Primers listed were used to amplify the sequence (Forward and Reverse primers) and to identify the SNP (Sequencing primer).

Acknowledgments

We would like to thank X. Cauchois and the UETM team from ENVA for their technical help; F. Pilot-Storck, J. Blondelle, G. Walmsley and R. Piercy for fruitful discussions; L. Transler, H. Battaglia and the ENVA Informatics staff for development of the CNM Project database. We acknowledge the numerous dog owners and veterinarians and the Retriever News for their contribution in providing samples.

Author Contributions

Conceived and designed the experiments: MM JM CH LT. Performed the experiments: MM JM LG MP CH. Analyzed the data: MM JM CH JJP LT. Contributed reagents/materials/analysis tools: MF TB NO JP GDS CH JLT IB SB GAH. Wrote the paper: MM LT. Critically revised the manuscript: GDS JJP NO JP CH JLT IB GAH SB.

References

1. Jungbluth H, Wallgren-Pettersson C, Laporte J (2008) Centronuclear (myotubular) myopathy. Orphanet J Rare Dis 3: 26.
2. Romero NB, Bitoun M (2011) Centronuclear Myopathies. Semin Pediatr Neurol 18: 250–256.
3. Laporte J, Hu LJ, Kretz C, Mandel JL, Kioschis P, et al. (1996) A gene mutated in X-linked myotubular myopathy defines a new putative tyrosine phosphatase family conserved in yeast. Nat Genet 13: 175–182.
4. Bitoun M, Maugenre S, Jeannet PY, Lacene E, Ferrer X, et al. (2005) Mutations in dynamin 2 cause dominant centronuclear myopathy. Nat Genet 37: 1207–1209.
5. Jungbluth H, Zhou H, Sewry CA, Robb S, Treves S, et al. (2007) Centronuclear myopathy due to a de novo dominant mutation in the skeletal muscle ryanodine receptor (RYR1) gene. Neuromuscul Disord 17: 338–345.
6. Nicot AS, Toussaint A, Tosch V, Kretz C, Wallgren-Pettersson C, et al. (2007) Mutations in amphiphysin 2 (BIN1) disrupt interaction with dynamin 2 and cause autosomal recessive centronuclear myopathy. Nat Genet 39: 1134–1139.
7. Tosch V, Rohde HM, Tronchere H, Zanoteli E, Monroy N, et al. (2006) A novel PtdIns3P and PtdIns(3,5)P2 phosphatase with an inactivating variant in centronuclear myopathy. Hum Mol Genet 15: 3098–3106.
8. Wilmshurst JM, Lillis S, Zhou H, Pillay K, Henderson H, et al. (2010) RYR1 mutations are a common cause of congenital myopathies with central nuclei. Ann Neurol 68: 717–726.
9. Bevilacqua JA, Monnier N, Bitoun M, Eymard B, Ferreiro A, et al. (2011) Recessive RYR1 mutations cause unusual congenital myopathy with prominent nuclear internalization and large areas of myofibrillar disorganization. Neuropathol Appl Neurobiol 37: 271–284.
10. Blot S, Tiret L, Devillaire AC, Fardeau M, Dreyfus PA (2002) Phenotypic description of a canine centronuclear myopathy. J Neurol Sci 199:S9.
11. Tiret L, Blot S, Kessler JL, Gaillot H, Breen M, et al. (2003) The *cnm* locus, a canine homologue of human autosomal forms of centronuclear myopathy, maps to chromosome 2. Hum Genet 113: 297–306. Epub 2003 Jul 2023.
12. Pelé M, Tiret L, Kessler JL, Blot S, Panthier JJ (2005) SINE exonic insertion in the PTPLA gene leads to multiple splicing defects and segregates with the autosomal recessive centronuclear myopathy in dogs. Hum Mol Genet 14: 1417–1427.
13. Kramer JW, Hegreberg GA, Bryan GM, Meyers K, Ott RL (1976) A muscle disorder of Labrador retrievers characterized by deficiency of type II muscle fibers. J Am Vet Med Assoc 169: 817–820.
14. McKerrell RE, Anderson JR, Herrtage ME, Littlewood JD, Palmer AC (1984) Generalised muscle weakness in the Labrador retriever. Vet Rec 115: 276.
15. Watson AD, Farrow BR, Middleton DJ, Smyth JB (1988) Myopathy in a Labrador retriever. Aust Vet J 65: 226–227.
16. Bley T, Gaillard C, Bilzer T, Braund KG, Faissler D, et al. (2002) Genetic aspects of labrador retriever myopathy. Res Vet Sci 73: 231–236.
17. Gortel K, Houston DM, Kuiken T, Fries CL, Boisvert B (1996) Inherited myopathy in a litter of Labrador retrievers. Can Vet J 37: 108–110.
18. Olby NJ, Sharp NJ, Anderson LV, Kunkel LM, Bonnemann CG (2001) Evaluation of the dystrophin-glycoprotein complex, alpha-actinin, dysferlin and calpain 3 in an autosomal recessive muscular dystrophy in Labrador retrievers. Neuromuscul Disord 11: 41–49.
19. McKerrell RE, Braund KG (1986) Hereditary myopathy in Labrador retrievers: a morphologic study. Vet Pathol 23: 411–417.
20. McKerrell RE, Braund KG (1987) Hereditary myopathy in Labrador Retrievers: clinical variations. J Small Anim Pract 28: 479–489.
21. Clark LA, Wahl JM, Rees CA, Murphy KE (2006) Retrotransposon insertion in SILV is responsible for merle patterning of the domestic dog. Proc Natl Acad Sci U S A 103: 1376–1381.
22. Xue Y, Wang Q, Long Q, Ng BL, Swerdlow H, et al. (2009) Human Y chromosome base-substitution mutation rate measured by direct sequencing in a deep-rooting pedigree. Curr Biol 19: 1453–1457.
23. Owczarek-Lipska M, Thomas A, Andre C, Holzer S, Leeb T (2011) [Frequency of gen defects in selected European Retriever-populations]. Schweiz Arch Tierheilkd 153: 418–420.
24. Lindblad-Toh K, Wade CM, Mikkelsen TS, Karlsson EK, Jaffe DB, et al. (2005) Genome sequence, comparative analysis and haplotype structure of the domestic dog. Nature 438: 803–819.
25. Knapp MC (1995) Retriver Field Trials. In: Ziessow BW, editor. The Official Book of the Labarador Retriever. Neptune City: T.F.H. Publications, Inc. pp. 181–204.
26. Dowling JJ, Gibbs EM, Feldman EL (2008) Membrane traffic and muscle: lessons from human disease. Traffic 9: 1035–1043.
27. Cowling BS, Toussaint A, Muller J, Laporte J (2012) Defective membrane remodeling in neuromuscular diseases: insights from animal models. PLoS Genet 8: e1002595.
28. Toussaint A, Cowling BS, Hnia K, Mohr M, Oldfors A, et al. (2011) Defects in amphiphysin 2 (BIN1) and triads in several forms of centronuclear myopathies. Acta Neuropathol (Berl) 121: 253–266.
29. Hnia K, Tronchere H, Tomczak KK, Amoasii L, Schultz P, et al. (2011) Myotubularin controls desmin intermediate filament architecture and mitochondrial dynamics in human and mouse skeletal muscle. The Journal of clinical investigation 121: 70–85.
30. Razzaq A, Robinson IM, McMahon HT, Skepper JN, Su Y, et al. (2001) Amphiphysin is necessary for organization of the excitation-contraction coupling machinery of muscles, but not for synaptic vesicle endocytosis in Drosophila. Genes & development 15: 2967–2979.
31. Al-Qusairi L, Weiss N, Toussaint A, Berbey C, Messaddeq N, et al. (2009) T-tubule disorganization and defective excitation-contraction coupling in muscle fibers lacking myotubularin lipid phosphatase. Proc Natl Acad Sci U S A 106: 18763–18768.
32. Shen J, Yu WM, Brotto M, Scherman JA, Guo C, et al. (2009) Deficiency of MIP/MTMR14 phosphatase induces a muscle disorder by disrupting Ca(2+) homeostasis. Nat Cell Biol 11: 769–776.
33. Dowling JJ, Vreede AP, Low SE, Gibbs EM, Kuwada JY, et al. (2009) Loss of myotubularin function results in T-tubule disorganization in zebrafish and human myotubular myopathy. PLoS Genet 5: e1000372.
34. Cowling BS, Toussaint A, Amoasii L, Koebel P, Ferry A, et al. (2011) Increased expression of wild-type or a centronuclear myopathy mutant of dynamin 2 in skeletal muscle of adult mice leads to structural defects and muscle weakness. The American journal of pathology 178: 2224–2235.
35. Blondeau F, Laporte J, Bodin S, Superti-Furga G, Payrastre B, et al. (2000) Myotubularin, a phosphatase deficient in myotubular myopathy, acts on phosphatidylinositol 3-kinase and phosphatidylinositol 3-phosphate pathway. Hum Mol Genet 9: 2223–2229.
36. Fidzianska A, Goebel HH (1994) Aberrant arrested in maturation neuromuscular junctions in centronuclear myopathy. J Neurol Sci 124: 83–88.
37. Dowling JJ, Joubert R, Low SE, Durban AN, Messaddeq N, et al. (2012) Myotubular myopathy and the neuromuscular junction: a novel therapeutic approach from mouse models. Disease models & mechanisms.
38. Denic V, Weissman JS (2007) A molecular caliper mechanism for determining very long-chain fatty acid length. Cell 130: 663–677.
39. Ikeda M, Kanao Y, Yamanaka M, Sakuraba H, Mizutani Y, et al. (2008) Characterization of four mammalian 3-hydroxyacyl-CoA dehydratases involved in very long-chain fatty acid synthesis. FEBS Lett 582: 2435–2440.
40. Posse de Chaves E, Sipione S (2010) Sphingolipids and gangliosides of the nervous system in membrane function and dysfunction. FEBS Lett 584: 1748–1759.
41. Kihara A, Sakuraba H, Ikeda M, Denpoh A, Igarashi Y (2008) Membrane topology and essential amino acid residues of Phs1, a 3-hydroxyacyl-CoA dehydratase involved in very long-chain fatty acid elongation. The Journal of biological chemistry 283: 11199–11209.
42. Beggs AH, Bohm J, Snead E, Kozlowski M, Maurer M, et al. (2010) MTM1 mutation associated with X-linked myotubular myopathy in Labrador Retrievers. Proc Natl Acad Sci U S A 107: 14697–14702.

7

A Frameshift Mutation within *LAMC2* Is Responsible for Herlitz Type Junctional Epidermolysis Bullosa (HJEB) in Black Headed Mutton Sheep

Stefanie Mömke[1], Andrea Kerkmann[1,2], Anne Wöhlke[1], Miriam Ostmeier[3], Marion Hewicker-Trautwein[3], Martin Ganter[2], James Kijas[4], for the International Sheep Consortium, Ottmar Distl[2]*

1 Institute for Animal Breeding and Genetics, University of Veterinary Medicine, Hannover, Germany, **2** Clinic for Swine and Small Ruminants, Forensic Medicine and Ambulatory Service, University of Veterinary Medicine, Hannover, Germany, **3** Institute for Pathology, University of Veterinary Medicine, Hannover, Germany, **4** Commonwealth Scientific and Industrial Research Organisation Livestock Industries, St. Lucia, Brisbane, Queensland, Australia

Abstract

Junctional epidermolysis bullosa (JEB) is a hereditary mechanobullous skin disease in humans and animals. A Herlitz type JEB was identified in German Black Headed Mutton (BHM) sheep and affected lambs were reproduced in a breeding trial. Affected lambs showed skin and mucous membranes blistering and all affected lambs died within the first weeks of life. The pedigree data were consistent with a monogenic autosomal recessive inheritance. Immunofluorescence showed a reduced expression of laminin 5 protein which consists of 3 subunits encoded by the genes *LAMA3*, *LAMB3* and *LAMC2*. We screened these genes for polymorphisms. Linkage and genome-wide association analyses identified *LAMC2* as the most likely candidate for HJEB. A two base pair deletion within exon 18 of the *LAMC2* gene (FM872310:c.2746delCA) causes a frameshift mutation resulting in a premature stop codon (p.A928*) 13 triplets downstream of this mutation and in addition, introduces an alternative splicing of exon 18 *LAMC2*. This deletion showed a perfect co-segregation with HJEB in all 740 analysed BHM sheep. Identification of the *LAMC2* deletion means an animal model for HJEB is now available to develop therapeutic approaches of relevance to the human form of this disease.

Editor: You-Qiang Song, The University of Hong Kong, Hong Kong

Funding: A. Kerkmann was supported by the FAZIT foundation Gemeinnützige Verlagsgesellschaft mbH, Frankfurt/Main. The funders had no role in study design, data collection and analysis, decision to publish, or preparation of the manuscript.

Competing Interests: The authors have declared that no competing interests exist.

* E-mail: ottmar.distl@tiho-hannover.de

Introduction

Epidermolysis bullosa (EB) is a heritable heterogeneous group of skin disorders affecting the integrity of the skin and mucosa. Abnormalities of macromolecules which anchor the dermis to the epidermis lead to diminished cohesion of the skin layers, blister formation, and fragility. The condition is triggered by frictional movement as well as minor trauma [1]. This mechanobullous disease is well known in several livestock species and in human. Based on the cleavage levels of skin, EB has been classified into the main groups EB simplex, dystrophic EB and junctional EB (JEB). JEB involves cleavage within the lamina lucida which is a component of the basement membrane [2]. Herlitz type JEB is a lethal condition, whereas non-Herlitz type JEB is rarely related to death. In human, three genes are known to be associated with HJEB including *laminin β3* (*LAMB3*), *laminin γ2* (*LAMC2*) and *laminin α3* (*LAMA3*). The defect is usually inherited in an autosomal recessive manner and also cases of compound heterozygosity were described [3]. In human, nonsense, splicing and deletion mutations of *LAMB3*, *LAMC2* and *LAMA3* have been reported as responsible for HJEB [4]. In domesticated animals, cases of JEB are described in horses [5–7], dogs [8–11] and cats [12]. In German Pointer dogs, a homozygous insertion of repetitive satellite DNA within intron 35 of *LAMA3* was shown to be causal for the defect [10]. Another study in a French subpopulation of this dog breed gave evidence for a non-conservative change of 14 amino acids within *LAMA3* causing JEB [11]. In Belgian draft horses, Comtois horses, and Breton horses affected by HJEB, a homozygous insertion of one nucleotide within exon 10 of *LAMC2* was detected [5,6]. Furthermore, in American Saddle-bred horses HJEB was reported to be caused by a homozygous deletion spanning exons 24–27 of *LAMA3* [7]. In sheep, cases of dystrophic EB have been described in the breeds Weisses Alpenschaf and Assaf sheep [13,14]. In German Black Headed Mutton (BHM) sheep ovine HJEB has been ascertained in several flocks and after performing a breeding trial with a sample of parents which gave birth to HJEB-affected lambs, a monogenic autosomal recessive inheritance was most likely [15].

In this study, we employed animals from farms and a breeding trial to identify the mutation causing ovine HJEB in German BHM sheep. The most likely candidate gene *LAMC2* was identified using the Illumina OvineSNP50 Beadchip and candidate gene-associated polymorphisms. We provide the complete ovine coding sequence of *LAMC2* and characterize the transcriptional effects of the *LAMC2*-mutation responsible for HJEB.

Results

Phenotype

The clinical examination of 21 HJEB affected lambs revealed typical signs as shedding of hoof horn, erosion and ulcers of the skin as well as the mucous membranes (Figure 1). All affected lambs had to be euthanised due to the progressive deterioration of their condition. Electron microscopy showed that the separations of the dermoepidermal junction were located in the lamina lucida of the basement membrane. Hemidesmosomes were present in reduced numbers. Immunofluorescence showed a markedly reduced expression of laminin 5 protein whilst expression of collagen VII appeared to be normal. Laminin 5 consists of three subunits encoded by the genes *LAMA3*, *LAMB2* and *LAMC2* [4], which consequently were chosen for scanning polymorphisms that could be used for linkage and association analyses.

Mapping the Causative Gene

The ovine genome assembly v2.0 (http://www.livestockgenomics.csiro.au/) located *LAMA3* on ovine chromosome (OAR) 23 at 34.8 Mb, *LAMB3* on OAR12 at 78.8 Mb and *LAMC2* also on OAR12 at 68.6 Mb. These genes were partly sequenced to detect polymorphisms, which were subsequently used for linkage analyses in the 21 affected sheep and their direct relatives. Within *LAMA3* (FM872294), seven single nucleotide polymorphisms (SNPs) and one microsatellite were detected (Table S1). Of these markers, five were in a common linkage group and the remaining two in another one. None of these markers showed linkage with HJEB in the data analysed here. Within *LAMB3* (FM872309), 15 SNPs distributed on seven linkage-disequilibrium blocks (Table S1) and within *LAMC2* (FM872310), five SNPs within four linkage-disequilibrium blocks were detected and analysed (Table 1). The chromosome-wide p-values for linkage with HJEB were at $p=0.004$ for *LAMB3*-associated SNPs and for *LAMC2*-associated SNPs at $p<0.00001$. Strong linkage disequilibrium among the markers within both genes obviated a further resolution among the two candidate genes. Thus, all these gene-associated SNPs were tested for association with HJEB. None of the markers within *LAMA3* and *LAMB3* showed a significant association with HJEB, while three of the five SNPs within *LAMC2* were significantly associated with HJEB ($p=0.0003$). In addition to the analysis of candidate gene-associated markers, we performed a genome-wide association study to validate linkage to *LAMC2* and determine if additional genomic regions displayed evidence of association. DNA from 12 HJEB-affected BHM lambs (cases), 6 HJEB-unaffected BHM sheep representing parents or full-sibs of the cases and 6 control samples from the whole BHM population were genotyped using the *ovine* Illumina 50 K beadchip. Quality control for genotyping was performed using two duplicates. Consistency of genotyping was >0.999. After filtering for a minor allele frequency >0.05 and genotyping rate >0.99, 43,130 SNPs (single nucleotide polymorphisms) were left for a genome-wide association analysis among cases and controls. After genome-wide permutation to correct for multiple testing, only 11 SNPs were genome-wide significant ($p<0.05$). All these hits were located on ovine chromosome (OAR) 12 in a region spanning 63.1–70.4 Mb which contains the *LAMC2* gene (at 68.8 Mb). The strongest association ($p=0.0001$) with HJEB was obtained for SNP *OAR12_65207540, OAR12_65811822, OAR12_66169798 and OAR12_s45876.* A mixed linear model analysis including the fixed effect of the sex of the animal and the random animal effect parameterized through the identical-by-state relationship matrix gave the highest hits at 67.333 Mb ($-\log_{10}$ p-value = 22.4) and at 68.951 Mb on OAR12 ($-\log_{10}$ p-value = 21.1) as shown in the Q-Q and Manhattan plots of the $-\log_{10}$ p-values (Figure S1). Therefore, *LAMC2* was confirmed through analysis of gene-associated SNPs and genome-wide SNPs as the most likely candidate harbouring the causal mutation for HJEB.

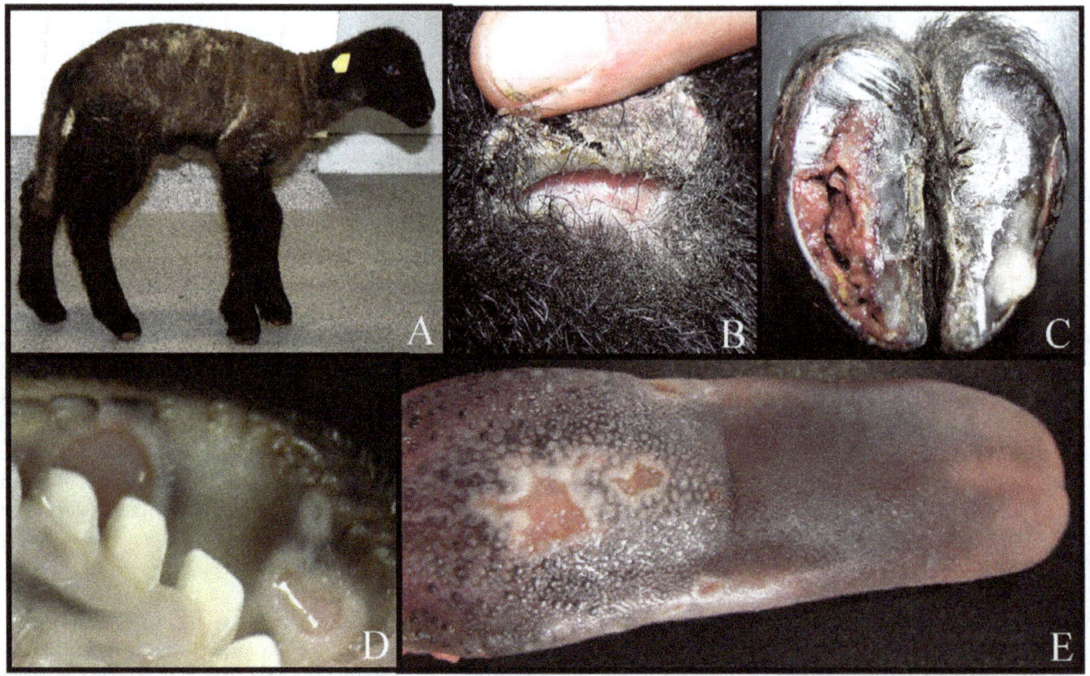

Figure 1. Clinical and pathomorphological feature of HJEB in German Black Headed Mutton sheep. Typical signs are a kyphotic attitude and severe lameness (A), detachment of the epidermis from the underlying dermis (B, dorsal carpal joint), detachment of hoof horn from the corium and accumulation of bloody fluid in the cavity (C), erosion of mucous membranes (D) and of the tongue (E).

Table 1. SNP motifs for the SNPs detected within *LAMC2*, their surrounding sequence, their effect on the protein sequence and their p-values of association with Herlitz type junctional epidermolysis bullosa (HJEB) in 73 Black Headed Mutton (BHM) sheep.

Polymorphism	Location within *LAMC2*	Wildtype sequence	Mutated sequence	Amino acid exchange	P-value ($-\log_{10}$)
FM872310:c.367C>T	exon 3	TTCCATACC**C**TCACCGAT	TTCCATACC**T**TCACCGAT	p.L123F	7.6
FM872310:c.570C>T	exon 5	GTTTTTGCTA**C**GGGCATT	GTTTTTGCTA**T**GGGCATT	-	
FM872310: c.1523G>A	exon 11	GGGGAAC**G**TGGTCCAGT	GGGGAAC**A**TGGTCCAGT	p.R508H	3.3
FM872310: c.1665T>C	exon 11	GTGCAAAGC**T**GGCTACT	GTGCAAAGC**C**GGCTACT	-	
FM872310: c.1878A>G	exon 13	GTTTATGCA**A**CAACTTGA	GTTTATGCA**G**CAACTTGA	-	
FM872310: c.1893T>C	exon 13	GAGAGCCTTGAGACACT	GAGAGCCT**C**GAGACACT	-	
FM872310: c.1923T>C	exon 13	CTCAGGCTGG**T**GGAGGA	CTCAGGCTGG**C**GGAGGA	-	
FM872310: c.2358T>C	exon 16	TGAAGACTA**T**TCCAAGCA	TGAAGACTA**C**TCCAAGCA	-	
FM872310: c.2546A>G	exon 17	ATAGTCTCC**A**CCTTCTCA	ATAGTCTCC**G**CCTTCTCA	p.H849R	0.4
FM872310: c.2746delCA	exon 18	AATGAGAGA**C**AGAAATCA	AATGAGAGA::GAGAAATCA	p.Q916EfsX13	14.8
FM872310: c.3000T>C	exon 20	TGCTGCTAC**T**GACGCCCA	TGCTGCTAC**C**GACGCCCA	-	
FM872310: c.3001G>A	exon 20	GCTGCTACT**G**ACGCCCA	GCTGCTACT**A**ACGCCCA	p.D1001N	10.1
FM872310: c.3258T>C	exon 22	AGCAGAGC**T**GAGAATGC	AGCAGAGC**C**GAGAATGC	-	
FM872310: c.3455G>A	exon 23	GCAGTGGG**G**CCACCTCC	GCAGTGGG**A**CCACCTCC	p.G1152D	9.9
FM872310: c.3483C>A	exon 23	ACAAGCAT**C**GATGGCATT	ACAAGCAT**A**GATGGCATT	-	
FM872310: c.3600T>C	3'UTR	TTTCCCAAC**T**GGGGTTCTT	TTTCCCAAC**C**GGGGTTCTT	-	
FM872310: c.2749+51A>G	intron 18	ATGGCTACC**A**GTAAGAAGA	ATGGCTACC**G**GTAAGAAGA	*	12.9

*Alternative splicing (only in combination with c.2746delCA deletion): p.Q916EfsX14.
The c.2746delCA mutation causes HJEB due to a premature stop codon.

Mutation Analysis

After transcription of mRNA into cDNA, the complete coding sequence of *LAMC2* was obtained in two unaffected and two HJEB-affected sheep. We identified a 3,576 bp open reading frame (ORF) in the healthy sheep, which corresponds to the bovine ORF of *LAMC2*. The ovine ORF sequence of the unaffected sheep had an identity of 96.8% with the orthologous bovine sequence. Comparing the sequences of unaffected and HJEB-affected sheep, we detected 14 SNPs and a 2-bp deletion. Of these polymorphisms, six were non-synonymous (c.367C>T, c.1523G>A, c.2546A>G, c.2746delCA, c.3001G>A, c.3455G>A) and led to an alternate amino acid sequence (p.L123F, p.R508H, p.H849R, p.Q916EfsX13, p.D1001N, p.G1152D) (Table 1). All non-conservative polymorphisms were analysed in all 21 HJEB-affected lambs and their relatives. The polymorphisms c.3001G>A and c.3455G>A were in the same linkage phase in all tested animals, while the other SNP alleles showed lower correlations with $r^2<0.8$ (Figure S2). Only the c.2746delCA mutation showed a perfect co-segregation with HJEB and allows detection of all affected individuals, unaffected wildtype individuals and heterozygous carriers of HJEB in BHM sheep (Table 2). The χ^2-values for genotypic and allelic distribution were at 68.0 and 50.4, respectively, and the corresponding p-values were at $p<0.00001$.

The c.2746delCA (p.Q916EfsX13) mutation causes a premature stop codon at position p.A928X and an alternative splicing of exon 18 (Figure S3). This deletion is located two base pairs upstream of the boundary between exon 18 and exon 19. The alternative splicing lead to an insertion of the first part of intron 18 into the alternatively spliced coding sequence of *LAMC2* and could be found in all affected animals and carriers. Overlapping cDNA sequences in HJEB-affected sheep were amplified using primer pairs from exon 17 to intron 18 and primer pairs from intron 18 to exon 20. Sequencing of these amplicons in both directions gave evidence of a 51-bp insertion from intron 18 into the alternatively spliced coding sequence and a SNP within intron 18 (c.2749+51A>G). This SNP activates a cryptic splice donor site and terminates the transcription of intron 18 (Figure S4). In order to proof the distribution of the c.2749+51A>G SNP, we genotyped all affected sheep and their relatives for this mutation. All HJEB-affected sheep were homozygous G/G, the heterozygous carriers were also heterozygous at c.2749+51A>G, except for three individuals which were homozygous G/G. The unaffected wildtype sheep were homozygous A/A at c.2749+51A>G, except for four individuals which were heterozygous. Of one of these four wildtype individuals, tissue samples were available for cDNA analysis. These samples were used for PCR with primer pairs spanning from exon 17 to intron 18, from intron 18 to exon 20, and from exon 17 to exon 20. While the amplicon including exon 17 to exon 20 was clearly visible on an agarose gel, the other PCR-products could not be amplified indicating an absence of the alternative splicing. Therefore, the c.2746delCA mutation seems to be necessary for the alternative splicing and the c.2749+51A>G mutation for the size of the alternatively spliced product. The alternatively spliced product contains a stop codon at c.2749+41 (Figure S5).

To estimate the distribution of the mutant allele in the BHM sheep population, 645 randomly sampled, unaffected individuals of this breed were genotyped for the c.2746delCA. An association analysis using all 717 BHM sheep genotyped in this study resulted in χ^2 values for genotypic and allelic distributions of 713 and 711, respectively. The corresponding p-values were $p = 1.49e^{-155}$ and $p = 1.08e^{-156}$. Of these sheep genotyped, no animal showed the homozygous mutant genotype and six individuals out of different flocks were heterozygous carriers of HJEB. These results allow the conclusion that about 0.9% of the BHM population are carriers for HJEB.

Table 2. Distribution of the *LAMC2* c.2746delCA mutation in Black Headed Mutton (BHM) sheep from the breeding experiment, random samples of HJEB-unaffected BHM, Suffolk, East Friesian and Leine sheep.

c.2746delCA genotype	BHM (breeding trial)		BHM	Suffolk	East Friesian	Leine
	HJEB-affected (n = 21)	Relatives of HJEB-affected (n = 52)	Random sample (n = 645)	Random sample (n = 175)	Random sample (n = 100)	Random sample (n = 62)
CA/CA		17	639	175	100	52
del/CA		35	6			
del/del	21					

Since Suffolk sheep have contributed to the foundation of the BHM breed, the deletion identified in BHM sheep was genotyped in 175 unaffected and randomly sampled Suffolk sheep. However, not any of the genotyped animals carried the c.2746delCA mutation. Furthermore, random samples of each 50 white and brown colour variants of the breed East Friesian and 62 Leine sheep were genotyped (Table 2). None of these animals showed the c.2746delCA mutation either.

Discussion

A 2-bp deletion within exon 18 of *LAMC2* (c.2746delCA) was identified as responsible for HJEB in BHM sheep. This c.2746delCA mutation causes a frameshift with a premature stop codon and an alternative splicing of exon 18. In all sheep exhibiting the c.2746delCA mutation, a second intronic c.2749+51A>G mutation could be shown. As the alternatively spliced RNA did also contain a stop codon 42 bp downstream of c.2746delCA, all HJEB-affected sheep in the present study will have a truncated *LAMC2* protein. The presence of c.2746delCA mutation is sufficient to introduce the alternative splicing process because for individuals alone with the c.2749+51A>G mutation alternatively spliced cDNA could not be shown. We assume that the deletion of CA changes the 5′ splice donor site from GACAG/GT to GAG/GT and due to the missing C, the splice site at the 5′ end of exon 18 is not recognized in each case [16]. The c.2749+51A>G SNP located in intron 18 creates a cryptic splice site by converting the sequence CCAGTAAGA to CCGG-TAAGA. Even if this splice site seems not to be perfect compared to the reported splice donor consensus sequences [16], the intronic insert was always terminated at this site. According to the splice site competition model, alternative splicing happens when one donor is sufficiently good to compete with the other donor for U1 snRNA binding [17]. In the case that both mutations are present, the splice sites are competitively used, which results in two different transcripts in sheep possessing these mutations.

LAMC2 encodes for laminin γ2, which is one of three distinct polypeptides that compose laminin 5. These laminin alpha, beta and gamma polypeptides generate a cruciform structure of three short arms formed by different chains and one long arm composed of all three chains. The long arm of laminin γ2, together with those of laminin α3 and laminin β3, spans the lamina lucida, ending right underneath the basal keratinocytes layer [18]. The short arm region contains the nidogen and fibulin binding sites, which integrate the laminin 5 protein into the basement membrane [19]. Mutations within laminin γ2 are most frequently located within the N-terminal LE domains and the L4 module, whereas mutations in the C-terminal α-helical domain are rare [4]. Compared with the human structure, the sheep mutation c.2746delCA (p.Q916EfsX13) is located within the α-helical domain and shortens the polypeptide chain by a premature stop codon 13 triplets downstream of the deletion. Therefore, this SNP mutation presumably influences the assembling of laminin γ2 with its partner chains leading to a non- or dysfunction of laminin 5.

The BHM breed has been introgressed by Suffolk sheep, which were reported to have shown signs of HJEB [20]. In order to confirm if the mutation was introduced by Suffolk sheep into the BHM breed, Suffolk from different flocks were randomly sampled and genotyped. However, none of the genotyped animals carried the HJEB mutation. This implies that either HJEB was not introduced into the BHM population by Suffolk sheep or the defect is more infrequent in the latter breed or maybe even eradicated. On the other hand, BHM sheep have been crossed into other breeds as white and brown colour variants of the breed East Friesian sheep and the Leine sheep. Therefore we checked random samples of these breeds for the presence of c.2746delCA. All individuals of these breeds were homozygous for the wild type sequence. This might indicate that HJEB has not been transmitted into these breeds or that the allele frequency is very low and the c.2746delCA mutation is limited to BHM. On the other hand, it should be noted that no symptomatic animals from these other breeds have been tested, which leaves open the possibility the c.2746delCA mutation is not confined to BHM or even more likely that other not yet known mutations within *LAMC2, LAMA3 or LAMB3* are causing HJED in other sheep breeds. Though HJEB is known in many species, and causal mutations within *LAMC2* have been identified in the human and horse [4,6], the c.2746delCA mutation was not reported before and can therefore be regarded as new in this regard (Table S2).

In conclusion, we identified the causal mutation for ovine HJEB in BHM sheep. This mutation (c.2746delCA) is located within *LAMC2* and leads to a frame shift of the ORF and a premature stop codon (p.Q916EfsX13) as well as induces an alternative splicing process for exon 18. The genetic test can be employed for eradication of this lethal mutation in the BHM sheep breed. Furthermore, this study provides a suitable animal model for therapeutic approaches of HJEB caused by a specific mutation. Due to the genetic complexity of HJEB, several animal models seem necessary to work out the specific effects caused by the different mutations within *LAMC2, LAMA3 or LAMB3* and the sheep model proposed allows therapeutic interventions for several weeks before HJEB becomes lethal and in particular, to study the factors causing lethality.

Materials and Methods

Ethics Statement

All animal work has been conducted according to the national and international guidelines for animal welfare. The breeding experiment at the University of Veterinary Medicine Hannover was under the supervision of the Lower Saxony state veterinary office Niedersächsisches Landesamt für Verbraucherschutz und Lebensmittelsicherheit, Oldenburg, Germany (registration number 33.42502-05/1023).

Animals

We obtained blood samples of a total of 21 HJEB affected BHM sheep, of which 19 were purebred and two were crossbred animals with German White Headed Mutton or Leine sheep relatives in second to fourth degree. The diagnosis of HJEB was ascertained by clinical, pathological and histological methods. In addition, immunofluorescence and electron microscopy were employed to distinguish HJEB from the non-Herlitz type of JEB. Fifteen of the HJEB affected lambs were born in three different flocks in Lower Saxony, Germany, and eight ewes from two farms and one ram which had already produced HJEB affected offspring were employed for a breeding experiment at the University of Veterinary Medicine Hannover and under the supervision of the state veterinary office (registration number 33.42502-05/1023). In this breeding experiment six HJEB affected lambs were born. Also 51 samples of unaffected sheep which were closely related with HJEB affected lambs were taken. Genome-wide association analyses were performed using DNA from 12 HJEB-affected BHM lambs (cases), 6 HJEB-unaffected BHM sheep representing parents and full-sibs of the cases and 6 control samples from the whole BHM population. We could not trace back the affected BHM lambs to a common founder due to missing information on some ancestors of the HJEB affected sheep (Figure S6). Furthermore, 645 samples of non-affected BHM sheep from 50 farms as well as 337 samples of non-affected sheep of other breeds as Suffolk sheep (175), East Friesian sheep (100), and Leine sheep (62) were used for genotyping. DNA was extracted from blood and tissue samples using the QIAamp 96 DNA Blood kit (Qiagen, Hilden, Germany). We used skin and lung tissue of each two unaffected, carrier and affected sheep for extraction of RNA. The samples were harvested immediately after euthanasia and asserved in RNAlater RNA Stabilization Reagent (Qiagen) for stabilization and protection of cellular RNA *in situ* and then stored at −20°C. The RNA was extracted from tissue samples using the Nucleospin RNAII-kit (Macherey-Nagel, Düren, Germany) and transcribed into cDNA using SuperScript III Reverse Transcriptase (Invitrogen, Karlsruhe, Germany).

Sequence and mutation analysis of the ovine *LAMA3*, *LAMB3* and *LAMC2* genes

For analysis of *LAMA3*, *LAMB3* and *LAMC2*, we designed primers with Primer3 software (http://frodo.wi.mit.edu/cgi-bin/primer3/primer3_www.cgi) using sequences derived from the ovine genome assembly v2.0 (http://www.livestockgenomics.csiro.au/) or, if ovine sequences were not available in the targeted region, we designed heterologous primers based on bovine sequences (Table S3). PCR products were sequenced on a MegaBACE 1000 capillary sequencer (GE Healthcare, Freiburg, Germany) and analysed using Sequencher 4.7 (GeneCodes, Ann Arbor, MI, USA). For the *LAMC2* mutation analysis we sequenced overlapping cDNA fragments spanning the entire open reading frame in each two affected and non-affected sheep. All detected polymorphisms were genotyped in the 21 samples of HJEB affected sheep and 51 samples of closely related unaffected sheep. After this, single- and multipoint non-parametric linkage analysis were performed using the Merlin software, version 1.1.2 [21]. The only polymorphism in complete concordance with HJEB in the genotyped animals was sequenced on cDNA and genomic DNA in each two affected, unaffected and carrier animals. Genotyping of c.2746delCA was performed by sequencing as well as by digestion of PCR products using the MnlI enzyme (NEB, Frankfurt, Germany).

Non-parametric linkage and association analyses

Non-parametric single- and multipoint linkage (NPL) analyses were employed for the HJEB-affected lambs and their closely relatives, which were from three different farms. Sheep from farm I and farm II were connected by common progeny born in the breeding trial (Figure S4) Linkage analysis was based on allele sharing by identical-by-descent methods and the MERLIN 1.1.2 software [21]. The NPL statistics Zmeans and the LOD (logarithm of the odds) scores were employed for detection of allele sharing among affected family members. The minimum (min) and maximum (max) achievable Zmeans and LOD scores were high enough to reach genome-wide significant linkage. For the genome-wide type I error probability (P_g), a Bonferroni correction was applied with $P_{genome\text{-}wide} = 1-(1-P_{chromosome\text{-}wide})^{1/r}$, where r = length of OAR12 (86.14 Mb) divided by the total ovine genome length in Mb (2647 Mb). Using this formula, the threshold for P_g of 0.05 and 0.01 is at a chromosome-wide p-value of 0.001668 and 0.000327. A significant co-segregation of a marker allele with the phenotypic expression of HJEB in the examined population was assumed for p-values <0.05.

Association of SNPs with HJEB was tested using the CASE-CONTROL procedure of SAS/Genetics (Statistical Analysis System, version 9.2, Cary, NC, USA, 2010) and PLINK, version 1.07 [22]. Genome-wide significance was obtained using 1,000,000 permutations with the max(T) permutation procedure of PLINK.

Statistical calculation of pairwise linkage disequilibrium (LD) was performed and pictured using HAPLOVIEW 4.0 [23]. We used the Tagger algorithm $r^2 \geq 0.8$ to detect SNPs with strong LD among alleles.

A mixed linear model (MLM) was employed to control for sex of the animals and the identity-by-state (IBS) kinship matrix among all individuals (K-matrix) using TASSEL [24]. The KIN option of TASSEL was used to create the K-matrix containing the IBS coefficients. Equations were solved via restricted maximum likelihood.

Supporting Information

Figure S1 Results of the genome-wide association analysis. (A) Q-Q plot of the $-\log_{10}$ p-values from a mixed linear model analysis for association of genome-wide SNPs with Herlitz type junctional epidermolysis bullosa (HJEB) in Black Headed Mutton (BHM) sheep. (B) Manhattan-plot of the $-\log_{10}$ p-values for the genome-wide association analysis of Herlitz type junctional epidermolysis bullosa (HJEB) in Black Headed Mutton (BHM) sheep. The peaks of the $-\log_{10}$ p-values are only on OAR12.

Figure S2 Linkage disequilibrium (LD) of six non-conservative SNPs within *LAMC2*. The r^2 values are shown for each SNP pair. The red square between the markers c.3001G>A and c.3455G>A indicates complete linkage.

Figure S3 cDNA sequence of an HJEB-unaffected lamb (A) in comparison with the cDNA sequence of an HJEB-affected lamb (B, C). The cDNA sequence of an HJEB-affected lamb is spanning from exon 17 to exon 19 (B) and the cDNA sequence of the same affected lamb is spanning from exon 17 to intron 18 (C). The vertical line marks the end of exon 18. In the affected individual (B/C), at the end of exon 18 two bases (CA) are missing and alternative splicing results in two transcripts with one of them including 51 bp of intron 18 (B). The presence of intronic DNA within the second transcript can be clearly shown by generating sequences starting from exon 17 and ending in intron 18 (C). The boundary between exon 17 and exon 18 of all products was smooth and used to verify that only cDNA was sequenced.

Figure S4 Cryptic intronic splice site in an HJEB-affected lamb. Section of the cDNA sequence of an HJEB-affected lamb showing the sequence of intron 18, which is spliced at the intronic base pair 51 to exon 19. The A>G mutation opening a cryptic splice site and therefore terminating this intronic insertion into the cDNA sequence is indicated.

Figure S5 Comparison of amino acid sequences among an unaffected and an HJEB-affected animal. Sequence labelled with 1 is from an unaffected lamb and sequences labelled 2 and 3 are from one HJEB-affected lamb. Sequence 2 demonstrates the transcript with correct and sequence 3 demonstrates the transcript with alternative splicing. Both variants (2 and 3) were present in every HJEB-affected lamb and both sequences lead to a premature stop codon and thus to a shortened, non-functional protein.

Figure S6 Pedigree of the HJEB-affected Black Headed Mutton sheep. Sheep from the three farms are marked by grey boxes in contrast to the progeny born in the mating experiment. Animals marked by an asterisk were genotyped on the ovine Illumina 50 K beadchip.

Table S1 Polymorphisms identified within ovine *LAMA3* and *LAMB3* used for linkage analysis and their location, polymorphism information content (PIC) and heterozygosity (HET).

Table S2 Mutations within *LAMC2* causing Herlitz and Non-Herlitz JEB in human and horse.

Table S3 Primer sequences with their product sizes (P) and annealing temperatures (AT) used for amplification of sequences within *LAMA3*, *LAMB3*, and *LAMC2* as well as the targeted regions within these genes.

Acknowledgments

We thank all members of the staff of the Institute for Animal Breeding and Genetics, Clinic for Small Ruminants and Swine, Forensic Medicine and Ambulatory Service and Institute for Pathology, University of Veterinary Medicine Hannover, Germany, who supported this study. We thank all breeders for the samples and the pedigree information of their sheep. We thank H. Klippert-Hasberg and S. Neander for their technical support during the work in the laboratory.

Author Contributions

Conceived and designed the experiments: MG OD. Performed the experiments: SM AK AW MO MH MG. Analyzed the data: SM AK MO MH MG OD. Contributed reagents/materials/analysis tools: MO MH MG JK OD. Wrote the paper: SM AK JK OD.

References

1. Nakano A, Chao SC, Pulkkinen L, Murrell D, Bruckner-Tuderman L, et al. (2002) Laminin 5 mutations in junctional epidermolysis bullosa: molecular basis of Herlitz vs. non-Herlitz phenotypes. Hum Genet 110: 41–51.
2. Bruckner-Tuderman L (1992) Pathogenesis of mechanobullous disorders. Exp Dermatol 1: 115–120.
3. Castiglia D, Posteraro P, Spirito F, Pinola C, Angelo P, et al. (2001) Novel mutations in the LAMC2 gene in non-Herlitz junctional epidermolysis bullosa: effects on laminin-5 assembly, secretion, and deposition. J Invest Dermatol 117: 731–739.
4. Schneider H, Mühle C, Pacho F (2007) Biological function of laminin-5 and pathogenic impact of its deficieny. Eur J Cell Biol 86: 701–717.
5. Spirito F, Charlesworth A, Linder K, Ortonne JP, Baird J, et al. (2002) Animal models for skin blistering conditions: absence of laminin 5 causes hereditary junctional mechanobullous disease in the Belgian horse. J Invest Dermatol 119: 684–691.
6. Milenkovic D, Chaffaux S, Taourit S, Guérin G (2003) A mutation in the LAMC2 gene causes the Herlitz junctional epidermolysis bullosa (H-JEB) in two French draft horse breeds. Genet Sel Evol 35: 249–256.
7. Graves KT, Henney PJ, Ennis RB (2009) Partial deletion of the LAMA3 gene is responsible for hereditary junctional epidermolysis bullosa in the American Saddlebred Horse. Anim Genet 40: 35–41.
8. Nagata M, Iwasaki T, Masuda H, Shimizu H (1997) Non-lethal junctional epidermolysis bullosa in a dog. Br J Dermatol 137: 445–449.
9. Dunstan RW, Sills RC, Wilkinson JE, Paller AS, Hashimoto KH (1988) A disease resembling junctional epidermolysis bullosa in a toy poodle. Am J Dermatopathol 10: 442–447.
10. Capt A, Spirito F, Guaguere E, Spadafora A, Ortonne JP, et al. (2005) Inherited junctional epidermolysis bullosa in the German Pointer: Establishment of a large animal model. J Invest Dermatol 124: 530–535.
11. Guaguere E, Capt A, Spirito F, Meneguzzi G (2003) L'Épidermolyse Bulleuse Jonctionnelle du Braque allemand: un modèle canin spontané de l'Épidermolyse Bulleuse Jonctionnelle de l'Homme. Bull Acad Vét France 157: 47–51.
12. Alhaidari Z, Olivry T, Spadafora A, Thomas RC, Perrin C, et al. (2006) Junctional epidermolysis bullosa in two domestic shorthair kittens. Vet Dermatol 16: 69–73.
13. Bruckner-Tuderman L, Guscetti F, Ehrensperger F (1991) Animal model for dermolytic mechanobullous disease: sheep with recessive dystrophic epidermolysis bullosa lack collagen VII. J Invest Dermatol 96: 452–458.
14. Pérez V, Benavides J, Herrera EL, Reyes LE, Ferreras MC, et al. (2005) Epidermolysis bullosa in Assaf lambs. Proceedings of the 23rd Meeting of the European Society of Veterinary Pathology, Naples, Italy 173.
15. Kerkmann A, Ganter M, Frase R, Ostmeier M, Hewicker-Trautwein M, et al. (2010) Epidermolysis bullosa in German black headed mutton sheep. Berl Münch Tierärztl Wochenschr 123: 413–421.
16. Zhang XHF, Heller KA, Hefter I, Leslie CS, Chasin LA (2003) Sequence information for the splicing of human pre-mRNA identified by support vector machine classification. Genome Res 13: 2637–2650.
17. Hiller M, Platzer M (2008) Widespread and subtle: alternative splicing at short-distance tandem sites. Trends Genet 24: 246–255.
18. Masunaga T, Shimizu H, Ishiko A, Tomita Y, Aberdam D, et al. (1996) Localization of laminin-5 in the epidermal basement membrane. J Histochem Cytochem 44: 1223–1230.
19. Sasaki T, Göhring W, Mann K, Brakebusch C, Yamada Y, et al. (2001) Short arm region of laminin-5 $\gamma2$ chain: Structure, mechanism of processing and binding to heparin and proteins. J Mol Biol 314: 751–763.
20. Alley MR, O'Hara JO, Middelberg A (1974) An epidermolysis bullosa of sheep. NZ Vet J 22: 55–59.
21. Abecasis GR, Cherny SS, Cookson WO, Cardon LR (2002) Merlin-rapid analysis of dense genetic maps using sparse gene flow trees. Nat Genet 30: 97–101.
22. Purcell S, Neale B, Todd-Brown K, Thomas L, Ferreira MAR, et al. (2007) PLINK: a toolset for whole-genome association and population-based linkage analysis. Am J Hum Genet 81: 559–575.
23. Barrett JC, Fry B, Maller J, Daly MJ (2005) Haploview: analysis and visualization of LD and haplotype maps. Bioinformatics 21: 263–265.
24. Bradbury PJ, Zhang Z, Kroon DE, Casstevens TM, Ramdoss Y, et al. (2007) TASSEL: software for association mapping of complex traits in diverse samples. Bioinformatics 23: 2633–2635.

8

Pharmacodynamics of Antimicrobials against *Mycoplasma mycoides mycoides* Small Colony, the Causative Agent of Contagious Bovine Pleuropneumonia

John D. Mitchell[1]*, Quintin A. McKellar[2], Declan J. McKeever[1]

1 Royal Veterinary College, Hatfield, Hertfordshire, United Kingdom, **2** University of Hertfordshire, Hatfield, Hertfordshire, United Kingdom

Abstract

Background: *Mycoplasma mycoides* subspecies *mycoides* Small Colony (*Mmm*SC) is the causative agent of Contagious Bovine Pleuropneumonia (CBPP), a disease of substantial economic importance in sub-Saharan Africa. Failure of vaccination to curtail spread of this disease has led to calls for evaluation of the role of antimicrobials in CBPP control. Three major classes of antimicrobial are effective against mycoplasmas, namely tetracyclines, fluoroquinolones and macrolides. Therefore, the objectives of this study were to determine the effector kinetics of oxytetracycline, danofloxacin and tulathromycin against two *Mmm*SC field strains in artificial medium and adult bovine serum.

Methods: Minimum inhibitory concentrations (MIC) were determined for oxytetracycline, danofloxacin and tulathromycin against *Mmm*SC strains B237 and Tan8 using a macrodilution technique, and time-kill curves were constructed for various multiples of the MIC over a 24 hour period in artificial medium and serum. Data were fitted to sigmoid E_{max} models to obtain 24 hour-area under curve/MIC ratios for mycoplasmastasis and, where appropriate, for mycoplasmacidal activity and virtual mycoplasmal elimination.

Results: Minimum inhibitory concentrations against B237 were 20-fold higher, 2-fold higher and approximately 330-fold lower in serum than in artificial medium for oxytetracycline, danofloxacin and tulathromycin, respectively. Such differences were mirrored in experiments using Tan8. Oxytetracycline was mycoplasmastatic against both strains in both matrices. Danofloxacin elicited mycoplasmacidal activity against B237 and virtual elimination of Tan8; similar maximum antimycoplasmal effects were observed in artificial medium and serum. Tulathromycin effected virtual elimination of B237 but was mycoplasmastatic against Tan8 in artificial medium. However, this drug was mycoplasmastatic against both strains in the more physiologically relevant matrix of serum.

Conclusions: Oxytetracycline, danofloxacin and tulathromycin are all suitable candidates for further investigation as potential treatments for CBPP. This study also highlights the importance of testing drug activity in biological matrices as well as artificial media.

Editor: Bernhard Kaltenboeck, Auburn University, United States of America

Funding: This study was funded by the Biotechnology and Biological Sciences Research Council (grant reference BB/H009450/1, http://www.bbsrc.ac.uk). The funders had no role in study design, data collection and analysis, decision to publish, or preparation of the manuscript.

Competing Interests: The authors have declared that no competing interests exist.

* E-mail: jdmitchell@rvc.ac.uk

Introduction

Mycoplasma mycoides subspecies *mycoides* Small Colony (*Mmm*SC) is the causative agent of Contagious Bovine Pleuropneumonia (CBPP), a major trans-boundary disease of livestock in sub-Saharan Africa [1] and an enduring threat to cattle in Europe. Indeed, CBPP is listed by the World Organisation for Animal Health as one of the diseases that it monitors on a global scale. The disease impacts farmers directly through mortality and poor productivity of their animals, and indirectly through missed opportunities for trade due to import bans and quarantine [1]. Contagious bovine pleuropneumonia manifests as a range of syndromes, from acute pneumonia to a protracted chronic phase, during which apparently recovered animals can harbour and shed the pathogen [2]. *Mmm*SC is spread by aerosol, primarily over only short distances [3], and therefore movement of cattle plays a key role in dissemination of the disease. Since livestock movement patterns in Africa are complex and difficult to control [4], state veterinary services have largely relied upon the use of live attenuated vaccines, in particular the $T_1/44$ strain, to control the disease. However, these are constrained by cold chain dependence, short-lived immunity and adverse events, including inoculation site reactions and occurrence of mild forms of the disease itself [5].

Several reports have suggested that antimicrobial therapy can improve the outcome of infection [6,7,8,9] and recent modelling studies suggest that co-deployment of antimicrobials would substantially enhance the impact of vaccination campaigns [4]. However, the use of antimicrobials in CBPP control has been discouraged largely because of the view that it favours the creation of chronic carriers [2]. Although there is no hard evidence for this, the use of antimicrobials to treat CBPP is not permitted in several countries where the disease is prevalent. Nevertheless, three major classes of antimicrobial are effective against mycoplasmas, namely tetracyclines, fluoroquinolones and macrolides [10]. Indeed, several antimicrobials have emerged on to the market since 1987, some of which show mycoplasmacidal activity *in vitro* [11,12]. The *in vivo* efficacy of such antimicrobials against *Mmm*SC remains to be fully determined, as studies have been few. In naturally affected cattle, treatment with danofloxacin, a fluoroquinolone, significantly reduced transmission of *Mmm*SC to healthy in-contact cattle but failed to improve the clinical outcome [9]. In contrast, long-acting oxytetracycline (OTC) improved clinical condition and, like danofloxacin, also prevented disease transmission to in-contact cattle; however, a bacteriological cure was not achieved in all treated animals [6].

Such partial efficacy may arise from sub-optimal dosage regimens. Increasingly, pharmacokinetic-pharmacodynamic (PK-PD) modelling is employed in veterinary medicine to determine antimicrobial dosages that result in bacteriological eradication, thereby reducing the risk of persistent carrier infections and development of resistance [13]. Indeed, such an approach led to a revision by the manufacturer of the dosage recommended for danofloxacin in the treatment of calf pneumonia [14]. As the first step towards defining dosage strategies for the treatment of CBPP, we investigated the *in vitro* killing profiles of OTC, danofloxacin and tulathromycin (tetracycline, fluoroquinolone and triamilide macrolide, respectively) against the virulent Kenyan *Mmm*SC strain B237 in artificial medium to assess antimicrobial efficacy. Because the composition of artificial medium differs from that of biological matrices, so that minimum inhibitory concentration (MIC) may differ between the two, we extended these studies to adult bovine serum, as a proxy for the 'shallow biophase,' namely plasma, interstitial fluid and well perfused tissues [15], which are the sites of most bacterial infections [16]. To determine whether findings were replicable in another *Mmm*SC strain, antimicrobial killing profiles in artificial medium and adult bovine serum were established for the Tanzanian field strain Tan8 [17]. We present preliminary pharmacodynamic modelling analysis of the data arising from these studies. Our observations are consistent with variation in efficacy between the drugs and illustrate the importance of evaluating drug function in biological matrices as well as artificial medium.

Materials and Methods

Materials

*Mmm*SC strains B237, originally isolated in Kenya [18], and Tan8 were provided by Joachim Frey, University of Bern, Switzerland, and the Animal Health and Veterinary Laboratories Agency, Weybridge, UK, respectively. Oxytetracycline hydrochloride and danofloxacin were obtained from Sigma-Aldrich (VETRANAL^{TM}, Poole, UK), and tulathromycin was supplied by Pfizer Ltd. (Kalamazoo, Michigan, US). Oxytetracycline hydrochloride was dissolved in double distilled water, danofloxacin in 0.01 M sodium hydroxide and tulathromycin in 0.0015 Mcitric acid. Artificial liquid and solid media were obtained from Mycoplasma Experience (Reigate, UK) and adult bovine serum from Sigma-Aldrich (Poole, UK). Liquid medium contained the pH indicator phenol red and was adjusted to pH 7.6 such that the indicator was red in colour.

Determination of MIC

Initially, MIC was determined using a microdilution technique, as described by Hannan [19]. To prepare the inoculum, mycoplasma were subcultured in liquid medium and diluted while in exponential phase to give the desired inoculum size. Briefly, series of doubling dilutions were prepared for each antimicrobial (final concentration ranges of 2×10^{-3} –8 mg/L for OTC and tulathromycin, and 0.03–8 mg/Lfor danofloxacin) in liquid medium. Triplicate 0.1 mL aliquots of each antimicrobial concentration were transferred to wells of a 96-well plate and supplemented with 0.1 mL of *Mmm*SC strain B237 diluted in liquid medium to give a final titre of 10^7 cfu/mL, the intended initial titre for subsequent time-kill studies. Growth controls (*Mmm*SC in absence of antimicrobials), end-point controls (blank medium set at pH 6.8), solvent controls (*Mmm*SC in presence of solvent at the concentration used to dissolve antimicrobials) and sterility controls (blank medium) were also included. After sealing with gas permeable film, plates were incubated at 37°C and assessed visually for any change in indicator colour at least three times daily until that of the growth control matched that of the end-point control. Minimum inhibitory concentration was defined as the lowest concentration of antimicrobial to show no change in the colour of the indicator. Since the error associated with establishing an MIC on doubling dilutions can be up to virtually 100% [20], five sets of overlapping doubling dilutions were used to define the MIC with greater accuracy.

For comparison, MICs were also determined by a macrodilution technique using volumes of 4 mL across the same range of antimicrobial concentrations and with an initial mycoplasmal titre of 10^7 cfu/mL. Cultures were incubated for 24 hours at 37°C and, at 0 and 24 hours, samples were removed and serially diluted tenfold down to 10^{-5}. Aliquots of each dilution were transferred to solid medium and incubated at 37°C in a humidified atmosphere of 5% carbon dioxide in air for at least 4 days. Minimum inhibitory concentration was defined as the lowest concentration of antimicrobial that prevented any increase in mycoplasma cfu/mL over the incubation period. Minimum inhibitory concentrations were also determined at initial inoculum sizes of 10^4, 10^5 and 10^6 cfu/mL to ascertain whether there was any inoculum effect (IE). For MIC determination in serum, five overlapping sets of doubling dilutions of antimicrobial were prepared and inoculated with exponential phase culture, such that the mycoplasmal titre was 10^6 cfu/mL in 2 mL volumes of 99:1 (v/v) serum:artificial medium.

Time-kill studies

Inocula for time-kill studies were prepared as described above. Liquid medium containing various concentrations of antimicrobial, which corresponded to multiples of the MICs given by the macrodilution technique, was inoculated with *Mmm*SC strain B237 to achieve an initial titre of 10^7 cfu/mL in a volume of 4 mL. Cultures were incubated at 37°C for 24 hours and, at 0, 2, 4, 8 and 24 hours, samples were removed and serially diluted down to 10^{-5}. Aliquots (10 μL) of each dilution were transferred to solid medium and incubated at 37°C in a humidified atmosphere of 5% carbon dioxide in air. Colonies were generally counted using the dilution which gave between 30 and 300 colonies per plate and values were converted to cfu/mL. Antimycoplasmal effect, defined as the change in $\log_{10}$ (cfu/mL) over a 24 hour time period, was determined for each concentration of antimicrobial in both matrices on at least two occasions. This was done to ensure reproducibility and data were averaged for subsequent pharmacodynamic analysis. The limit of detection was 2 $\log_{10}$ (cfu/mL) units. Parallel studies were conducted in the absence of antimicrobials and in the presence of solvents at concentrations used to dissolve antimicrobials for control purposes. Time-kill studies in adult bovine serum were performed as for those in artificial medium, except that initial titres of 10^6 cfu/mL in 2 mL volumes of serum were used. Initial inoculum size was smaller than in studies using artificial medium as *Mmm*SC attained a maximum titre of only 10^7 cfu/mL in serum. For comparison, studies to determine MIC (macrodilution technique with a single set of doubling dilutions) and time-kill assays were repeated using *Mmm*SC strain Tan8 in artificial medium and adult bovine serum.

Pharmacodynamic analysis

Twenty-four hour-area under curve (AUC):MIC ratios were calculated for each antimicrobial concentration. Using Phoenix WinNonlin 6.2 professional software (Pharsight Corporation, Mountain View, CA, USA), data were subsequently fitted to a sigmoid E_{max} model given by the equation,

$$E = E_0 + \frac{((E_{max} - E_0)C_e^N)}{(EC_{50}^N + C_e^N)}$$

where E is the antimycoplasmal effect, E_0 is the difference in $\log_{10}$ (cfu/mL) after 24 hours compared to the initial titre when no antimicrobial is present, E_{max} is the maximum antimycoplasmal effect, EC_{50} is the AUC:MIC ratio for an antimicrobial that gives rise to 50% of the maximal response, C_e is the AUC:MIC ratio of the antimicrobial in the effect compartment (i.e. artificial medium or serum) and N is the Hill coefficient, which reflects the slope of the relationship between antimycoplasmal effect and AUC:MIC. From the resulting graph, AUC:MIC ratios were obtained for mycoplasmastatic (E = 0, no change in mycoplasmal count after 24 hours) and mycoplasmacidal (E = −3, 99.9% reduction of original inoculum count after 24 hours) activity of antimicrobials, and for virtual mycoplasmal elimination (E = −4, 99.99% reduction of original inoculum count after 24 hours).

Results

Determination of MIC for antimicrobials against MmmSC strain B237

Minimum inhibitory concentration values obtained for danofloxacin and tulathromycin in artificial medium were comparable using microdilution and macrodilution techniques (figure 1). However, the MIC value obtained for OTC by microdilution was approximately ten-fold lower than that obtained by macrodilution. This suggested that visual inspection for a change in indicator colour was not sufficiently sensitive to detect small increases in mycoplasmal growth. Minimum inhibitory concentrations obtained using the macrodilution technique were therefore used for subsequent studies. These were 0.40, 0.15 and 0.02 mg/L for OTC, danofloxacin and tulathromycin, respectively. Errors arising from the use of a single set of doubling dilutions for establishing MIC values were 25%, 67% and 50% for OTC, danofloxacin and tulathromycin, respectively, highlighting the importance of using overlapping dilution series.

Minimum inhibitory concentrations were also determined at different inoculum sizes to evaluate the effect of this parameter on the MIC value obtained (figure 2). Whereas IEs were observed for tulathromycin and OTC, the largest of which was an 8-fold increase in MIC for OTC when inoculum size increased from 10^5 to 10^7 cfu/mL, no IE was evident for danofloxacin.

Minimum inhibitory concentrations determined in adult bovine serum were 2.0 mg/L, 0.3 mg/L and 0.06 µg/L for OTC, danofloxacin and tulathromycin, respectively. These values were 20-fold higher (OTC), 2-fold higher (danofloxacin) and approximately 330-fold lower (tulathromycin) than those determined in artificial medium at the equivalent inoculum size of 10^6 cfu/mL.

Time-kill curves and pharmacodynamic analysis

Representative graphs of the *in vitro* killing profiles of OTC, danofloxacin and tulathromycin against *Mmm*SC strain B237 in artificial medium and adult bovine serum are presented in figure 3, with sigmoid E_{max} models shown in figure 4. Twenty-four hour-AUC:MIC ratios for ycoplasmastasis and, where appropriate, mycoplasmacidal activity and virtual mycoplasmal elimination are provided in table 1. Oxytetracycline had a mycoplasmastatic action in artificial medium, eliciting a maximum antimycoplasmal effect of only −0.61 $\log_{10}$ (cfu/mL) units (table 1). Danofloxacin was mycoplasmacidal with a maximum antimycoplasmal effect of −3.71 $\log_{10}$ (cfu/mL) units and tulathromycin elicited virtual mycoplasmal elimination with a maximum antimycoplasmal effect of −4.36 of $\log_{10}$ (cfu/mL) units. The presence of solvents at concentrations used to dissolve antimicrobials had no effect on mycoplasmal growth.

As in artificial medium, OTC was mycoplasmastatic and danofloxacin was mycoplasmacidal in adult bovine serum, producing maximum antimycoplasmal effects of −0.25 and

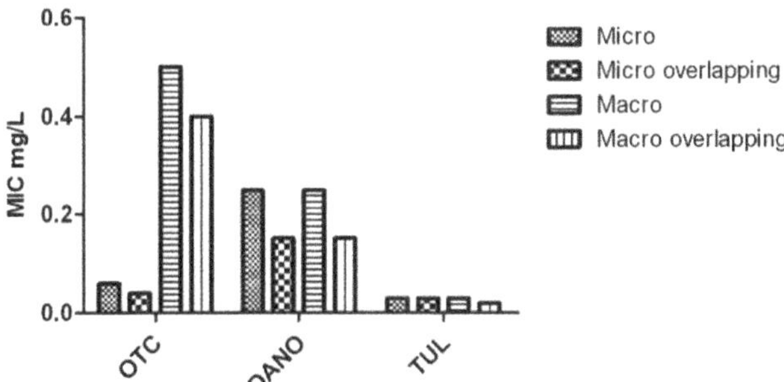

Figure 1. Minimum inhibitory concentrations. Minimum inhibitory concentrations for oxytetracycline (OTC), danofloxacin (DANO) and tulathromycin (TUL) against *Mmm*SC strain B237 in artificial medium using microdilution and macrodilution techniques (inoculum size 10^7 cfu/mL). Values were based on either just one set of doubling dilutions (micro, macro) or five overlapping sets of doubling dilutions (micro overlapping, macro overlapping).

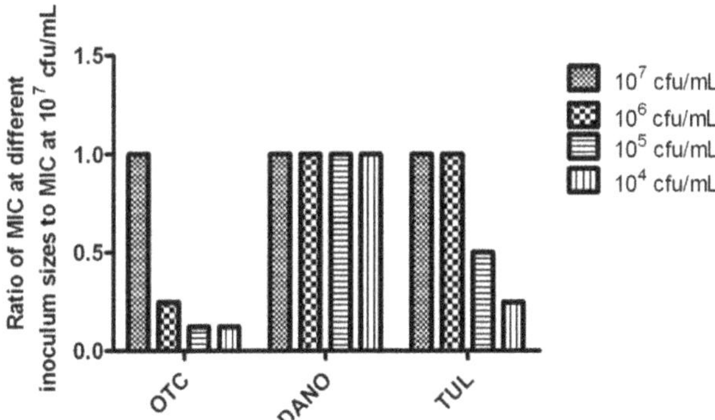

Figure 2. Effect of inoculum size on MIC. Ratio of MIC at different inoculum sizes to MIC at 10^7 cfu/mL for oxytetracycline (OTC), danofloxacin (DANO) and tulathromycin (TUL) against *Mmm*SC strain B237 in artificial medium.

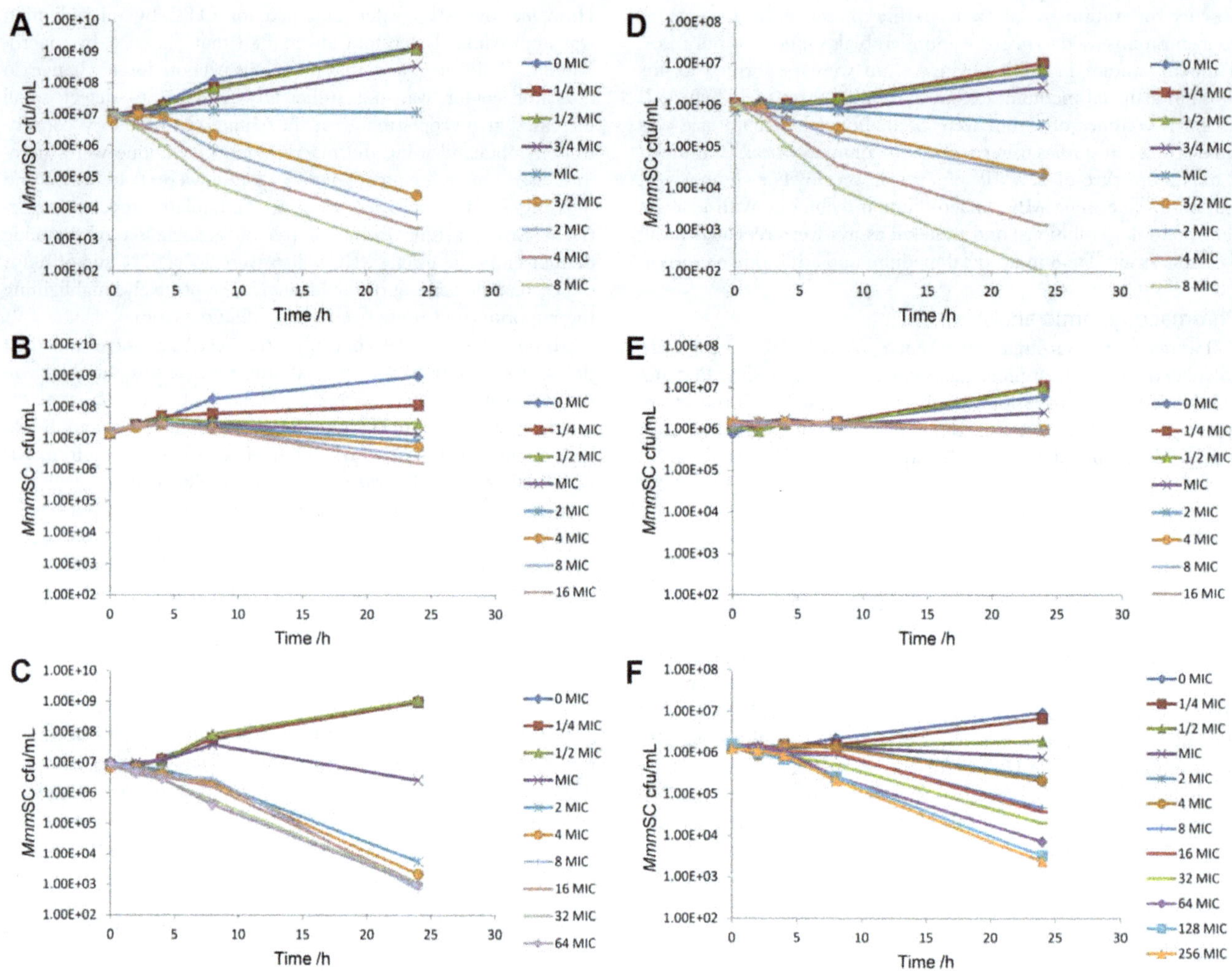

Figure 3. Time-kill curves. Representative time-kill curves for (A) danofloxacin, (B) oxytetracycline and (C) tulathromycin in artificial medium, and (D) danofloxacin, (E) oxytetracycline and (F) tulathromycin in adult bovine serum against *Mmm*SC strain B237.

-3.74 $\log_{10}$ (cfu/mL) units, respectively. However, in marked contrast to artificial medium, tulathromycin was mycoplasmastatic in serum with a maximum antimycoplasmal effect of only -2.63 $\log_{10}$ (cfu/mL) units.

Killing profiles of antimicrobials against MmmSC strain Tan8

Using just one set of doubling dilutions to define MIC, values for danofloxacin, OTC and tulathromycin against *Mmm*SC strain Tan8 were 0.125, 0.25 and 0.016 mg/L in artificial medium, and 0.5, 1 and 3×10^{-5} mg/L in adult bovine serum. Danofloxacin elicited virtual mycoplasmal elimination in both matrices (E_{max}, $\log_{10}$ (cfu/mL) units: -4.08, artificial medium; -4.19, serum), while OTC (E_{max}, $\log_{10}$ (cfu/mL) units: -1.22, artificial medium; -1.09, serum) and tulathromycin (E_{max}, $\log_{10}$ (cfu/mL) units: -2.80, artificial medium; -0.72, serum) were mycoplasmastatic in both.

Discussion

A large swathe of antimicrobials can be ruled out for the treatment of diseases caused by mycoplasmas because they lack a cell wall. Nevertheless, the fluoroquinolones, tetracyclines and macrolides have shown efficacy against these organisms [10], although few studies have specifically addressed the potential of these drugs for the treatment of CBPP. The aim of the present study was to determine the killing kinetics of three antimicrobial agents against the virulent Kenyan B237 strain of *Mmm*SC in both artificial medium and adult bovine serum. This forms part of a longer term goal to use the PK-PD modelling approach outlined by Lees *et al.* [21] to determine optimised dosage strategies for the treatment of this disease. The approach has a major advantage over classical dose titration studies; whereas dose titration is generally focused on clinical outcome and is not informative of bacteriological cure, PK-PD modelling allows optimisation of antimicrobial dose towards a desired bacteriological outcome, reducing the risks of persistent carrier infections and development of resistance. Indeed, dose titration studies are confounded by the 'Pollyanna effect,' whereby the efficacy of a drug giving a good bacteriological response is often underestimated while that of a drug with a poor bacteriological response is over-estimated [15,22].

Danofloxacin, OTC and tulathromycin were selected as representatives of the three classes of antimicrobial known to have efficacy against mycoplasmas. Minimum inhibitory concentrations were initially determined for each drug against *Mmm*SC

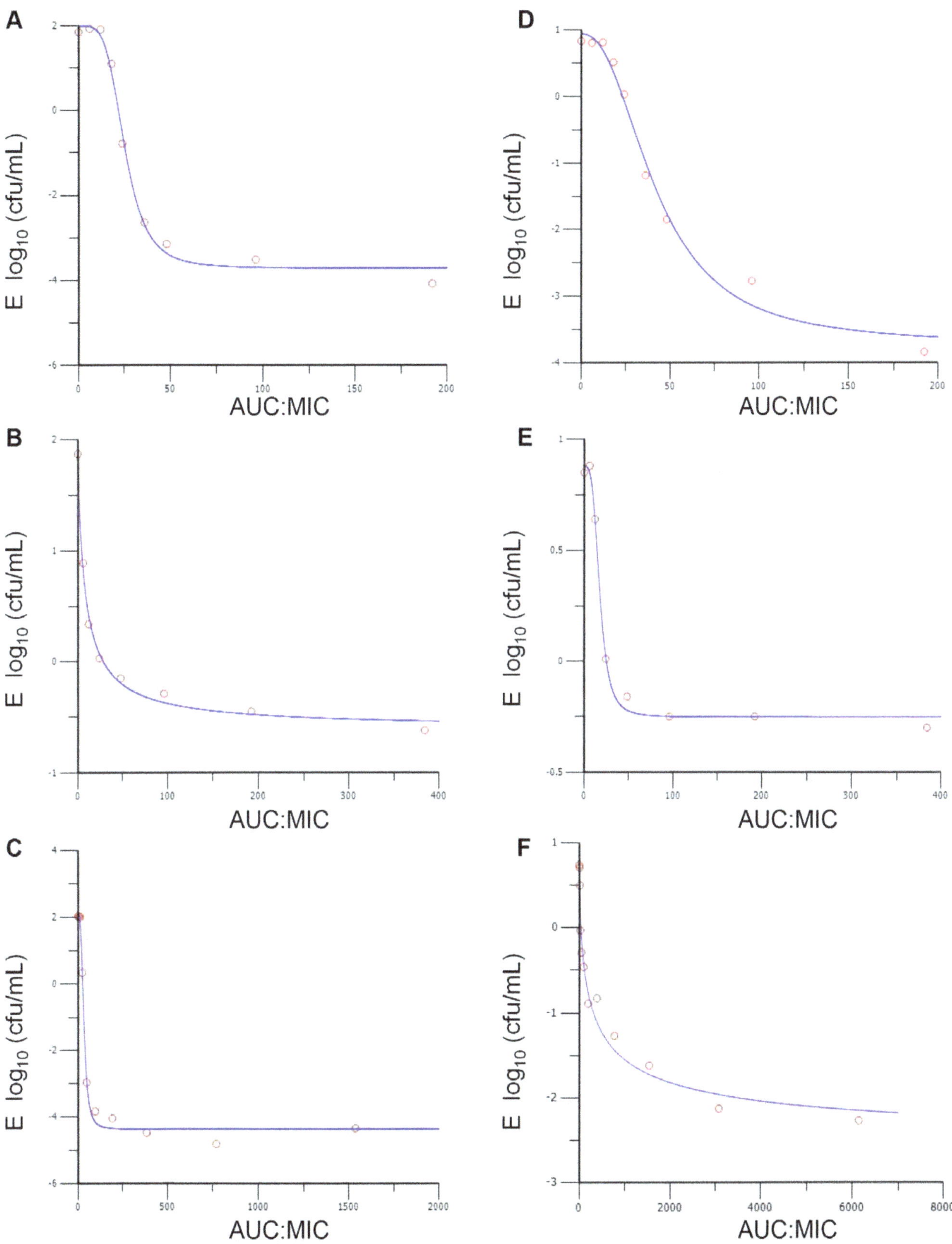

Figure 4. Sigmoid E_{max} models. Sigmoid E_{max} relationships for antimycoplasmal effect (E, log_{10} (cfu/mL)) versus *in vitro* AUC:MIC ratio, derived from data obtained from time-kill curves for (A) danofloxacin (B) oxytetracycline and (C) tulathromycin in artificial medium, and (D) danofloxacin, (E) oxytetracycline and (F) tulathromycin in adult bovine serum against *Mmm*SC strain B237.

Table 1. Pharmacodynamic analysis of data obtained from *in vitro* time-kill studies in artificial medium and adult bovine serum for oxytetracycline (OTC), danofloxacin (DANO) and tulathromycin (TUL) against *Mmm*SC strain B237.

	Artificial Medium			Adult Bovine Serum		
Variable	**DANO**	**OTC**	**TUL**	**DANO**	**OTC**	**TUL**
E_0	2.00	1.88	2.12	0.94	0.88	0.88
E_{max}	−3.71	−0.61	−4.36	−3.74	−0.25	−2.63
MS	21.80	28.36	26.00	23.12	24.80	35.00
MC	39.78	-	50.01	86.63	-	-
VME	-	-	81.01	-	-	-
EC_{50}	25.23	8.29	32.69	42.04	17.41	239.99
N	4.27	0.92	3.11	2.31	3.53	0.57

E_0 is the difference in $\log_{10}$ (cfu/mL) units after 24 hours compared to the initial titre when no antimicrobial is present, E_{max} is the maximum antimycoplasmal effect in $\log_{10}$ (cfu/mL) units, EC_{50} is the twenty-four hour-area under curve:minimum inhibitory concentration ratio (AUC:MIC) of antimicrobial that gives rise to 50% of the maximum response and N is the Hill coefficient. AUC:MIC ratios are provided for mycoplasmastatic activity (MS) and, where appropriate, mycoplasmacidal activity (MC) and virtual mycoplasmal elimination (VME).

strain B237 to define a concentration range over which time-kill assays should be performed. To date, MICs have been published for only OTC and danofloxacin against a number of *Mmm*SC isolates, with MIC ranges of 0.125–4 mg/L and <0.06–0.5 mg/L for OTC and 0.125–1 mg/L and 0.12–0.5 mg/L for danofloxacin in artificial medium [11,12]. Minimum inhibitory concentrations against *Mmm*SC have not been reported for tulathromycin, although Godinho *et al.* [23] reported MICs of <0.004–0.125 mg/L against *Mycoplasma hyopneumoniae* isolates. However, because standardised conditions are lacking for *in vitro* susceptibility testing of veterinary mycoplasmas, the MIC is potentially a crude measure of antimicrobial activity. Indeed, MIC can vary widely between the strains within a species and methodological factors, such as medium composition, inoculum size and reading of the test, can influence the value obtained [24]. Minimum inhibitory concentrations obtained from the present study are therefore not directly comparable with those from previous studies.

Minimum inhibitory concentrations were determined using both microdilution and macrodilution techniques. Whereas the latter is based on post-incubation changes in colony counts relative to the original inoculum, the former relies upon visual assessment of pH indicator colour change to represent mycoplasmal growth. Although these two methods produced comparable MIC values for danofloxacin and tulathromycin, the MIC for OTC was ten-fold lower when the microdilution technique was followed, suggesting that visual observation of a colour change was not sufficiently sensitive to detect small increases in mycoplasmal growth. It is likely that this issue was only encountered for OTC because both danofloxacin and tulathromycin had steeper relationships between AUC:MIC and antimycoplasmal effect, with Hill coefficients of 4.27 and 3.11 for danofloxacin and tulathromycin, respectively, versus 0.92 for OTC.

Inoculum size can also have considerable impact on MIC and the IE, defined as a significant increase in the MIC of an antimicrobial when the number of organisms inoculated is increased [25], has been well documented for some combinations of antimicrobial and mycoplasma species [19]. Although recommendations state that MIC should be determined at a mycoplasma inoculum of 10^3–10^5 cfu/mL [19], MICs were initially established at 10^7 cfu/mL in artificial medium; this was the intended initial titre for time-kill assays, which needed to be sufficiently high to demonstrate maximal antimycoplasmal effects of drugs. In fact, it can be speculated that a larger inoculum size more closely resembles the bacterial density at the site of infection [26]. However, when MICs were determined at smaller inoculum sizes, a significant IE (i.e. ≥8-fold rise in MIC at a higher inoculum compared to a lower inoculum) was observed for OTC, although no effect was evident for danofloxacin. This is consistent with previous observations that inoculum size has a less dramatic effect on MIC for fluoroquinolones than for than for other antimicrobial classes [27,28]. Nonetheless, a large body of evidence suggests that the occurrence and magnitude of an IE depend on the combination of pathogen and antimicrobial under scrutiny [25]. Inoculum size may also influence bactericidal activity. For example, Morrissey and George [29] showed that as inoculum size of *Streptococcus pneumoniae* was increased, bactericidal activity of fluoroquinolones declined to the extent that they were only bacteriostatic at 10^{13} cfu/L. The clinical relevance of IE is controversial. While Craig *et al.* [30] refute that *in vitro* inoculum effects have a bearing on *in vivo* antimicrobial efficacy, at least for β-lactams, Soriano *et al.* [31] found that higher serum concentrations relative to the MIC were required to reduce mortality of rats infected with *Escherichia coli* for drugs with a pronounced IE when compared to those with little or no IE. Furthermore, higher effective doses of fluoroquinolones and, to a greater extent, carbapenems were observed in mice infected with large inocula of either *Staphylococcus aureus* or *Pseudomonas aeruginosa* compared to those infected with smaller inocula [32]. Finally, an IE may result in over-estimation of the dosage by PK-PD modelling approaches, particularly if the *in vivo* inoculum size is smaller than that used in *in vitro* studies [33].

Minimum inhibitory concentrations were also affected by matrix composition, as highlighted by the differences observed in artificial medium and bovine serum. Minimum inhibitory concentrations for danofloxacin and OTC were respectively two-fold and 20-fold greater in serum than artificial medium at an inoculum size of 10^6 cfu/mL. Since only the free fraction of drugs is active in plasma and total protein concentration in serum was higher than in artificial medium (data not shown), the higher MICs in serum may be explained, at least in part, by protein binding. In this regard, danofloxacin and OTC exhibit plasma protein binding of 49% [34] and 71.7% [35], respectively. In addition, the calcium ion concentration was higher in serum than in artificial medium and it can be speculated that this resulted in increased chelation of OTC in serum [36]. In marked contrast to danofloxacin and OTC, the MIC of tulathromycin was approximately 330-fold lower in serum. Such a low MIC (0.06 μg/L) is not unprecedented; Devine and Hagerman [37] reported an MIC of 0.1 μg/L for coumermycin A_1 against *Neisseria meningitidis*. The potency of the weak base tulathromycin in acidic conditions is expected to be lower due to ionisation and the consequent inability to penetrate cell membranes. It has been shown previously that acidification of culture medium with carbon dioxide resulted in higher MICs for tulathromycin against *Actinobacillus pleuropneumoniae* and *Haemophilus somnus*, while the presence of serum reduced the MICs [38]. It was noted that the pH of adult bovine serum and also fresh sterile-filtered calf serum was higher than that of artificial medium (approximately pH 8 versus pH 7.6). The MIC of tulathromycin against *Mmm*SC in artificial medium set at pH 8 was 0.008 mg/L at a 10^6 cfu/mL inoculum size, i.e. 2.5-fold lower than at pH 7.6 (data not shown). Such a pH difference may therefore contribute, at least in part, to the MIC difference observed between artificial medium and adult bovine serum. In addition, it is plausible that acidification arising from the release of carbon dioxide from *Mmm*SC resulted in reduced drug potency in artificial medium. Under these circumstances, lower MIC values observed in serum would arise from its natural buffering capacity. However, despite this apparent enhanced potency and the smaller inoculum size used for time-kill assays, tulathromycin was only mycoplasmastatic in this matrix, whereas it elicited virtual mycoplasmal eradication in artificial medium. This conflicts with previous reports of serum enhancement of the antibacterial effect of tulathromycin against *H. somnus* and a shortening of the time to exert bactericidal effects against *A. pleuropneumoniae* [38]. However, we have observed that tulathromycin elicits only mycoplasmastatic effects against lag phase *Mmm*SC in artificial medium (data not shown). The observed discrepancy between serum and artificial medium may therefore relate to the longer lag phase that occurs in serum after mycoplasma culture is diluted to obtain the desired inoculum size for time-kill assays.

Although the aim of the current study was to provide antimicrobial dosage protocols specifically for cattle infected with *Mmm*SC strain B237, MIC and time-kill assays were repeated using the Tanzanian field strain Tan8 to determine whether the effects observed were replicable in a different strain. The MIC values (based on one set of doubling dilutions) against B237 and Tan8 were comparable, being at most only two-fold lower against Tan8. In addition, the differences between MIC values obtained in artificial medium and serum against Tan8 mirrored those observed against B237. Regarding antimicrobial activity, OTC behaved similarly against B237 and Tan8, as did danofloxacin, with differences of less than 1 $\log_{10}$ (cfu/mL) unit between E_{max} values against each strain. However, whereas tulathromycin effected virtual elimination of B237 in artificial medium, it was only mycoplasmastatic against Tan8. Despite this, in the physiologically more relevant matrix of serum, this drug was mycoplasmastatic against both strains.

Pharmacodynamic analysis allows estimations of dosages that would be required *in vivo* for either mycoplasmastatic or mycoplasmacidal activity using the formula,

$$DO = \frac{CL \times \frac{AUC}{MIC} \times MIC_{90}}{F \times f_u \times 24h}$$

where DO is the optimal dose (mg/kg/day), CL is the body clearance (L/kg/day), AUC/MIC is the breakpoint surrogate marker for the required effect (h), MIC_{90} is the MIC for 90% of strains of a species (mg/L), F is the bioavailability (from 0 to 1) and f_u is the free drug fraction (from 0 to 1). This formula can be simplified if time-kill assays are performed in serum as no correction is necessary for protein binding and, in the case of the present study, since we are aiming to provide dosage regimens for cattle infected with the virulent strain B237, MIC_{90} can be replaced by the strain-specific MIC. If the drug can be administered by intravenous (i.v.) route, F can also be excluded [20]. This gives

$$DO = CL \times \frac{AUC}{MIC} \times MIC$$

where clearance is expressed as L/kg/h.

Using the AUC:MIC ratios generated in serum and previously published data for body clearance and bioavailability, dosages for mycoplasmastasis can be calculated for OTC and tulathromycin, and a mycoplasmacidal dosage can be estimated for danofloxacin. A meta-analysis of PK data for long-acting OTC gave a clearance of 0.115 L/kg/h [39] and bioavailability has been recorded at 78.5% via the intramuscular route in male cattle [40]. Together with an AUC:MIC ratio of 24.80 and MIC of 2 mg/L in serum, a predicted dosage of 7.3 mg/kg/day is obtained for mycoplasmastasis of strain B237. Based on an AUC:MIC ratio of 26.40 and MIC of 1 mg/L in serum, a lower dosage of 3.9 mg/kg/day is obtained for mycoplasmastasis of strain Tan8. Both are below the licensed dose of 20 mg/kg. It is believed that OTC is one of the most widely used drugs to treat CBPP in Africa [12]. However, information regarding current dosing practice is not available.

The clearance of tulathromycin in beef calves was 0.181 L/kg/h and the bioavailability was 91.3% by the subcutaneous (s.c.) route [41]. Given an AUC:MIC ratio of 35.00 and an MIC of 0.06 μg/L, a dosage of at least 0.4 μg/kg/day is estimated to achieve mycoplasmastasis of strain B237. To obtain the same effect against Tan8, a dosage of 0.15 μg/kg/day is predicted to be required (AUC:MIC ratio, 24.88; MIC, 3×10^{-5} mg/L). Again both are far below the licensed dosage of 2.5 mg/kg. Furthermore, the *in vivo* distribution of this drug is particularly advantageous; lung concentrations have been measured at 11–325 times higher than those concurrently in serum and the half-time for elimination from lung was 184 hours, giving rise to a potentially prolonged exposure of respiratory pathogens to tulathromycin [41]. However, a disadvantage of using this drug to treat CBPP at its current licensed dosage is the contra-indication of treating cattle whose milk is intended for human consumption. However, it may be possible to revise the datasheet for this drug if the lower dosage suggested by the current study can be adopted.

For danofloxacin, bioavailability was 94% if administered via the s.c. route and plasma clearance was 0.468 L/kg/h in cross-bred calves [42]. Given an AUC:MIC ratio of 86.63 for mycoplasmacidal activity and an MIC of 0.30 mg/L, the optimal dosage would be 12.9 mg/kg/day to treat cattle infected with strain B237. A similar dosage of 14.7 mg/kg/day is predicted to elicit mycoplasmacidal activity against strain Tan8 (AUC:MIC ratio, 59.19; MIC, 0.5 mg/L). Furthermore, a dosage of 44.4 mg/kg/day is estimated for virtual elimination of strain Tan8 (AUC:MIC ratio, 178.34; MIC, 0.5 mg/L) but this is over seven-fold greater than the licensed dosage (6 mg/kg, single injection, s.c. or i.v.) and side-effects may be encountered. At the licensed dosage, only mycoplasmastasis would occur. This may explain the lack of effect of 2.5 mg/kgdanofloxacin on the clinical score of CBPP-affected cattle reported by Huebschle *et al* [9]. However, it is important to remember that the PK-PD modelling approach does not take into account the immune response of the animal. This may act additively or synergistically with the antimicrobial agent, and the predicted dosage may therefore be an over-estimate. In addition, a limitation of the dosage prediction stems from the fact that previously published PK data are derived from studies on calves, albeit ruminating in the majority of cases. Although most changes in PK seem to occur between newborn pre-ruminant and ruminating stages [43,44], it is possible that age-related PK changes exist between calves and adult cattle, as observed in the human population [45]. Furthermore, PK parameters may be influenced by gender [46], physiological status [47], breed of cattle [48], or indeed the species (i.e. *Bos taurus* versus *Bos indicus*).

The results of this study show efficacy for danofloxacin, OTC and tulathromycin against virulent *Mmm*SC strain B237 *in vitro*, providing evidence that all three may be suitable candidates for the treatment of CBPP caused by this strain. Similar observations were made for strain Tan8, suggesting the findings of this study may apply across the species. Although dosages can be estimated from fixed concentration pharmacodynamic models, these do not account for the decline in concentration as drug is cleared from the body. The next stage will be to develop *in vitro* dynamic concentration models [49] to simulate *in vivo* antimicrobial PK, enabling not only determination of post-antibiotic-sub-MIC inhibitory effects of antimicrobials but also assessment of concentration and/or time dependence of antimicrobial activity through administration of drug by bolus and infusion. Finally, this study highlights the importance of susceptibility testing in biological fluids in addition to artificial media, as demonstrated by marked differences in MICs between the two matrices.

Acknowledgments

We thank Joachim Frey at the University of Bern for supplying *Mmm*SC strain B237, the Mycoplasma Group at the Animal Health and Veterinary Laboratories Agency for providing *Mmm*SC strain Tan8 and Pfizer Ltd. for donating tulathromycin.

Author Contributions

Conceived and designed the experiments: JDM QAM DJM. Performed the experiments: JDM. Analyzed the data: JDM QAM DJM. Wrote the paper: JDM QAM DJM.

References

1. Thomson GR (2005) Contagious bovine pleuropneumonia and poverty: A strategy for addressing the effects of the disease in sub-Saharan Africa. Research report, DFID Animal Health Programme, Centre for Tropical Veterinary Medicine, University of Edinburgh, UK.
2. Provost A, Perreau P, Breard A, le Goff C, Martel JL, et al. (1987) Contagious bovine pleuropneumonia. Rev Sci Tech Oie 6: 625–679.
3. Regalla J, Caporale V, Giovannini A, Santini F, Martel JL, et al. (1996) Manifestation and epidemiology of contagious bovine pleuropneumonia in Europe. Rev Sci Tech 15: 1309–1329.
4. Mariner JC, McDermott J, Heesterbeek JA, Thomson G, Roeder PL, et al. (2006) A heterogeneous population model for contagious bovine pleuropneumonia transmission and control in pastoral communities of East Africa. Prev Vet Med 73: 75–91.
5. Rweyemamu MM, Litamoi J, Palya V, Sylla D (1995) Contagious bovine pleuropneumonia vaccines: the need for improvements. Rev Sci Tech Oie 14: 593–601.
6. Niang M, Sery A, Cisse O, Diallo M, Doucoure M, et al. (2006) Effect of antibiotic therapy on the pathogenesis of CBPP. CBPP control: antibiotics to the rescue? FAO-OIE-AU/IBAR-IAEA Consultative Group Meeting on CBPP in Africa 6–8 November 2006. Rome. pp. 25–32.
7. Niang M, Sery A, Doucoure M, Kone M, N'Diaye M, et al. (2010) Experimental studies on the effect of long-acting oxytetracycline treatment in the development of sequestra in contagious bovine pleuropneumonia-infected cattle. J Vet Med Anim Health 2: 35–45.
8. Yaya A, Wesonga H, Thiaucourt F (2004) Use of long-acting tetracycline for CBPP: preliminary results. FAO-OIE-AU/IBAR-IAEA Consultative Group on Contagious Bovine Pleuropneumonia Third Meeting.
9. Huebschle OJ, Ayling RD, Godinho K, Lukhele O, Tjipura-Zaire G, et al. (2006) Danofloxacin (Advocin) reduces the spread of contagious bovine pleuropneumonia to healthy in-contact cattle. Res Vet Sci 81: 304–309.
10. Cooper AC, Fuller JR, Fuller MK, Whittlestone P, Wise DR (1993) In vitro activity of danofloxacin, tylosin and oxytetracycline against mycoplasmas of veterinary importance. Res Vet Sci 54: 329–334.
11. Ayling RD, Baker SE, Nicholas RA, Peek ML, Simon AJ (2000) Comparison of in vitro activity of danofloxacin, florfenicol, oxytetracycline, spectinomycin and tilmicosin against Mycoplasma mycoides subspecies mycoides small colony type. Vet Rec 146: 243–246.
12. Ayling RD, Bisgaard-Frantzen S, March JB, Godinho K, Nicholas RA (2005) Assessing the in vitro effectiveness of antimicrobials against Mycoplasma mycoides subsp. mycoides small-colony type to reduce contagious bovine pleuropneumonia infection. Antimicrob Agents Chemother 49: 5162–5165.
13. McKellar QA, Sanchez Bruni SF, Jones DG (2004) Pharmacokinetic/pharmacodynamic relationships of antimicrobial drugs used in veterinary medicine. J Vet Pharmacol Ther 27: 503–514.
14. Sarasola P, Lees P, AliAbadi FS, McKellar QA, Donachie W, et al. (2002) Pharmacokinetic and pharmacodynamic profiles of danofloxacin administered by two dosing regimens in calves infected with Mannheimia (Pasteurella) haemolytica. Antimicrob Agents Chemother 46: 3013–3019.
15. Toutain PL, del Castillo JR, Bousquet-Melou A (2002) The pharmacokinetic-pharmacodynamic approach to a rational dosage regimen for antibiotics. Res Vet Sci 73: 105–114.
16. Shojaee Aliabadi F, Lees P (2003) Pharmacokinetic-pharmacodynamic integration of danofloxacin in the calf. Res Vet Sci 74: 247–259.
17. March JB, Clark J, Brodlie M (2000) Characterization of strains of Mycoplasma mycoides subsp. mycoides small colony type isolated from recent outbreaks of contagious bovine pleuropneumonia in Botswana and Tanzania: evidence for a new biotype. J Clin Microbiol 38: 1419–1425.
18. Jores J, Nkando I, Sterner-Kock A, Haider W, Poole J, et al. (2008) Assessment of in vitro interferon-gamma responses from peripheral blood mononuclear cells of cattle infected with Mycoplasma mycoides ssp. mycoides small colony type. Vet Immunol Immunopathol 124: 192–197.
19. Hannan PC (2000) Guidelines and recommendations for antimicrobial minimum inhibitory concentration (MIC) testing against veterinary mycoplasma species. International Research Programme on Comparative Mycoplasmology. Vet Res 31: 373–395.
20. Lees P, Concordet D, AliAbadi FS, Toutain PL (2006) Drug selection and optimization of dosage schedules to minimize antimicrobial resistance. In: Aarestrup FM, editor. Antimicrobial Resistance in Bacteria of Animal Origin. 1 ed. Washington DC: ASM Press. pp. 49—71.
21. Lees P, AliAbadi FS, Toutain PL (2004) PK-PD modelling: an alternative to dose titration studies for antimicrobial drug dosage selection. Journal of Regulatory Affairs 15: 175–180.
22. Marchant CD, Carlin SA, Johnson CE, Shurin PA (1992) Measuring the comparative efficacy of antibacterial agents for acute otitis media: the "Pollyanna phenomenon". J Pediatr 120: 72–77.
23. Godinho KS (2008) Susceptibility testing of tulathromycin: interpretative breakpoints and susceptibility of field isolates. Vet Microbiol 129: 426–432.
24. Frimodt-Moller N (2002) How predictive is PK/PD for antibacterial agents? Int J Antimicrob Agents 19: 333–339.
25. Brook I (1989) Inoculum effect. Rev Infect Dis 11: 361–368.
26. Levison ME (2004) Pharmacodynamics of antimicrobial drugs. Infect Dis Clin North Am 18: 451–465, vii.
27. Firsov AA, Vostrov SN, Kononenko OV, Zinner SH, Portnoy YA (1999) Prediction of the effects of inoculum size on the antimicrobial action of trovafloxacin and ciprofloxacin against Staphylococcus aureus and Escherichia coli in an in vitro dynamic model. Antimicrob Agents Chemother 43: 498–502.
28. Konig C, Simmen HP, Blaser J (1998) Bacterial concentrations in pus and infected peritoneal fluid–implications for bactericidal activity of antibiotics. J Antimicrob Chemother 42: 227–232.
29. Morrissey I, George JT (1999) The effect of the inoculum size on bactericidal activity. J Antimicrob Chemother 43: 423–425.
30. Craig WA, Bhavnani SM, Ambrose PG (2004) The inoculum effect: fact or artifact? Diagn Microbiol Infect Dis 50: 229–230.
31. Soriano F, Ponte C, Santamaria M, Jimenez-Arriero M (1990) Relevance of the inoculum effect of antibiotics in the outcome of experimental infections caused by Escherichia coli. J Antimicrob Chemother 25: 621–627.
32. Mizunaga S, Kamiyama T, Fukuda Y, Takahata M, Mitsuyama J (2005) Influence of inoculum size of Staphylococcus aureus and Pseudomonas aeruginosa on in vitro activities and in vivo efficacy of fluoroquinolones and carbapenems. J Antimicrob Chemother 56: 91–96.
33. Martinez M, Toutain PL, Walker RD (2006) The Pharmacokinetic-Pharmacodynamic (PK/PD) Relationship of Antimicrobial Agents. In: Giguere S, Prescott JF, Baggot JD, Walker RD, Dowling PM, editors. Antimicrobial Therapy in Veterinary Medicine. 4 ed. Iowa: Blackwell Publishing. pp. 81—106.
34. Friis C (1993) Penetration of danofloxacin into the respiratory tract tissues and secretions in calves. Am J Vet Res 54: 1122–1127.
35. Nouws JF, Breukink HJ, Binkhorst GJ, Lohuis J, van Lith P, et al. (1985) Comparative pharmacokinetics and bioavailability of eight parenteral oxytetracycline-10% formulations in dairy cows. Vet Q 7: 306–314.
36. Martin SR (1979) Equilibrium and kinetic studies on the interaction of tetracyclines with calcium and magnesium. Biophys Chem 10: 319–326.
37. Devine LF, Hagerman CR (1970) Spectra of susceptibility of Neisseria meningitidis to antimicrobial agents in vitro. Appl Microbiol 19: 329–334.
38. Evans NA (2005) Tulathromycin: an overview of a new triamilide antibiotic for livestock respiratory disease. Vet Ther 6: 83–95.
39. Craigmill AL, Miller GR, Gehring R, Pierce AN, Riviere JE (2004) Meta-analysis of pharmacokinetic data of veterinary drugs using the Food Animal Residue Avoidance Databank: oxytetracycline and procaine penicillin G. J Vet Pharmacol Ther 27: 343–353.
40. Davey LA, Ferber MT, Kaye B (1985) Comparison of the serum pharmacokinetics of a long acting and a conventional oxytetracycline injection. Vet Rec 117: 426–429.
41. Nowakowski MA, Inskeep PB, Risk JE, Skogerboe TL, Benchaoui HA, et al. (2004) Pharmacokinetics and lung tissue concentrations of tulathromycin, a new triamilide antibiotic, in cattle. Vet Ther 5: 60–74.

42. Giles CJ, Magonigle RA, Grimshaw WT, Tanner AC, Risk JE, et al. (1991) Clinical pharmacokinetics of parenterally administered danofloxacin in cattle. J Vet Pharmacol Ther 14: 400–410.
43. Burrows GE, Barto PB, Martin B (1987) Comparative pharmacokinetics of gentamicin, neomycin and oxytetracycline in newborn calves. J Vet Pharmacol Ther 10: 54–63.
44. Guard CL, Schwark WS, Friedman DS, Blackshear P, Haluska M (1986) Age-related alterations in trimethoprim-sulfadiazine disposition following oral or parenteral administration in calves. Can J Vet Res 50: 342–346.
45. Mangoni AA, Jackson SH (2004) Age-related changes in pharmacokinetics and pharmacodynamics: basic principles and practical applications. Br J Clin Pharmacol 57: 6–14.
46. Witkamp RF, Yun HI, van't Klooster GA, van Mosel JF, van Mosel M, et al. (1992) Comparative aspects and sex differentiation of plasma sulfamethazine elimination and metabolite formation in rats, rabbits, dwarf goats, and cattle. Am J Vet Res 53: 1830–1835.
47. Bengtsson B, Jacobsson SO, Luthman J, Franklin A (1997) Pharmacokinetics of penicillin-G in ewes and cows in late pregnancy and in early lactation. J Vet Pharmacol Ther 20: 258–261.
48. Sallovitz J, Lifschitz A, Imperiale F, Pis A, Virkel G, et al. (2002) Breed differences on the plasma availability of moxidectin administered pour-on to calves. Vet J 164: 47–53.
49. Gloede J, Scheerans C, Derendorf H, Kloft C (2010) In vitro pharmacodynamic models to determine the effect of antibacterial drugs. J Antimicrob Chemother 65: 186–201.

Movements and Habitat Use of an Endangered Snake, *Hoplocephalus bungaroides* (Elapidae): Implications for Conservation

Benjamin M. Croak[1]*, Mathew S. Crowther[1], Jonathan K. Webb[2], Richard Shine[1]

1 School of Biological Sciences A08, University of Sydney, Camperdown, New South Wales, Australia, **2** School of the Environment, University of Technology Sydney, Broadway, New South Wales, Australia

Abstract

A detailed understanding of how extensively animals move through the landscape, and the habitat features upon which they rely, can identify conservation priorities and thus inform management planning. For many endangered species, information on habitat use either is sparse, or is based upon studies from a small part of the species' range. The broad-headed snake (*Hoplocephalus bungaroides*) is restricted to a specialized habitat (sandstone outcrops and nearby forests) within a small geographic range in south-eastern Australia. Previous research on this endangered taxon was done at a single site in the extreme south of the species' geographic range. We captured and radio-tracked 9 adult broad-headed snakes at sites in the northern part of the species' distribution, to evaluate the generality of results from prior studies, and to identify critical habitat components for this northern population. Snakes spent most of winter beneath sun-warmed rocks then shifted to tree hollows in summer. Thermal regimes within retreat-sites support the hypothesis that this shift is thermally driven. Intervals between successive displacements were longer than in the southern snakes but dispersal distances per move and home ranges were similar. Our snakes showed non-random preferences both in terms of macrohabitat (e.g., avoidance of some vegetation types) and microhabitat (e.g., frequent use of hollow-bearing trees). Despite many consistencies, the ecology of this species differs enough between southern and northern extremes of its range that managers need to incorporate information on local features to most effectively conserve this threatened reptile.

Editor: Ulrich Joger, State Natural History Museum, Germany

Funding: Australian research council Linkage grant: number LP0776647 awarded to professor Richard Shine. Linkage Contributors: NSW National parks and wildlife: http://www.nationalparks.nsw.gov.au/; Forests NSW: http://www.forests.nsw.gov.au/; The Hawkesbury/Nepean catchment authority: http://www.hn.cma.nsw.gov.au/; Zoos Victoria: http://www.zoo.org.au/; The Australian Reptile Park: http://www.reptilepark.com.au/. The funders had no role in study design, data collection and analysis, decision to publish, or preparation of the manuscript.

Competing Interests: The authors have read the journal's policy and have the following conflicts. Australian Reptile Park provided funding for this study.

* E-mail: bencroak@gmail.com

Introduction

Human-induced fragmentation of landscapes and habitats can lead to a reduction in biodiversity [1,2]. Although species that are able to exploit a variety of habitats may be relatively insensitive to habitat disturbance [3], species that have evolved behaviors or physical traits that facilitate reliance on specialized habitat use may find altered habitats difficult or impossible to occupy [3–5]. For such species, disturbance of critical habitat can lead to endangerment or extinction [3]. Life history traits also influence a species' ability to tolerate degradation of preferred habitat type; for example, taxa with small population sizes and low rates of reproduction and dispersal may be at particular risk [6,7].

To conserve highly specialized animals, we need detailed information on habitat use, dispersal and movement patterns [8]. Unfortunately, such data often are laborious to collect, especially for endangered species – both because they are rare, and because research methods must not inflict additional stress [9]. As a result, our knowledge on many endangered taxa is based on studies that have been performed at only a single site (where researchers can most easily obtain and study animals: [10,11]). Often, such sites are atypical of conditions that pertain over most of the species' range [10,11]. Indeed, a disproportionate reliance on studies on a small and unrepresentative series of populations is a general problem in ecological research: much of what we know about even widely-distributed lineages is based upon multiple studies on a small number of populations (e.g., gartersnakes in Manitoba: [12]). This is especially worrying for endangered-species research, because logistics may make studies elsewhere almost impossible.

One such species is the broad-headed snake (*Hoplocephalus bungaroides*), an elapid species that has drastically declined since European settlement of Australia [13–16]. Broad-headed snakes rely on specific habitat attributes; they shelter beneath thin, sun-exposed exfoliated rocks on sandstone rock outcrops with western or north-western aspects [17]. These retreat sites allow snakes to thermoregulate during winter and spring. *Hoplocephalus bungaroides* also exhibit other life history traits that render them vulnerable to disturbance e.g., dependence on high rates of adult survival, infrequent breeding (every 3 to 4 years), low fecundity (3 to 4 offspring per litter), late maturity (up to 6 years), low rates of dispersal and a small geographic range. All of these traits contribute to the endangered status of *H. bungaroides* [18]. Also, the habitat of *H. bungaroides* has become fragmented, and subject to vegetation overgrowth [19–21] and removal of shelter-sites (exfoliated rock) for landscaping and gardening [15,22–24].

To date, most research on *H. bungaroides* has been conducted on a single population in the extreme south of the species' range [17,18,23–25]. Genetic data show that this intensively-studied population belongs to a genetically distinct clade, with another isolated, evolutionarily significant unit identified in the north of the species range. Those two clades diverged approximately 800 000 years ago [26]. Vegetation, temperatures and potential prey species differ between the northern and southern parts of the species' range [27]. In the current paper, we describe habitat use and movements of snakes from the previously unstudied northern clade.

Materials and Methods

Ethics Statement

The University of Sydney Animal Care and Ethics Committee specifically approved this study and provided permits specifically for this project (L04/12-2008/3/4927). All work with live animals followed the approved ethical protocols. Snakes were collected by hand, and returned to the laboratory in clean cloth bags (individually) in insulated containers. They were maintained in individual enclosures with access to heating, shelter and food (see below). All surgical procedures were performed by trained veterinary surgeons, and snakes were carefully monitored post-operatively prior to release into the field at their original capture site. Prior to surgery snakes were administered morphine to relieve pain. No snakes were killed during the study, and all were alert and active when released at the conclusion of the work.

Study Species

Hoplocephalus bungaroides are medium sized (to 90 cm: [27]), brightly colored ambush predators [28]. During winter the snakes live in thermally suitable crevices that form between thin, exfoliated rock and parent bedrock that is exposed to afternoon sun [17]. During the warmer parts of the year, these exposed rock exfoliations become too hot and snakes move into tree hollows in adjacent woodlands [21]. This habitat specificity means that *H. bungaroides* are restricted to areas that provide access both to sun exposed rock-on-rock exfoliations, and to suitable areas of surrounding forest [17,21].

Study Sites

Yengo and Wollemi National Parks are 100 km north-west of Sydney. We radio-tracked snakes at one study site inside Wollemi National Park (NP), and at two study sites inside Yengo NP. All sites were approximately 2 km apart, and consisted of exposed Hawkesbury sandstone outcrops surrounded by open eucalypt woodland dominated by Sydney peppermint (*Eucalyptus urceolaris*), narrow-leafed stringy-bark (*Eucalyptus sparsifolia*), yellow bloodwood (*Corymbia eximia*), red bloodwood (*Corymbia gummifera*), grey gum (*Eucalyptus punctata*), and scribbly gum (*Eucalyptus haemastoma*).

Capturing Snakes

To track *H. bungaroides* in the spring/summer period of 2010/2011 and 2011/2012 we captured nine snakes during late winter of 2010 and 2011. Snakes are accessible at this time of year because they shelter beneath thin rock exfoliations that are easily lifted and replaced. We captured seven snakes in Wollemi NP and two snakes in Yengo NP. We tracked two of the snakes caught in Wollemi NP and the two snakes caught in Yengo NP over the spring/summer of 2010/2011 (20/10/2010 to 07/02/2011). We tracked one of the snakes from Yengo NP, one of the snakes from Wollemi NP and an additional snake captured in Wollemi NP during the winter of 2011 from 10/05/2011 to 11/08/2011. We tracked the remaining four snakes in Wollemi NP over the spring/summer of 2011/2012 (16/11/2011 to 16/01/2012: see Table 1). We captured all snakes by hand and placed them in cotton bags for transportation to the laboratory. We housed snakes individually in plastic containers (31×22 cm, 10 cm high, containing a shelter and water dish) in a 12:12 light:dark regime and constant temperature of 19°C. We placed a heat mat under one end of the enclosure to allow snakes to thermoregulate. We fed the snakes fortnightly on frozen-then-thawed laboratory mice. We transported snakes to an approved veterinarian as per animal ethics protocol L04/12-2008/3/4927 for surgical implantation of transmitters (BD-2T, Holohil Systems, Carp, Ontario, Canada). We recaptured snakes prior to signal failure so that we could surgically remove the transmitters.

Surgical Methods

All surgeries were carried out by a qualified veterinarian. Each snake was examined and weighed, then pre-medicated with morphine 1 mg. kg^{-1} intramuscularly 10 min prior to induction. Snakes were induced with alfaxan 10 mg. kg^{-1} (intramuscular, or injected into the tail vein). Once the snake was anesthetized, a mask made from a 10 ml syringe was placed over the snake's head (held in place with transpore tape) to provide a mixture of isoflourane and oxygen for anesthesia. Transmitters were cold-sterilized in a solution of F10 and water, and scales/skin were prepared using chlorhexidine scrub followed by an iodine spray. The transmitter aerial was trimmed to fit within the snake's body.

A scalpel was used to make a small incision 20 mm above the vent, and then alligator forceps were used to blunt-dissect against the body wall up to a point two-thirds of the way up the snake's body. A second incision was made over the tip of the alligator forceps and the transmitter antenna was grasped with the forceps and pulled through the coelom such that the aerial sat flat within

Table 1. Home ranges of radio-tracked broad-headed snakes, *Hoplocephalus bungaroides*, at sites in the extreme north of the species' range.

ID	Site	Sex	SVL (mm)	Mass (g)	Season	Home Range (ha)
Snake 1	Y	M	550	50.5	S10/11	9.43
Snake 3	Y	F	565	52.0	S10/11	6.36
Snake 4	W	F	565	51.5	S10/11	9.89
Snake 5	W	F	670	62.0	S10/11	1.39
Snake 3	W	F	565	52.0	W 11	0.09
Snake 5	W	F	670	62.0	W 11	0.83
Snake 7	W	M	555	51.0	W 11	0.57
Snake 6	W	F	672	63.5	S11/12	1.22
Snake 9	W	F	554	50.0	S11/12	0.01
Snake 11	W	M	570	52.0	S11/12	2.43
Snake 12	W	M	650	62.0	S11/12	0.24

"Season" shows season and year: for example, "S10/11" = spring and summer of 2010–2011. SVL = snout to vent length; M = male; F = female; W = Wollemi National Park; Y = Yengo National Park; S10/11 = spring/summer tracking period of 2010–2011; S11/12 = spring/summer tracking period of 2011–2012; W11 = winter tracking period of 2011. Home ranges were estimated using the minimum convex polygon method in ARC GIS 9.3.

the body cavity. The transmitter body was then introduced into the coelom. Both incisions were closed with 3-0 premilene non-absorbable suture material. A mixture of 41% warm water, 9% saline and 50% Hartmann's fluids were then injected subcutaneously at a dose of 3% body mass. To remove transmitters, the above procedure was reversed. No adverse effects were noted from surgery, and we released all snakes within one week after surgery.

Tracking Snakes

We tracked snakes twice per week during spring and summer in 2010–2011 (October to February) and 2011–2012 (November to February). We tracked snakes once per week during winter 2011. We used a hand-held UHF tracking receiver (Australis 26K, Titley Scientific, QLD, Australia) fitted with a Yagi antenna, and recorded location data using a hand-held global positioning system (GPS) device (GPSMAP 76, Garmin International, Olathe, KS, USA). We quantified attributes of trees used by snakes as retreat sites in spring/summer, plus five randomly chosen nearby trees (see analysis of microhabitat use by snakes). We also quantified the thermal regime of rocks used by snakes in winter (see seasonal shifts in thermal regimes within retreat sites).

Analyses of Snake Movements

We used ARC GIS 9.3 (Esri, Redlands, CA, USA) to calculate the total distances moved by snakes throughout the study (m), the mean distance per move (displacement <1 m) and the time interval between moves (moves. day^{-1}). We also calculated moves per tracking day; that is, the number of displacements divided by the number of radio-tracking days. We used a two-factor analysis of variance (2-way ANOVA) to test the effect of year and sex on these variables.

Analyses of Snake Home Ranges

We imported GPS points of snake retreat sites into ARC GIS 9.3 and estimated home range sizes using the minimum convex polygon method [29,30], to allow comparison with previous studies [17]. We imported layers (on vegetation types, elevation, waterways and roads and access points) to facilitate visual interpretation of habitat types.

Analyses of Macrohabitat Use by Snakes

Using Student's two sample *t*-tests, we compared tree characteristics (number of hollows, tree diameter at breast height [DBH; mm]) and tree height (m) in the vegetation structure types most often used by snakes ("Hawkesbury–Hornsby plateau exposed woodland" and "Mellong sandmass dry woodland"; see home ranges in Results section 3.2) to those in a widespread adjacent but non-used vegetation type ("Hawkesbury sheltered dry forest"; see home ranges in results section).

Analyses of Microhabitat Use by Snakes

We compared the following characteristics of trees used by snakes to those of five nearby (unused) trees: species, alive or dead, DBH (mm), tree height (m), the number of visible hollows large enough to accommodate snakes, and height above-ground of the lowest hollow (m).

We used a generalized mixed effects model (GLMM: [31]) in the R package 'nlme' [32] with a binomial distribution to compare the characteristics of used trees to nearby trees, with individual snake being the random variable. GLMMs account for the non-independence of multiple measurements from each snake in resource selection models [33]. To assess which models best fitted the data, we ranked models, using all combinations of the variables, by the AICc. Any model with a ΔAICc <4 was considered a good fit to the data [34].

Some arboreal retreat-sites were inaccessible to us, but where feasible we measured thermal regimes inside used and unused hollows by attaching thermal data loggers (iButtons, Maxim Integrated, Sunnyvale, CA, USA) to lengths of wire, and inserting these as far as possible (typically, 10–50 cm) into hollows. We compared thermal data collected from used versus unused hollows with a repeated-measures ANOVA, with time of day as the repeated measure, and year and "used or not" as factors. We also compared maximum temperatures experienced within hollows of used versus unused trees using a Student's paired *t*-test.

Seasonal Shifts in Thermal Regimes within Retreat-Sites

Our radio-tracked snakes consistently used crevices beneath sun-warned rocks as winter retreat-sites, and hollows within trees as spring/summer retreat-sites. Thus, we compared thermal regimes under rocks with those in tree hollows (in both summer and winter), to compare the conditions that are available to snakes inside these types of shelter-sites at different times of year. We used thermal data loggers to measure temperatures under five rocks and four tree hollows (see above) used by *H. bungaroides* throughout 2010, 2011 and early 2012. We used one-way ANOVA to compare the total number of hours over both summers that 17 tree hollows and 16 rocks exceeded 32°C, the VTMax (Voluntary Maximum Temperature) for *H. bungaroides* [18]. The CTMax (Critical Maximum Temperature) has not been determined for *H. bungaroides*, so our analyses of this parameter were based on an estimate for the closely-related tiger snake, *Notechis scutatus* (38.0°C: [35,36]).

Spatial Ecology in the North *versus* the South of the Species' Range

We compared home range size, mean distance per move and total distance moved of snakes tracked in the north to those of snakes tracked in the south during a study conducted over the spring/summer of 1992–93, 1993–94 and 1994–95 [17].

Results

Analyses of Snake Movements

We found no significant effect of sex or year on total distances moved by our radio-tracked snakes (sex: $F_{1,5} = 1.64$, $P = 0.26$; year: $F_{1,5} = 2.71$, $P = 0.16$; Fig. 1a), nor on mean distance per move (sex: $F_{1,5} = 3.59$, $P = 0.12$; year: $F_{1,5} = 0.37$, $P = 0.57$; Fig. 1b), interval between successive moves (sex: $F_{1,5} = 0.24$, $P = 0.65$; year: $F_{1,5} = 0.10$, $P = 0.77$; Fig. 1c) or moves per tracking day (sex: $F_{1,5} = 0.05$, $P = 0.83$; year: $F_{1,5} = 0.44$, $P = 0.54$; Fig. 1d). No interactions between year and sex were statistically significant (i.e., all $P > 0.05$) in any of the above analyses.

Analyses of Snake Home Ranges

The mean home range of snakes throughout this study was 2.97±1.14 ha. Home range sizes differed between seasons: mean summer home range was 4.42±1.54 ha, and mean winter home range was 0.50±0.22 ha (see Table 1 for home range size for individual snakes and Fig. 2 for home range plots), although this difference was not significant due to low winter sample size.

Analyses of Macrohabitat Use by Snakes

During summer, our radio-tracked snakes remained within two specific macrohabitat types: the "Hawkesbury–Hornsby plateau exposed woodland" and "Mellong sandmass dry woodland"

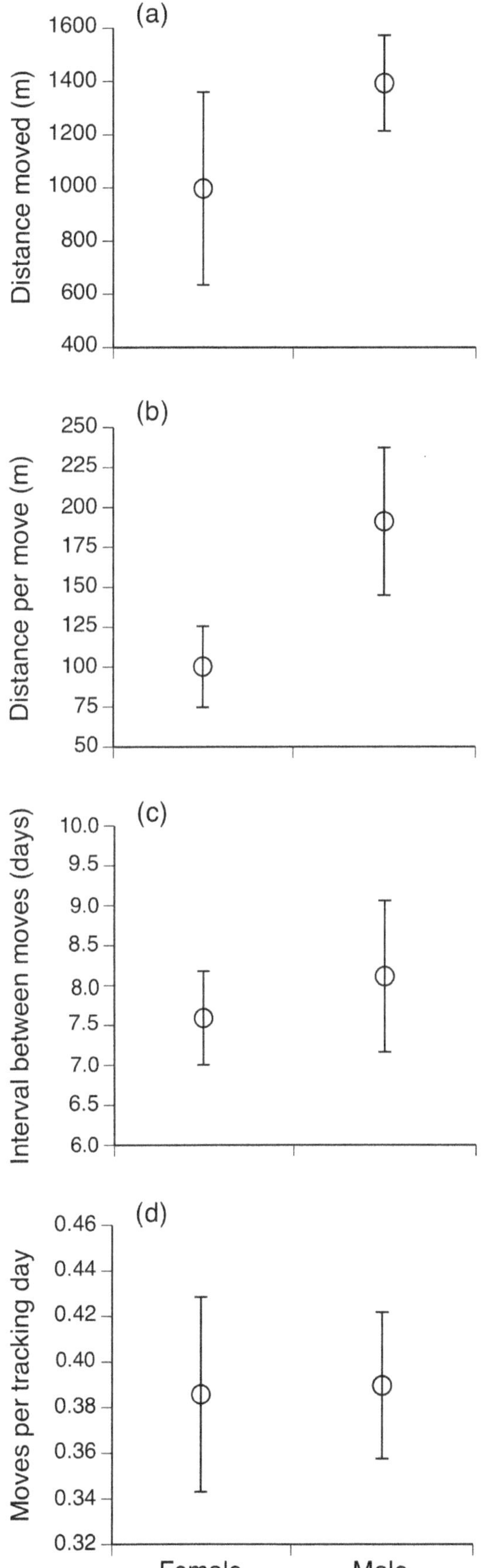

Figure 1. Movement data for broad-headed snakes collected over the Australian spring and summer seasons of 2010/2011 and 2011/2012. (a) mean total distance (in meters) moved by male and female snakes, (b) mean distance moved in meters per location shift by male and female snakes, (c) mean number of days between location shifts by male and female snakes and (d) the number of moves per tracking day for male and female snakes. All graphs show mean values and associated standard errors.

(Fig. 2) where they used hollows in a variety of tree species, most notably red bloodwood, yellow bloodwood, grey gum, scribbly gum, narrow-leaved stringy bark and stags (standing dead trees). The snakes avoided the adjacent "Hawkesbury sheltered forest" (Fig. 2) which contained thinner trees (based on DBH, $t = 5.44$, $df = 270$, $P < 0.001$; Fig. 3b) with fewer hollows per tree ($t = 8.16$, $df = 218$, $P < 0.001$; Fig. 3a), but which were similar in mean height ($t = 0.146$, $df = 247$, $P = 0.884$; Fig. 3c) to those in the preferred habitat types.

Analyses of Microhabitat Use by Snakes

A comparison between used and adjacent unused trees (all within the same habitat type) showed that snakes sheltered within a non-random subset of trees with respect to several variables. Our analysis of all combinations of variables produced 65 models, with 7 in the 95% confidence set ($\Sigma w_i = 0.95$). Only 4 models had a ΔAICc <4. Compared to availability, snakes selectively used dead trees that were wider at the diameter at breast height, shorter and had many hollows relatively close to ground level (Table 2). The species of tree appeared to be less important than these structural features, with tree species not appearing in any of the highly-ranked models.

We found no significant difference in mean temperatures between used versus unused tree hollows ($F_{1,36} = 0.10$, $P = 0.75$), and no significant thermal difference between years ($F_{1,36} = 0.65$, $P = 0.43$; interaction NS also). Temperatures within a tree hollow shifted with time of day ($F_{11,26} = 19.31$, $P < 0.001$; Fig. 4), with a significant interaction between time of day and year ($F_{11,26} = 7.63$, $P < 0.001$: the summer of 2011–2012 was cooler than that of 2010–2011; Fig. 4). Maximum temperatures were higher in unused tree hollows than in hollows of used trees ($t = 2.25$, $df = 15.9$, $P = 0.02$).

Seasonal Shifts in Thermal Regimes within Retreat Sites

Mean temperatures under rocks differed from those inside tree hollows ($F_{1,13} = 22.01$, $P < 0.001$; Fig. 5) and were higher in summer than in winter ($F_{1,13} = 442.40$, $P < 0.001$; Fig. 5). Temperatures also differed with time of day ($F_{1,13} = 106.932$, $P = 0.001$; Fig. 5), but with no significant interaction between time of day and habitat type or time of day and season (all $P > 0.05$). The number of hours during summer that CTMax ($F_{1,33} = 20.12$, $P < 0.001$) and VTMax ($F_{1,33} = 32.19$, $P < 0.001$) were exceeded was higher under rocks than in tree hollows, with rocks often exceeding those thermal limits (Fig. 6).

Spatial Ecology in the North *versus* the South of the Species' Range

Home range size did not differ significantly between northern and southern populations of *H. bungaroides* ($F_{1,33} = 0.035$, $P = 0.852$), nor did mean distance per move ($F_{1,33} = 0.813$, $P = 0.375$), nor total distances moved ($F_{1,33} = 0.518$, $P = 0.476$).

Discussion

Our data reveal many similarities between *H. bungaroides* in southern populations (as previously studied) and those in the north

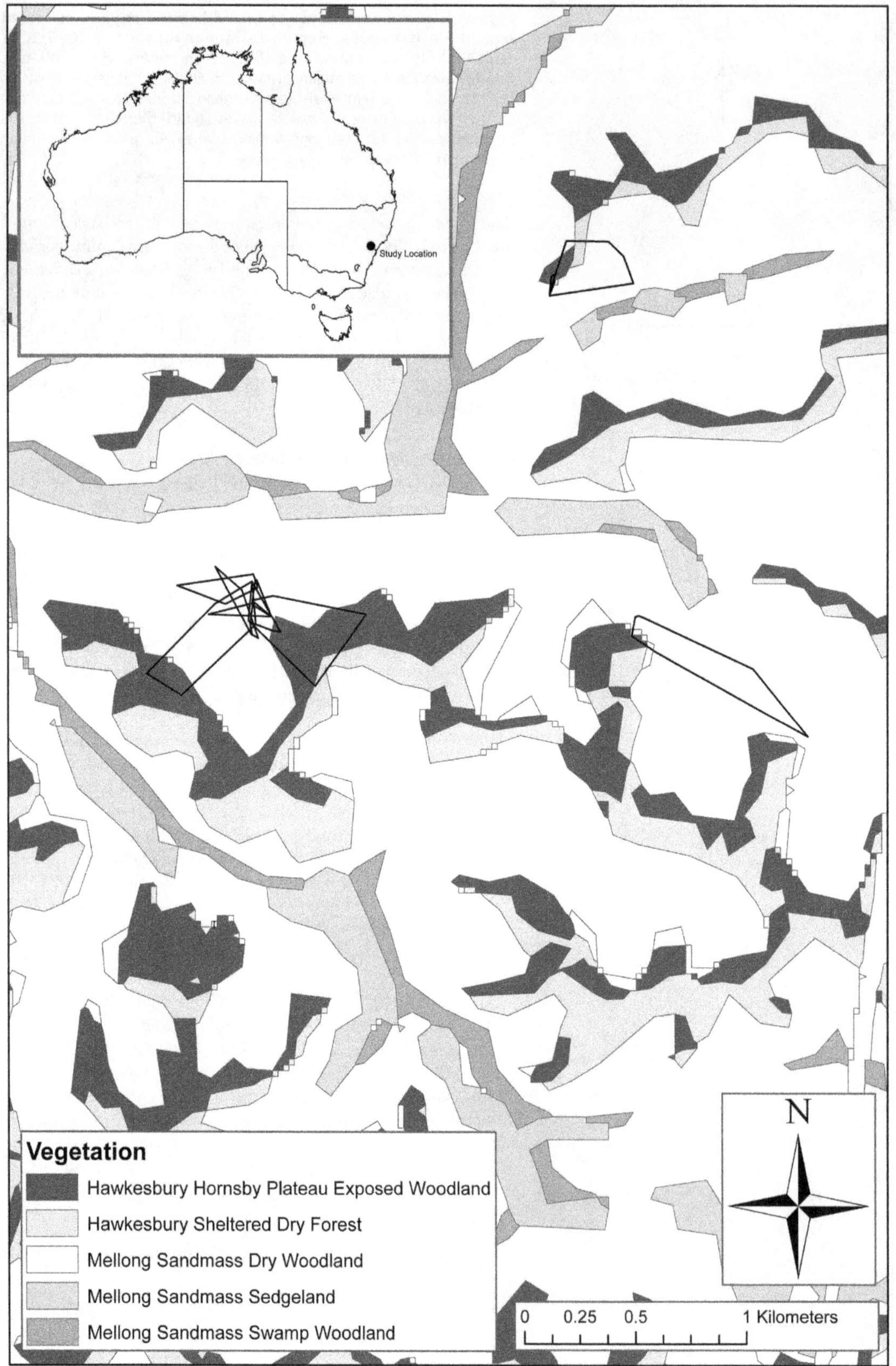

Figure 2. Home ranges of five adult female and three adult male broad-headed snakes that we radio-tracked. The home range boundaries were estimated using the minimum convex polygon method, with vegetation layer overlaid. All snakes that were tracked remained within "Mellong sandmass dry woodland" and "Hawkesbury–Hornsby plateau exposed woodland" and avoided all other vegetation types.

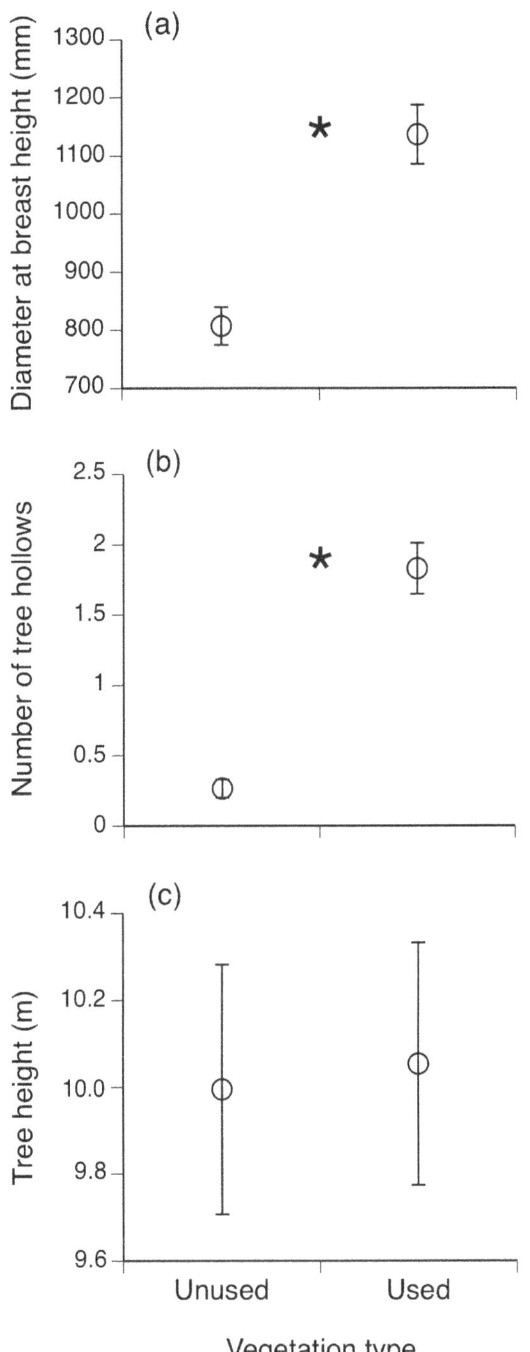

Figure 3. Characteristics of trees in vegetation types that were either used by radio-tracked broad-headed snakes ("Mellong sandmass dry woodland" and "Hawkesbury-Hornsby plateau exposed woodland") or were not used by our snakes ("Hawkesbury sheltered dry forest"). In the preferred macrohabitat types, tree diameter at breast height (a) was greater and trees had more hollows (b). Mean tree height (c) did not differ between used and unused vegetation types. Graphs show mean values and associated standard errors. * indicates a statistically significant difference.

of the range (the subject of our current work). For example, our radio-tracked snakes showed the same seasonal shift in habitat types, from rock crevices in winter to tree hollows in summer. Our data on thermal regimes within those habitat types support the hypothesis that these seasonal shifts are driven by temperature [17]. By moving between these habitat types seasonally, the snakes had access to relatively consistent thermal conditions inside refuges year-round (Fig. 5). Trees (summer habitat) are too cool to allow snakes to thermoregulate in winter, whereas sun-exposed rock crevices (winter habitat) attain lethally high temperatures in summer (see Figs 5 and 6). During the entire summer of 2010/2011, ambient temperatures in crevices (both under randomly-chosen rocks, and those actually used by *H. bungaroides* as winter retreat sites) exceeded the broad-headed snake VTMax for an average of 162.6 hours, and exceeded the snakes' estimated CTMax for an average of 97.6 hours. In contrast, the temperatures that we measured inside randomly-chosen and used tree hollows exceeded VTMax for an average of only 28.3 hours, and exceeded CTMax for 9.8 hours (Fig. 6). Trees that were used by snakes never exceeded CTMax, and exceeded VTMax for only 9 hours throughout the summer. The hollows used by snakes were cooler then nearby unused hollows during the hottest parts of the day (see Fig. 4). We observed snakes basking outside tree hollows, and signal directions suggested that snakes moved up and down hollow limbs and trunks depending on ambient temperature. That mobility suggested active temperature selection by snakes within tree-hollows, similar to southern populations of the same species [21] and the more northerly-distributed congener, Stephen's banded snake (*H. stephensii*: [37]). The smaller size of rocks precludes this kind of active behavioral thermoregulation, so the snakes' shift to tree hollows in the warmer months of the year may reflect the advantages of greater accessible spatial thermal heterogeneity, as well as lower mean temperatures [21].

In terms of spatial ecology, the snakes we tracked in the extreme north of the species' range were similar to conspecifics in southern populations. As well as the thermally-driven shifts in habitat noted above, mean home range sizes were similar for snakes in both regions (3.3 ha versus 3.0 ha: [17]), as were mean movement distances between successive displacements (134 m versus 159 m: [17]), the active selection of trees with many hollows and relatively large DBH [21], and fidelity for specific trees [21]. Like the southern snakes (J. K. Webb, unpublished data), our radio-tracked northern snakes sometimes were encountered under bushes and in hollow logs on the forest floor.

However, our data also identify some points of difference between snakes from the northern versus southern clades. In summer, southern conspecifics used trees on top of plateaus and below cliffs [17] whereas snakes in our northern study areas moved into shallow valleys away from rock outcrops, and occupied specific vegetation types while avoiding others. No such selectivity at this macrohabitat level has been recorded for the southern population, perhaps reflecting more homogeneous forest-habitat types in that region. The northern snakes showed several points of similarity with *H. stephensii*, an arboreal congeneric species that occurs north of the range occupied by *H. bungaroides* [27,37]. Our study sites were close to the southern limit of *H. stephensii* distribution, and thus experience climatic conditions more similar to those encountered by southern *H. stephensii* populations than southern *H. bungaroides* populations. Thermal regimes may drive similarities such as occasional rock use by *H. stephensii* [38], as well as similar periods of sequestration inside retreat sites (mean of 7.9 days for *H. bungaroides* versus 8 days for *H. stephensii*: [39]). The southern *H. bungaroides* studied by Webb and Shine [17] moved much more frequently (mean of 2.9 days: [17]), suggesting that higher ambient temperatures may restrict the frequency of movement. Some specific trees were used by different individual snakes (both simultaneously and at different times) in our study, and snakes also used leaf litter as

Table 2. Coefficients of the four best generalized mixed models and standard errors, with AICc values, change in AICc values (ΔAICc) and Akaike weight (w_i).

Intercept	Alive or Dead	DBH	Hollow Height	# Hollows	Tree Height	AICc	ΔAICc	w_i
−4.114	+	0.002±0.001	-	0.415±0.145	−0.198±0.102	94.499	0	0.425
−4.223	+	0.002±0.001	−0.086±0.124	0.451±0.154	−0.185±0.104	96.169	1.670	0.184
−5.425	+	0.001±0.001	-	0.327±0.134	-	96.672	2.173	0.143
−5.495	+	0.002±0.001	−0.134±0.123	0.394±0.148	-	96.934	2.435	0.126

retreat sites. Both of these patterns were noted for *H. stephensii* [40], but rarely for southern *H. bungaroides* [17,21]. In combination, these trends suggest that suitable arboreal shelter-sites may be more limiting in the north, such that in hot weather snakes may re-use a limited set of tree hollows, or else abandon arboreal sites for the cooler leaf litter.

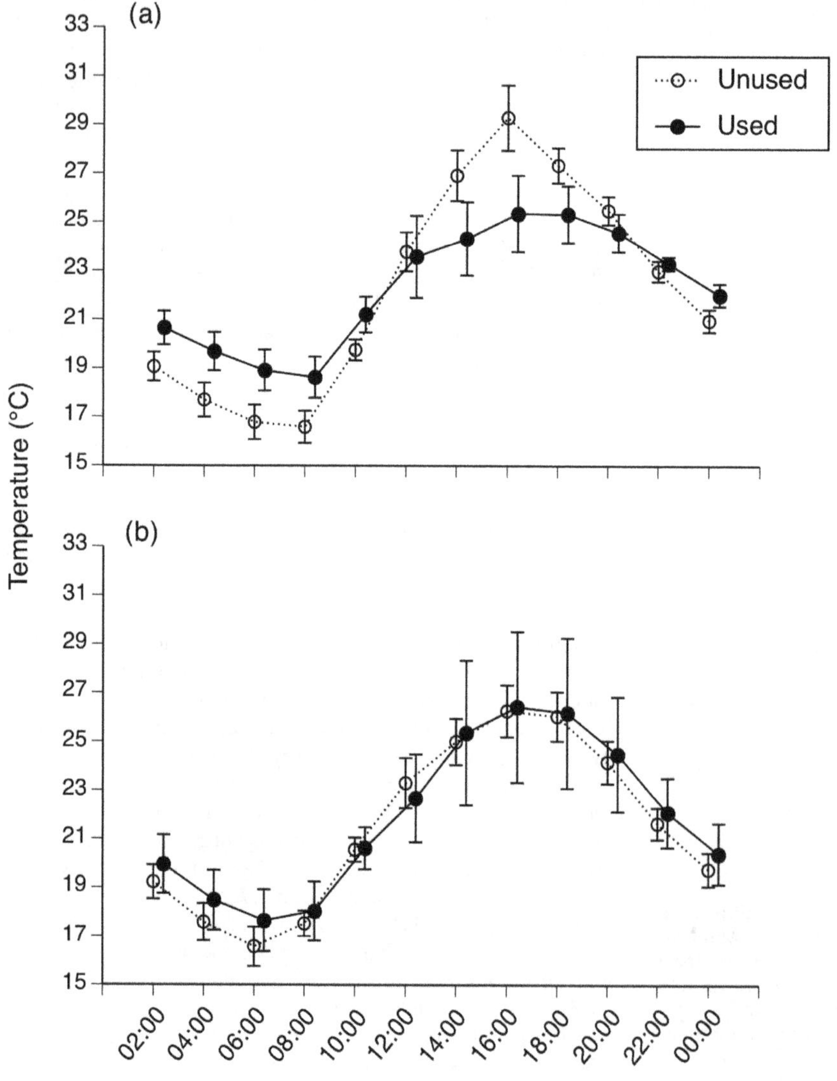

Figure 4. Thermal regimes in retreat-sites and potentially available retreat-sites. Panel (a) shows the temperature cycle on a hot day in the summer of 2010/2011 and (b) shows the same cycle on a hot day in the (cooler) summer of 2011/2012. Graphs show mean values and associated standard errors.

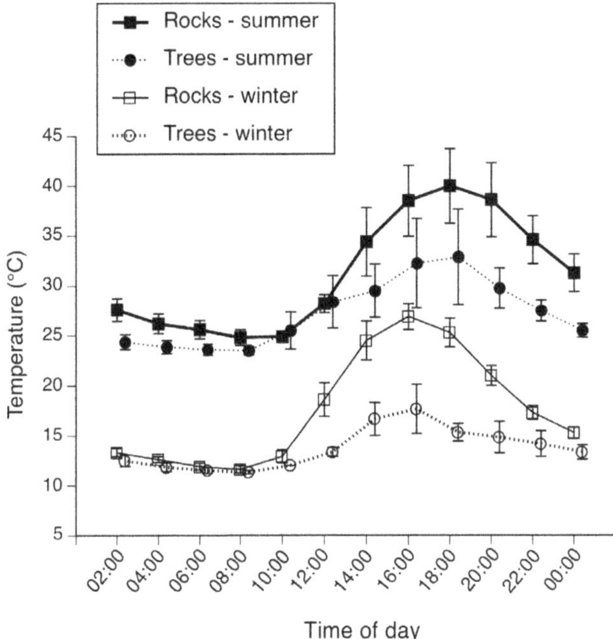

Figure 5. Mean maximum ambient temperatures experienced under rocks (winter habitat for broad-headed snakes) and in tree hollows (summer habitat for broad-headed snakes) during winter and summer. By shifting habitat between winter and summer, these snakes experience relatively stable thermal regimes and avoid extreme temperatures.

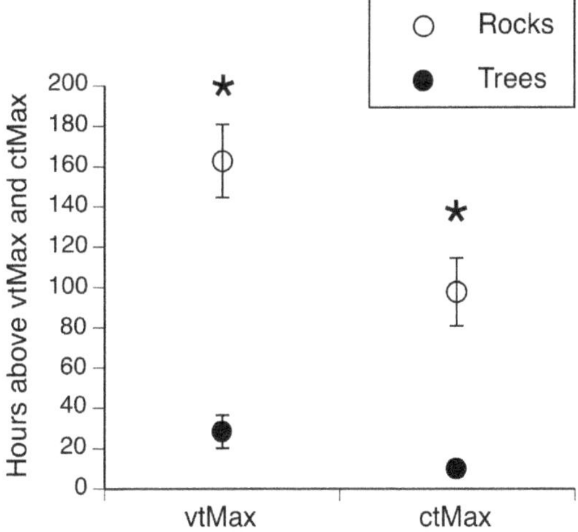

Figure 6. Thermal extremes in snake retreat-sites during the summer (1 December to 28 February) of 2010/2011. The graph shows the total number of hours at which retreat-site temperatures were above the voluntary thermal maximum (VTMax, 32.5°C) and estimated critical thermal maximum (CTMax, 38.0°C) of broad-headed snakes. Data are shown separately for two habitat types used by those snakes: those used in summer (tree hollows) and in winter (under rocks). Rocks often exceeded both VTMax and CTMax in summer, whereas tree hollows exceeded these limits only rarely. * indicates a statistically significant difference.

The snakes that we radio-tracked used different species of trees for shelter than did the previously-studied southern population of *H. bungaroides* or *H. stephensii*, but this difference is most parsimoniously attributed to geographic differences in forest composition. In support of that inference, tree species seemed to have less effect than tree structure in determining frequency of use by snakes. The four generalized mixed models with best fit to our data (Table 2) suggested that snakes prefer trees that were dead, with a large DBH but were also fairly short with many hollows close to the ground. In contrast, the tallest available trees were preferred by both southern-clade *H. bungaroides* and more northern *H. stephensii* [21,40]. That difference in tree height may explain an otherwise-puzzling discrepancy between our study and the earlier work: that is, we saw snakes basking in exposed positions on trees a total of 9 times (including 5 different snakes), whereas this behavior was rarely observed in the studies on other *Hoplocephalus* [21,40]. Overt basking may be more likely on shorter trees (because they tend to be mostly in shade due to adjacent taller trees); and also, basking may be easier to observe if the snakes are closer to the ground (and thus, to the observer).

During our study, three trees were used by more than one snake, with up to four individual snakes using the same tree throughout both summers and the winter tracking period. Two of these trees were inhabited by two snakes simultaneously, a phenomenon also observed (albeit rarely) in *H. stephensii* [40] but not in southern clade *H. bungaroides*. Northern clade *H. bungaroides* showed strong site fidelity, as also reported in southern clade *H. bungaroides* and *H. stephensii*. We observed five snakes return to the same trees, with one snake using the same tree on four occasions throughout the summer of 2010/2011. Such re-use suggests that trees with suitable hollows a limiting resource for snakes in this system.

Broadly, the habitats used by our northern-clade *H. bungaroides* were similar to those used by southern-clade conspecifics in winter. The reliance on hollow-bearing trees during summer is shared not only by the two *H. bungaroides* clades, but also by two congeneric arboreal taxa (*H. stephensii* and *H. bitorquatus*, the pale-headed snake: [39,40]). Although detailed studies are lacking, arboreality and tree-hollow use also are likely to be important for the most closely related outgroup taxa to *Hoplocephalus* – *Tropidechis carinatus* (the rough-scaled snake) and *Paroplocephalus atriceps* (the Lake Cronin snake: [36,41,42]. Phylogenetic reconstructions suggest that *H. bitorquatus* most closely resembles the ancestral *Hoplocephalus* species [41]; hence, year-round arboreality may be an ancestral trait for this lineage. The expansion of the southernmost taxon (*H. bungaroides*) into cooler areas rendered local tree-hollows too cool for foraging in winter, plausibly stimulating a behavioral shift towards rock-crevice use during cooler times of year.

Our results have direct implications for conservation and management of the genetically distinct northern clade of *H. bungaroides*. First, the population that we studied relies upon both rock outcrops (in winter) and nearby forests (in summer), so management needs to conserve that combination of habitat types in close proximity. That requirement is similar to that for southern conspecifics, whereas rock crevices appear to play only a minor role in the ecology of the other *Hoplocephalus* species [40]. In terms of conserving rock-outcrop habitats, attention needs to focus not only on human disturbance to local areas (especially, rock theft for landscaping, and illegal collection of animals for the pet trade: [15,16]) but also on broader landscape-scale processes. Analyses of historical photographs, and long-term field studies, have shown that vegetation overgrowth imperils *H. bungaroides* at the southern study sites [20]. Removal of shading vegetation significantly enhanced habitat quality for *H. bungaroides* in this area [19]. We have no equivalent data for the northern-clade populations, but they may well be under similar threats (e.g., illegal rock collection is rife: B. Croak, unpublished data). Thus, management should prioritize retention of existing surface rock, and mitigation of processes that facilitate vegetation overgrowth [14,15,19,20,22].

Because *H. bungaroides* show such a profound seasonal shift in habitat use, we also need to maintain large forest blocks that contain hollow-bearing trees, in areas adjacent to sandstone outcrops [21,37]. For the northern population, that forested area should lie within vegetation types such as "Hawkesbury–Hornsby plateau exposed woodland" and "Mellong sandmass dry woodland", rather than other locally occurring forest types. The preferred macrohabitats may be distinctive because they contain a relatively high number of trees with large hollows suitable for retreat-site use by *H. bungaroides*. The same types of hollows are used by many other arboreal taxa, emphasizing the importance of this critical habitat for a wide variety of species [43,44]. Thus, forestry management plans should aim to conserve tree hollows. In Australia, managed landscapes generally support less than half the number of hollow-bearing trees as occur in natural stands [43]. This issue may be especially critical for the northern populations of *H. bungaroides*, because their frequent re-use of the same tree hollows, and use of those hollows by multiple animals, suggests that such trees may be a limiting resource in this system.

The spatial extent of reserves to protect northern-clade *H. bungaroides* is likely to be similar to that needed for their southern-clade conspecifics. Movement patterns of northern *H. bungaroides* were broadly similar to those of their southern conspecifics. Rates of gene flow also are likely to be similar in the two clades [45], with a complex metapopulation structure that includes unidirectional gene flow from source to peripheral sink populations [45]. Identification of source and sink populations through genetic investigation within the northern range of this endangered species would facilitate effective conservation and/or habitat restoration [45–47].

Acknowledgments

We thank David Vella and Michelle Bingley for performing surgeries. We thank numerous volunteers, in particular Reid Tingley, Ryan Fraser, George Madani, Cissy Ballen, Rebecca Stutz and especially Matt Greenlees for assistance with fieldwork. Melanie Elphick provided assistance with figures and proof reading. Meagan Hinds provided encouragement. Paul Godfrey, Anthony Horwood and especially Richard Colbourne facilitated site access. All research was conducted under NPWS Scientific Licence SL100472.

Author Contributions

Conceived and designed the experiments: BC MC JW RS. Performed the experiments: BC. Analyzed the data: BC MC JW RS. Contributed reagents/materials/analysis tools: RS. Wrote the paper: BC RS.

References

1. Dirzo R, Raven PH (2003) Global state of biodiversity and loss. Annu Rev Env Resour 28: 137–167.
2. Gibson L, Lee TM, Koh LP, Brook BW, Gardiner TA, et al. (2011) Primary forests are irreplaceable for sustaining tropical biodiversity. Nature 478: 378–383.
3. Bonin MC (2012) Specializing on vulnerable habitat: *Acropora* selectivity among damselfish recruits and the risk of bleaching-induced habitat loss. Coral Reefs 31: 287–297.
4. Julliard R, Jiguet F, Couvet D (2003) Common birds facing global changes: what makes a species at risk? Glob Change Biol 10: 148–154.
5. Munday PL (2004) Habitat loss, resource specialization and extinction on coral reefs. Glob Change Biol 10: 1642–1647.
6. Gaston KJ (1994) Rarity. Chapman and Hall, London.
7. Webb JK, Brook BW, Shine R (2002) What makes a species vulnerable to extinction? Comparative life-history traits of two sympatric snakes. Ecol Res 17: 59–67.
8. Cooke SJ (2008) Biotelemetry and biologging in endangered species research and animal conservation: relevance to regional, national, and IUCN red list threat assessments. Endangered Species Res 4: 168–185.
9. Caughley G, Gunn A (1995) Conservation Biology in Theory and Practice. 1st Edition. Wiley, New York.
10. Hucke-Gaete R, Osman LP, Moreno CA, Findlay KP, Ljungblad DK (2003) Discovery of a blue whale feeding and nursing ground in southern Chile. Proc R Soc B 271: S170–S173.
11. Mills MGL, Broomhall LS, du Toit JT (2004) Cheetah *Acinonyx jubatus* feeding ecology in the Kruger National Park and a comparison across African savanna habitats: is the cheetah only a successful hunter on open grassland plains. Wildl Biol 10: 177–186.
12. Shine R (2012) Sex at the snake den: lust, deception and conflict in the mating system of red-sided gartersnakes. Adv Study Behav 44: 1–51.
13. Krefft G (1869) The Snakes of Australia: An Illustrated and Descriptive Catalogue of All the Known Species. Thomas Richards, Government Printer, Sydney.
14. Shine R, Fitzgerald M (1989) Conservation and reproduction of an endangered species: the broad-headed snake, *Hoplocephalus bungaroides* (Elapidae). Aust Zool 25: 65–67.
15. Shine R, Webb JK, Fitzgerald M, Sumner J (1998) The impact of bush-rock removal on an endangered snake species, *Hoplocephalus bungaroides* (Serpentes: Elapidae). Wildl Res 25: 285–295.
16. Webb JK, Brook BW, Shine R (2002) Collectors endanger Australia's most threatened snake, the broad-headed snake, *Hoplocephalus bungaroides*. Oryx 36: 170–181.
17. Webb JK, Shine R (1997) A field study of the spatial ecology and movements of a threatened snake species, *Hoplocephalus bungaroides*. Biol Conserv 82: 203–217.
18. Webb JK, Shine R (1998) Thermoregulation by a nocturnal elapid snake (*Hoplocephalus bungaroides*) in southeastern Australia. Physiol Zool 71: 680–692.
19. Pike DA, Webb JK, Shine R (2011) Chainsawing for conservation: ecologically informed tree removal for habitat management. Ecol Manag Restor 12: 110–118.
20. Pringle RM, Webb JK, Shine R (2003) Canopy structure, microclimate, and habitat selection by a nocturnal snake, *Hoplocephalus bungaroides*. Ecology 84: 2668–2679.
21. Webb JK, Shine R (1997) Out on a limb: conservation implications of tree-hollow use by a threatened snake species (*Hoplocephalus bungaroides*: Serpentes, Elapidae). Biol Conserv 81: 21–33.
22. Croak BM, Pike DA, Webb JK, Shine R (2008) Three-dimensional crevice structure affects retreat site selection by reptiles. Anim Behav 76: 1875–1884.
23. Webb JK, Shine R (1998) Ecological characteristics of a threatened snake species, *Hoplocephalus bungaroides* (Serpentes: Elapidae). Anim Conserv 1: 185–193.
24. Webb JK, Shine R (2000) Paving the way for habitat restoration: can artificial rocks restore degraded habitats of endangered reptiles? Biol Conserv 92: 93–99.
25. Webb JK, Shine R (2008) Differential effects of an intense wildfire on survival of sympatric snakes. J Wildl Manage 72: 1394–1389.
26. Sumner J, Webb JK, Shine R, Keogh JS (2010) Molecular and morphological assessment of Australia's most endangered snake, *Hoplocephalus bungaroides*, reveals two evolutionarily significant units for conservation. Conserv Genet 11: 747–758.
27. Cogger HG (2000) Reptiles and Amphibians of Australia. 6th Edition. Reed New Holland, Sydney.
28. Webb JK, Brook BW, Shine R (2003) Does foraging mode influence life history traits? A comparative study of growth, maturation and survival of two species of sympatric snakes from south-eastern Australia. Austral Ecol 28: 601–610.
29. Harris S, Cresswell WJ, Forde PG, Trewhella WJ, Woollard T, et al. (1990) Home-range analysis using radio-tracking data – a review of problems and techniques particularly as applied to the study of mammals. Mammal Rev 20: 97–123.
30. White GC, Garrott RA (1990) Analysis of Wildlife Radio-Tracking Data. Academic Press, San Diego, California.
31. McCulloch CE, Searle SR (2001) Generalized, Linear and Mixed Models. John Wiley & Sons, New York.
32. Pinheiro J, Bates D, DebRoy S, Sarkar D, R Development Core Team (2011) nlme: Linear and Nonlinear Mixed Effects Models. R Package Version 3.1–102, Austria.
33. Gillies CS, Hebblewhite M, Nielsen SE, Krawchuk MA, Aldridge CL, et al. (2006) Application of random effects to the study of resource selection by animals. J Anim Ecol 75: 887–898.
34. Burnham KP, Anderson DR (2002) Model Selection and Multimodel Inference: A Practical Information-Theoretic Approach. 2nd Edition. Springer, New York.
35. Greer A (1997) The Biology and Evolution of Australian Snakes. Surrey, Beatty and Sons, Sydney.
36. Keogh JS, Scott IAW, Scanlon JD (2000) Molecular phylogeny of viviparous Australian elapid snakes: affinities of *Echiopsis atriceps* (Storr, 1980) and *Drysdalia coronata* (Schlegel, 1837), with a description of a new genus. J Zool 252: 317–326.
37. Fitzgerald M, Shine R, Lemckert F, Towerton A (2005) Habitat requirements of the threatened snake species *Hoplocephalus stephensii* (Elapidae) in eastern Australia. Austral Ecol 30: 465–474.

38. Wilson S, Swan G (2010) A Complete Guide to the Reptiles of Australia. 2nd Edition. Reed New Holland, Sydney.
39. Fitzgerald M, Shine R, Lemckert F (2002) Spatial ecology of arboreal snakes (*Hoplocephalus stephensii*, Elapidae) in eastern Australian forest. Austral Ecol 27, 537–545.
40. Fitzgerald M, Shine R, Lemckert F (2002) Radiotelemetric study of habitat use by the arboreal snake *Hoplocephalus stephensii* (Elapidae) in eastern Australia. Copeia 2002: 321–332.
41. Keogh JS, Scott IAW, Fitzgerald M, Shine R (2003) Molecular phylogeny of the Australian venomous snake genus *Hoplocephalus* (Serpentes, Elapidae) and conservation genetics of the threatened *H. stephensii*. Conserv Genet 4: 57–65.
42. Sanders KL, Lee MSY, Leys R, Foster R, Keogh JS (2008) Molecular phylogeny and divergence dates for Australian elapids and sea snakes (Hydrophiinae): evidence from seven genes for rapid evolutionary radiations. J Evol Biol 21: 882–895.
43. Gibbons P, Lindenmayer DB, Barry SC, Tanton MT (2002) Hollow selection by vertebrate fauna in forests of southeastern Australia and implications for forest management. Biol Conserv 103: 1–12.
44. Gibbons P, Lindenmayer DA (2002) Tree Hollows and Wildlife Conservation in Australia. CSIRO Publishing, Melbourne.
45. Dubey S, Sumner J, Pike DA, Keogh JS, Webb JK, et al. (2011) Genetic connectivity among populations of an endangered snake species from southeastern Australia (*Hoplocephalus bungaroides*, Elapidae). Ecol Evol 2: 218–227.
46. Croak BM, Pike DA, Webb JK, Shine R (2010) Using artificial rocks to restore nonrenewable shelter sites in human degraded systems: colonisation by fauna. Restor Ecol 18: 428–438.
47. Croak BM, Pike DA, Webb JK, Shine R (2012) Habitat selection in a rocky landscape: experimentally decoupling the influence of retreat-site attributes from that of landscape features. PLoS ONE 7: e37982.

The Frontal Eye Fields Limit the Capacity of Visual Short-Term Memory in Rhesus Monkeys

Kyoung-Min Lee*, Kyung-Ha Ahn

Department of Neurology, Seoul National University Hospital, Seoul, Republic of Korea

Abstract

The frontal eye fields (FEF) in rhesus monkeys have been implicated in visual short-term memory (VSTM) as well as control of visual attention. Here we examined the importance of the area in the VSTM capacity and the relationship between VSTM and attention, using the chemical inactivation technique and multi-target saccade tasks with or without the need of target-location memory. During FEF inactivation, serial saccades to targets defined by color contrast were unaffected, but saccades relying on short-term memory were impaired when the target count was at the capacity limit of VSTM. The memory impairment was specific to the FEF-coded retinotopic locations, and subject to competition among targets distributed across visual fields. These results together suggest that the FEF plays a crucial role during the entry of information into VSTM, by enabling attention deployment on targets to be remembered. In this view, the memory capacity results from the limited availability of attentional resources provided by FEF: The FEF can concurrently maintain only a limited number of activations to register the targets into memory. When lesions render part of the area unavailable for activation, the number would decrease, further reducing the capacity of VSTM.

Editor: Maurice Ptito, University of Montreal, Canada

Funding: Supported by a grant from the National Research Foundation of Republic of Korea (Grants No. 800-20100003 and 800-20110005). The funders had no role in study design, data collection and analysis, decision to publish, or preparation of the manuscript.

Competing Interests: The authors have declared that no competing interests exist.

* E-mail: kminlee@snu.ac.kr

Introduction

Primates process visual information with remarkable efficiency, yet can hold only a limited number of discrete locations or objects in memory at one time [1–3]. This limit is easily demonstrable, for instance, by situations evoking change blindness, i.e., the failure to detect obvious differences between images when separated by time or space, and by neuropsychological tests probing the visual short-term memory (VSTM). The capacity limit in VSTM has been estimated to be three or four items in both human [4–8] and non-human primates [2,9,10].

The frontal eye fields (FEF) seems to play an important role in VSTM [11]. A majority of neurons in the area respond to visual events and visual responses in some outlast the stimulus [12], potentially subserving the short-term memory. In fact, when the FEF is temporarily inactivated by chemicals such as muscimol, a GABA agonist, or lidocaine, a local anesthetic, memory-guided saccades are impaired: Saccades directed to a briefly flashed target can no longer made, whereas those to a visible target are much less affected [13–16]. However, many details still remain unanswered regarding the nature of short-term memory carried out by FEF, and in this study we addressed the following two specific questions.

First, we asked whether or not FEF inactivation would affect the VSTM capacity. Recent works demonstrated the bilateral advantage in visual tracking [17] and visual working memory [18]: Bilateral presentations of visual stimuli lead to an increased probability of storage in memory and better performance in tracking than unilateral presentations. The bilateral advantage implies that these functions are carried out in the left and right hemifields independently, imposing a constraint on the potential neural substrates for the functions [19]. Since the FEF surely meets this requirement of hemifield independence, we asked whether rendering FEF unavailable for activation would reduce the behavioral capacity of VSTM.

Second, numerous studies have implicated the FEF in attention shift [20–25], and we wondered how the short-term memory function by this area would relate to the deployment of spatial attention by the same area. We designed task conditions where the distribution of saccade targets and the bottom-up visual attention prompted by the targets would vary between contralesional and ipsilesional sides during memory encoding. Analysis of memory-guided saccades as a function of target distribution indeed revealed an interaction between visual attention and the effect of FEF inactivation on VSTM. The interaction, consistent with the retinotopic mapping in FEF, was observable only when the two functions are taxed with multiple targets.

Materials and Methods

Ethics Statement

All experimental procedures were approved by the Seoul National University Hospital Animal Care and Use Committee (IACUC No: 09-0166, Project Title: Neural mechanisms of saccade choice in primate frontal cortex), and followed the US Public Health Service Policy on the humane care and use of laboratory animals. All animals used in this study were cared for at a temperature- and humidity-controlled room in the Primate Center of Seoul National University Hospital. While they were housed in individual cages, social contacts were encouraged by regularly opening a retractable door between cages. Environmental enrichment was also provided with a variety of toys. The animals were provided with a regular chow for monkeys, supplemented by fresh fruits. The health status of the animals was monitored daily by care-givers and by regular physical examinations and blood tests by the staff veterinarian. At the end of experiments, each animal was euthanized by deep anesthesia with zoletil chloride (10 mg/kg IM) and sodium pentobarbital (100 mg/kg, IV). After confirming total lack of a corneal reflex as an indication of adequate level of anesthesia, the animal was perfused with a liter of 0.1% phosphate buffered saline followed by several liters of fixative solution (10% buffered formalin). This procedure is consistent with the recommendations of the Panel on Euthanasia of the American Veterinary Medical Association [26].

Subjects and Surgical Preparation

Two adult female rhesus monkeys (*Macaca mulatta*, M9 and M10) weighing between 4 and 5 kg were prepared for chemical inactivation experiments. They were the same animals previously used in another study [27]. A head-restraint post and recording cylinders were implanted under isoflurane anesthesia and sterile surgical conditions. The recording cylinders (20 mm, internal diameter) were positioned over craniotomies centered on the right arcuate sulcus in all animals.

Procedures to Minimize Animal Discomfort, Distress, Pain and Injury

Three situations existed in which a monkey might experience discomfort, distress and/or pain in our experimental protocols: a) survival surgery; b) restraint for handling or routine testing and c) training and experimental recording sessions. The following steps were taken to ameliorate animal suffering in each situation. **a) Survival surgery.** The purpose of the surgical procedures was to implant recording chambers and a head restraint device for neurophysiological experiments. All surgeries were carried out in the animal surgical suite at the Primate Center of Seoul National University Hospital. Animals were prepared with sterile, anesthetic surgical procedures. A licensed veterinarian was present throughout the surgical procedures and the recovery period for anesthetic induction and for monitoring and recording all measured physiological variables. Animals were allowed free access to water but no food the night prior to scheduled surgery. One hour before the surgery the animal was given atropine sulfate (0.08 mg/kg, IM) to prevent excessive salivation during the surgery. One-half hour later it was sedated with zoletil chloride (10 mg/kg, IM), intubated, and placed under isoflurane anesthesia. A saline drip was maintained through an intravenous catheter placed into a leg vein. Throughout the surgery, core body temperature, heart rate, blood pressure, oxygen saturation and respiratory rate was continuously monitored. The animal was returned to its home cage after waking from the anesthesia and allowed to recover fully from the effects of surgery before behavioral training started. During the period of post-surgical recovery the animal was monitored closely and given injections of an analgesic agent (meloxicam 0.4 mg/kg IM) and antibiotics (cephazolin, 25/mg/kg IM) in consultation with the veterinarian for 3 days post-op. **b) Restraint for handling or routine testing.** Restraint for certain procedures, such as physical examination or blood sampling for health check, was accomplished with zoletil chloride (10 mg/kg IM). **c) Training and experimental recording sessions.** After recovery from the surgical procedure the animal was trained to be held by the arms and moved into a large plastic primate chair. This was done by supplying the animal with rewards of fruit and juice. The chair had a perch with an adjustable height for each animal's comfort. Wastes fell into a collection pan below the animal, and thus, did not cause the animal discomfort. The animals were trained by the delivery of water or fruit juice rewards in daily sessions during which time they received their entire liquid intake in the experimental apparatus. When the animal was fully trained the experiments began. During the experimental sessions the animal's head was painlessly restrained through the use of the implanted head post which mated to a vertical rod attached to the primate chair. The animals did not show any sign of discomfort by the head restraint device: They continued to train steadily for the period of time that they were in restraint and often fell asleep as they sat in the darkened room between blocks of trials.

Behavioral Tasks

1) The multi-target memory-guided saccade task (MEM, Figure 1A, upper panel). A trial began with the appearance of a white 1.0-degree square at the center of visual field. Four hundred milliseconds after the animal started fixation at the square, a four-by-three matrix of circular discs was presented. The color of discs distinguished targets (red) from non-targets (green), and the animal was trained to make saccades to the targets. Now, as soon as the first saccade was initiated, the targets were rendered green and indistinguishable from non-targets. The animal therefore had to rely on memory in order to make subsequent saccades to the second target and onwards. A drop of water reward was given after all targets were visited by at least one saccade.

The location of targets varied randomly across trials, but the target number, ranging from one to four, remained constant in a block of 40 trials. Blocks were randomly ordered and counterbalanced in terms of the target number, so that blocks of the same target number were run twice in a session.

Each disc was 1.0 degree in diameter with luminance of 124 cd/m^2 with the black background of 1.70 cd/m^2 (measured by a chromameter, CS-100; Minolta Photo Imaging, Mahwah, NJ). The rows and columns of discs were separated by 15 degrees, such that the matrix covered a visual field of 45 degrees horizontally and 30 degrees vertically.

The purpose of using the matrix-form arrangement of target locations, instead of a more traditional circular array, was to explore a wider range of visual fields with targets evenly spaced. In the circular array, the vector relationship between the first and the second saccades is biased to roughly opposite directions. In contrast, the matrix formation has the advantage that the target array remains similar for successive saccades in a series. For instance, after the first saccade to the nearest left or right target from the central fixation, a similar target array becomes available for the second saccade. This will result in a more even mixture of contra- and ipsilesional saccades in series. Thus, the matrix array would be better in general for studying saccade sequences such as in saccade remapping. By the same token, it would also be useful in examining the eye-position effect on visual or oculomotor functions, for instance, with respect to eye- versus head-centered coordinates.

The task for the animal was to make at least one saccade to each target, and water reward was delivered as soon as all targets had been visited. The order of visits was left up to the animal. Repeated saccades to the same target was permitted, as was saccades to non-targets. Constraints were set on the response period such that a trial would be terminated if the total number of saccades exceeded two times that of targets (i.e., two saccades in trials with a single target, four with two targets, etc.) or the total elapsed time after the matrix onset surpassed 400 ms times the

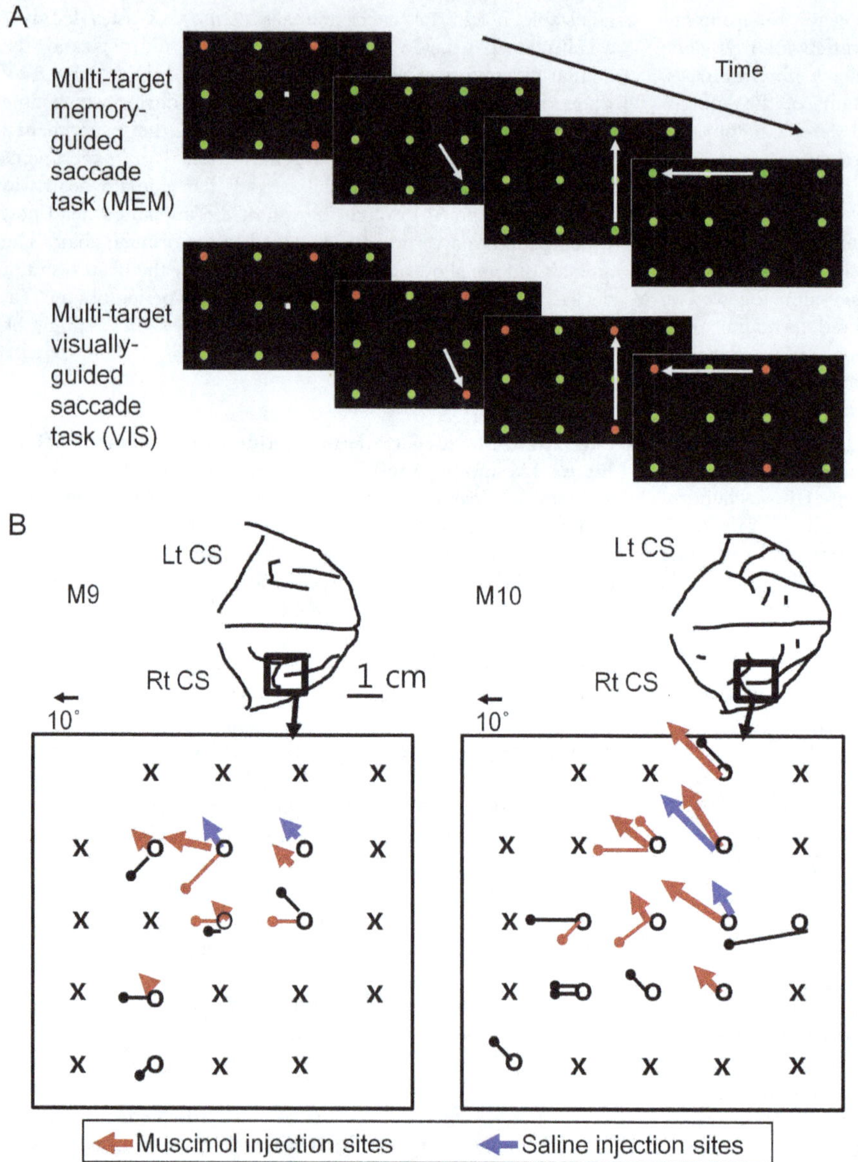

Figure 1. The behavioral tasks and the FEF inactivation sites are schematically depicted. (**A**) The multi-target visual short-term memory and pop-out search tasks. After fixation at the central square, a set of discs were shown in either red or green. The red discs were saccade targets defined by the color contrast. In the multi-target memory-guided saccade task (MEM, upper panel), the targets were rendered indistinguishable from non-targets as soon as the first saccade was initiated. The animal therefore had to rely on short-term memory for subsequent saccades. In the visually-guided saccade task (VIS, lower panel), the targets were visible while the animal made a series of saccades to each target, obviating the need for memory. (**B**) Sites in the FEF are shown where saccades were evoked by electrical stimulation (black circles). X's denote sites with no saccade evoked with the current level up to 300 microampere, and colored lines indicate that the current threshold of saccade evocation was lower than or equal to 50 microampere. Red and blue arrowheads mark the penetrations with injection of muscimol (red) or normal saline (blue), whereas a circular head indicates sites that were tested but not infused. Each arrow coming from a circle represents the vector of saccades evoked at the site and depth of injections. Some sites were penetrated more than once, and the lines were slightly shifted for clarity.

target number (for instance, 400 ms in single-target trials and 1600 ms in trials with four targets). However, once trained, the animals rarely reached these constraints, and the saccades formed an efficient and specific trajectory, stopping only on targets and once at each target.

Given these behavioral requirements, the chance levels in the memory task were calculated using a bootstrap method: Serial saccades to twelve target locations were numerically simulated using MATLAB (The Mathworks, Natick, MA, USA). Ten thousand blocks of forty sample-trials each were generated and trials were counted where the random series of saccades met the behavioral constraints for reward described above. According to this simulation, the chance levels of trial success rates are 16.6, 7.9, 5.7, and 5.1% for the target number of one through four, respectively, when the saccades were sequenced with the possibility of revisit to targets. When inhibition of return was imposed, the chance levels were higher at 16.6, 9.1, 9.0, and 14.1% for one to four targets, respectively.

2) The multi-target visually-guided saccade task (VIS, Figure 1A, lower panel). Events in this task were the same as in the MEM task above, except one feature that the red targets remained visible throughout the trial. Therefore, the animals did not need to rely on short-term memory to reach the second target and onwards. When there was only one target, VIS was identical to MEM.

VIS served as a baseline condition in comparison with MEM. In both tasks, saccade targets were selected based on salient color contrast. While VIS did not require memory of the targets, the planning and execution of sequential saccades was comparable with MEM. Other details, such as constraints on the response period and behavioral measures were the same in both.

Eye Tracking Data Acquisition

Eye movements were monitored by infrared video-oculography with a sampling rate of 500 Hz (Eyelink2, SR Research Ltd, Kanata, Ontario, Canada). Events in the tasks were controlled and saccade behavior measured on-line by custom-made applications written in MATLAB (The Mathworks, Natick, MA, USA). Markers were set for all experimental events for off-line analysis. The onset and offset of saccades were determined by velocity criteria (30°/s radial velocity for onset and 10°/s for offset). This was performed on-line to control the events in the behavioral tasks, such as detecting the first saccade and hiding targets in MEM. Correct detection of saccade onsets was confirmed during off-line data analysis.

Given the matrix arrangement of the visual stimuli, saccades were judged as directed to the nearest disc, regardless of the absolute distance from the disc to the saccade end-point. In other words, a saccade was judged as directed to a disc if it ended within a square window of 15-degree width and height centered at the disc.

Muscimol Inactivation

To identify and map the FEF (Figure 1B), tungsten electrodes (FHC Co., USA) were introduced through a guide tube positioned by a grid system (Crist Instruments Co., USA). A cortical sites of electrode penetration was regarded as within the FEF if a saccade was evoked with a probability greater than 0.5 by electrical stimulation (ES) with a current less than or equal to 50 microampere (negative-first biphasic pulses with 0.1 ms in each phase, 100 Hz train frequency, and 200 ms train duration). For each track of penetration, the electrode was slowly lowered by a electrical microdrive (NAN Instruments Ltd, Nazareth, Israel) and responses to ES were checked at every 0.5 mm interval in depth. The depth with the lowest threshold of ES-evoked saccades was marked on the way into the cortex and confirmed again on the way out.

An injectrode constructed using a 33-gauge hypodermic cannula was inserted at the same site as the electrode, and lowered slowly until its tip was located at the depth marked as having the minimal ES threshold. Muscimol (or saline in control experiments) was injected using a minipump (Aladdin 1000, World Precision Instruments, Sarasota, FL, USA). The muscimol concentration was five mg/ml, and the injected volume was one microliter over about two minutes. Following the injection, the cannula was left in place for about five minutes before it was withdrawn. Data collection began immediately before the injection and continued up to three hours. Data were also collected in the following day, and full recovery was always noted. The injection experiments including the saline control were separated by at least two days.

In order to obtain homogenous behavioral effects, muscimol injections were made at FEF sites where ES-evoked saccades were directed to the left either horizontally or with an upward component and the current threshold was lower than or equal to 50 microampere (penetrations marked by red arrows shown in Figure 1B, five sites in M9, and six in M10). For control experiments, two sites in each monkey were tested by injecting saline (penetrations marked by blue arrows in Figure 1B).

Behavioral Measures and Statistical Analysis

Two behavioral measures were assessed from the eye traces: (1) the trial success rate, or the proportion of trials rewarded, reflecting the overall performance in the tasks, and (2) the saccade proportion rate to each target location, i.e., the proportion of trials where at least one saccade was made to the location over trials in which a target was shown at that location. This measure was used to assess the spatial distribution of effects by FEF inactivation.

Two-way analysis-of-variance (ANOVA) was used to test statistical significance of the main effects of time after an injection and task type (i.e., with or without memory requirement) or target number. Interactions between post-injection time and task type or between post-injection time and target number were also tested. The Kruskal-Wallis test (a non-parametric one-way ANOVA) was used for comparisons over categorical variables. A threshold of $p<0.05$ was regarded as evidence of statistical significance, and the p values reported. All statistical analyses were conducted using MATLAB (Mathworks, Natick, MA).

Results

Performance in the MEM Task was Impaired during FEF Inactivation, but not in VIS

After a few months of training on the VIS and MEM tasks (Figure 1A), the performance of two rhesus monkeys (*Macaca mulatta*, M9 and M10) reached an asymptote. For both animals, the trial success rate (TSR) in four-target MEM was consistently lower than 50%. Since the animals often got frustrated with the low yield of reward and refused to work, MEM was tested only up to three targets in inactivation experiments. To use the reward sparingly, the VIS task was administered only with one or three targets, skipping the two-target condition. Mean TSR before FEF inactivation were: in VIS with one target and three targets, >99% for both animals; in MEM with two targets, 89% by M9 and 93% by M10; and in MEM with three targets, 67% by M9 and 79% by M10 (pre-injection data shown in Figure 2).

During reversible inactivation of the right FEF (sites with red arrows in Figure 1B) by muscimol, the performance in MEM was impaired (Figure 2): TSR declined over time following muscimol injection in the two- and three-target memory conditions (○ and •, respectively). The TSR data in MEM were tested using two-way ANOVA for two main factors: time after injection (a continuous variable) and number of targets per trial (NT, two versus three memory targets). Both main effects were significant as well as their interaction in both monkeys (two-way ANOVA, the time effect $F=62.7$, $p=3.9\times10^{-7}$, the NT effect $F=25.2$, $p=4.2\times10^{-8}$, the interaction $F=22.7$, $p=1.4\times10^{-7}$ for M9; time effect $F=29.9$, $p=2.9\times10^{-6}$, NT effect $F=12.3$, $p=7.1\times10^{-5}$, interaction $F=12.6$, $p=5.9\times10^{-5}$ for M10).

In contrast, the performance in VIS was unaffected by FEF inactivation. For both animals, the TSR in the one- and three-target search tasks (∇ and x in Figure 2, respectively) stayed close to one with no significant change after injection, regardless of target number (two-way ANOVA, time effect $F=2.8$, $p=0.10$, NT effect between one and three targets $F=0.3$, $p=0.57$, interaction $F=2.8$, $p=0.10$ for M9; time effect $F=1.4$, $p=0.24$, NT effect $F=0.05$, $p=0.83$, interaction $F=1.4$, $p=0.24$ for M10).

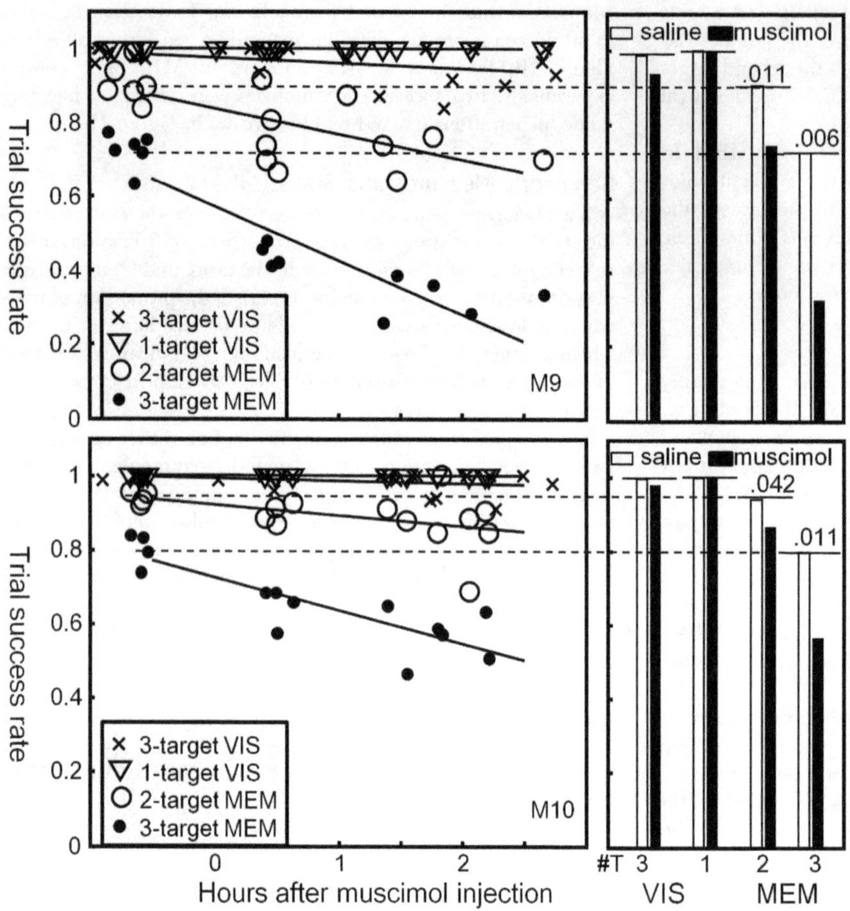

Figure 2. Effects of FEF inactivation on the overall performance of the multi-target memory- and visually-guided saccade tasks (MEM and VIS, respectively) are shown. The trial success rate, i.e., the ratio of rewarded trials over total trials, is plotted as a function of time after muscimol injection with regression lines. Shown are search conditions with one or three targets (▽ and x, respectively) and memory conditions with two or three targets (○ and ●, respectively). Data were pooled over five and six experiments with M9 and M10, respectively. Location of the inactivated FEF sites is given in Figure 1B. The bar graphs on the right represent the TSR more than one hour after muscimol (black bars) or saline injections (white bars). A significant difference ($p<0.05$) by the Kruskal-Wallis test between the two injection types was indicated by the p value above the bars. Horizontal dashed lines indicate the pre-injection TSR levels. #T: number of targets.

A direct comparison between the three-target MEM and VIS tasks confirmed the task effect (two-way ANOVA, time effect $F=70.1$, $p=7.1\times10^{-10}$, task effect between MEM and VIS $F=51.4$, $p=2.3\times10^{-8}$, interaction $F=47.0$, $p=5.9\times10^{-8}$ for M9; time effect $F=58.6$, $p=4.6\times10^{-7}$, task effect $F=47.8$, $p=4.3\times10^{-8}$, interaction $F=43.5$, $p=1.1\times10^{-7}$ for M10).

The specificity of muscimol injection was demonstrated in comparison with saline injection (Bar graphs on the right side in Figure 2): The performance after saline injection remained at the same level as before the injection (not different from the pre-injection levels indicated by horizontal lines in the figure), while it declined after muscimol injections. TSR more than one hour after muscimol (black bars) and saline injections (white bars) were statistically significantly different in the two- and three-target MEM conditions in both monkeys (p values given in the figure by the Kruskal-Wallis test).

The Impairment in MEM was not Attributable to Changes in Saccade Behavior

Minor changes in saccade latency and end-point accuracy were observed during FEF inactivation (Figures 3 and 4). There was an appreciable increase in dispersion of saccade endpoints around discs during the inactivation (Figure 3A), and the latency of first saccades in a series was delayed during inactivation by about 30 ms when they were directed contralesionally (Figure 3B). While consistent with previous observations [14,15,21], the slight increase in saccade inaccuracy and latency would not account for the decline in TSR in the MEM tasks, because the saccade dispersions were within the window boundaries set for detecting correctly targeted saccades (Figure 3A).

To delve into the reasons underlying the worse performance of MEM during FEF inactivation, saccade behavior was examined in detail. Specifically three aspects were considered as possible explanations for the TSR decline: overall frequency of generating saccades, relative frequency of saccades during rewarded and error trials, and target discriminability by individual saccades (Table 1).

First, we hypothesized that perhaps the animals became less prudent in saccade generation during FEF inactivation. Too many non-discriminatory saccades would have negatively affected the task performance, resulting in lower TSR. However, this hypothesis was not supported by the data: Both animals actually made significantly fewer saccades per trial when the FEF on one side was inactivated. As shown in the table, the total number of saccades per trial decreased by approximately 10%, in three-target

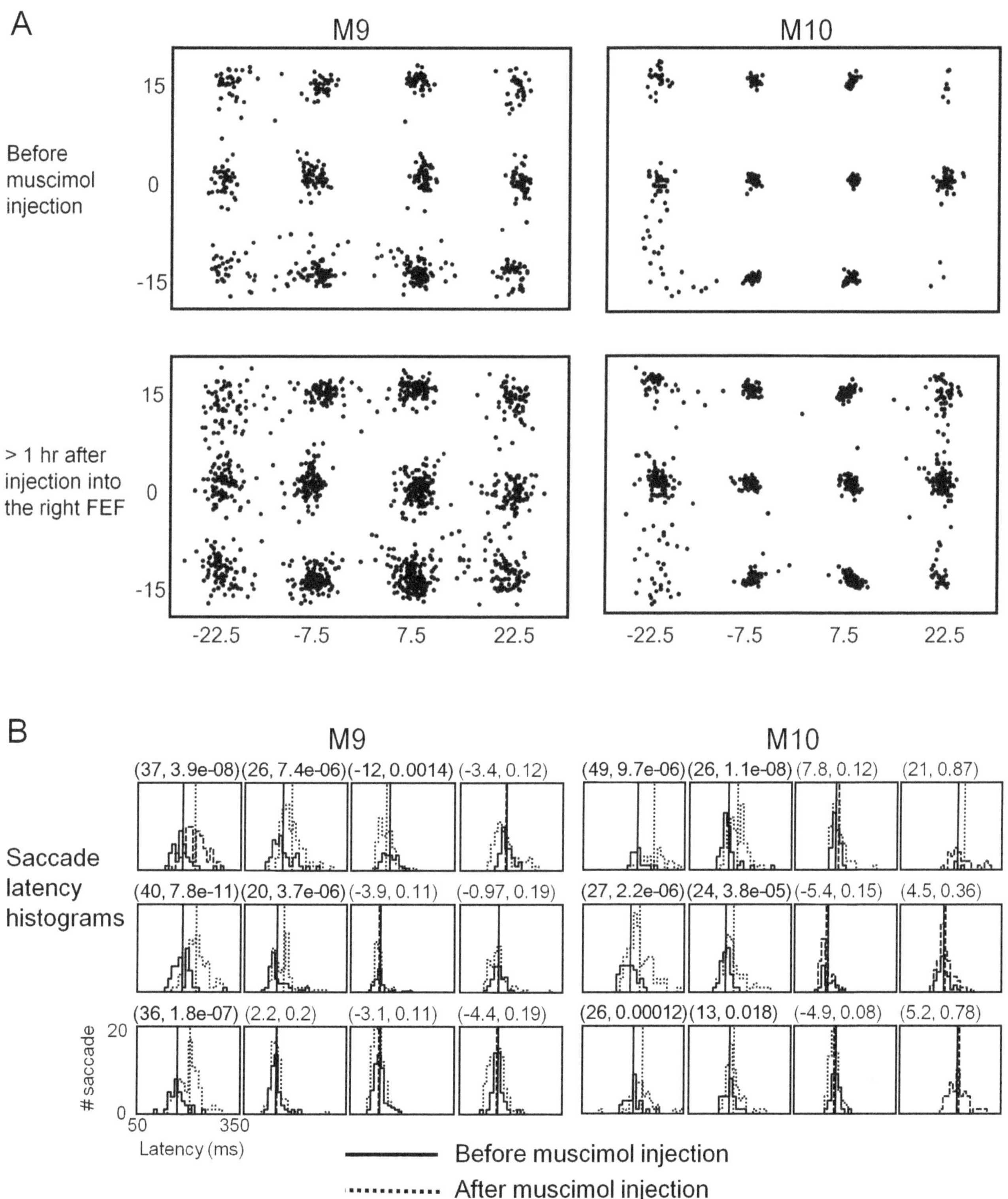

Figure 3. Minor effects on saccade parameters are observed during FEF inactivation. (**A**) The effect of FEF inactivation on the accuracy of saccades. End-points are shown of all saccades in three-target MEM sessions, before muscimol infusion into the right FEF (upper panels) and more than one hour after (lower panels). The post-muscimol data are pooled from multiple sessions to show approximately equal number of saccades to the contralesional locations. (**B**) FEF inactivation effect on saccade latency. The latency of the first, presumably visually-driven saccades are plotted in histograms, with the solid and broken curves representing data before and during inactivation, respectively. In each panel, the x axis indicates the latency in milliseconds, and the y axis the saccade count. Twelve panels in a set are arranged according to the target locations. The first number in a pair above each panel indicate the difference of median saccade latency (in ms) between pre- and post-injection data and the second the p value of the difference by the Kruskal-Wallis test. Significant differences ($p<0.05$) are printed in bold face. The latency increased by about 30 ms for contralesionally-directed visually-guided saccades during FEF inactivation.

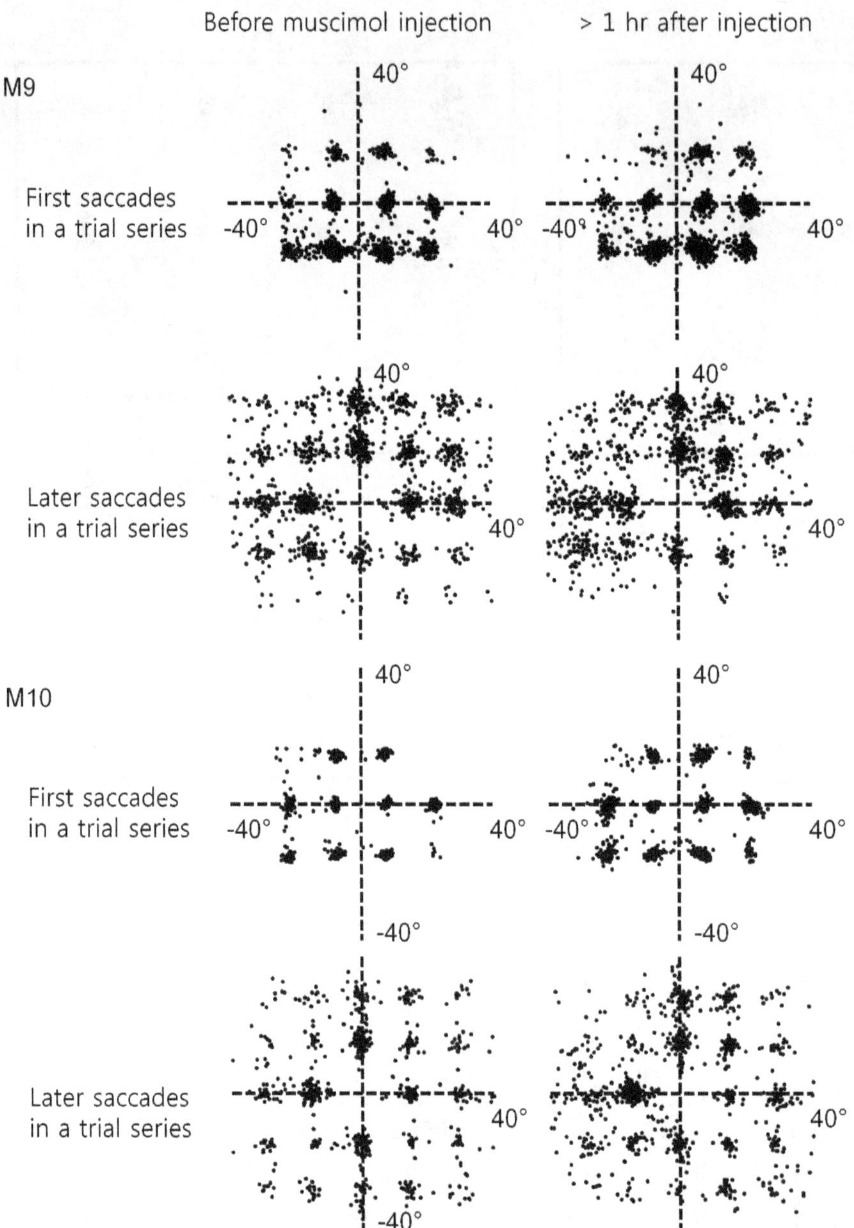

Figure 4. Saccade vectors for the three-target MEM task were comparable before and during FEF inactivation by muscimol. The first and later saccades of the saccade sequence in the trials were separately displayed. The data for M9 and M10 are shown in upper and lower sections, respectively. Both monkeys made downward saccades more often as the first saccade in the series. Note that later saccades driven by short-term memory tended to be multiples of 15 degrees in amplitude in both horizontal and vertical directions, which corresponded to the separation of discs in the matrix array. No obvious changes occurred during FEF inactivation, other than slight reduction in saccade frequency and increase in saccade vector variability when the saccade were directed contralesionally.

MEM. The data also showed that the reduction was more prominent with saccades directed contralateral to the inactivated FEF for both animals (the second column in Table 1). Therefore, the decrease in TSR did not appear to result from less prudent saccade behavior, but rather from a reduction of contralesionally-directed saccades. Now, the reduction in saccade counts occurred only in situations requiring a high-load of short-term memory, i.e., in three-target MEM, and not in three-target VIS where the animals made as many saccades to both hemifields after muscimol injections as before them (saccades per trial in 3-target VIS: from 3.82 to 3.78 with muscimol injection in M9, $p = 0.71$, paired t-test; 3.63–>3.65 in M10, $p = 0.56$). Thus, it appeared that FEF inactivation specifically affected the memory of saccade targets, rather than visual or oculomotor aspects in saccade behavior.

Second, we compared the number of saccades between rewarded and unrewarded trials. If indiscriminate saccade behavior was responsible for the failure in unrewarded trails, the saccade count would be higher in these trials. To the contrary, there was fewer saccades in unrewarded in both animals, consistent with our impression that the animals were skilled enough on the tasks to refrain from making unnecessary saccades when unsure of where the targets had been. The animal apparently maintained this strategy during FEF inactivation, making fewer saccades in unrewarded trials. Presumably, the

Table 1. The FEF inactivation effect on the number of saccades per trial in the three-target memory task.

M9	Total saccades per trial	Contralesional saccades	Rewarded trials	On-target sac	1.41 → 1.15*
	2.97 → 2.59**	1.52 → 1.08**	1.63 → 1.36*	Not on-target	0.21 → 0.21
				TDI (%)	87.0 → 84.6
			Unrewarded trials	On-target sac	0.92 → 0.67*
			1.30 → 0.90*	Not on-target	0.38 → 0.23*
				TDI (%)	71.5 → 74.8
		Ipsilesional saccades	Rewarded trials	On-target sac	1.50 → 1.78*
		1.45 → 1.51	1.60 → 1.90*	Not on-target	0.10 → 0.12
				TDI (%)	93.8 → 93.8
			Unrewarded trials	On-target sac	0.94 → 1.12**
			1.10 → 1.28**	Not on-target	0.16 → 0.16
				TDI (%)	85.0 → 87.7
M10	Total saccades per trial	Contralesional saccades	Rewarded trials	On-target sac	1.46 → 1.32
	3.10 → 2.84*	1.54 → 1.31*	1.65 → 1.53	Not on-target	0.19 → 0.21
				TDI (%)	88.4 → 86.6
			Unrewarded trials	On-target sac	0.88 → 0.76
			1.11 → 0.99	Not on-target	0.22 → 0.23
				TDI (%)	80.6 → 76.9
		Ipsilesional saccades	Rewarded trials	On-target sac	1.49 → 1.64*
		1.57 → 1.53*	1.67 → 1.78*	Not on-target	0.18 → 0.14
				TDI (%)	89.4 → 92.1
			Unrewarded trials	On-target sac	1.06 → 1.08
			1.17 → 1.18	Not on-target	0.11 → 0.11
				TDI (%)	90.9 → 91.2

The values are the averages over five and six muscimol-injection experiments for M9 and M10, respectively. The first number in an arrowed pair is the saccade count before the inactivation and the second that during inactivation. Statistically significant differences between the two counts were marked by asterisks (*: $p<0.05$; **: $p<0.01$, by two-tailed paired t test). TDI: target discrimination index (= on-target saccades/all saccades ×100).

mnemonic representation of saccade targets was weakened by the inactivation.

Third, target discrimination by saccades was unaffected by FEF inactivation. As given in Table 1, there was no change in the target discrimination index (TDI), or the ratio of on-target saccades over all saccades. Even when the overall performance was impaired by FEF inactivation, the animals made saccades very selectively to the targets, and avoided non-targets as successfully as before the inactivation. Therefore, the decline in TSR was not attributable to indiscriminate saccade behavior. By the same token, increased scatter in saccade end-points during inactivation (Figure 3) could not account for the TSR decline either. Despite the saccade motor errors, TDI remained high (Table 1), i.e., saccades discriminated targets from non-targets very well during inactivation.

The above analyses on saccade behavior together made it rather unlikely that abnormalities in saccade execution could account for the impairment in MEM during FEF inactivation.

The Impairment in MEM was Visual-field Specific and Load-dependent

To explore the relationship between spatial coding in the inactivated FEF sites and the memory impairment, we measured the saccade proportion to each target location, i.e., the proportion of trials in which at least one saccade was made to a location over all trials in which a target was shown at that location. Note that, per location, a target were shown $N * m/12$ times on average (N: the total number of trials, m: the target number on each trial), such that, if a total of 120 trials were administered, for each location, ten trials were expected to have a target at that location in the one-target VIS or MEM task, 20 trials in the two-target task, and so on. Therefore, the denominator of the saccade proportion varied depending on the target number in the tasks. On the other hand, the numerator in the saccade proportion was trials in which at least one saccade was made to a location on each trial. For this calculation, even if multiple saccades was made to a location on a single trial, the trial was counted only once. In this way, the saccade proportion was designed to quantify the saccade responses as a function of target location, normalizing the saccade behavior with respect to the target appearance in multi-target search and memory.

To evaluate the effect of FEF inactivation, the saccade proportion was compared before versus during FEF inactivation by a ratio (i.e., the saccade proportion ratio, SPR). Now, SPR close to one indicated no change in the saccade proportion, while zero meant complete disruption of memory saccades to a specific target location by the inactivation. (In theory, SPR can be higher than one, meaning better performance with FEF inactivation. However, no such case was observed in our experiments, likely because of the near-perfect performance before the inactivation.).

In the grayscale images of Figure 5A, SPRs were shown in a 3×4 matrix corresponding to 12 target locations in the visual fields. No

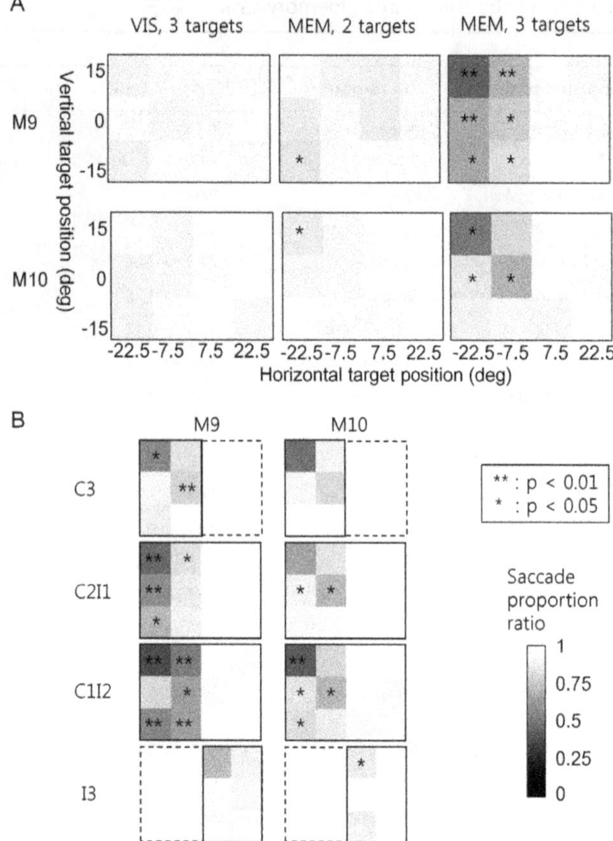

Figure 5. VSTM impairment during FEF inactivation was visual-field specific and dependent on target distribution. (**A**) Effects of FEF inactivation on the saccade behavior on each target location. The saccade proportion ratio (SPR) before and during inactivation is shown by grayscale images representing the layout of target locations. The saccade proportion is the proportion of trials in which a saccade was made to a target location over those where the target had appeared therein. Target locations in horizontal and vertical dimensions are marked in visual angle (degree). The saccade proportion decreased (SPR <1) during inactivation of the right FEF at target locations in the left upper visual fields, especially with the three-target memory (MEM) task. No decline of saccade proportion was observed with the multi-target search task (VIS). (**B**) FEF inactivation effects on the SPR as a function of the target distribution in the visual fields. The saccade proportion impairment was influenced by the layout of other accompanying targets in the three-target memory task. Trials were categorized into three groups by target distribution across the visual fields: C3 where all three targets were in the fields contralateral to muscimol infusion, C2I1 with two targets in contra- and one in ipsilateral fields, and so on. Visual fields in which the saccade proportion decreased during FEF inactivation were larger when more targets appeared in the ipsilateral fields (C3> C2I1> C1I2> I3). Asterisks indicate the p-values of paired t-tests comparing the saccade proportions before and during FEF inactivation: **, p<0.01; *, p<0.05. The grayscale bar is given at the bottom right, with the SPR ranging between zero and one.

changes in the saccade proportion were observed (SPR of about one) for three-target VIS (the left column in Figure 5A).

In contrast, in the two- and three-target MEM (middle and right panels, respectively, in Figure 5A), the SPR was less than one, especially at location on the left-top quadrant, indicating that the saccade proportion decreased during FEF inactivation at these locations. This indicated that the impairment of overall memory performance (as indicated by the TSR data in Figure 2) resulted from the failure to make memory-guided saccades to these specific visual fields, which matched with the direction of electrically evoked saccades before muscimol infusion (Figure 1B).

The Impairment of Multi-target Memory Depended on the Spatial Distribution of Targets

Given the spatially specific impairment in MEM, we next asked whether the memory failure was related to the deployment of visual attention at the time of target presentation. To investigate this possibility, we analyzed SPR as a function of spatial distribution of targets (Figure 5B). Trials were grouped according to the number of targets in the contra- or ipsi-lateral hemifields to the inactivated FEF: C3 (all three targets in the contralateral fields), C2I1 (two targets in contra- and one in ipsilateral fields), C1I2 (one contralateral and two ipsilateral targets), and I3 (all three targets in the ipsilateral fields). The rationale behind this grouping was that the accompanying targets would either boost or hinder attention to a target depending on where they were. For instance, a target in the inactivated field might be better remembered if other targets were on the same side, because attention drawn by these targets might enhance memory of the target. This was in fact what apparently happened in both animals: SPR at contralateral target locations (on the left side in each image in Figure 5B) decreased as a function of the number of targets in the opposite, ipsilateral hemi-field (C3> C2I1> C1I2). By the same token, the visual fields where the saccade proportion was negatively affected by FEF inactivation were larger, when more targets appeared in the ipsilateral fields (C3< C2I1< C1I2< I3). In the case of I3, the SPR decrease was observed even at the ipsilateral locations.

To check an alternative explanation for this target-distribution effect that the animals made more guessing saccades to the contralateral locations when targets had clustered on this side, the TDIs were compared across the trial groups. No significant difference was observed, regardless of the target distribution or the FEF inactivation.

Discussion

FEF Inactivation Reduced VSTM Capacity

FEF inactivation led to impairment of the multi-target memory-guided saccade task without significantly affecting serial saccades over the targets using salient color contrast. The impairment in MEM was load-dependent, and behaviorally speaking, the VSTM capacity was reduced by the inactivation. Based on the maximum number of targets that could be remembered in the MEM task, the VSTM capacity before FEF inactivation was estimated to be about three items. (This estimate included the first target which for sure was reached visually. However, whether this target entered and occupied a slot in the VSTM was not determinable in our experiments and tangential to the main findings in the study regarding the effect of FEF inactivation. Also, the estimate was obtained with the TSR of 50% regarded as the threshold. With a lower threshold, the estimate would be larger, without significantly altering our interpretations.) During the inactivation, the capacity was reduced to less than three in both animals: The performance in the three-target memory condition dropped to the chance level in M9, and to a significantly lower level in M10.

At the same time, the memory impairment was visual-field specific: it occurred only when a target was presented in the upper left visual fields, which matched with the direction of saccades electrically evoked at the inactivated FEF sites. Therefore, the FEF inactivation effect was conditional on both requirements, that is, high memory load and location of targets in the visual fields. Note in this regard that, while depicted in spatial coordinates of target locations, the memory deficit was in fact retinotopic since the animal fixated at the center when the targets were shown in the MEM task. The conjunction of visual-field specificity and memory-load dependence points to specific behavioral situations where the FEF are crucially required. This indicates that this cortical area is the neural structure where visual attention and VSTM interact with each other.

Only minor abnormalities in visually-guided saccades were observed during FEF inactivation previously (Figure 3) [13–16]. In keeping with this, normal performance was maintained in our multi-target search task (VIS in Figure 2), indicating that the inactivation did not significantly impinge on target detection and selection. On the other hand, serial saccades based on VSTM was impaired when the memory load approached the capacity limit. Given these findings, one may speculate that the size of neural population required for detecting and remembering the targets was different. Perhaps, a smaller population of FEF neurons would suffice for target detection than for short-term memory. Neurons that were relatively spared from inactivation could signal the targets for immediate saccades, but were unable to maintain the activity long enough over two saccades. Yet another possibility is that different neural elements are responsible for search versus memory: It is possible that visuo-movement neurons with sustained activity in the FEF [12] are crucial for the maintenance of target information, and inactivation of these neurons specifically would weaken the memory trace and hence impair the VSTM. Consistent with this notion of cell-type specific functions are the recent observations that shifts of gaze and shifts of attention may be carried out by different cell types [28] and even by different dopaminergic receptors [29] within this cortical area.

Implications on FEF's Role in Visual Attention and Short-term Memory

Current findings have a number of implications on the role played by the FEF in visual attention and VSTM [13–15,22,24,30]. First, the fact that FEF inactivation did not affect the performance in visual search was consistent with the previous demonstration that posterior parietal neurons signaled the target location earlier than those in the frontal cortex in a visual search task similar to ours [22] and also in the change detection paradigm [31]. Given the selective impairment of VSTM, the FEF seemed more crucially involved in maintaining the saliency information after it was coded. In keeping with this distinction, a recent human fMRI study reported that the FEF, but not the parietal cortices, showed sustained delay-period activity for both the short-term memory and the attention tasks [32].

Second, our findings implicate the FEF as a neural substrate for the VSTM capacity. The inactivation effect on the MEM performance was load-dependent, which in behavioral terms amounted to a reduction in the VSTM capacity. Location memory has long been modeled as consisting of storage slots that are discrete in the sense that the entry into the slots is in an approximately all-or-none manner and does not critically depend on attentional effort during encoding [33,34]. However, recently mounting evidence supports alternative views that the memory storage is not so discrete or fixed as previously assumed [35–37]. Whether entered into discrete slots [34] or encoded with variable precision [37], memory trace would first be established based on perceptual saliency which determines the priority of entry into the storage [38], and then sustained by FEF neurons.

The importance of the interaction between FEF and visual cortices for the VSTM capacity has been emphasized by a recent study where VSTM of location and object identity were investigated with functional MRI. FEF as well as parietal regions including the intraparietal sulcus exhibited activity related to the location VSTM [39]. Here, we demonstrated that FEF inactivation resulted in a reduction of VSTM capacity for target locations, and whether similar results will be obtained after inactivation of the parietal areas is certainly worth future investigation.

Third, the current results suggest that there is a dynamic competition during memory encoding of target locations, consistent with recent neurophysiological investigations using human [40] and non-human [31] subjects. In our study, the deficit in memory-guided saccades to the inactivated fields was exacerbated by accompanying targets in the opposite hemi-field, suggesting that concurrent neural activities encoding the targets inhibited one another. Furthermore, the competition was not confined to one FEF, but involved bilateral FEF's at the same time. Cross-hemispheric interaction must be at play, given that activation of the intact FEF by a target(s) contralateral to the affected fields worsened the memory failure, whereas co-activation of the inactivated FEF by additional targets near the affected fields ameliorated it.

These considerations are consistent with the following neural model on how the FEF normally functions in visual attention and VSTM: Being spatially coded and provided with visual signals from posterior cortices, FEF neurons may determine the entry of visual information into storage. As targets and non-targets are distinguished by color contrast, ensembles of FEF neurons get activated by neurons at more posterior parts of the brain, and a competition will start among the ensembles. The entry into VSTM storage will then depend on whether an ensemble grows beyond a size large enough to establish a self-sustaining activation. Important insights from our study are 1) that the size of FEF matters in this process: That is, the cortical area can concurrently support only a limited number of such large ensembles, and the entry into VSTM is allowed only up to this number. 2) Our data also suggest that the neuronal ensembles encoding saccade targets compete to recruit from the limited population of FEF neurons. The extent and the activity level of the competing ensembles of active neurons might represent the averaged sum of discrete resources assigned to slots in the slots-plus-averaging model [34] or correspond to the mnemonic representation of stimuli with variable gain and precision in the variable-precision model [37]. When a chemical lesion renders part of the FEF unexcitable, the number of self-sustainable ensembles will further decline resulting in a reduction of VSTM capacity. In this sense, the VSTM capacity is a behavioral manifestation of the limited expanse of neural tissue in FEF.

Limits of Our Experiments in Investigating VSTM

Our results alone could not determine whether the effect of FEF inactivation was on the memory trace *per se* or on updating the memory after saccades [41,42]. With this distinction in mind, we analyzed error trials and compared TSR as a function of the first-saccade direction: If our monkeys had behaved like a human patient with a right frontoparietal lesion who was impaired in double-step saccades only when the first saccade was contralesionally directed [43], the idea would be supported that FEF inactivation disrupted space remapping after the saccade by corollary discharge. However, there was no difference in TSR regardless of the direction of the first saccades: In the three-target memory condition and two-hours after muscimol injection, TSR of M9 were 0.36 and 0.37 with the first saccade directed contralesionally and ipsilesionally, respectively ($p = 0.65$, two-tailed paired t-test). Likewise, TSR of M10 was 0.61 and 0.57 ($p = 0.27$). Moreover, given the preserved performance in the two-target memory condition, it was clear that the mnemonic representation of the target for the second saccades was normally updated after the first saccades despite FEF inactivation, at least under low memory-load. Obviously, this finding does not necessarily rule out the FEF's role in saccade remapping: In fact, the muscimol effect might have accumulated over a sequence of saccade and hence the deficit was seen only with high memory-load. Given that human patients with remapping impairments between saccades had lesions involving the parietal lobe [43,44], inactivation experiments on the parietal oculomotor areas in monkeys might prove more elucidating in this regard.

Neither was determinable by our experiments whether mnemonic representations of the saccade target were rendered weaker in strength or fewer in number by FEF inactivation. Behaviorally, either situation would result in the same TSR decline, because we probed the memory trace by saccade responses and consequently the probing was stretched over time. With more targets to remember, the time taken by the saccade series also lengthened. Therefore, we cannot tell whether FEF inactivation have affected the memory by limiting the number of targets encoded, or by accelerating the memory decay over time.

An issue may be raised regarding the short and variable retention times in our memory task: Saccades were made immediately after visual encoding of the targets and the retention time for each target was variable because the saccade responses were made in sequence. Thus, our task might have tapped on the iconic memory [45], and the mnemonic representations of saccade targets might not have been stabilized when the saccade responses were triggered. This would not, however, invalidate our view that the deployment of spatial attention, as enacted by FEF, plays a pivotal role in the stabilization (i.e., encoding) process. In our opinion, whether the visual short-term memory capacity is imposed at the encoding stage or during stable retention is of some theoretical importance but probably indistinguishable in neural terms, given the highly dynamic nature of neural activity underlying the mnemonic representations [31].

Author Contributions

Conceived and designed the experiments: KML. Performed the experiments: KML KHA. Analyzed the data: KML KHA. Contributed reagents/materials/analysis tools: KML. Wrote the paper: KML.

References

1. Marois R, Ivanoff J (2005) Capacity limits of information processing in the brain. Trends Cogn Sci 9: 296–305.
2. Wright AA (2007) An experimental analysis of memory processing. J Exp Anal Behav 88: 405–433.
3. Heyselaar E, Johnston K, Paré M (2011) A change detection approach to study visual working memory of the macaque monkey. J Vis 11: 11.
4. Todd JJ, Marois R (2004) Capacity limit of visual short-term memory in human posterior parietal cortex. Nature 428: 751–754.
5. Vogel EK, Machizawa MG (2004) Neural activity predicts individual differences in visual working memory capacity. Nature 428: 748–751.
6. Luck SJ, Vogel EK (1997) The capacity of visual working memory for features and conjunctions. Nature 390: 279–281.
7. Cowan N (2001) The magical number 4 in short-term memory: a reconsideration of mental storage capacity. Behav Brain Sci 24: 87–114; discussion 114–185.
8. Wheeler ME, Treisman AM (2002) Binding in short-term visual memory. J Exp Psychol Gen 131: 48–64.
9. Elmore LC, Ma WJ, Magnotti JF, Leising KJ, Passaro AD, et al. (2011) Visual short-term memory compared in rhesus monkeys and humans. Curr Biol 21: 975–979.
10. Lara AH, Wallis JD (2012) Capacity and precision in an animal model of visual short-term memory. J Vis 12.
11. Inoue M, Mikami A, Ando I, Tsukada H (2004) Functional brain mapping of the macaque related to spatial working memory as revealed by PET. Cereb Cortex 14: 106–119.
12. Bruce CJ, Goldberg ME (1985) Primate frontal eye fields. I. Single neurons discharging before saccades. Journal of Neurophysiology 53: 603–635.
13. Dias EC, Kiesau M, Segraves MA (1995) Acute activation and inactivation of macaque frontal eye field with GABA-related drugs. Journal of Neurophysiology 74: 2744–2748.
14. Sommer MA, Tehovnik EJ (1997) Reversible inactivation of macaque frontal eye field. Exp Brain Res 116: 229–249.
15. Dias EC, Segraves MA (1999) Muscimol-induced inactivation of monkey frontal eye field: effects on visually and memory-guided saccades. J Neurophysiol 81: 2191–2214.
16. Keller EL, Lee KM, Park SW, Hill JA (2008) Effect of inactivation of the cortical frontal eye field on saccades generated in a choice response paradigm. J Neurophysiol 100: 2726–2737.
17. Alvarez GA, Cavanagh P (2005) Independent resources for attentional tracking in the left and right visual hemifields. Psychol Sci 16: 637–643.
18. Umemoto A, Drew T, Ester EF, Awh E (2010) A bilateral advantage for storage in visual working memory. Cognition 117: 69–79.
19. Alvarez GA, Gill J, Cavanagh P (2012) Anatomical constraints on attention: hemifield independence is a signature of multifocal spatial selection. J Vis 12: 9.
20. Schall JD, Hanes DP (1993) Neural basis of saccade target selection in frontal eye field during visual search. Nature 366: 467–469.
21. Wardak C, Ibos G, Duhamel JR, Olivier E (2006) Contribution of the monkey frontal eye field to covert visual attention. J Neurosci 26: 4228–4235.
22. Buschman TJ, Miller EK (2007) Top-down versus bottom-up control of attention in the prefrontal and posterior parietal cortices. Science 315: 1860–1862.
23. Monosov IE, Thompson KG (2009) Frontal eye field activity enhances object identification during covert visual search. J Neurophysiol 102: 3656–3672.
24. Buschman TJ, Miller EK (2009) Serial, covert shifts of attention during visual search are reflected by the frontal eye fields and correlated with population oscillations. Neuron 63: 386–396.
25. Wardak C, Vanduffel W, Orban GA (2010) Searching for a salient target involves frontal regions. Cereb Cortex 20: 2464–2477.
26. AVMA Panel on Euthanasia (2001) 2000 Report of the AVMA Panel on Euthanasia. J Am Vet Med Assoc 218: 669–696.
27. Lee KM, Ahn KH, Keller EL (2012) Saccade generation by the frontal eye fields in rhesus monkeys is separable from visual detection and bottom-up attention shift. PLoS One 7: e39886.
28. Gregoriou GG, Gotts SJ, Desimone R (2012) Cell-type-specific synchronization of neural activity in FEF with V4 during attention. Neuron 73: 581–594.
29. Noudoost B, Moore T (2011) Control of visual cortical signals by prefrontal dopamine. Nature 474: 372–375.
30. Moore T, Fallah M (2004) Microstimulation of the frontal eye field and its effects on covert spatial attention. J Neurophysiol 91: 152–162.
31. Buschman TJ, Siegel M, Roy JE, Miller EK (2011) Neural substrates of cognitive capacity limitations. Proc Natl Acad Sci U S A 108: 11252–11255.
32. Offen S, Gardner JL, Schluppeck D, Heeger DJ (2010) Differential roles for frontal eye fields (FEFs) and intraparietal sulcus (IPS) in visual working memory and visual attention. J Vis 10: 28.
33. Rouder JN, Morey RD, Cowan N, Zwilling CE, Morey CC, et al. (2008) An assessment of fixed-capacity models of visual working memory. Proc Natl Acad Sci U S A 105: 5975–5979.
34. Zhang W, Luck SJ (2008) Discrete fixed-resolution representations in visual working memory. Nature 453: 233–235.
35. Bays PM, Husain M (2008) Dynamic shifts of limited working memory resources in human vision. Science 321: 851–854.
36. Cowan N, Rouder JN (2009) Comment on "Dynamic shifts of limited working memory resources in human vision". Science 323: 877; author reply 877.
37. van den Berg R, Shin H, Chou WC, George R, Ma WJ (2012) Variability in encoding precision accounts for visual short-term memory limitations. Proc Natl Acad Sci U S A 109: 8780–8785.
38. Spence C, Parise C (2010) Prior-entry: a review. Conscious Cogn 19: 364–379.
39. Harrison A, Jolicoeur P, Marois R (2010) "What" and "where" in the intraparietal sulcus: an FMRI study of object identity and location in visual short-term memory. Cereb Cortex 20: 2478–2485.
40. Vogel EK, McCollough AW, Machizawa MG (2005) Neural measures reveal individual differences in controlling access to working memory. Nature 438: 500–503.
41. Colby CL, Goldberg ME (1999) Space and attention in parietal cortex. Annu Rev Neurosci 22: 319–349.
42. Bays PM, Husain M (2007) Spatial remapping of the visual world across saccades. Neuroreport 18: 1207–1213.
43. Duhamel JR, Goldberg ME, Fitzgibbon EJ, Sirigu A, Grafman J (1992) Saccadic dysmetria in a patient with a right frontoparietal lesion. The importance of corollary discharge for accurate spatial behaviour. Brain 115 (Pt 5): 1387–1402.
44. Pisella L, Mattingley JB (2004) The contribution of spatial remapping impairments to unilateral visual neglect. Neurosci Biobehav Rev 28: 181–200.
45. Lu ZL, Neuse J, Madigan S, Dosher BA (2005) Fast decay of iconic memory in observers with mild cognitive impairments. Proc Natl Acad Sci U S A 102: 1797–1802.

11

Integrating Fasciolosis Control in the Dry Cow Management: The Effect of Closantel Treatment on Milk Production

Johannes Charlier[1]*, Miel Hostens[2], Jos Jacobs[3], Bonny Van Ranst[4], Luc Duchateau[5], Jozef Vercruysse[1]

1 Department of Virology, Parasitology and Immunology, Faculty of Veterinary Medicine, Ghent University, Merelbeke, Belgium, **2** Department of Reproduction, Obstetrics and Herd Health, Faculty of Veterinary Medicine, Ghent University, Merelbeke, Belgium, **3** Elanco Animal Health, Vosselaar, Belgium, **4** Uniform-Agri BV, Assen, The Netherlands, **5** Department of Physiology and Biometrics, Faculty of Veterinary Medicine, Ghent University, Merelbeke, Belgium

Abstract

The liver fluke *Fasciola hepatica* is a parasite of ruminants with a worldwide distribution and an apparent increasing incidence in EU member states. Effective control in dairy cattle is hampered by the lack of flukicides with a zero-withdrawal time for milk, leaving the dry period as the only time that preventive treatment can be applied. Here, we present the results of a blinded, randomized and placebo-controlled trial on 11 dairy herds (402 animals) exposed to *F. hepatica* to 1) assess the effect of closantel treatment at dry-off (or 80–42 days before calving in first-calving heifers) on milk production parameters and 2) evaluate if a number of easy-to-use animal parameters is related to the milk production response after treatment. Closantel treatment resulted in a noticeable decrease of anti-*F. hepatica* antibody levels from 3–6 months after treatment onwards, a higher peak production (1.06 kg) and a slightly higher persistence (9%) of the lactation, resulting in a 305-day milk production increase of 303 kg. No effects of anthelmintic treatment were found on the average protein and fat content of the milk. Milk production responses after treatment were poor in meagre animals and clinically relevant higher milk production responses were observed in first-lactation animals and in cows with a high (0.3–0.5 optical density ratio (ODR)), but not a very high (≥0.5 ODR) *F. hepatica* ELISA result on a milk sample from the previous lactation. We conclude that in dairy herds exposed to *F. hepatica*, flukicide treatment at dry-off is a useful strategy to reduce levels of exposure and increase milk production in the subsequent lactation. Moreover, the results suggest that treatment approaches that only target selected animals within a herd can be developed based on easy-to-use parameters.

Editor: Bernhard Kaltenboeck, Auburn University, United States of America

Funding: The research of JC was supported by the Agency for Innovation by Science and Technology of Flanders (IWT Vlaanderen, www.iwt.be, projectOZM090697). Additional financial support for this study was received from the E.U. (FP7 GLOWORM project - Grant agreement no 288975CP-TP-KBBE.2011.1.3-04, http://cordis.europa.eu/fp7) and Elanco Animal Health. The funders IWT Vlaanderen and EU FP7 had no role in study design, data collection and analysis, decision to publish, or preparation of the manuscript. Elanco Animal Health played a role in the study design and the writing of the paper and no role in the data collection and analysis and decision to publish.

Competing Interests: BVR is affiliated to Uniform-Agri BV. JJ is affiliated to Elanco Animal Health. This study was co-financed by Elanco Animal Health. Seponver® is a marketed product of Elanco Animal Health. Dairy Datawarehouse® is a marketed product of Uniform-Agri BV. There are no other patents, products in development or other marketed products to declare.

* E-mail: johannes.charlier@ugent.be

Introduction

The liver fluke *Fasciola hepatica* is a parasite of cattle and sheep with a worldwide distribution. The infection is transmitted by freshwater snails of the family Lymnaeidae. In Europe, the principal intermediate host for *F. hepatica* is the amphibious snail *Galba truncatula*. Under optimal conditions, it takes 6 weeks before an infected snail starts to shed infective cercariae. These cercariae encyst to metacercariae on grass, which are ingested by the final host during grazing. Within the cow, it takes approximately 12 weeks for the parasite to mature to the adult stage and produce eggs that are released via the cow's faeces on pasture [1]. In western Europe, the main period where cattle acquire new infections is the autumn [2].

Because the completion of the life cycle depends on the presence of suitable habitats for the intermediate host, the disease is characterized by a focal distribution [3,4]. Nonetheless, herd-level prevalences in cattle of 30% to 80% are commonly encountered across Western Europe [5,6,7]. Moreover, several studies report increasing incidences of fasciolosis in EU member states and this trend has been primarily attributed to climatic changes, supporting the overwintering of the intermediate host and of the metacercariae [7,8,9,10].

Fasciolosis in cattle is generally subclinical and the negative impact of infections on milk yield is well accepted [11]. Nonetheless, already in 1987 Dargie expressed his concern on the lack of studies to quantify this effect [12]. Very few properly controlled trials to assess the impact of flukicide treatment on milk yield were conducted since then. With the abolition of the E.U. milk quota regulations in 2015, European dairy producers face a future situation with more volatile output prices and competition [13]. In this context, quantification of the production impact of enzootic animal diseases and their control measures is crucial for supporting managerial decisions.

Traditionally, the anthelmintic control of fasciolosis is based on whole-herd treatments with flukicides during the winter period. These treatment schemes have been recommended because most flukicides only have a good activity against the adult stages of *F. hepatica*, which are present during the winter period [14,15]. However, with the disappearance of flukicides with a zero-withdrawal time for milk in most EU member states, such treatment schemes are no longer economically justifiable and the only period when flukicides can still be administered in lactating animals is during the dry period [16]. To date, no studies are available that evaluate the efficacy or impact on production of flukicide treatment during the dry period. Only few flukicides are registered for use in cows whose milk is used for human consumption, but recently the European Medicines Agency (EMA) recommended a provisional maximum residue limit (MRL) for closantel in milk of bovine and ovine species (EMA/CVMP/846853/2011) to avoid the creation of a therapeutic vacuum.

The objectives of this study were 1) to assess the effect of closantel treatment at dry-off on milk production parameters using a randomized and placebo-controlled study and 2) to evaluate if a number of easy-to-use animal parameters is related to the production response after treatment, allowing a more selective use of flukicides in the future.

Materials and Methods

Farm selection criteria

The study was conducted on 12 dairy herds located in Flanders (Belgium). The herds were selected based on the following criteria: (a) herds were naturally exposed to *F. hepatica* based on bulk tank milk ELISA result (≥0.8 optical density ratio (ODR)) indicative for economic losses induced by the infection [6] at the beginning of the trial (September 2010); (b) the animals involved did not receive flukicide treatment ≤6 months before the experimental treatment; (c) application of an average dry period ≥42 days in order to respect the provisional withdrawal period for milk of closantel and (d) storage of herd information and production data in UNIFORM-Agri software (Assen, The Netherlands) enabling standardized collection of the data.

Study design

This study was a blinded, randomized and controlled clinical trial evaluating the effect of treatment with closantel on milk production parameters and anti-*F. hepatica* antibody levels in milk samples. Animals were drenched with closantel 5% oral solution (Seponver®, Elanco Animal Health) or a placebo (the vehicle liquid of the drug without the active compound) at a dosage of 0.2 ml per kg bodyweight at dry-off. First-calf heifers were drenched between 80 and 42 days before the expected calving date. The active compound and the placebo were dispensed in identical bottles, uniquely labelled with a study and letter code. Nor the farmer, nor the herd veterinarian, nor the principle investigator (JC) knew which letter code corresponded to the active product or placebo. The key was stored at Janssen Animal Health (now Elanco Animal Health) and only revealed after data-analysis.

Treatments (closantel/placebo) were randomly assigned according to Taves' minimization method [17] assuring a proportional assignment of the treatments within herd, infection level (based on pre-treatment *F. hepatica* ELISA result), lactation number and production level.

The study was approved by the Federal Agency for Medicines and Health Products of Belgium, provided a provisional withdrawal time for milk of 42 days was respected (File number 09 VN 1617).

On farm measurements

The treatment assignments were communicated to the farmer through a hard copy list mentioning cow identification, expected calving date, target date of experimental treatment administration and treatment code. Treatments were performed by the farmer based on estimated bodyweight. At timing of treatment, the farmer was requested to complete the hard copy list with the body condition score (BCS) (according to [18]), estimated bodyweight, administered dose and date of treatment. The progress and compliance to the study was monitored through monthly telephonic contacts and three-monthly farm visits by the principal investigator.

Collection of milk samples and *Fasciola hepatica* milk ELISA

Bulk tank milk samples were collected with monthly intervals from the beginning of the study (September 2010) until July 2011. Individual milk samples from all lactating animals were collected with three-monthly intervals from July 2010 onwards. The samplings occurred as part of the routine samplings for quality control and milk production registration programmes in cooperation with Milk Control Centre Flanders (Lier, Belgium) and CRV (Arnhem, The Netherlands). The samples were immediately kept on ice during transport and stored at −20°C in the laboratory until analysis.

The collected milk samples were subjected to a *F. hepatica* ELISA as previously described [19]. This ELISA quantifies IgG antibodies binding to the excretory-secretory products of *F. hepatica* and the test results are expressed as ODR. The ELISA is based on the protocol as described by Salimi-Bejestani et al. [20] who reported a sensitivity and specificity when compared to serum ELISA results of 92% and 88%, respectively. The sensitivity and specificity of the ELISA applied on serum when compared to worm counts was estimated at 87% and 90%, respectively [21]. Animals with an ODR≥0.30 are considered positive for *F. hepatica*. In our study, the aim was to evaluate whether *F. hepatica* ELISA applied on individual milk samples in the previous lactation could be used to identify which animals would benefit most in terms of production responses to anthelmintic treatment.

Collection of production records and data processing

Production records from the participating herds were extracted from the Dairy Data Warehouse (UNIFORM-Agri, Assen, The Netherlands). The extracted variables were: kg milk, fat concentration (g/kg), protein concentration (g/kg), somatic cell count (SCC)/1000, breed, days in milk and lactation number. Depending on the production registration programme of the farm, milk production records were recorded on a daily, 4-weekly or 6-weekly basis.

Next, the milk production records were subjected to the MilkBot® lactation model (DairySight LLC, Argyle, New York) in order to obtain one aggregate measure of 305 day-milk production per cow lactation. This lactation model is designed for detecting and quantifying effects of disease or management interventions on milk production. The functional form of the MilkBot® lactation model was described by Ehrlich [22]. The model has been previously used to assess the effect of metabolic diseases on milk production [23] and demonstrated higher accuracy and precision than the current dairy herd improvement associations' method for calculating lactation yields in the United

States [24]. The model quantifies both the shape and magnitude of lactation curves as a set of parameter values, each of which is associated with a single aspect of lactation curve shape. The parameter "scale" is a measure of magnitude, without changing the shape of the curve. The parameter "ramp" measures the steepness of the post-parturient rise in production. The parameter "decay" is used to measure the rate of decline in production after the peak in milk production. Lactation curve analysis allows detecting changes in the distribution of production that are not apparent when only totals are analyzed.

Statistical data-analysis

The effect of closantel treatment on anti-*F. hepatica* antibody levels in individual milk samples was investigated by a linear mixed model with herd and cow as random effects and treatment (closantel/placebo), days after treatment and an interaction term between treatment and days after treatment as fixed effects. Because the herds were sampled at 3-monthly intervals, the variable 'days after treatment' was categorized in 3 intervals: '0–3 months', '3–6 months', '>6 months'.

The effect of closantel treatment on milk production parameters was investigated by a linear mixed model with the production parameter as outcome variable, herd as random effect and treatment (closantel/placebo) as fixed effect. Lactation number ('1st', '2nd', '3rd or higher'), breed and the natural logarithm of SCC/1000 were introduced as additional fixed effects because they were considered as potential confounding factors. One herd was excluded from the analysis because no SCC data were available. In addition, two cows with breed Brown Swiss and one with breed Friesian Red and White were removed from the analysis because they all belonged to the closantel group without counter parts in the placebo group. The evaluated production parameters were (predicted) 305 day milk production, the different lactation curve parameters (scale, ramp, decay), average fat content (g/kg), average protein content (g/kg) and Ln(SCC/1000). Cows were only included in the analysis if at least 3 separate production records over a time period of >3 months were available.

The relationship of animal parameters with the production response after treatment was evaluated using the model to estimate the effect of treatment of 305-day milk production. Continuous potential decision parameters (anti-*F. hepatica* antibody level and BCS) were categorized according to their quartiles. If more than one anti-*F. hepatica* antibody measurement was available pre-treatment, the average value was used for categorization. The treatment effect was estimated within each category of the pre-treatment anti-*F. hepatica* antibody level, BCS centred to the herd mean, year quarter of treatment and lactation number.

All statistical analyses were carried out with the PROC MIXED command in the software package SAS version 9.3 (SAS institute Inc., Cary, NC, USA). Normality of the residuals was checked by Q-Q plots. Heteroscedasticity was checked by plots of the residuals vs. predicted values. Additional diagnostic plots were performed to assess independence of the residuals and linearity of the means. Variance component estimation was based on restricted maximum likelihood and statistical significance of fixed effects was based on F-statistics.

Results

Herd characteristics before treatment and treatment allocation

Treatment records and ELISA results to analyse the effect of treatment on anti-*F. hepatica* antibody levels were available for 475 cows from 12 herds. The closantel and placebo group in this analysis consisted of 246 and 229 animals, respectively. The average anti-*F. hepatica* antibody level in individual milk samples in the period before treatment administration was similar in both treatment groups (Table 1).

Table 1. Number of cows, average ± standard deviation of anti-*F. hepatica* antibody levels before treatment and 305-day milk production in the lactation before treatment and distribution of breed, parity and year quarter of treatment in the 2 treatment groups.

Parameter	Closantel	Placebo
N° of cows	208	194
Anti-*F. hepatica* antibody level (ODR)	0.36±0.26	0.40±0.27
305-day milk production (kg)	9,012±1,661	9,059±1,742
Breed:		
Holstein Friesian	45.3	43.0
Dutch Friesian	6.5	5.2
Parity (%):		
1st	11.2	10.5
2nd	16.7	13.7
≥3rd	23.9	24.1
Year quarter:		
Jan–Mar	12.4	11.9
Apr–Jun	5.2	4.7
Jul–Sep	16.9	15.7
Oct–Dec	17.2	15.9

The analysis of the effect of treatment on milk production parameters was based on data from 402 cows from 11 herds. Table 1 shows the characteristics of the cows included in the analysis of the effect of treatment on milk production parameters: the 305-day milk production in the period before treatment was similar and the number of cows in the treatment groups, parity, breed and year quarter in which the treatment was performed was evenly distributed between the 2 treatment groups, indicating a successful treatment allocation.

Anti-*Fasciola hepatica* antibody levels in milk

The course of anti-*F. hepatica* antibody levels in bulk-tank milk during the study period is shown in Fig. 1A. Two months after the start of the trial, the mean bulk-tank milk antibody level showed a substantial decrease and subsequently remained at a more or less stable level. The course of anti-*F. hepatica* antibody levels in individual milk samples relative to the time post-treatment is shown Fig. 1B. The anti-*F. hepatica* antibody levels decreased after treatment in both the closantel and the placebo-group ($P<0.001$) with significantly lower antibody levels in the closantel group than in the placebo group ($P=0.05$). The interaction term between treatment and days after treatment was not significant ($P=0.11$). The proportion of the total variation in anti-*F. hepatica* antibody levels that resided at the herd, cow and residual level was 7, 51 and 42% respectively, indicating that there was a great variation in anti-*F. hepatica* antibody levels between cows within a herd.

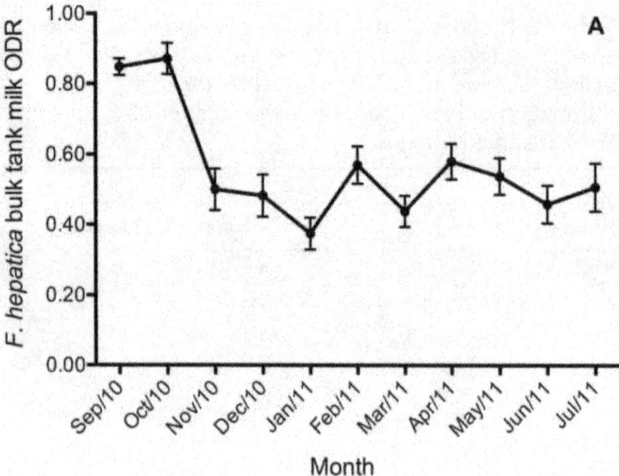

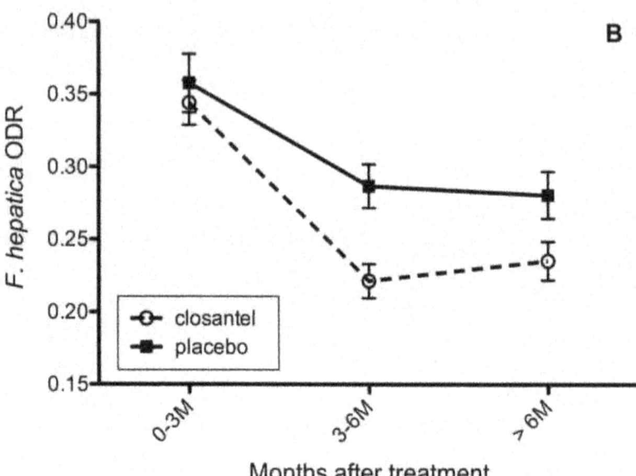

Figure 1. The course of anti-*F. hepatica* antibody levels (ODR) during the study period in bulk-tank milk samples from the 12 studied herds (A) and relative to the months after experimental treatment in individual milk samples of 475 cows in the 12 herds (B). Bars represent standard error of the mean.

Overall treatment effect on milk production

The results of the linear mixed model to evaluate the effect of closantel treatment on 305-day milk production are given in Table 2. After controlling for the factors lactation number, breed and somatic cell count, the 305-day milk production in the closantel group was increased by 303 kg ($P=0.026$), which corresponds to a milk production response of 0.99 kg/day per cow. No significant effects of anthelmintic treatment were found on the average protein ($P=0.93$) and fat content ($P=0.58$) of the milk produced or on somatic cell counts ($P=0.45$). Least square means of these variables in both treatment groups are given in Table 3. Finally, the MilkBot® parameters (scale, ramp, decay) in Table 3 and the resulting lactation curve in Fig. 2 show how the shape of the lactation curve was modified by treatment. The results suggest that closantel treatment resulted in a higher peak production and a slightly higher persistence (9%) of the lactation.

The relationship between animal parameters and the milk yield response after anthelmintic treatment

The effect of closantel treatment on milk production according to several potential decision parameters is given in Fig. 3. The

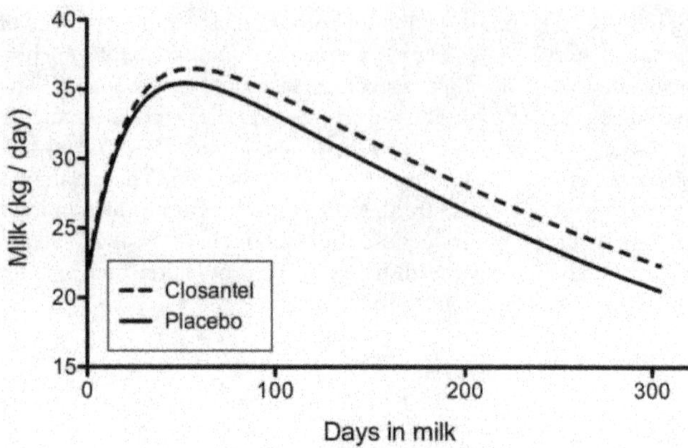

Figure 2. The average lactation curve of cows following treatment with closantel or a placebo at dry-off (Curves represent the data for Holstein Friesian cows in ≥3rd lactation).

highest treatment effect was found in cows with a pre-treatment *F. hepatica* ELISA result between 0.30 and 0.48 ODR (3rd quartile). In this category, the 305-day milk production was increased by 823 kg (95% confidence interval: 164, 1482). No treatment effect was observed in the highest *F. hepatica* ODR category (4th quartile). Other potential trends were greater milk production responses after closantel treatment in cows with increasing BCS, in cows treated during the third year quarter and in first-lactation cows. However, the 95%-confidence intervals of these categories all included 0.

Discussion

To our knowledge, this is the first blinded, randomized placebo-controlled study on the effect of fasciolicide treatment on milk yield. Previous studies only investigated associations between *F. hepatica* infection status and milk yield [19,25], or assessed the effect of chemotherapy but lacked a placebo-administered control group, randomization and follow-up during a whole lactation [26,27,28]. The anthelmintic treatments and the recording of potential decision parameters were performed by the farmers, therefore the results of this study are considered repeatable under field circumstances.

Previously, we showed that an increase in the anti-*F. hepatica* level in bulk tank milk over the interquartile range was associated with a drop in the annual average milk yield of 3% [19]. Here, we show that these losses are to a large extent recoverable by anthelmintic treatment. Closantel treatment at dry-off resulted in a 3.3% increase in milk yield (1 kg/cow per day) in the subsequent lactation. This effect was mainly due to a better start-off of the lactation with a steeper rise in production and a higher peak production, suggesting it is induced by an improved liver metabolism post-partum. The observed effect of 3.3% increase in milk yield is considerably lower than in previous studies where milk production responses up to 8 and 15% after flukicide treatment are reported [26,27]. However, these authors failed to monitor milk production over a whole lactation and such production responses may thus be realistic on a short term or in individual animals as observed here in animals with a *F. hepatica* ODR between 0.3 and 0.5, but not on an average basis. Nonetheless, compared with the cost of an anthelmintic dose, a treatment response of 3.3% increase in milk yield represents approximately a 10-fold return on investment [29].

Table 2. The results of a linear mixed model to estimate the effect of closantel treatment at dry-off (or approximately 42 days before calving for heifers) on 305-day milk production in 11 herds exposed to *F. hepatica* (based on 402 cows).

Variable	β	S.E.	P
Intercept	10,685	544	<0.001
Closantel (vs. placebo)	303	135	0.026
Lactation number (baseline = 3rd and higher):			<0.001
First	−2,522	189	
Second	−543	163	
Breed (baseline = Holstein Friesian):			
Dutch Friesian	−256	259	0.324
Ln (SCC[a]/1000)	−158	61	0.009
Random effects	**Variance**	**S.E.**	**Proportion of total variance (%)**
Herd	2,007,621	924,635	53
Residual	1,812,943	130,498	47

[a]Somatic cell count.

In contrast to previous studies, we could not observe an effect of flukicide treatment on the fat content of the milk [28,30]. Because we investigated the effect of treatment on the average fat concentration over the whole lactation, such effect may still have been present on a short term after treatment, which was not detectable in our analysis.

We must recognize that probably not all of the observed effects on milk yield can be ascribed to reduction in the *F. hepatica* burden. Closantel is also active against other blood-feeding parasites of cattle such as *Haemonchus* spp. and *Hypoderma bovis* [31]. However, the prevalence of these parasites in dairy cows in the study area is low [32,33,34]. Moreover, the significant drop in anti-*F. hepatica* levels post-treatment suggests that the majority of the effect of closantel treatment on milk yield is caused by its activity against *F. hepatica*.

As reported in other studies [35,36], the difference in anti-*F. hepatica* antibody level between the 2 treatment groups could only be clearly observed >3 months post-treatment. The significant drop in anti-*F. hepatica* antibody levels suggests that treatment at dry-off resulted in a successful reduction of the worm burden, even if these treatments were applied throughout the year when immature stages of *F. hepatica* are present. Closantel has only a partial activity against immature stages (<9 weeks old) of *F. hepatica* in the cow [15,37]. However, in our study the population of immature stages may have been small. This is suggested by the decrease in anti-*F. hepatica* antibody levels that was observed in the placebo-treated animals and in the bulk-tank milk during the study. Low levels of reinfection may be attributed to the treatment of part of the herd and the climatic conditions that were considered unfavourable for the development of free-living stages of *F. hepatica* during the study period (2010–2011) (Based on the reports of the Prognosis Commission on liver fluke of the Netherlands; L. Moll, personal communication).

Table 3. Least square means[a] (standard error of the mean) of average protein and fat concentration and milk production parameters following treatment in the closantel and placebo group.

Variable	Closantel	Placebo	P
Average protein content (g/kg)	31.8 (0.6)	31.8 (0.6)	0.93
Average fat content (g/kg)	38.7 (0.9)	38.4 (0.9)	0.58
Ln (SCC[b]/1000)	5.05 (0.15)	4.96 (0.15)	0.45
Scale	43.59 (2.26)	42.53 (2.27)	0.14
Ramp	24.98 (0.89)	23.69 (0.91)	0.05
Decay	0.0022 (0.00009)	0.0024 (0.00009)	0.10

P-values evaluate the difference between the 2 treatment groups.
[a]Least square means for Holstein Friesian Cows in ≥3rd lactation.
[b]Somatic cell count.

It is of major concern to food safety organisations and dairy cooperatives to prevent the presence of medicine residues above the MRL in commercialized milk. Selective use of flukicides will therefore become of increasing importance to reduce the consumer's risk of exposure to residues in milk. Moreover, selective use of anthelmintics is considered to reduce the development of anthelmintic resistance [38]. In this context, treatment at dry-off where only few individuals are treated at a given moment is a safer strategy than the traditional whole-herd treatments. Moreover, our results suggest that it is possible to identify animals within a herd that will benefit most from anthelmintic treatment by easy-to use animal parameters, thus enabling a more selective use of anthelmintics. The animal parameters were evaluated based on a randomized study. Therefore, observed differences are likely to have a causal relationship with the treatment.

Clinically relevant higher production responses after treatment were observed in animals with a pre-treatment ODR between 0.3 to 0.5, in animals with a higher BCS at dry-off (3rd quartile), in first-lactating animals and treatments administered in the 3rd year quarter. Higher treatment responses in the 3rd year quarter may be explained by the fact that this was in the beginning of the trial when the levels of infection were considered highest (see discussion above). Higher treatment responses in animals with a pre-treatment ODR >0.3 could be expected because animals above this threshold are considered infected with *F. hepatica.* However, the lack of milk yield response after treatment in the highest pre-treatment ODR category (0.5–1.5) is striking. There is no reason

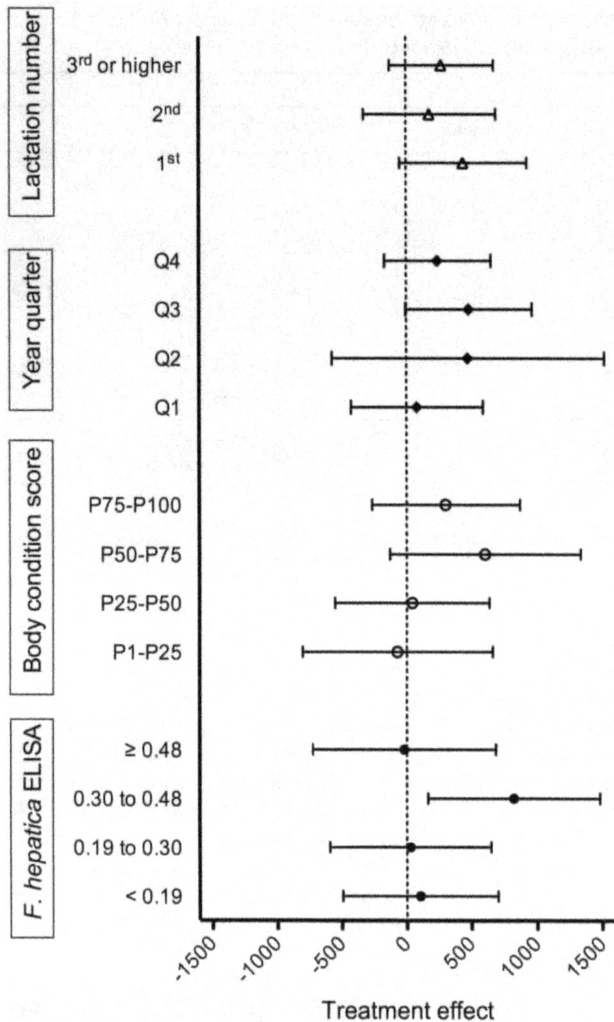

Figure 3. The estimated effect of closantel treatment at dry-off (or approximately 42 days before calving for heifers) on 305-day milk production according to several potential decision parameters for selective anthelmintic treatment. Error bars represent the 95%-confidence interval of the treatment-effect. Categories for *F. hepatica* ELISA results and body condition score represent quartiles.

to believe that this is related to lack of anthelmintic efficacy. However, it has been shown that *F. hepatica* ODR is correlated with infection intensity and extent of liver pathology [21,39,40] suggesting that remaining liver pathology after treatment prevented the occurrence of a clear production response in these animals. This was also suggested as the reason for lack of production response in retired dairy cows where closantel treatment efficiently removed the worm burden, but did not induce increased weight gain [41]. Alternatively, lack of production responses in very high-ODR animals could also be caused by a-specific reactions in the *F. hepatica* ELISA such as those that can occur in milk samples from mastitis-affected udders [42]. The observed relationship between BCS and milk yield response after treatment appears highly similar as the documented quadratic relationship between BCS around partus and subsequent milk production with an optimum milk production in cows with a BCS (on a 5-point scale) of 3.5 [43]. In our study poor production responses were observed in animals in the first and second quartile of BCS and highest production responses in animals in the third quartile of BCS. The greater milk yield with increasing BCS to an optimum is considered to be the result of a greater availability of energy for the cow. By comparison, the reduction in milk yield when the optimum calving BCS is surpassed is considered as the result of lower dry-matter intake in overconditioned cows [43]. BCS may thus be an important parameter for selective flukicide treatment, but our study did not look into potential weight gain responses after treatment in low BCS animals. Finally, the higher treatment responses in 1st lactation animals can be explained by the typical different quality of pastures grazed by heifers compared to milking cows. The better pastures are typically preserved for the milking cows; heifer pastures being more humid and displaying more vegetation diversity thus exhibiting a greater transmission potential for *F. hepatica* infection [4,44].

In conclusion, in this randomized controlled field study, we demonstrated that in dairy herds exposed to *F. hepatica*, closantel treatment at dry-off is a useful strategy to reduce the levels of infection with *F. hepatica* and increase milk production in the subsequent lactation. Production responses were highest in first-lactating animals and in animals with a high (0.3–0.5 ODR), but not very high (>0.5 ODR) anti-*F. hepatica* antibody level in pre-treatment milk samples, while they remained poor in meagre animals. We propose to use age and anti-*F. hepatica* antibody level in pre-treatment milk samples as easy-to-use animal parameters for selective treatment within a herd. This will likely reduce the risk of unwanted flukicide residues in milk. Further research is required to assess the economic impact of our findings and of selective treatment approaches.

Acknowledgments

We are very grateful to the participating farmers and their veterinarians; Stany Lens, Leo Van Leemput and Marcel Willemsen (Elanco Animal Health); Harm-Jan van der Beek and Jan De Pestel (UNIFORM-Agri); Luc De Meulemeester and Jean-Marie Van Crombrugge (Milk Control Centre Flanders) and Hugo Verstraeten (CRV) without whose support this study would not have been possible. Jim Ehrlich is thanked for the provision of the MilkBot® lactation model.

Author Contributions

Conceived and designed the experiments: JC BVR LD JJ JV. Performed the experiments: JC. Analyzed the data: JC MH LD. Contributed reagents/materials/analysis tools: JJ. Wrote the paper: JC MH JJ LD JV.

References

1. Andrews SJ (1999) The life cycle of *Fasciola hepatica*. In: Dalton JP editor. Fasciolosis. Oxon: CABI Publishing. pp. 1–20.
2. Gaasenbeek CPH, Over HJ, Noorman N, de Leeuw WA (1992) An epidemiological study of *Fasciola hepatica* in The Netherlands. Vet Quart 14: 140–144.
3. Zukowksi SH, Wilkerson GW, Malone JB (1993) Fasciolosis in cattle in Louisiana. II. Development of a system to use soil maps in a geographic information system to estimate disease risk on Louisiana coastal marsh rangeland. Vet Parasitol 47: 51–65.
4. Charlier J, Bennema SC, Caron Y, Counotte M, Ducheyne E, et al. (2011) Towards assessing fine-scale indicators for the spatial transmission risk of *Fasciola hepatica* in cattle. Geospatial Health 5: 239–245.
5. Mezo M, González-Warleta M, Castro-Hermida JA, Ubeira FM (2008) Evaluation of the flukicide treatment policy for dairy cattle in Galicia (NW Spain). Vet Parasitol 157: 235–243.
6. Bennema S, Vercruysse J, Claerebout E, Schnieder T, Strube C, et al. (2009) The use of bulk-tank milk ELISAs to assess the spatial distribution of *Fasciola hepatica, Ostertagia ostertagi* and *Dictyocaulus viviparus* in dairy cattle in Flanders (Belgium). Vet Parasitol 165: 51–57.

7. McCann CM, Baylis M, Williams DJL (2010) Seroprevalence and spatial distribution of *Fasciola hepatica*-infected dairy herds in England and Wales. Vet Rec 166: 612–617.
8. van Dijk J, Sargison ND, Kenyon F, Skuce PJ (2010). Climate change and infectious disease: helminthological challenges to farmed ruminants in temperate regions. Animal 3: 377–392.
9. Fox NJ, White PCL, McClean CJ, Marion G, Evans A, et al. (2011) Predicting impacts of climate change on *Fasciola hepatica* risk. Plos One, e16126.
10. Fairweather I (2011) Reducing the future threat from (liver) fluke: realistic prospect or quixotic fantasy? Vet Parasitol 180: 133–14
11. Torgerson P, Claxton J (1999) Epidemiology and Control. In: Dalton JP editor. Fasciolosis. Oxon: CABI Publishing. pp. 113–149.
12. Dargie JD (1987) The impact on production and mechanisms of pathogenesis of trematode infections in cattle and sheep. Int J Parasitol 17: 453–463.
13. Jongeneel RC, van Berkum S, de Bont C, van Bruchem C, Helming J, et al. (2010) European dairy policy in the years to come: Quota abolition and competitiveness. LEI, The Hague, Report N°. 2010-017.
14. Bossaert K, Lonneux J-F, Losson B, Peeters J (1999) Fasciolosis incidence forecasts in Belgium by means of climatic data. Ann Méd Vét 143: 201–210.
15. Fairweather I, Boray JC (1999) Fasciolicides: efficacy, actions, resistance and its management. Vet J 158: 81–112.
16. O' Brien B, Jordan K, Danaher M (2010) Update on the use of flukicides. Irish Vet J 63: 702–704.
17. Staquet M, Dalesio O (1990) Designs for phase III trials. In: Buyse ME, Staquet MJ, Sylvester RJ editors. Cancer Clinical Trials Methods and Practice. Oxford: Oxford University Press. pp. 260–275.
18. Edmonson AJ, Lean IJ, Weaver LD, Farver T, Webster G (1989) A body condition scoring chart for holstein dairy-cows. J Dairy Sci 72: 68–78.
19. Charlier J, Duchateau L, Claerebout E, Williams D, Vercruysse J (2007) Associations between anti-*Fasciola hepatica* antibody levels in bulk-tank milk samples and production parameters in dairy herds. Prev Vet Med 78: 57–66.
20. Salimi-Bejestani MR, Daniel R, Cripps P, Felstead S, Williams DJL (2007) Evaluation of an enzyme-linked immunosorbent assay for detection of antibodies to *Fasciola hepatica* in milk. Vet Parasitol 149: 290–293.
21. Charlier J, De Meulemeester L, Claerebout E, Williams D, Vercruysse J (2008) Qualitative and quantitative evaluation of coprological and serological techniques for the diagnosis of fasciolosis in cattle. Vet Parasitol 153: 44–51.
22. Ehrlich J (2011) Quantifying shape of lactation curves, and benchmark curves for common dairy breeds and parities. Bovine Practioner 45: 88–95.
23. Hostens M, Ehrlich J, Van Ranst B, Opsomer G (2012) On farm evaluation of the effect of metabolic diseases on the shape of the lactation curve in dairy cows through the Milkbot lactation model. J Dairy Sci 95: 2988–3007.
24. Cole JB, Ehrlich JL, Null DJ (2012) Projecting milk yield using best prediction and the milkbot lactation model. J Dairy Sci 95: 4041–4044.
25. Mezo M, González-Warleta M, Castro-Hermida JA, Muiño L, Ubeira FM (2011). Association between anti-*F. hepatica* antibody levels in milk and production losses in dairy cows. Vet Parasitol 180: 237–242.
26. Ross JG (1970) The economics of *Fasciola hepatica* infections in cattle. Br Vet J 126: 13–15.
27. Randell WF, Bradley RE (1980) Effects of hexachlorethane on the milk yields of dairy cows in North Florida infected with *Fasciola hepatica*. Am J Vet Res 41: 262–263.
28. Khan MK, Sajid MS, Khan MN, Iqbal Z, Arshad M, et al. (2011) Point prevalence of bovine fascioliasis and the influence of chemotherapy on the milk yield in a lactating bovine population from the district of Toba Tek Singh, Pakistan. J Helminthol 85: 334–338.
29. Charlier J, Van der Voort M, Hogeveen H, Vercruysse J (2012) ParaCalc® - a novel tool to estimate the costs of worm infections on the dairy herd. Vet Parasitol 184: 204–211.
30. Black NM, Froyd G (1972) The possible influence of liver fluke infestation on milk quality. Vet Rec 90: 71–72.
31. Guerrero J (1984) Closantel: a review of its antiparasitic activity. Prev Vet Med 2: 317–327.
32. Agneessens J, Claerebout E, Dorny P, Borgsteede FHM, Vercruysse J (2000) Nematode parasitism in adult dairy cows in Belgium. Vet Parasitol 90: 83–92.
33. Borgsteede FHM, Tibben J, Cornelissen JBWJ, Agneessens J, Gaasenbeek CPH (2000) Nematode parasites of adult dairy cattle in the Netherlands. Vet Parasitol 89: 287–296.
34. Haine D, Boelaert F, Pfeiffer DU, Saegerman C, Lonneux J-F, et al. (2004) Herd-level seroprevalence and risk-mapping of bovine hypodermosis in Belgian cattle herds. Prev Vet Med 65: 93–104.
35. Levieux D, Levieux A, Mage C, Garel J-P (1992) Immunological detection of chemotherapeutic success in bovine fasciolosis using the specific antigen f2. Vet Parasitol 45: 81–88.
36. Boulard C, Carreras F, Van Gool F (1995) Evaluation of nitroxynil and closantel activity using ELISA and egg counts against *Fasciola hepatica* in experimentally and naturally infected cattle. Vet Res 26: 249–255.
37. Hanna REB, Cromie L, Taylor SM, Couper A (2006) The effect of a parenteral ivermectin/closantel injection on the growth and reproductive development of early immature *Fasciola hepatica* in cattle. Vet Parasitol 142: 79–90.
38. van Wyk JA, Hoste H, Kaplan RM, Besier RB (2006) Targeted selective treatment for worm management – How do we sell rational programs to farmers? Vet Parasitol 139: 336–346.
39. Marcos LA, Yi P, Machicado A, Andrade R, Samalvides F, et al. (2007) Hepatic fibrosis and *Fasciola hepatica* in cattle. J Helminthol 81: 381–386.
40. Salimi-Bejestani MR, Cripps P, Williams DJL (2008) Evaluation of an ELISA to assess the intensity of *Fasciola hepatica* infection in cattle. Vet Rec 162:109–111.
41. Mage C, Levieux D, Bernabe P, Degez P (1993) Liver fluke therapy by closantel in culled dairy cows. Revue Méd Vét 144: 425–429.
42. Charlier J, Duchateau L, Vangroenweghe F, Claerebout E, Burvenich C, et al. (2006) The effect of an experimentally induced acute mastitis on the test results of an *Ostertagia ostertagi* ELISA. Vet Parasitol 136: 161–165.
43. Roche JR, Friggens NC, Kay JK, Fisher MW, Stafford KJ, et al. (2009) Invited review: Body condition score and its association with dairy cow productivity, health, and welfare. J Dairy Sci 92: 5769–5801.
44. Rondelaud D, Hourdin P, Vignoles P, Dreyfuss G, Cabaret J (2011) The detection of snail host habitats in liver fluke infected farms by use of plant indicators. Vet Parasitol 181: 166–173.

Experimental Feeding of *Hydrilla verticillata* Colonized by Stigonematales Cyanobacteria Induces Vacuolar Myelinopathy in Painted Turtles (*Chrysemys picta*)

Albert D. Mercurio[1,2]*, Sonia M. Hernandez[1,2], John C. Maerz[1], Michael J. Yabsley[1,2], Angela E. Ellis[3], Amanda L. Coleman[1], Leslie M. Shelnutt[4], John R. Fischer[2], Susan B. Wilde[1]

1 D. B. Warnell School of Forestry and Natural Resources, University of Georgia, Athens, Georgia, United States of America, **2** Southeastern Cooperative Wildlife Disease Study (SCWDS), Department of Population Health, Wildlife Health Building, College of Veterinary Medicine, University of Georgia, Athens, Georgia, United States of America, **3** The Athens Veterinary Diagnostic Laboratory, College of Veterinary Medicine, University of Georgia, Athens, Georgia, United States of America, **4** The University of Georgia College of Veterinary Medicine, University of Georgia, Athens, Georgia, United States of America

Abstract

Vacuolar myelinopathy (VM) is a neurologic disease primarily found in birds that occurs when wildlife ingest submerged aquatic vegetation colonized by an uncharacterized toxin-producing cyanobacterium (hereafter "UCB" for "uncharacterized cyanobacterium"). Turtles are among the closest extant relatives of birds and many species directly and/or indirectly consume aquatic vegetation. However, it is unknown whether turtles can develop VM. We conducted a feeding trial to determine whether painted turtles (*Chrysemys picta*) would develop VM after feeding on *Hydrilla* (*Hydrilla verticillata*), colonized by the UCB (*Hydrilla* is the most common "host" of UCB). We hypothesized turtles fed *Hydrilla* colonized by the UCB would exhibit neurologic impairment and vacuolation of nervous tissues, whereas turtles fed *Hydrilla* free of the UCB would not. The ability of *Hydrilla* colonized by the UCB to cause VM (hereafter, "toxicity") was verified by feeding it to domestic chickens (*Gallus gallus domesticus*) or necropsy of field collected American coots (*Fulica americana*) captured at the site of *Hydrilla* collections. We randomly assigned ten wild-caught turtles into toxic or non-toxic *Hydrilla* feeding groups and delivered the diets for up to 97 days. Between days 82 and 89, all turtles fed toxic *Hydrilla* displayed physical and/or neurologic impairment. Histologic examination of the brain and spinal cord revealed vacuolations in all treatment turtles. None of the control turtles exhibited neurologic impairment or had detectable brain or spinal cord vacuolations. This is the first evidence that freshwater turtles can become neurologically impaired and develop vacuolations after consuming toxic *Hydrilla* colonized with the UCB. The southeastern United States, where outbreaks of VM occur regularly and where vegetation colonized by the UCB is common, is also a global hotspot of freshwater turtle diversity. Our results suggest that further investigations into the effect of the putative UCB toxin on wild turtles *in situ* are warranted.

Editor: Mónica V. Cunha, INIAV, I.P.- National Institute of Agriculture and Veterinary Research, Portugal

Funding: Funding was provided by The University of Georgia Graduate School, The D. B. Warnell school of Forestry and Natural Resources, The National Institutes of Health (NIH R15 #1R15AI089565-01), The United States Army Corps of Engineers (W912HZ-12-2-0013), and The United States Fish and Wildlife Service (F11AC00889). The funders had no role in study design, data collection and analysis, decision to publish, or preparation of the manuscript.

Competing Interests: The authors have declared that no competing interests exist.

* E-mail: mercurad@uga.edu

Introduction

Vacuolar myelinopathy (VM) is a neurologic syndrome that primarily affects birds associated with freshwater habitats. The effects of VM on wild birds are documented for American coots (*Fulica americana*), bald eagles (*Haliaeetus leucocephalus*), mallards (*Anas platyrhynchos*), ring-necked ducks (*Aythya collaris*), buffleheads (*Bucephala albeola*), Canada geese (*Branta canadensis*), great horned owls (*Bubo virginianus*), and killdeer (*Charadrius vociferus*) in approximately 20 southeastern U.S. reservoirs ranging from Texas to North Carolina [1,3–5]. It is thought that birds develop VM by directly or indirectly consuming aquatic vegetation colonized by a novel species of epiphytic cyanobacteria in the order Stigonematales (hereafter "UCB" for "uncharacterized cyanobacterium") that produces a yet to be described toxin(s) [6,7]. The UCB grows in high abundance on *Hydrilla* (*Hydrilla verticillata*), a widespread invasive exotic plant, although it can also grow on several native aquatic plant species [6]. Birds may acquire the toxin(s) directly by ingesting plants that are colonized with the UCB or indirectly by feeding on herbivorous prey such as invertebrates [8] or other bird species that have fed on plants that are colonized with the UCB [9]. Affected birds develop microscopic vacuoles in the white matter of the central nervous system. Lesions tend to be most prominent in the optic tectum but can occur in the cerebrum, cerebellum, brain stem, or spinal cord. Degenerative lesions in peripheral nerves have rarely been reported. Ultrastructurally, vacuolation is due to splitting of myelin lamellae at the intraperiod line, consistent with intramyelinic edema. These lesions result in variable neurologic dysfunction that in severe cases can result in death within a few days [2–4,10].

A number of studies stress the need to evaluate the risk that consumption of vegetation colonized by the UCB poses to other taxa [11,12]. Previous work showed that grass carp (*Ctenopharyngodon idella*) experimentally fed *Hydrilla* colonized with the UCB developed vacuolations consistent with avian models, yet domestic pigs (*Sus domesticus*) and laboratory mice did not [5,13,14]. To date, there are no reports for any species representing the remaining major vertebrate lineages (amphibians or reptiles).

Freshwater turtles have a number of characteristics that, if susceptible to the putative UCB toxin(s), make them likely candidates to develop vacuolar myelinopathy. Turtles and crocodilians are members of the Archosauria and therefore are the closest extant relatives to birds [15]. The southeastern United States, the current location of VM outbreaks, is a global hotspot of freshwater turtle diversity with ~10% of the world's turtle species occurring in the region [16]. The vast majority of these turtles occur in freshwater, many species are omnivorous or herbivorous, and several feed extensively on submerged aquatic vegetation including *Hydrilla*, or on invertebrates that graze on epiphytic algae [17]; and turtles are known to be susceptible to other food chain-linked cyanotoxins [18]. Therefore, the objective of this study was to test the hypothesis that turtles fed *Hydrilla* colonized by the UCB and verified to be neurotoxic to birds would develop clinical signs of neurologic disease and histologic lesions similar to those of described in birds with vacuolar myelinopathy.

Focal turtle species

We selected painted turtles (*Chrysemys picta*) as our focal species for this study. Painted turtles are one of the most thoroughly studied turtle species in the world, and their husbandry protocols are well established [17,19]. They are abundant and readily available in regions where they occur and adapt well to captivity [20]. As a member of Emydidae, they are related to most of the turtle species in the southeastern U.S., and they are omnivorous but highly herbivorous as adults. We have documented *Hydrilla* in the gut contents of painted turtles in reservoirs experiencing VM epornitics (Mercurio et al. unpublished data) and they are known to feed on invertebrates that graze on epiphytic algae [17].

Materials and Methods

Ethics statement

All procedures were approved by the University of Georgia's Institutional Animal Care and Use Committee (A2012 02-001-Y2-A4). Field studies did not involve endangered or protected species and wildlife collections were permitted by the U.S. Fish and Wildlife Service (MB779238-0) and the Georgia Department of Natural Resources (29-WBH-12-95), which allow for the collection of wildlife from Georgia public state lands. In addition, the Henry County Water and Sewerage Authority provided permission to access Upper Towaliga Reservoir (33.3472°,−84.2145°). The University of Georgia Golf Course permitted access to a pond in Athens, GA (33.9041°, −83.3674°).

First *Hydrilla* collection

Approximately enough *Hydrilla* to fill three, 50 gallon coolers was collected from J. Strom Thurmond Reservoir (33.6972°,−82.2540°) on the border of Georgia and South Carolina during a VM epornitic and Lake Seminole on the Georgia-Florida border in December 2011. *Hydrilla* was transported within clean zip top plastic bags (3.79 l) on ice to the University of Georgia [12]. VM positive birds have been recovered in late fall from J. Strom Thurmond Reservoir annually since 1998 and *Hydrilla* in this reservoir is consistently colonized by the UCB [1,6]. Lake Seminole has never experienced a VM case, and the UCB has never been detected at this site [6]. Light and epifluorescent microscopy were used to confirm the presence/absence of the UCB following established methods [6,7]. Briefly, 5 representative leaves were wet mounted on a glass slide. Light microscopy and a rhodamine filter set were used to visualize cyanopigments on *Hydrilla* leaves and the presence/absence of the UCB colonies were documented via visual assessment. The rest of the *Hydrilla* was frozen at −20°C for 48 hours. To lyophilize the material, one gallon sized paper bags of frozen *Hydrilla* were then placed in the lyophilizing chamber of a Labconco Freeze Dryer 5 (Labconco, Kansas City, MO) at ~5 mm Hg for 48 hours or until completely dry. Once dry, *Hydrilla* was stored in sealed plastic bags in a temperature controlled facility at 26.6°C.

Validation of the toxicity of the first *Hydrilla* collection

Because some plant samples with the UCB do not induce VM when consumed, a feeding trial was conducted to determine the toxicity of the *Hydrilla* [21]. Domestic chickens (*Gallus gallus domesticus*) are susceptible to VM through dietary exposure of aquatic vegetation collected from sites where VM has been documented in wild birds [5]. A chicken feeding trial was conducted as previously described with the first collection of *Hydrilla* to assess its potential to induce VM [5]. Briefly, 4-week-old specific pathogen free leghorn chickens (0.8–1.5 kg, n = 10) were housed at the University of Georgia Poultry Diagnostic and Research Center in Horsfal (isolation) units. Once a week, chickens were weighed and received a full physical and neurologic exam consistent with previous trials [5,22,23]. Mentation, posture, attitude, movement, gait, postural reactions, spinal reflexes, and cranial nerve function were assessed. Limbs were palpated to evaluate asymmetry, masses, tenderness, contour, and tone. Birds were also weighed and observed for any superficial injuries. Chickens were allowed to acclimate to laboratory conditions for four days and were fed a non-medicated starter feed produced by the University of Georgia feed mill *ad libitum* (~30 g/kg bw/day) out of ceramic bowls. All chickens were in good body condition and no physical or neurologic abnormalities were noted at the beginning of the trial. Chickens were then randomly assigned to two treatment groups. Five treatment group birds were fed 30 g/kg bw/day of poultry starter feed and 2 g/kg bw/day of lyophilized *Hydrilla* colonized with the UCB from J. Strom Thurmond Reservoir for 28 days. The other five control group birds were fed the same volume of poultry starter feed and lyophilized *Hydrilla* free of the UCB from Lake Seminole. Each bird was monitored twice daily for clinical signs of VM (difficulty standing or ambulating, ataxia, loss of balance, limb paresis and/or head droop) and were weighed twice a week [10].

All chickens were humanely euthanized on day 28 with CO_2 followed by cervical dislocation. Calvaria were opened and partially removed with rongeurs to expose the dorsal surface of the brain. Brains were removed intact from the calvaria using a scalpel and/or scissors and immediately placed into 10% neutral buffered formaldehyde. Following ten days of fixation, brains were halved longitudinally. A single longitudinal section was then made 1–2 mm lateral to midline and an additional 1–2 transverse sections were made through the optic lobe. Resulting sections were placed whole into a cassette. These sections were routinely processed, embedded in paraffin, sectioned at 5 µm, and stained with hematoxylin and eosin prior to light microscopic examination by a veterinary pathologist [3]. All treatment chickens fed *Hydrilla* from J. Strom Thurmond Reservoir were bright, alert, responsive and eating well throughout the entire trial but developed very mild neurologic clinical signs (mild ataxia beginning on day seven until the end of the trial) and developed vacuolations consistent with VM, whereas none of the control birds fed *Hydrilla* from Lake Seminole developed clinical signs or vacuolations.

In December 2012, we collected more fresh *Hydrilla* (same volume) from Upper Towaliga Reservoir in Henry County, GA and from Lake Seminole (30.7428°,−84.8776°). Like J. Strom Thurmond Reservoir, Upper Towaliga Reservoir undergoes annual VM outbreaks and *Hydrilla* in this reservoir is routinely colonized by the UCB. This *Hydrilla* was collected during a VM epornitic at Upper Towaliga Reservoir and was transported on ice to the University of Georgia as previously described. The presence/absence of the UCB was verified via light and epifluorescent microscopy as previously described. VM lesions were verified in coots recovered from Upper Towaliga Reservoir during the fall of 2012 (Fischer et al. unpublished data). *Hydrilla* was frozen at−20°C in zip top plastic bags (3.79 l) and was thawed as needed.

Turtle feeding trial

Adult painted turtles (*Chrysemys picta*, straight carapace length >7 cm: 7 females, 3 males) were collected using canned sardine (Crown Prince, City of Industry, CA) baited hoop traps (model TN210; Memphis Net and Twine Co, Inc., Memphis, TN) from a pond in Athens, GA where an VM outbreak has never been documented and the UCB has never been documented. Turtles were individually transported in clean plastic bins to the Whitehall Herpetology Laboratory, a climate controlled facility, where we completed physical and neurologic exams as described below. The ten turtles were selected from a larger sample and were determined to be neurologically and physically normal. The turtles were housed individually in 37.8 l (50.8 cm×25.4 cm×30.48 cm) glass tanks following standard husbandry protocols [19]. Briefly, incandescent lights provided a 12 hour light cycle, the ambient temperature was maintained in the room at 26.6°C, water temperature at 24.4°C, and basking surfaces (clay bricks) at ~32.2°C. Fresh city water was supplied as needed to maintain a depth of 20 cm. Water quality was maintained using aquarium filters (Fluval Nano; Rolf C. Hagen Corp, Mansfield, MA). Each week the water was removed, the gravel was rinsed, the tank was scrubbed with a mild dish detergent and rinsed thoroughly, one half of the old water was replaced, and the tank was filled up to 20 cm with fresh water. Turtles were monitored daily for gross appearance, behavior, food consumption, mentation, and were allowed to acclimate to laboratory conditions and to our feeding delivery method for a minimum of 15 days. During this time they were fed ReptoMin floating turtle sticks (Spectrum Brands Inc., Melle, Germany) homogenized into a uniform powder and packed into transparent gelatin capsules (Capsuline Corporation, Pompano Beach, FL and Torpac Inc., Fairfield, NJ) at 0.02 kcal/g body weight/day, calculated using an allometric food calculator developed by the University of Georgia College of Veterinary Medicine Teaching Hospital [24].

Five turtles were randomly assigned into either a treatment *Hydrilla* or a control *Hydrilla* group. *Hydrilla* was fed to turtles in two ways to maximize consumption. The *Hydrilla* from the first collection with confirmed UCB toxicity status was packed into transparent gelatin capsules. To increase palatability and provide additional nutrition, capsules were coated in a mixture of sardine oil and ReptoMin prior to feeding. Each turtle was offered ~6 g/kg bw/day of their assigned *Hydrilla* diet in floating gelatin capsules. ReptoMin was also provided as needed to maintain each turtle's body weight relative to the start of the study. Starting on day 30 of the feeding trial, 50 g of intact floating *Hydrilla* from the second collection with confirmed UCB toxicity status was added to each tank each day to maximize *Hydrilla* consumption by turtles. The amount of the floating *Hydrilla* consumed each day was measured to the nearest 10 g. More accurate monitoring of material consumed was not possible because the turtles shredded *Hydrilla* during normal feeding activities.

Physical and neurologic exams

Turtles underwent a complete physical and neurologic exam once per week. Turtles were weighed and were observed for any obvious injuries, lesions, dysecdysis, or abrasions. A neurologic exam as described for reptiles in [25] and [24] was performed to assess the mental status, attitude, general activity, head and body posture, limb movement and coordination, gait, position in the water while swimming, and sensory and motor responses. Briefly, the turtles were first observed from a distance within their tanks for coordination while swimming, posture, and mentation prior to handling. The turtles were then removed from their tanks and held by the observer. The limbs were palpated to determine musculoskeletal symmetry, tone, strength, and tenderness. Reflexes were described as absent, reduced, normal, or clonus (where applicable) unless otherwise stated. Leg and head withdrawal reflexes and the ability to maintain their head position in a horizontal plane while rotated and listed in midair were assessed. The function of cranial nerves II, IV, and VII was assessed by inciting a menace response in a standard manner by obscuring the vision in one eye and making a slow threatening hand gesture to the other eye [24]. Cranial nerves III, IV, and VI functions were assessed by observing for strabismus (present/absent). Cranial nerve V function was evaluated by assessing mandibular movement during feeding (normal/abnormal). Cranial nerve VIII function was assessed by observing for nystagmus by moving the turtle's head side to side in a horizontal plane and observing the resulting movement of eyes. The presence/absence of nystagmus when the turtle was held stationary was also assessed. Cranial nerve VIII function was also assessed by observing for head tilting, rolling, and the righting reflex. The function of cranial nerves IX, XI, and XII was assessed by looking for signs of dysphagia. The turtles were then allowed to ambulate to evaluate symmetry of movement, gait, and posture.

Detection of vacuolations

At the conclusion of the trial (97 days) or if an individual developed neurologic signs, humane euthanasia was performed using an injection of sodium pentobarbital (100 mg/kg) [24] with a 22 gauge needle into the subcarapacial vein followed immediately by complete necropsy. Briefly, the plastron was removed using a striker saw to expose the coelomic cavity. Representative samples of liver, lungs, kidney, heart, spleen, gonads, stomach, and intestine were excised and placed into 10% neutral buffered formalin. An approximately 5 mm segment of skeletal muscle and peripheral nerve was excised from a rear leg. Brains were removed in a fashion similar to that previously described for the chickens with the exception that the proximal 2–5 mm of the spinal cord was also removed with the brain. The brain was halved longitudinally and halves were immediately placed into fixative (either 10% buffered formaldehyde for histopathology or chilled 2% glutaraldehyde, 2% paraformaldehyde, and 0.2% picric acid in a 0.1 M cacodylate buffer (pH 7.2) for transmission electron microscopy (EM). Following a fixation time of approximately 30 days, the formalin fixed half of the brain was sectioned transversely at approximately 2 mm intervals, resulting in 5 total sections that were placed into a divided cassette. Spinal cord was also sectioned transversely, resulting in 3–5 sections that were placed into a second cassette. Formalin fixed tissues were routinely processed, embedded, and stained as previously described for the chickens and were subsequently examined by a pathologist with experience in chelonian histopathology following previously described methods [9]. Subsequently one treatment and one control turtle were randomly selected for EM examination at the Electron Microscopy Laboratory at the University of Georgia [5]. Transmission electron microscopy specimens were post-fixed in 1% osmium tetroxide, serially dehydrated, infiltrated in an acetone/epoxy plastic, and then embedded in a plastic mold. Plastic blocks were cut with an ultramicrotome, and thick sections were stained with toluidine blue to identify optimal areas for thin sectioning. Thin sections were cut at 55–60 nm, placed on copper grids, and stained with uranyl acetate and lead citrate.

Statistical analysis

A Student's t-test for paired samples was used to determine if all turtles increased in weight from the beginning of the trial to the end. A Student's t-test was then used to determine if the change in weight over time significantly varied between treatment groups. An Analysis of Covariance was also used to determine if the average amount of *Hydrilla* consumed per day varied between treatment groups while accounting for body mass [26]. Statistical analyses were completed in IBM SPSS Version 21.

Results

Turtle feeding trial

The weight of the turtles increased significantly throughout the trial ($t_{\alpha\ 0.05,\ 9} = -2.788$, $p = 0.021$) with no difference between the treatment and control groups ($t_{\alpha\ 0.05,\ 7} = -0.030$, $p = 0.977$). Control turtles consumed an average of 2.76 g of lyophilized *Hydrilla*/kg bw/day (SE±0.73 g) and turtles fed *Hydrilla* with UCB consumed an average of 1.58 g of lyophilized *Hydrilla*/kg bw/day (SE±0.13 g). The main effect of treatment group was not significant, $F(1,6) = 0.65$, $p = 0.45$, $\eta p^2 = 0.10$, nor was body mass, $F(1,6) = 0.52$, $p = 0.49$, $\eta p^2 = 0.08$, nor was the interaction between mass and treatment group, $F(1,6) = 0.39$, $p = 0.55$, $\eta p^2 = 0.06$. For floating *Hydrilla*, control turtles consumed an average of 14.5 g/kg bw/day (SE±3.22 g) whereas turtles fed *Hydrilla* with UCB consumed an average of 8.55 g/kg bw/day (SE±1.03 g). The main effect of treatment group was not significant, $F(1,6) = 1.11$, $p = 0.33$, $\eta p^2 = 0.156$, nor was body mass, $F(1,6) = 0.27$, $p = 0.63$, $\eta p^2 = 0.04$, nor was the interaction between mass and treatment group, $F(1,6) = 0.71$, $p = 0.43$, $\eta p^2 = 0.11$.

All turtles appeared healthy until day 82 of the trial. Between days 82–89, the five treatment turtles began displaying neurologic dysfunction, including, but not limited to, various degrees of ataxia (mild gait asymmetry to severe limb dragging- Video S1) and inability to right themselves, in addition to performing poorly on one or more aspects of the neurologic exam (Table 1). Three of the turtles were euthanized on day 82. Two turtles (#85 and 119) only displayed mild neurologic deficits on day 89, the first observation of deficits. We maintained these turtles, which were still alert and eating well, until day 97 to observe the progression of clinical signs. During this time, the feeding volume decreased to anorexia in #85, however, its gait improved to normal by day 94. Turtle 119 continued to eat and intermittently displayed mild neurologic deficits. Both turtles were subsequently euthanized on day 97. Control turtles appeared healthy throughout the entire trial.

Diagnostic findings

No gross abnormalities were observed for any turtles at necropsy. All turtles were in good body condition and contained food in the gastrointestinal tract, with the exception of the three turtles in the treatment group that displayed anorexia or reduced feed intake towards the end of the trial. Significant histologic abnormalities were not observed in any of the controls. However, all turtles in the treated group had severe, diffuse vacuolation of white matter throughout the entire brain, including cerebrum, cerebellum, and brain stem, and spinal cord with no single area appearing to be consistently more or less affected than other areas. Mild multifocal inflammatory lesions consisting of lymphocytic perivascular cuffing were noted in peripheral nerves. However, these were present and similar in both the control and treatment groups and may have been related to schistosomes which were an incidental finding in several turtles. Significant lesions were not present in any of the other examined organs (kidney, liver, heart, lung, spleen, gonad, and gastrointestinal tract) in both treatment groups. Light microscopic changes were present throughout the white matter of the brain and spinal cord of treatment group turtles and consisted of coalescing, round to ovoid, clear vacuoles that were approximately 5–40 µm in diameter (Figure 1). Similar but less widespread vacuolation was also noted in the Purkinje and inner granular cell layers of the cerebellum. However, perikarya were unaffected. In the cerebral gray matter, scattered vacuoles, either individually or in small clusters, were also observed but this tended to occur at white matter interfaces. Electron microscopic findings in the brain of the treatment group turtle consisted of axonal swelling and degeneration with splitting of myelin at the intraperiod line (Figure 2). No significant histologic (Figure 3) or electron microscopic abnormalities were noted in the brain of the control turtles.

Discussion

Our study demonstrates that a common freshwater turtle species, the painted turtle, can develop neurologic signs and

Table 1. Clinical signs observed in the treatment group turtles after the first observed deficits on day 82 of the experiment.

ID #	Anorexic?	Gait and movement Normal?	Able to Swim?	Mentation	Spinal and other Reflexes Normal?	Could keep head in horizontal plane when rotated and listed?
107	Yes	Would not ambulate	Floating upside down	Stupor	No attempt to right itself	Yes
104	Yes	Ataxia	No	Stupor	Unable to right itself	Reduced ability
118	No	Ataxia	Yes	Depressed	No head withdrawal, no attempt to right itself	Reduced ability
85	Yes	Ataxia	Yes	Alert	Unable to right itself and head withdrawal reflex was reduced	Yes
119	No	Ataxia	Yes	Alert	Unable to right itself	Yes

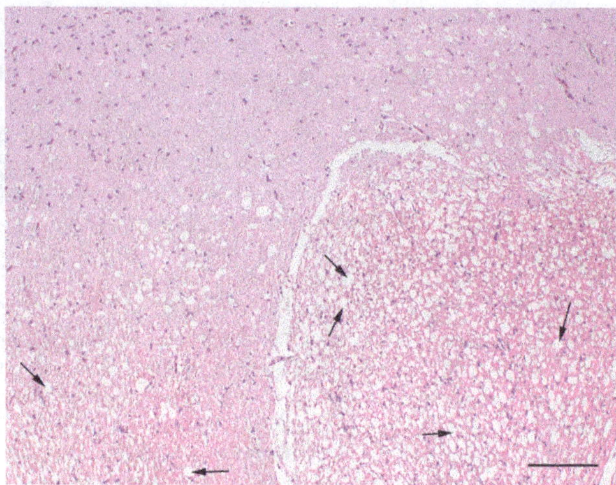

Figure 1. Histopathological slide of the optic tectum of a painted turtle fed toxic *Hydrilla* material. Painted turtle (*Chrysemys picta*), brain: Numerous clear vacuoles (black arrows) representing myelin degeneration and dilation of axonal sheaths are present in the white matter of a turtle treated with toxic hydrilla. H&E, 100X. Scale bar is 100 μm.

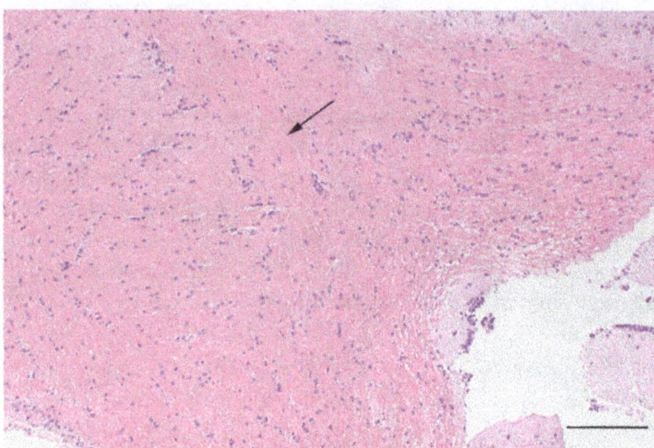

Figure 3. Histopathological slide of the optic tectum of a normal turtle. Painted turtle (*Chrysemys picta*), brain: white matter, indicated by black arrows, appears normal with no evidence of vacuolation or myelin degeneration. H&E, 100X. Scale bar is 100 μm.

vacuolations consistent with VM from consuming *Hydrilla* with UCB. Clinical signs in turtles were consistent with avian models, presenting as varying degrees of neurologic and physical impairment [5,10]. A subjective attempt was made to correlate lesions with neurologic severity and/or type of neurologic signs. However, with the exception of the cerebellar lesions, all affected turtles appeared to have similar, severe, widespread lesions and no such correlations could be identified. While some variation in distribution and severity was present among the cerebellar lesions, this did not appear to correlate with any differences in the clinical signs. These findings are similar to those described in birds with VM [3,10].

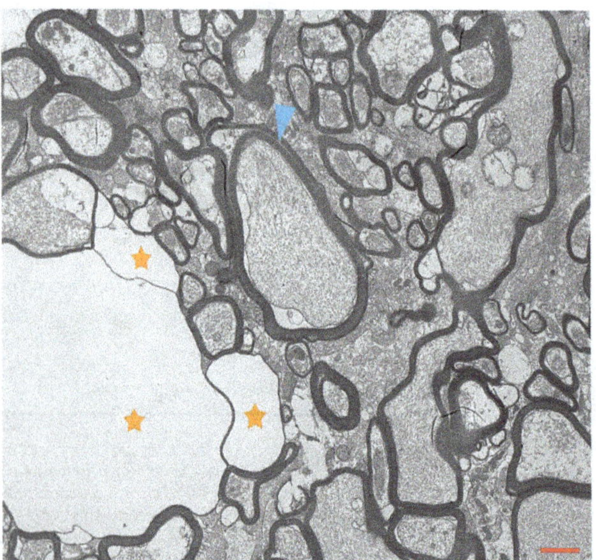

Figure 2. Electron Micrograph of central nervous tissue of a painted turtle fed toxic *Hydrilla* material. Electron Microscopy, painted turtle (*Chrysemys picta*), brain: Axons are swollen and degenerate and myelin sheaths are frequently disrupted by large, clear, intramyelinic vacuoles (orange stars). In less severely affected axons, splitting can be seen to occur at the intraperiod lines (blue arrow). Scale bar is 2 μm.

Though the specific agent or agents that cause VM have not been identified, we believe that our results provide strong evidence that the same active agent(s) that induce VM in birds and are associated with ingestion of the UCB induce the lesions and associated neurologic disease in painted turtles. There might be a generalized effect among these two closely related taxa. A previous study demonstrated that grass carp fed toxic *Hydrilla* also developed vacuolations, suggesting the toxin(s) produced by the UCB may have broad neurologic effects among vertebrates [10]. Although two studies of domestic pigs and one study of laboratory mice fed toxic *Hydrilla* failed to find evidence of neurologic signs or detectable vacuolations, the authors of those studies emphasize the dose and/or duration of toxin(s) exposure may vary among taxa and experimental design, and may not have been sufficient to induce disease [5,13,14]. Our results support the hypothesis that taxa may vary in the required dosage or exposure duration to induce neurologic lesions. Standard avian trials are less than 30 days in length, and birds are often symptomatic within a few days. Grass carp euthanized 37 days post exposure to colonized *Hydrilla* had vacuolations, although no clinical signs were noted [10]. In our study, chickens fed *Hydrilla* colonized by the UCB exhibited mild neurologic signs within 7 days; however, turtles fed the same *Hydrilla* did not exhibit detectable clinical signs until 82 days. Possible explanations for this difference are the slower metabolism of ectotherms when compared to endotherms, differences in digestive efficiency, different metabolic pathways, an innate resistance to the toxin, or some other unknown factor.

We caution that while turtles may be sensitive to the UCB toxin, it remains to be determined whether turtle populations are vulnerable to the UCB's spread and invasions of freshwaters. Vulnerability incorporates both sensitivity and exposure. Many ponds and reservoirs in the southeastern U.S. have dense *Hydrilla* or native submerged aquatic vegetation that supports abundant concentrations of the UCB [1,6]. In those systems, a diet consisting of large amounts of *Hydrilla* may be biologically realistic, particularly for highly herbivorous turtles (e.g., *Trachemys* and

Pseudemys spp.) [27,28]. However, VM epornitics occur during late fall-winter, leading some to suggest that toxin production is related to season [2]. Most turtle species in the southeastern U.S. exhibit limited activity in the late fall to winter and may limit feeding during the cooler months of peak VM epornitics. To date, no large-scale die offs of aquatic turtles have been reported in reservoirs where VM die offs were reported for birds. Dead turtles may sink, decompose, or become scavenged in the water, which may contribute to low detection rates of impaired turtles. Moreover, our observations were that impaired turtles could show some motor recovery despite significant lesions in the brain. Turtles that have lesions but are not clearly distressed may not be reported [9], and the dominant effects of ingesting the UCB may be subacute and not associated with high mortality. It is also not known whether turtles can recover longer term from the neurologic damage associated with ingesting the UCB. Clearly, more studies will be needed to elucidate important details on the epidemiology and vulnerability of the UCB to turtles and other wildlife. We propose a near term need for sensitivity studies of wider suites of taxa including those feeding directly or indirectly on UCB host plants, and studies of the seasonality of toxin production relative to seasonal variation in foraging rates of exposed taxa to determine potential population level vulnerabilities.

Acknowledgments

Numerous graduate, undergraduate students, and staff in the Wilde, Maerz, Yabsley and Hernandez laboratories at the University of Georgia, the University of Georgia Herpetological Society, and various University of Georgia College of Veterinary Medicine students contributed to laboratory work. The Southeastern Cooperative Wildlife Disease Study (SCWDS) provided logistical support and facilities for necropsies. The Poultry Diagnostic Research Center in Athens, GA and the University of Georgia Golf Course provided technical and logistical assistance. We would like to thank the U.S. Army Corps of Engineers for collecting *Hydrilla* samples from J. Strom Thurmond Reservoir. In particular, we would like to thank Bridget Altman, Kristin Hinkson, and Matthew Walter for their assistance with collecting turtles, providing husbandry, and assisting in feeding trials.

Author Contributions

Conceived and designed the experiments: ADM SMH JCM MJY SBW. Performed the experiments: ADM LMS ALC. Analyzed the data: ADM. Wrote the paper: ADM SMH JCM MJY AEE ALC LMS JRF SBW. Principal pathologist for this study: AEE. Secondary pathologist for this study: JRF.

References

1. Fischer JR, Lewis-Weis LA, Tate CM, Gaydos JK, Gerhold RW, et al. (2006) Avian vacuolar myelinopathy outbreaks at a southeastern reservoir. J Wildl Dis 42: 501–510.
2. Rocke TE, Miller K, Augspurger T, Thomas NJ (2002) Epizootiologic studies of avian vacuolar myelinopathy in waterbirds. J Wildl Dis 38: 678–684.
3. Thomas NJ, Meteyer CU, Sileo L (1998) Epizootic vacuolar myelinopathy of the central nervous system of bald eagles (*Haliaeetus leucocephalus*) and American coots (*Fulica americana*). Vet Pathol 35: 479–487.
4. Augspurger T, Fischer JR, Thomas NJ, Sileo L, Brannian RE, et al. (2003) Vacuolar myelinopathy in waterfowl from a North Carolina impoundment. J Wildl Dis. 39: 412–417.
5. Lewis-Weis LA, Gerhold RW, Fischer JR (2004) Attempts to reproduce vacuolar myelinopathy in domestic swine and chickens. J Wildl Dis 40: 476–484.
6. Wilde SB, Murphy TM, Hope CP, Habrun SK, Kempton J, et al. (2005) Avian vacuolar myelinopathy linked to exotic aquatic plants and a novel cyanobacterial species. Environ Toxicol 20: 348–353.
7. Williams SK, Kempton J, Wilde SB, Lewitus A (2007) A novel epiphytic cyanobacterium associated with reservoirs affected by avian vacuolar myelinopathy. Harmful Algae 6: 343–353.
8. Robertson SM (2012) Potential threats of the exotic apple snail *Pomacea insularum* to aquatic ecosystems in Georgia and Florida. Thesis, University of Georgia 74 p.
9. Fischer JR, Lewis-Weis LA, Tate CM (2003) Experimental vacuolar myelinopathy in red-tailed hawks. J Wildl Dis 39: 400–406.
10. Larsen RS, Nutter FB, Augspurger T, Rocke TE, Tomlinson L, et al. (2002) Clinical features of avian vacuolar myelinopathy in American coots. J Am Vet Med Assoc 221: 80–85.
11. Birrenkott AH, Wilde SB, Hains JJ, Fischer JR, Murphy TM, et al. (2004) Establishing a food-chain link between aquatic plant material and avian vacuolar myelinopathy in mallards (*Anas platyrhynchos*). J Wildl Dis 40: 485–492.
12. Wiley FE, Twiner MJ, Leighfield TA, Wilde SB, Van Dolah FM, et al. (2009) An extract of *Hydrilla verticillata* and associated epiphytes induces avian vacuolar myelinopathy in laboratory mallards. Environ Toxicol 24: 362–368.
13. Rocke TE, Thomas NJ, Meteyer CU, Quist CF, Fischer JR, et al. (2005) Attempts to identify the source of avian vacuolar myelinopathy for waterbirds. J Wildl Dis 41: 163–170.
14. Haynie RS, Bowerman WW, Williams SK, Morrison JR, Grizzle JM, et al. (2013) Triploid grass carp susceptibility and potential for disease transfer when used to control aquatic vegetation in reservoirs with avian vacuolar myelinopathy. J Aquat Anim Health 25: 252.
15. Chiari Y, Cahais V, Galtier N, Delsuc F (2012) Phylogenomic analyses support the position of turtles as the sister group of birds and crocodiles (Archosauria). BMC Biol 10: 65–65.
16. Buhlmann KA, Akre TSB, Iverson JB, Karapatakis D, Mittermeier RA, et al. (2009) A global analysis of tortoise and freshwater turtle distributions with identification of priority conservation areas. Chelonian Conserv Biol 8: 116–149.
17. Ernst CH, Lovich JE (2009) Turtles of the United States and Canada. Baltimore: Johns Hopkins University Press, 2nd ed. 840 p.
18. Kozlowsky-Suzuki B, Wilson AE and Ferrão Filho AdS (2012) Biomagnification or biodilution of microcystins in aquatic foodwebs? Meta-analyses of laboratory and field studies. Harmful Algae 18: 47–55.
19. Johnson JH (2004) Husbandry and medicine of aquatic reptiles. Semin Avian Exot Pet 13: 223–228.
20. Davis KM, Burghardt GM (2007) Training and long-term memory of a novel food acquisition task in a turtle (*Pseudemys nelsoni*). Behav Processes 75: 225–230.
21. Williams BJ, Puchulutegui C, Landsberg JH, Williams SK (2009) The cyanobacterium (order stigonematales) suspected of causing avian vacuolar myelinopathy is confirmed in Florida fresh waters. J Freshwat Ecol 24: 309–314.
22. Clippinger TL, Bennett RA, Platt SR (2007) The avian neurologic examination and ancillary neurodiagnostic techniques: a review update. Vet Clin North Am Exot Anim Pract 10: 803–836.
23. Lightfoot TL, Harrison GJ (2006) Clinical avian medicine. Palm Beach, FL: Spix Publishing. 1007 p.
24. Mader DR (2006) Reptile medicine and surgery. St. Louis, MO: Saunders Elsevier. 2nd ed. 1242 p.
25. Mariani CL (2007) The neurologic examination and neurodiagnostic techniques for reptiles. Vet Clin North Am Exot Anim Pract 10: 855–891.
26. Quinn GP, Keough MJ (2002) Experimental design and data analysis for biologists. New York: Cambridge University Press. 556 p.
27. Bjorndal KA, Bolten AB, Lagueux CJ, Jackson DR (1997) Dietary overlap in three sympatric congeneric freshwater turtles (*Pseudemys*) in Florida. Chelonian Conserv Biol 2: 430–433.
28. Fields JR, Simpson TR, Manning RW, Rose FL (2003) Food habits and selective foraging by the Texas river cooter (*Pseudemys texana*) in Spring Lake, Hays County, Texas. J Herpetol 37: 726–729.

Using Hormones to Manage Dairy Cow Fertility: The Clinical and Ethical Beliefs of Veterinary Practitioners

Helen M. Higgins[1]*, Eamonn Ferguson[2], Robert F. Smith[3], Martin J. Green[1]

1 Population Health and Welfare Group, School of Veterinary Medicine and Science, University of Nottingham, Sutton Bonington, United Kingdom, **2** Personality, Social Psychology, and Health Research Group, School of Psychology, University of Nottingham, Nottingham, United Kingdom, **3** Division of Livestock Health and Welfare, School of Veterinary Science, University of Liverpool, Neston, United Kingdom

Abstract

In the face of a steady decline in dairy cow fertility over several decades, using hormones to assist reproduction has become common. In the European Union, hormones are prescription-only medicines, giving veterinary practitioners a central role in their deployment. This study explored the clinical and ethical beliefs of practitioners, and provides data on their current prescribing practices. During 2011, 93 practitioners working in England completed a questionnaire (95% response rate). Of the 714 non-organic farms they attended, only 4 farms (0.6%) never used hormones to assist the insemination of lactating dairy cows. Practitioners agreed (>80%) that hormones improve fertility and farm businesses profitability. They also agreed (>80%) that if farmers are able to tackle management issues contributing to poor oestrus expression, then over a five year period these outcomes would both improve, relative to using hormones instead. If management issues are addressed instead of prescribing hormones, practitioners envisaged a less favourable outcome for veterinary practices profitability ($p<0.01$), but an improvement in genetic selection for fertility ($p<0.01$) and overall cow welfare ($p<0.01$). On farms making no efforts to address underlying management problems, long-term routine use at the start of breeding for timing artificial insemination or inducing oestrus was judged "unacceptable" by 69% and 48% of practitioners, respectively. In contrast, practitioners agreed (≥90%) that both these types of use are acceptable, provided a period of time has been allowed to elapse during which the cow is observed for natural oestrus. Issues discussed include: weighing quality versus length of cow life, fiscal factors, legal obligations, and balancing the interests of all stakeholders, including the increasing societal demand for food. This research fosters debate and critical appraisal, contributes to veterinary ethics, and encourages the pro-active development of professional codes of conduct.

Editor: Bernhard Kaltenboeck, Auburn University, United States of America

Funding: This research was funded by the Wellcome Trust[087797/Z/08/Z], www.wellcome.ac.uk. The funder had no role in study design, data collection and analysis, decision to publish, or preparation of the manuscript.

Competing Interests: The authors have declared that no competing interests exist.

* E-mail: helen.higgins@nottingham.ac.uk.

Introduction

Post World War II, scientific and technological advances enabled the industrialization and intensification of agriculture. Concurrently, this has generated a multitude of ethical issues concerning the use of technologies in food production and how farm animals *ought* to be cared for [1,2]. It is perhaps surprizing, therefore, that veterinary ethics has only recently emerged as an academic discipline; the paucity of literature and lack of any devoted research journal negates an important subject that presents unique challenges, inherently distinct from medical ethics [3]. To start to address this gap in the literature this research concerns the use of a reproductive technology, the prescription of synthetic hormones to manage and improve dairy cow fertility.

There has been a steady decline in the reproductive performance of dairy cows over several decades [4,5]. Over this time period market forces have driven efficiency savings and lead to genetic selection for production traits, especially higher milk yield. As a result, the specialist dairy Holstein breed is now a substantial component of the UK national herd, managed predominately in a 'high input high output' farming system [6]. It is widely accepted that the modern Holstein cow displays less overt signs of oestrus behaviour and for a reduced period of time relative to her lower yielding predecessors [7]. Hence todays farming and veterinary communities are challenged with managing the fertility of an animal that inherently has poorer reproductive performance. Currently in the UK, the annual culling rate for dairy herds is 23% and poor fertility is the commonest reason for culling [8]. In the face of this decline in fertility performance, hormones have been advocated [9] and increasingly been deployed to assist breeding, although to the authors' knowledge there are no data quantifying the scale of such use currently, nor that has charted this use over time. Hormones, along with all veterinary medicines, are paid for by the farmer.

This study concerned three hormones (progesterone, prostaglandin and gonadotrophin releasing hormone), when prescribed to adult lactating dairy cows, *without* reproductive pathology. Two types of use were considered. Firstly, using hormones to induce oestrus - if the farmer knows when to expect to see the cow in oestrus he will observe her more closely and this increases the probability of the cow being served either by the bull or by artificial insemination (AI); this is subsequently referred to as 'oestrus induction'. Secondly, using hormones over a period of time (often referred to as a synchronization programme) to enable

AI on a known date and time; this is subsequently referred to as 'fixed-time AI'. Oestrus induction requires less hormonal treatments but the farmer must observe the cows several times per day for oestrus (oestrus detection); fixed-time AI involves more hormonal treatments but removes the need for oestrus detection completely. In both cases, hormones can either be used as soon as the cow becomes eligible for breeding after calving, or alternatively, they may only be used if the cow has not been inseminated by the end of a certain period of time, during which she is observed for natural oestrus by the farmer. There are therefore four main ways to assist breeding, as summarised in Figure 1, with (a) involving the greatest quantities of hormones, decreasing in order to (d) with the least. The entire eligible cow population would receive hormones in (a) and (c) but a smaller proportion, depending on the success of natural oestrus detection, in (b) and (d). We focused on the acceptability of use in these four contexts when management problems exist. The acceptability in other scenarios was not explored, such as when unpredictable events occur (e.g. crop failures due to poor weather) which can have a major and unavoidable impact on fertility.

Importantly, in the public eye, the word 'hormone' in the context of food production may have negative connotations; historically there has been considerable societal controversy over the prescription of certain hormones to cattle [10]. However 'hormone' is a term that classifies a very diverse group of physiological signalling compounds, and the effect and acceptability of use rests entirely on the specific drug and prescribing context. Moreover, in the European Union, all hormones are legally categorised as 'Prescription Only Medicines Veterinarian' (POM-V) [11], making them subject to stringent control under legislation contained within Directive 2001/82/EC (as amended) [12]. In the UK this legislation is enforced by the Veterinary Medicines Directorate (VMD), an executive government agency [13,14]. In particular, manufacturers must prove that any medicine residues in edible tissues are below the statutory 'maximum residue limits' and hence safe for consumers health [15,16]. The VMD monitors on-going safety by continually testing produce for residues [13,17].

Several stakeholders have vested interests in the debate over the use of this reproductive technology in the context described. This paper explores the issue primarily from the perspective of veterinary practitioners working in private practice in England. As POM-V medicines, administration legally requires prescription from a veterinarian, giving them a central and influential role with respect to how and when these medicines are deployed. Understanding the clinical and ethical beliefs of a range of veterinary practitioners, and any divergence, is important. However to our knowledge, there are no published data on this, or their current prescribing practices. The main aims of this study were therefore: (i) to report the current prescription of hormones to assist breeding by a sample of veterinary practitioners in England, (ii) to explore their clinical beliefs and ethical stance.

Methods

Instrument Design

Purposive sampling was used to select two veterinary academics from the University of Nottingham, one veterinary academic from the University of Liverpool and two private veterinary practitioners. Individual semi-structured interviews were conducted by the first author, and the information gathered (see Figure 2) was used to inform and design a questionnaire that was subsequently piloted on two veterinary academics, one psychologist and three veterinary practitioners. The final document comprised a mixture of question formats, and was delivered to a sample of veterinary practitioners (see next section). The questionnaire is available in Appendix S1 and subsequent references to question numbers relate to this Appendix.

Recruitment of Veterinary Practitioners

Eligible practitioners were those providing healthcare to dairy cattle in England during their normal working hours, and working within a veterinary practice that contained at least one practitioner possessing post-graduate cattle qualifications – specifically, the Royal College of Veterinary Surgeons (RCVS) post-graduate Certificate in Cattle Health and Production or the Diploma in Bovine Reproduction. A two-stage cluster design stratified by geographic location was used. Veterinary practices were selected first, using a 'without-replacement systematic method' [19], that involved randomly selecting a starting point and then systematically selecting practices with probability proportional to the number of practitioners they contained. Once 20 practices had consented to take part, five practitioners were then randomly selected from within each practice by using the random number generator function in the software programme 'R' version 2.13.1 [18] to pick numerical identifiers; all pracitioners were recuirted in practices that contained less than five eligible practitioners. With this sampling strategy, every individual had approximately the same probability of being selected, irrespective of the size of the practice they worked in. The online database (http://www.rcvs.org.uk/) supplied by RCVS provided a sampling frame of veterinary practices. Practitioners were provided with an inconvenience allowance of £100 per hour (pro-rata). Data were collected from the 8th June to 1st September 2011.

Data Analysis

The data was initially entered into Excel (Version 2010, Microsoft Corporation). To compare how practitioners' opinions

a) Immediate fixed-time AI. Artificial insemination on a known date and time to be used immediately a cow becomes eligible for breeding, post-calving

b) Delayed fixed-time AI. Artificial insemination on a known date and time to be used if a cow is not inseminated by some defined point after calving, but not as soon as she is eligible for breeding

c) Immediate oestrus induction. Inducing oestrus immediately a cow becomes eligible for breeding, post-calving

d) Delayed oestrus induction. Inducing oestrus to be used if a cow is not inseminated by some defined point after calving, but not as soon as she is eligible for breeding

Figure 1. The four main ways to assist breeding in lactating dairy cattle using hormones.

Potential Advantages

- Facilitates regular veterinary visits to farms.
- Strengthens veterinary-farmer relationship.
- Generates opportunities for vets to identify and address other health/welfare issues on farm.
- Quick and practical to implement.
- Fertility may rapidly improve for relatively low investment; fewer cattle may be culled.
- May reduce future health/welfare problems related to prolonged calving intervals.
- The improved fertility is easily attributable to the action taken (i.e. the use of hormones).
- Provides vets with revenue.
- Farmers may be unable to afford the labour/time for oestrus detection.
- Farmers may be unable to make the capital investment needed to address any underlying causes of poor fertility.
- Improved job satisfaction for vets.
- Positive perception of the veterinary profession as providers of 'innovative technical solutions'.

Potential Disadvantages

- May mask underlying management and health/welfare problems.
- May diminish the need/urgency to tackle the underlying cause(s) of the problem
- May be over-prescribed; alternative (and possibly cheaper) approaches may be over-looked.
- Efficacy/cost-effectiveness may be falsely assumed if outcomes are not monitored.
- Potential for misuse exists.
- Economic benefits have not been proven against alternative approaches.
- Long-term use involves on-going costs to farmers.
- Widespread use may mean that genetic selection for improved fertility may be more difficult in the long term.
- There is a welfare cost to cows from administration
- Negative perception of the veterinary profession as providers of 'hormones' not 'expertise'.

Figure 2. Potential advantages/disadvantages of prescribing hormones from a veterinary perspective. The context relates to the use of hormones to assist breeding in lactating dairy cattle without reproductive pathology. The lists provide a summary of interviews with three veterinary academics and two veterinary practitioners. There is no significance attached to the vertical order of items.

changed between related categorical questions, two-sided marginal tests of homogeneity were performed [20] (an extension of McNemar's test for categorical variables) using the software programme SPSS Statistics (Version, 20, IBM); the significance level was <0.05.

Factor analysis was performed using the 'fa' function in the 'psych' package in the software programme R [18]. The number of factors to extract was based on a combination of: (i) Cattell's scree plot [21] (ii) eigenvalues greater than 1.0 [22] (iii) interpretability of extracted factors [23] and (iv) chi squared goodness of fit statistic for the maximum likelihood extraction (for a good fit $p>0.05$) [24]. Sensitivity of the results to the method of analysis was assessed with respect to two different extraction methods (maximum likelihood and principal axes) combined with two different rotations, varimax [25] and promax [26]. A final check on goodness of fit was assessed by the Root Mean Square Error of Approximation (RMSEA); an RMSEA ≤ 0.06 indicated acceptable fit [27]. Only variables with absolute loading values of ≥ 0.3 were included in the interpretation of a factor [28]. Variables with little or no variance were excluded from the interpretation. Factor scores (based on all items) for each practitioner were estimated using regression; the distribution of factor scores was assessed to establish majority views across survey questions.

Three logistic regression models were fitted to identify factors associated with responses to three questions in the questionnaire:

i. Practitioners reporting concern (yes/no) over the prescription of hormones to assist breeding (question 5).
ii. Practitioner judgement regarding the acceptability (yes/no) of the long term routine use of immediate fixed-time AI as a substitute for good management i.e. in herds with underlying management problems that are not being addressed (question 16a).
iii. Practitioner judgement regarding the acceptability (yes/no) of the long term routine use of immediate oestrus induction as a substitute for good management (question 16c).

Questions 16a and 16c carried a 'don't know' option and observations falling in this category were omitted from the analysis. MLwiN software [29] was used and veterinary practice was included as a normally distributed random effect to account for the clustered nature of the data. All models used a logit link function and a penalized quasi-likelihood method for estimation [30]. There were 30 (level 1) covariates available (see Appendix S2). For questions 16a and 16c, factors identified from the factor analysis were also included as covariates. Univariate analysis was conducted and covariates with a P-value of ≤ 0.05 are reported. Covariates that achieved $P\leq 0.1$ were carried forward for model building, and were retained in the final model if they achieved $P\leq 0.05$, having adjusted for the other covariates.

The study was approved in full by the Research and Ethics committee, School of Veterinary Medicine and Science, University of Nottingham.

Results

Response Rates and Characteristics of Participants

Veterinary practice response rate was 95% (19/20). Non-participation of one practice was due to a failure for all eligible practitioners within it to agree to participate. Another practice was selected and consented, from the same region. These 20 practices contained 95 eligible practitioners, 93 of whom replied, giving a practitioner response rate of 98% (93/95).

Table 1. Characteristics of veterinary practitioners (n = 94).

Characteristic	Result	
Gender	Male: 59 (63%)	Female: 34 (37%)
Employment status	Partner: 37 (40%)	Assistant: 56 (60%)
Post-graduate cattle qualifications	Yes: 23 (25%)	No: 70 (75%)
Years qualified	Median: 7	Range: 0–37

Of the 20 practices, 6 were located in the North, 3 in the Midlands, and 11 in the South of England. Table 1 summarises practitioner characteristics.

Current Prescribing Practices of Veterinary Practitioners in England

Of the 93 respondents, 81 conducted dairy cow fertility work at least once per month on one or more farms; between these practitioners this tallied to 753 farms in total, 39 (5.2%) of which operated under organic regulations that prohibit the use of hormones to assist breeding. Of the 714 non-organic farms, 4 (0.6%) never used hormones to assist breeding, 56 (7.8%) used hormones for immediate fixed-time AI on the majority of cows, 193 (27.0%) used hormones for delayed fixed-time AI on the majority of cows. The remaining 461 farms (64.6%) used hormones to induce oestrus to varying extents, and/or for occasional fixed-time AI.

Practitioners' Clinical Beliefs

A key clinical question was whether prescribing hormones contributes to making any underlying causes of poor oestrus expression, better or worse (Q11). Responses by category were: better 9 (9.8%), no effect 32 (34.7%), worse 33 (35.9%), don't know 18 (19.6%). With respect to underlying causes, practitioners were asked to list the three most important issues that they believed contributed most often to the problem of poor oestrus expression on dairy farms, see Figure 3.

Practitioners also answered a pair of questions, each concerning five key outcomes. The first question asked what effect prescribing hormones would have on each outcome (Q8), and the second question asked what effect tackling the root causes of poor oestrus

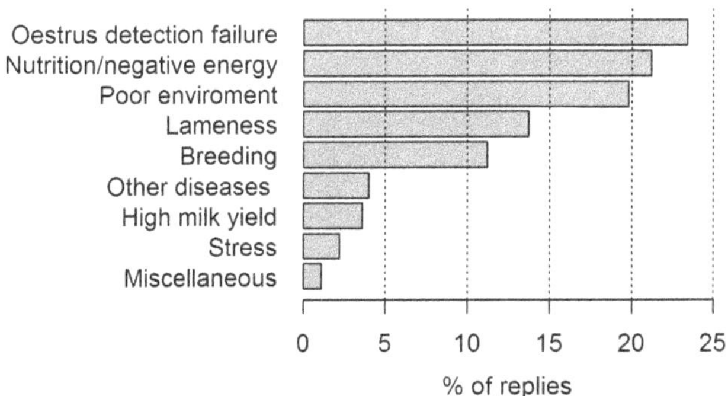

Figure 3. Factors believed to contribute to poor oestrus expression on dairy farms (n = 278 replies). Practitioners' replies to question 13a were categorized to reflect the answers given, but overlap existed in terms of concepts (e.g. high yield, breeding and lameness are related). The raw data are available in Appendix S3.

expression would have after a five year period, if this approach was taken instead of using hormones (13b); the latter was conditional on a crucial assumption, namely that farmers were in a position to make the necessary management changes, including any capital investments required. Responses to the two questions are compared in Figure 4. A two-sided marginal test of homogeneity on this data showed that if underlying management issues are addressed instead of prescribing hormones, practitioners envisaged a less favourable outcome for veterinary practices profitability ($p<0.01$), but an improvement in genetic selection for fertility ($p<0.01$) and overall dairy cow welfare ($p<0.01$).

Practitioners' responses to the remaining clinical questions are given in Figure 5, whilst their perceptions of other stakeholders are illustrated in Figure 6. With regard to decision-making, the main influence over practitioners' decision to prescribe (Q12) was: veterinarians 46 (51%), farmers 32 (35%), both 13 (14%). Theoretically speaking, if practitioners only had to please themselves and the dairy cow (Q10), then 55 (60%) would use hormones, versus 37 (40%) who would not.

Practitioners' Ethical Beliefs

Practitioners' responses to the question "Does the use of fertility drugs to get dairy cows served give you any cause for concern?" were divided: 48 (52%) yes, 45 (48%) no. Positive respondents were asked to describe their concerns. Their answers have been categorised in Figure 7, the raw data are available in Appendix S4. The logistic regression results for factors associated with practitioners reporting concern are reported in Table 2.

Practitioners' ethical beliefs regarding the acceptability in the different prescribing contexts are provided in Table 3. Acceptability was subject in each case to two important conditions: (i) long term routine use, i.e. involving the majority of cows, (ii) prescribing when underlying problems definitely exist that are causing the problem but are *not* being addressed.

Factor analysis identified two factors accounting for 30% of the variance. Technical details of this analysis, including the rotated factor matrix are included in Appendix S5. Factor 1 was interpreted as a 'positive attitude towards the outcomes of prescribing hormones to assist breeding'. Factor 2 was interpreted as a 'positive attitude towards outcomes if underlying causes of poor oestrus expression are tackled'. Distribution of factor scores suggested that for those variables where there was diversity in opinion, the majority of practitioners tended overall towards both a negative attitude towards the outcomes of using pharmaceutical intervention and a positive attitude towards outcomes that could be achieved if the underlying causes of poor oestrus expression can be addressed.

Logistic regression revealed that only one covariate, years qualified, was positively associated with practitioners judging long term routine use of immediate fixed-time AI acceptable in the face of unaddressed management issues ($p = 0.03$, $OR = 1.05$ per extra year, 95% CI 1.04 to 1.11).

Practitioner acceptability of long term routine use of immediate oestrus induction in the face of unaddressed management issues was positively associated with two covariates: (i) the number of farms for which the practitioner was personally currently prescribing hormones for the purpose of any form of oestrus induction ($p = 0.02$, $OR = 1.10$ per extra farm, 95% CI 1.02 to 1.24), and (ii) practitioners scores for factor 1 i.e. a positive attitude towards using hormones to assist breeding ($p = 0.02$, $OR = 2.1$ per unit increase in score, 95% CI 1.1 to 3.7). It was also negatively associated with one covariate: practitioners score for factor 2 i.e. a positive attitude towards outcomes if underlying causes of poor oestrus expression are tackled ($p = 0.02$, $OR = 0.54$ per unit

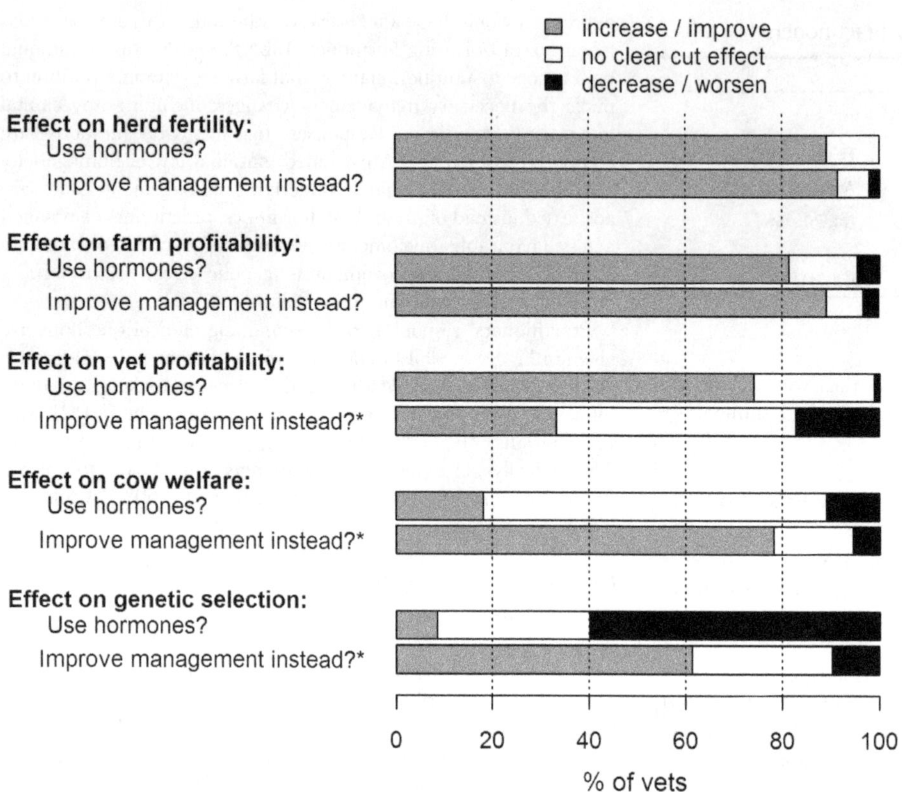

Figure 4. The effect of prescribing hormones versus addressing underlying causes instead over 5 years (n = 93 vets). *denotes a statistically significant change in the distribution of responses between categories, from the outcome if hormones are used to the outcome if management issues are improved instead ($p < 0.01$).

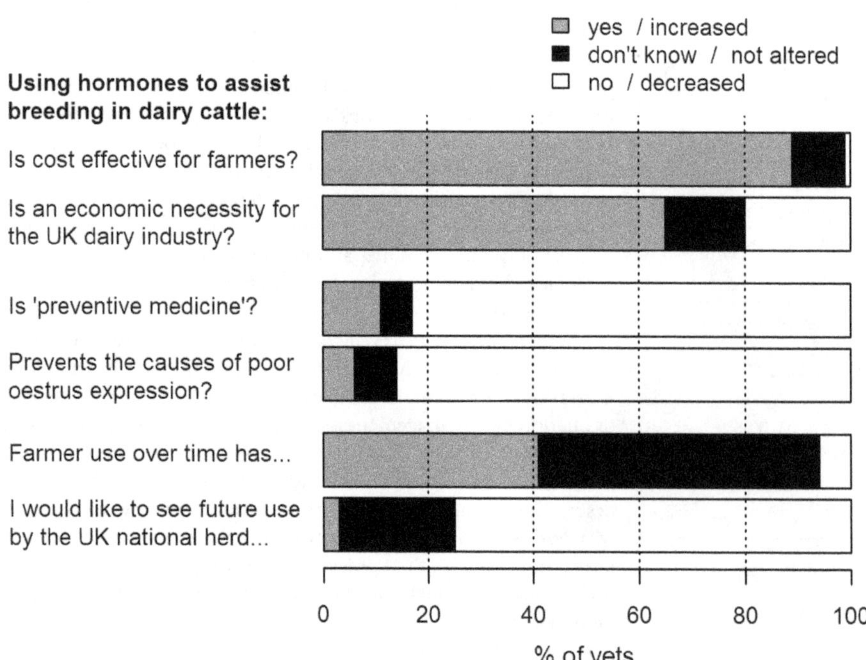

Figure 5. Practitioners' responses to clinical questions (n = 93). All questions relate to use in lactating dairy cattle, without reproductive pathology. As listed in the figure, these relate to questions 2, 17, 7, 9, 6, and 14 of the questionnaire.

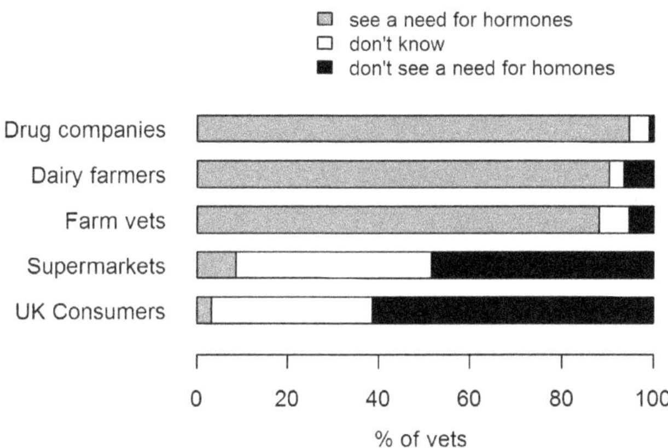

Figure 6. Practitioners' perceptions of other stakeholders (n = 93). Question 15(a-e) asked practitioners to state whether they believe other stakeholders see a need to prescribe hormones to assist breeding in lactating dairy cattle.

increase in score, 95% CI 0.31 to 0.92). The final multivariate model contained all three covariates with negligible alterations to their parameter estimates or standard errors.

Finally, participants were invited to make additional comments; 25/93 (27%) did so, and some practitioners wrote additional comments throughout the questionnaire (see Appendix S6).

Discussion

With regard to the acceptability of using hormones to assist breeding in lactating dairy cattle, our results show that even when management problems exist that are causing poor fertility and are not being addressed, the majority of veterinary practitioners judged any type of long term routine use acceptable, provided it was not straight after the start of the breeding period. This may reflect a deontological stance, related to the economic necessity for cows to become pregnant quickly after calving to avoid culling; practitioners' may consider it wrong to let animals be culled that could be saved, especially given they have a sworn an oath to 'ensure the health and welfare of animals committed to my care' [31]. There is also a clinical argument to re-breed cows quickly, since this may reduce the risk of future health problems [32]. Hormonal treatments are quick and easy to implement, however if routine use diminishes the need to tackle root causes, this may have health and welfare implications for the herd. Clinically, there is also the question of whether using hormones contributes towards making any underlying causes of poor oestrus expression better or worse. Veterinary opinion here was ambiguous and divided but not positive, and it is worth noting that time devoted to oestrus detection is also time devoted to disease detection. A utilitarian analysis of 'do the greatest good for the greatest number' over a long period may be less supportive of use, although importantly, tackling the root causes may require large capital investment, sustained changes in human behaviour, and take time to resolve; the latter also has implications for sustaining farmer motivation. Two veterinary ethical issues reside here that need advancement. First, how to define and measure a cow's quality of life, and second how to weigh length versus quality of cow life. In human medicine, the quandary of weighing length versus quality of life has seen 'quality adjusted life years' (QALY) used for healthcare resource allocation by organizations such as The National Institute for Health and Clinical Excellence; although QALY is controversial [33] and in need of further research [34]. No equivalent practical decision making tool exists for veterinary practitioners, and the issues involved in developing any such measure are different and arguably even more complex.

Although this survey did not specifically explore how practitioners arrived at their answers with regards to the acceptability of using hormones, some insight can be gained from the additional comments they made. In particular, one practitioner commented "it is [acceptable] in humans", however there are difficulties with attempting to make reference to seemingly analogous prescribing contexts in the humans. In women the decision to undergo hormonal fertility treatment is a conscious choice, based on knowledge of the advantages and disadvantages of doing so. It is impossible to know if a cow, given the same knowledge (which we cannot impart to them) would make a similar choice to the one that we make for them - and this is assuming that cows can reason. Moreover, the reasons for use and outcomes are very different. Hormones are used to facilitate pregnancy in both fertile and non-fertile animals for reasons related, at least in part, to profitability and human convenience, and non-pregnancy results in culling for human management reasons. In contrast, hormones are only used to facilitate pregnancy in infertile humans, for the sole reason of improving fertility per se, and within a guaranteed non-fatal outcome.

Our results showed that some practitioners did consider it unacceptable to use hormones routinely when management problems are not addressed, especially if conducted at the start of the breeding period. However in reality, the line that separates 'reasonable assistance to breed' from 'a substitute for good management' may not always be clear-cut. This raises the

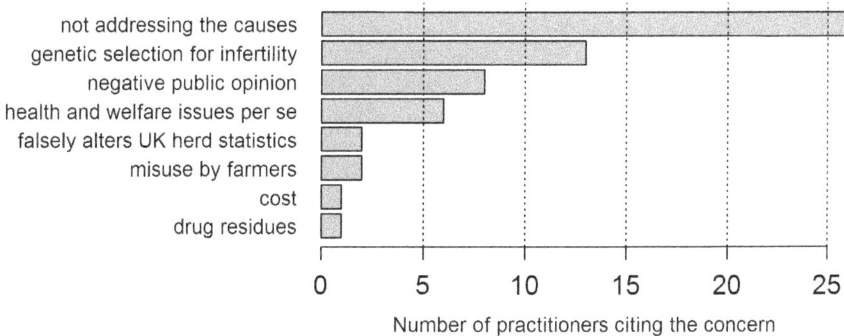

Figure 7. Practitioners' concerns regarding the use of hormones to assist breeding in lactating dairy cattle (n = 48). Note: some practitioners cited more than one concern.

Table 2. Logistic regression results for practitioner characteristics associated with reporting concern over the prescription of hormones to assist breeding.

	Univariable analysis		Multivariable analysis	
Practitioner characteristic+	**Odds Ratio(95% CI)**	**P-value**	**Odds Ratio(95% CI)**	**P-value**
Currently prescribes hormones for delayed fixed-time AI*?	3.66(1.4–10.3)	0.01		
Attended professional training event on dairy cattle fertility within 2 years?	3.89(1.52–9.94)	<0.01	3.72(1.41–9.83)	<0.01
Reports reading the journal 'UK Vet'?	3.41(1.31–8.85)	0.01		
Number of journals read (odds ratio per additional journal).	1.54(1.09–2.17)	0.01	1.47(1.04–2.08)	0.03

+ The full list of covariates available is provided in Appendix S2.
*fixed-time artificial insemination to be used if a cow has not been inseminated by some defined point after calving, but not as soon as she is eligible to be bred from.

question of whether veterinary practitioners with a business contract to provide services to a farmer, have a legal obligation to prescribe if requested by a paying client. Legally, as POM-V medicines, the decision to prescribe is the practitioners alone [35]. A farmer who disagreed could attest to a breach of business contact and claim for loss of earnings through a civil court, or in the UK, they could claim professional misconduct to the RCVS. However no precedent has been set and speculating on the outcome is difficult; ordinarily a farmer would terminate the business contract and employ the services of another. By demonstrating the diversity in clinical beliefs and ethical acceptability amongst practitioners, our results suggest that finding someone else to prescribe would not be difficult. Furthermore, veterinarians have professional obligations not only to the animals under their care, but also to farmers and to themselves. Indeed it is postulated that some of the diversity in practitioners' beliefs related to their empathy towards the various stakeholders which was not directly captured in our survey; this may partly explain why the factor analysis accounted for only one third of the observed variation. In this regard, in the Code of Professional Conduct for Veterinary Surgeons [36], produced by the RCVS, it states: "...veterinary surgeons should balance the professional responsibilities, having regard first to animal welfare." However, taking an ethical stance as an individual working in private veterinary practice is complicated by the conflicting interests - there is the potential for a substantial loss in revenue. Practitioners have both a need and a right to earn a living, and there are consequences not only for themselves, but also for the support staff that they employ.

Table 3. Practitioner acceptability of long-term routine prescription of hormones to assist breeding when management problems are not addressed (questions 16 and 18).

Prescribing context	Number of practitioners		
	Acceptable	**Unacceptable**	**Don't know**
Immediate fixed-time AI	25(31%*)	56(69%)	12
Delayed fixed-time AI	81(90%)	9(10%)	3
Immediate oestrus induction	44(52%)	41(48%)	8
Delayed oestrus induction	87(98%)	2(2%)	4
In general	75(82%)	8(9%)	9

*Percentages relate to the definitive replies.

Our results suggest that the use of hormones to assist breeding in England is widespread, and the majority of practitioners we surveyed wanted to see future national use decreased. However this represents a challenge for the profession, especially given the conflicting interests described in the previous paragraph. Thus, our results lend support to the *pro-active* development of professional ethical codes of conduct by the RCVS that all veterinarians should abide to. Pursuing a reactive approach is unlikely to be sufficient in the future; the challenge for the 21st century is to provide the rapidly rising world population with a sustainable supply of food, in the context of an increasing demand for animal products, global climate change and declining resources. One practitioner justified their replies in the context of the wider perspective: "all my acceptable answers are making the assumption that the Holstein and its genetics and increased yield and decreased fertility is here to stay to satisfy the need for dairy produce to feed the population." How to weigh the interests of all stakeholders in the wider context is a crucial question, but currently it is consumers who have the defining influence; in a market-driven playing field it is consumers who collectively, although perhaps unwittingly, drive the efficiency savings and set the economic boundaries within which farmers and veterinary surgeons work. Furthermore, few would argue that it is important for the UK to be able to compete on global market.

With regard to consumers and the public, some practitioners had concerns over negative public perception and the majority believed that UK consumers would not see a need for hormones. It is speculated that these concerns may in part be based on beliefs that the public are not well informed on the issue and that prima facie they would perceive it negatively because it involves hormones, a word that already holds negative connotations for many in the context of food production. However, the actual view of the well informed public is unknown, and needs to be quantified so that the veterinary profession can respond accordingly. In this respect, it is worth noting that in the UK the VMD has a strong track record for ensuring the responsible and safe use of POM-V veterinary medicines and enforcing the legislation contained within the EU Directive [17]. Furthermore there are numerous examples were financial remuneration by doctors has been perceived negatively by the public and adversely affected the level of trust between the public and the medical profession [37]. The inherent financial conflict of interests that inevitably arise from exclusively private veterinary practice will always have the potential to serve as a basis for undermining faith in veterinary expertise. This highlights the importance of studies such as these, which aim in part to inform stakeholders, as well as professional codes of conduct which provide reassurance to the public.

This study has explored some of the issues surrounding the use of one reproductive technology in a given context, but it is not difficult to envisage that veterinary ethical and clinical issues of the type debated here will become more numerous in the future. A key UK government policy for livestock production is 'sustainable intensification' [38], and it is proposed that this will be achieved through new scientific and technological advances; thus it is highly probable that, as occurred post World War II, these will bring with them an upsurge in new ethical challenges. Indeed several, such as cloning, are already upon us [3,4]. There is an urgent need to advance veterinary ethics as a subject and to ensure that it is firmly embedded in undergraduate veterinary curricula. Society has bestowed a considerable responsibility to the veterinary profession for both farm animals and their keepers. In return, society expects us to be acutely aware of the major ethical issues we are part of, to be pro-active and consistent in our approach to tackling them, and to keep the public informed; failure to do so runs the serious risk of loss of autonomy [1,3].

Supporting Information

Appendix S1 The questionnaire. This file contains the three page questionnaire which was delivered to a sample of veterinary practitioners working in England, UK.

Appendix S2 Covariate definitions and descriptions. This file contains details of all the covariates used in the statistical analysis.

Appendix S3 Factors believed to contribute to poor oestrus expression on dairy farms. This file contains the free text relies from the 93 practitioners in response to the question: Please list the 3 most important areas that you believe contribute most often to the problem of poor heat expression on dairy farms.

Appendix S4 Practitioners' concerns regarding the prescription of hormones to assist breeding in lactating dairy cattle. This file contains the free text replies detailing the concerns raised by 48 (of 93) practitioners who responded yes to the question: Does the use of fertility drugs to get dairy cows served give you any cause for concern?

Appendix S5 Factor analysis. This file contains technical details of the factor analysis.

Appendix S6 Veterinary practitioners' additional comments. This file contains (i) the free text relies detailing the additional comments made by 25 (of the 93) practitioners, in response to the question: If you have other comments about any aspect of the use of fertility drugs to get dairy cows served, or this questionnaire in general, please write them below or overleaf. (ii) additional comments made for any question posed in the questionnaire.

Acknowledgments

Thanks go to the practitioners and academics who participated, and the three reviewers for their helpful comments.

Author Contributions

Critically appraised the paper: EF RFS MJG. Conceived and designed the experiments: HMH EF RFS MJG. Performed the experiments: HMH. Analyzed the data: HMH EF MJG. Wrote the paper: HMH.

References

1. Rollin BE (2006) An introduction to veterinary medical ethics: theory and cases. Hoboken, NJ: Wiley-Blackwell.
2. Thompson PB (2007) Food biotechnology in ethical perspective. Berlin: Springer.
3. Legood G (2000) An introduction to veterinary ethics. London: Continuum.
4. Moore K, Thatcher WW (2006) Major advances associated with reproduction in dairy cattle. J Dairy Sci 89: 1254–1266.
5. Royal MD, Darwash AO, Flint APE, Webb R, Woolliams JA (2000) Declining fertility in dairy cattle: changes in traditional and endocrine parameters of fertility. Animal Science 70: 487–501.
6. van Arendonk JAM, Liinamo A (2003) Dairy cattle production in Europe. Theriogenology 59: 563–569.
7. Dobson H, Walker SL, Morris MJ, Routly JE, Smith RF (2008) Why is it getting more difficult to successfully artificially inseminate dairy cows? Animal 2: 1104–1111.
8. Orpin PG, Esslemont RJ (2010) Culling and wastage in dairy herds: an update on incidence and economic impact in dairy herds in the UK. Cattle Pract 18: 163–172.
9. Thatcher WW, Drost M, Savio JD, Macmillan KL, Entwistle KW, et al. (1993) New clinical uses of GnRH and its analogues in cattle. Anim Reprod Sci 33: 27–49.
10. Johnson R, Hanrahan CE (2010) The U.S.-EU beef hormone dispute. Congressional Research Service Report for Congress. Available: http://www.nationalaglawcenter.org/assets/crs/R40449.pdf. Accessed 30 November 2012.
11. Veterinary Medicines Directorate (2011) Controls of veterinary medicines. Available: http://www.vmd.defra.gov.uk/pdf/vmgn/VMGNote01.pdf. Accessed 30 November 2012.
12. Directive 2001/82/EC of the European parliament and of the council (2001) The community code relating to veterinary medicinal products. Available: http://ec.europa.eu/health/files/eudralex/vol-5/dir_2001_82_cons2009/dir_2001_82_cons2009_en.pdf. Accessed 30 November 2012.
13. Veterinary Medicines Directorate (2012) The work of the VMD. Available: http://www.vmd.defra.gov.uk/pdf/leaflet_workVMD.pdf. Accessed 30 November 2012.
14. The Veterinary Medicines Regulations (2011) No.2159. Available: http://www.legislation.gov.uk/uksi/2011/2159/pdfs/uksi_20112159_en.pdf. Accessed 30 November 2012.
15. Veterinary Medicines Directorate (2009) How to determine withdrawal periods. Available: http://www.vmd.defra.gov.uk/pdf/leaflet_withdrawalperiod.pdf. Accessed 30 November 2012.
16. Veterinary Medicines Directorate (2009) Avoiding veterinary residues in food–maintaining consumer confidence. Available: http://www.vmd.defra.gov.uk/pdf/leaflet_residues.pdf. Accessed 30 November 2012.
17. Dyer F, Diesel G, Cooles S, Tait A (2012) Suspected adverse reaction surveillance scheme: suspected adverse events, 2011. Vet Rec 170: 640–643.
18. R Development Core Team (2011) R: A language and environment for statistical computing. R foundation for statistical computing, Vienna, Austria. Available: http://www.R-project.org/. Accessed 4 April 2013.
19. Kalton G (1987) Introduction to survey sampling. Thousand Oaks, CA: Sage Publications.
20. Agresti A (2002) Categorical data analysis. New York: Wiley-Interscience.
21. Cattell RB (1966) The scree test for the number of factors. Multivariate Behav Res 1: 245–276.
22. Nunnally JC (1978) Psychometric theory. New York: McGraw-Hill.
23. Thompson B (2004) Exploratory and confirmatory factor analysis: understanding concepts and applications. Washington, DC: American Psychological Association.
24. Kim J, Mueller CW (1978) Factor Analysis: Statistical methods and practical issues. Thousand Oaks, CA: Sage Publications.
25. Kaiser HK (1958) The varimax criterion for analytic rotation in factor analysis. Psychometrika 23: 187–200.
26. Hendrickson AE, White PO (1964) Promax: A quick method for rotation to oblique simple structure. Br J Math Stat Psychol 17: 65–70.
27. Hu L, Bentler PM (1999) Cutoff criteria for fit indexes in covariance structure analysis: conventional criteria versus new alternatives. Struct Equ Modeling 6: 1–55.
28. Kline P (1994) An easy guide to factor analysis. London: Routledge.

29. Rasbash J, Charlton C, Browne WJ, Healy M, Cameron B (2011) MLwiN version 2.24. Centre for multilevel modelling, University of Bristol.
30. Goldstein H (2010) Multilevel statistical models. Hoboken, NJ: Wiley-Blackwell.
31. RCVS (2012) Guide to Profesisonal Conduct. Available: http://www.rcvs.org.uk/advice-and-guidance/code-of-professional-conduct-for-veterinary-surgeons/#declaration. Accessed 30 November 2012.
32. Green MJ, editor (2012) Dairy Herd Health. Wallingford, UK: CABI Publishers.
33. Hoey R (2007) Experts disagree over NICE's approach for assessing drugs. Lancet 370: 643–644.
34. Longworth L, Sculpher MJ, Bojke L, Tosh JC (2011) Bridging the gap between methods research and the needs of policy makers: A review of the research priorities of the National Institute for Health and Clinical Excellence. Int J Technol Assess Health Care 27: 180–187.
35. Veterinary Medicines Directorate (2011) Guidance for retailers. Available: http://www.vmd.defra.gov.uk/pdf/vmgn/VMGNote03.pdf. Accessed 30 November 2012.
36. RCVS (2012) Code of profesisonal conduct for veterinary surgeons. Available:http://www.rcvs.org.uk/advice-and-guidance/code-of-professional-conduct-for-veterinary-surgeons/#declaration. Accessed 30 November 2012.
37. Hobson-West P (2007) Trusting blindly can be the biggest risk of all: organised resistance to childhood vaccination in the UK. Sociol Health Illn 29: 198–215.
38. Foresight (2011) The future of food and farming executive summary. The Government Office for Science, London. Available: http://www.bis.gov.uk/assets/foresight/docs/food-and-farming/11-547-future-of-food-and-farming-summary. Accessed 30 November 2012.

14

Globus Pallidus External Segment Neuron Classification in Freely Moving Rats: A Comparison to Primates

Liora Benhamou, Maya Bronfeld, Izhar Bar-Gad, Dana Cohen*

The Leslie and Susan Gonda Multidisciplinary Brain Research Center, Bar-Ilan University, Ramat-Gan, Israel

Abstract

Globus Pallidus external segment (GPe) neurons are well-characterized in behaving primates. Based on their firing properties, these neurons are commonly divided into two distinct groups: high frequency pausers (HFP) and low frequency bursters (LFB). However, no such characterization has been made for behaving rats. The current study characterizes and categorizes extracellularly recorded GPe neurons in freely moving rats, and compares these results to those obtained by extracellular recordings in behaving primates using the same analysis methods. Analysis of our data recorded in rats revealed two distinct neuronal populations exhibiting firing-pattern characteristics that are similar to those obtained in primates. These characteristic firing patterns are conserved between species although the firing rate is significantly lower in rats than in primates. Significant differences in waveform duration and shape were insufficient to create a reliable waveform-based classification in either species. The firing pattern analogy may emphasize conserved processing properties over firing rate per-se. Given the similarity in GPe neuronal activity between human and non-human primates in different pathologies, our results encourage information transfer using complementary studies across species in the GPe to acquire a better understanding of the function of this nucleus in health and disease.

Editor: Thomas Boraud, Centre national de la recherche scientifique, France

Funding: This study was funded in part by Israel Science Foundation (ISF) grants 861/06 (DC) and 327/09 (IBG), and by the Legacy Heritage Biomedical Program of ISF grant 981-10 (IBG). The funders had no role in study design, data collection and analysis, decision to publish, or preparation of the manuscript.

Competing Interests: The authors have declared that no competing interests exist.

* E-mail: danacoh@gmail.com

Introduction

Current thinking emphasizes the role played by the basal ganglia in channeling information from limbic to cognitive and to motor circuits by a parallel and integrative circuit architecture [1]. The central position of the BG network in a neuronal loop connecting most cortical areas primarily to the frontal cortex [2,3] gives the basal ganglia the potential ability to participate in complex behaviors. However, the role of this structure remains elusive, thus emphasizing the importance of observation of the information flow from the cortex through these nuclei. The primate basal ganglia consist of multiple nuclei: two main input structures – the Striatum (Str) and Subthalamic nucleus (STN) – which are reciprocally connected to the Globus Pallidus external segment (GPe). These three structures converge onto two output structures: the Globus Pallidus internal segment (GPi) and the Substantia Nigra pars reticulata (SNr). Despite differences in terminology (Globus pallidus (GP) and Entopeduncular nucleus (EP) in rats, and GPe and GPi in primates, respectively) and a few structural differences, the rodent and primate basal ganglia roughly share similar cell types and connectivity, suggesting that comparative studies could provide valuable insights. For simplification, we will use the primate terminology also for rodents.

The GPe, located in the core of the basal ganglia, was classically viewed as a relay station along the indirect pathway [4]. Anatomical evidence as well as electrophysiological studies now suggest a more central function for the GPe in the basal ganglia network [5,6,7]. The strong reciprocal connections to all basal ganglia input nuclei endow the GPe with capacities to modulate the flow of information through the basal ganglia and its examination should shed light on basal ganglia function in general.

An early electrophysiological study in primates classified GPe neurons into two types based on their distinct *in-vivo* discharge patterns: (1) high-frequency discharge with pauses (85%), and (2) low frequency discharge with bursts (15%) neurons [8]. These two populations are now broadly known as high frequency pausers (HFP) and low frequency bursters (LFB). In addition, a third type dubbed border cells has been described and is believed to represent an extension of the cholinergic neurons of the substantia innominata or nucleus basalis of Meynert [8,9]. Similar GPe neuronal groups have been reported in humans [10]. Later studies in primates classified GPe neurons based on LFB and HFP firing patterns divergences [11,12,13,14,15]. In the rodent GPe, the distinction between subpopulations is more controversial. *In-vitro* electrophysiological [16,17,18,19] and anatomical studies [5,20,21] have reported conflicting data, with two to three GPe neuron types in each field. A physiological and computational study has suggested that GPe neuron properties are spread over a continuous space, making differentiation into subgroups impossible [22].

Chronic recording is well-developed in rats and permits stable recording of neurons from deep structures for prolonged periods of time. Thus, investigating the GPe in behaving rats could supply further information on the function of the GPe to supplement existing findings in the primate. Creating a common mapping of rat and primate GPe neurons would enable complementary studies within both species. This would allow researchers to benefit from findings on each species while minimizing the limitations inherent to each. Given the interest in observing the information flow through basal ganglia nuclei and the lack of consensus regarding the categorization of rat GPe neurons and their relation to categorization in primates, the current study was designed to provide a classification of GPe cells in rats by drawing parallels between extracellularly recorded GPe neurons in behaving primates and freely moving rats.

Methods

Surgical Procedures and Data Collection

Rats. All procedures were in accordance with the National Institutes of Health Guide for the Care and Use of Laboratory Animals and the Bar-Ilan University Guidelines for the Use and Care of Laboratory Animals in Research. All procedures were approved and supervised by the Institutional Animal Care and Use Committee (IACUC). This procedure was approved by the National Committee for Experiments in Laboratory Animals at the Ministry of Health (permit number 01-01-10). Activity of Globus Pallidus neurons was recorded in three freely moving adult male Long-Evans rats alternating between periods of immobility and exploration of the recording cage. The surgical procedure has been described previously [23,24]. In brief, adult male Long-Evans rats (Harlan) weighing 435 g on average, (range: 415 to 445 g) were sedated with 5% isoflurane and then injected i.m. with ketamine HCl and xylazine HCl (100 and 10 mg/kg, respectively). Supplementary injections of xylazine and ketamine were administered as required. The rat's head was fixed in a stereotaxic frame (Kopf Instruments, USA). After sterilization of the skin, an incision was made in order to expose the skull surface. Connective tissue was removed and the skull surface cleaned. Two craniotomies, slightly larger than the electrode, were made bilaterally above the GPe (AP: −1.4, ML: 3.6, DV: −6.6). 2×8 electrode arrays made with isonel coated tungsten microwires (50 microns diameter – California Fine Wire Company) or 27 gauge cannulae filled with 8 Formvar coated Nichrome wires (coated: 0.0015″, A–M Systems, Inc.) were slowly introduced into the GPe (impedance 0.1–0.2 MΩ at 1 kHz). Electrodes were fixed in place using dental cement, leaving the upper part of the connectors exposed.

At the end of the experiment, the rats were anesthetized with ketamine HCl, xylazine HCl and morphine (100 and 10 mg/kg and 0.15 ml/kg, respectively), and electrolytic lesions were made before perfusion with 10% formalin, brain fixation with 20% sucrose and formalin followed by cryostat sectioning of 60 μm thick slices. Electrode placement was confirmed histologically with a microscope (Nikon Eclipse E400, 1×/0.04).

Following about 10 days of recovery from surgery the animals were connected to the recording system. Neural activity was amplified, band-pass filtered at 150–8000 Hz and sampled at 40 KHz using a multichannel acquisition processor system (MAP system; Plexon Inc, Dallas, TX, USA). All waveforms exceeding a selected threshold were saved and offline sorted for later analysis. Most of the channels containing neurons were also recorded continuously at the same sampling rate to enable additional assurance of single neurons' quality. Offline sorting was performed on all continuously recorded units (OfflineSorter V2.8.8; Plexon, Dallas, TX) and the data were analyzed using custom-written MATLAB software (R2010b, MathWorks Inc., Natick, MA). The animals' activity was continuously monitored in the chamber to ensure that throughout recordings they remain awake.

Monkeys. All procedures followed the National Institutes of Health Guide for the Care and Use of Laboratory Animals, Bar-Ilan University Guidelines for the Use and Care of Laboratory Animals in Research and in accordance with the recommendations of the Weatherall Report. All procedures were approved and supervised by the Institutional Animal Care and Use Committee (IACUC). This procedure was approved by the National Committee for Experiments in Laboratory Animals at the Ministry of Health (permit number 18-07-08). Data were obtained from two male cynomolgus monkeys (Macaca fascicularis). The monkeys were kept in an enriched environment under fixed day/night light cycle. During the training and recording periods the animals had free food and were under water restriction. They received their daily water during the experimental session and were supplemented as required following the session. The monkeys' water, food consumption and weight were measured daily and their health was monitored by a veterinarian. Full details of the surgery and recording procedures have been provided previously [25]. Briefly, the monkeys underwent a surgical procedure to attach a recording chamber to the skull allowing access to the GPe and other cortical and basal ganglia structures. The surgical procedure was performed under aseptic conditions and general anesthesia induced by intramuscular ketamine-HCl (10 mg/kg) and Domitor (0.1 mg/kg) and maintained by isoflurane (1–3%), N_2O (1%) and oxygen (1%) ventilation delivered through tracheal intubation. Appropriate analgesics and antibiotics were given during surgery and postoperatively as required. All surgeries and follow-ups were under the supervision of a veterinarian. All efforts were made to minimize suffering. Recording sessions began after recovery from surgery. The monkeys were seated in a primate chair with their head fixed during the recording sessions. Using a cylindrical guide, eight glass-coated tungsten microelectrodes (impedance 0.2–0.7 MΩ at 1 kHz) were advanced separately into the GP. The electrode signal was continuously sampled at 40 kHz (Alphamap 10.10, Alpha-Omega Engineering), amplified (×1000) and wide bandpass filtered (2–8000 Hz four-pole Butterworth filter) (MCP-Plus 4.10, Alpha-Omega Engineering). Action potentials of individual neurons were sorted offline (OfflineSorter V2.8.7; Plexon, Dallas, TX). The external (GPe) and internal (GPi) segments were distinguished online based on characteristics of neuronal activity and the existence of border cells and white matter between the two segments. Only high-frequency pausers (HFP) and low-frequency bursters (LFB) from the GPe, identified as single neurons using off-line sorter, were included in this study. The average recording time per neuron was 120±47 seconds (mean±STD).

Following the end of the experiment, animals were anesthetized with ketamine (10 mg/kg) and stereotactic marking microlesions (DC current 60 μA for 30 s) were made. The lesions were targeted to dorsal white matter tracts at the anatomical plane that was derived from electrophysiological mapping to be consistent with the anterior commissure (AC0) position. Animals were then deeply anesthetized using sodium pentobarbital (50 mg/kg) and transcardially perfused with 1 liter of physiological saline, followed by 1 liter of 4% paraformaldehyde. The whole brain was removed and buffered in graded sucrose solution 10–30% over 7 days. The brain was then frozen at −25°C and cut in the coronal plane using a cryostat (Leica Mycrosystems). Each section of interest was mounted onto glass slides and Nissl stained. Contours of brain structures were traced using the digitized images and the anteroposterior position of each injection site was plotted on coronal planes, taking AC0 as the origin of the system axes.

Data Analysis

Statistical analysis. All the data are presented as the mean ± SEM. Analysis was structured as 2×2 interactions of animals (primates vs. rats) and cell type (HFPs vs. LFBs) evaluated by a N-way analysis of variance (ANOVAN). Multiple comparisons based on a non-parametric test (Kruskal-Wallis test) provided similar results. Comparison of two groups that did not follow a normal distribution was evaluated by the non-parametric Mann-Whitney U-test.

Waveform parameters. Waveform parameters consisted of valley width, peak to valley ratio, peak to valley duration, peak and valley amplitudes and zero-cross. The valley is the minimal amplitude time point and the peak is the maximal amplitude time point coming after the valley. Briefly, valley width describes the duration of the extracellular waveform at its half amplitude, the peak to valley ratio is the absolute value of the peak amplitude divided by the valley amplitude and zero-cross describes the time elapsed between the two time points around the valley in which the amplitude equals zero.

Firing parameters. Firing parameters including Coefficient of Variation (CV), Fano Factor (FF), firing rate, mode Inter-Spike Interval (ISI) and peri-modal width were calculated. The term coefficient of variation defines the standard deviation of the ISI distribution divided by its mean. The Fano Factor is the variance of the spike count distribution calculated in non-overlapping time windows, divided by its mean (window duration equals the median ISI of every single neuron). The firing rate is the total number of spikes divided by the total recording time (spike count rate). Mode ISI describes the mode value of the ISI distribution using 1 ms precision bins. In addition, in order to estimate the variability of ISIs values around the mode ISI and thereby measure the ISI distribution width, we calculated the peri-modal width which represents the width of the ISI distribution at an ordinate that equals the mode ISI divided by two.

Auto- and Cross-Correlations. Autocorrelations and cross-correlation functions were calculated for latencies of 1000 ms (bin equals 1 ms).

The post-spike suppression (PSP) [26] was defined as the earliest latency at which the rate equaled the average firing rate in the autocorrelation.

An Autocorrelation-Form based Category (AFC) was calculated by applying a low-pass filter on the autocorrelation function and counting the number of peaks. If the low-pass autocorrelation function presented one peak, it was identified as a burster and if two peaks were observed it was identified as a pauser. We validated this parameter by comparing the obtained categorization with a classification used in previous studies on primates.

For the cross-correlation functions, upper and lower confidence levels were calculated as follows: mean and standard deviation of the cross-correlograms at time ±4–5 s were calculated. The probability that the signal crosses a specified limit in 1% of the bins over one second in every bin according to the Bonferroni correction for multiple comparisons was calculated in the following manner: $p = \frac{0.01}{Nbins}$. Assuming a normal distribution, we obtained the number of standard deviations (Z-value) required to attain the probability p and drew the lower and upper confidence levels at the ordinates corresponding to the mean ± Z standard deviations.

Burst analysis. In order to identify bursts in the spike trains, we used the Poisson surprise method [27]. Briefly, the Poisson surprise (S) represents the degree to which the occurrence of n spikes in time T surprises us given the neuron firing rate and assuming a Poisson process. The Poisson surprise is computed in the following manner: $S = -\log P$, where P is the probability that, in a random spike train having the same firing rate (r), a given time interval of length T contains n or more spikes.

$$P = e^{-rT} \cdot \sum_{i=n}^{\infty} \frac{(rT)^i}{i!}$$

A time interval T was determined for each neuron depending on its firing rate as described below. Initially, an ISI shorter than T was detected. If the following ISI increased the Poisson surprise, it was added to the previously selected ISI until the Poisson surprise did not increase with an additional consecutive ISI. After burst identification, the first spike in the burst was deleted if the Poisson surprise increased by its removal from the burst. Bursts had to contain a minimum of three spikes. The burst percentage counts the number of spikes in bursts compared to the total spikes emitted by the neuron. For example, a neuron containing 20% of its spikes in bursts will obtain a burst percentage of 20%.

The Poisson surprise method requires a criterion for the time interval T to prevent faulty identification of regular ISIs occurring after a long ISI as bursts. The time interval T providing the most reliable identification of bursts by avoiding over or under-inclusion of ISIs [28] was the mean firing rate divided by 2.

Pause analysis. In order to identify pauses, the pause surprise method was used [13]. This method calculates how improbable it is that a number n of spikes or less appears in a defined period T given the average firing rate r and assuming a Poisson process. The Poisson surprise is computed in the following manner: $S = -\log P$, where P is the probability that in a random spike train having the same firing rate (r), a given time interval of length T contains n or fewer spikes. $P = e^{-rT} \cdot \sum_{i=0}^{n} \frac{(rT)^i}{i!}$. From all the possible segments formed from the same core interval, the segment that maximizes the pause surprise is called a pause. First, ISIs greater than ten times median ISI were detected (core interval). Then a maximal number of 5 ISIs (upper limit of added intervals) were added one by one before or after each identified long ISI and the pause surprise was calculated. If the addition of an ISI increased the pause surprise, it was included in the pause period. In primates, according to Elias et al. (2007), only periods with a duration greater than 300 ms (minimal length of the final pause) were considered as pauses. Because rat neurons have a significantly lower mean firing rate and the probability of encountering a period of silence of 300 ms is greater than in primates, we increased the minimal duration of the final pause proportionally to the decrease in the mean firing rate compared to primates and set it at 900 ms. Two adjacent pauses were merged if the number of spikes between them did not exceed three (maximal number of spikes enabling merging of adjacent pauses). In rats, the pause fraction represents the number of minutes in which two or more pauses were observed divided by the total recording minutes. Thus, neurons were defined as pausers if they had a minimal pause fraction of 80%. Recordings in primates were shorter (120±47 seconds; average duration ± STD), so a neuron was defined categorically as a pauser if it displayed at least two pauses in the available recording minute without the definition of a pause fraction.

Results

In order to explore the similarities and differences in rat and primate GPe activity, we characterized and compared the activity of 49 GPe neurons recorded in three rats and 63 GPe neurons recorded in two primates. The position of all electrodes used for recording GPe neurons in rats was verified by electrolytic lesions and histological slice observation (see Methods). An example of electrode positioning in rats is shown in Figure 1A and its corresponding coronal slice is shown in Fig. 1B. A summary of all electrode positioning in rats is shown in Figure 1 C. Initial observation of the recorded spike trains revealed that, on average, firing rates recorded in rats (20.07±2.87 spikes/s) were significantly lower than those recorded in primates (73.37±4.27 spikes/s; Mann Whitney U-test; $p<0.001$). Nonetheless, two main firing patterns could be distinguished in both species: one consisting of tonic Poisson firing and the other consisting primarily of bursts. Some of the tonically firing neurons also presented periods of silence or pauses. Interestingly, in rats, we did not record neuron with firing patterns resembling border neurons. Autocorrelations and spike trains of rat and primate GPe neurons representative of the three firing patterns types (i.e. low frequency with bursts, higher frequency with and without pauses) are shown in figure 2. We observed a remarkable similarity between rat and primate firing patterns belonging to the same group (compare traces in Fig. 2A & D; 2B & E; and 2C & F). Therefore, we decided to categorize rat GPe neurons based on firing properties, as commonly done in primates. To that end, we measured and calculated a variety of neuronal firing properties such as the coefficient of variation (CV), the Fano factor (FF) and post-spike suppression, and tested whether the two observed populations were also distinct in rats. We found that a data presentation based on firing properties of post-spike suppression, FF and the autocorrelation-form based category (AFC) parameter created two distinct clusters in both rats and primates (Fig. 3A & B). Comparison of the current primate classification into HFPs and LFBs with that obtained earlier on the same data [29] showed a complete match with one exception (~2%) that exhibited a relatively high value of FF and AFC value of one. Based on the similarity in primate and rat cluster shapes, rat GPe neurons were classified into HFP and LFB. This classification generated 5 outlier neurons that exhibited higher FF values compared to other neurons sharing a similar AFC. By analogy to primate neuronal classification these 5 outliers (5 out of 49; 10%) were also classified as HFP. According to this classification, we obtained 8 (13%) LFB and 55 (87%) HFP neurons in primates and 13 (27%) LFB and 36 (73%) HFP neurons in rats. Based on this classification, similar fraction of pausers was identified within cells classified as HFP neuronal population in rats and primates; 10 out of 36 (28%) HFPs in rats were identified as pausers by the pause analysis and 16 out of 55 (29%) in primates.

Based on the preceding classification, different parameters were calculated and compared between the different GPe neuronal populations (HFP and LFB) found in both species in order to characterize the similarities and differences among these neuronal populations. First, we examined the average firing rates of the identified groups. Primate HFPs exhibited a significantly higher firing rate compared to the LFBs (HFP: 80.28±4.88 spikes/s; LFB: 18.09±1.67 spikes/s; $p<0.001$; Fig. 3C) whereas in rats the differences in firing rates between HFP and LFB were not significant (HFP: 22.39±3.11 spikes/s; LFB: 13.63±2.56 spikes/s; $p = 0.2623$; Mann-Whitney U-test; Fig. 3C). By contrast to the firing rates, all parameters characterizing firing patterns properties showed similar statistically significant differences between the two classes of neurons, HFP and LFB, in the two species. These firing pattern differences were maintained between the two species. First, we looked at the parameters used for neuron classification: LFB neurons presented larger FF (rats: 2.17±0.17; primates: 3.37±0.35), a shorter post-spike suppression (rats: 5.47±2.53 ms; primates: 2.43±0.11 ms) and different AFC values than HFP neurons (rats: FF = 0.80±0.07; primates: FF = 0.73±0.11; rats: post-spike suppression = 42.21±5.64 ms; primates: post-spike suppression = 6.91±0.24 ms) in both species (FF: $p<0.001$; and post-spike suppression: $p<0.001$; Fig. 3 D & E). In addition, rat neurons exhibited longer post-spike suppressions than primates (rats: 16.53±1.88 ms; primates: 6.41±2.23 ms; ANOVAN; $p<0.001$) as can be seen in the representative autocorrelations in Fig. 2 and in Fig. 3E.

Next, we compared additional firing pattern characteristics such as burst fraction, pause fraction, mode ISI and the width of ISI distribution. As expected by their description as bursters, the LFB burst percentage was significantly higher than that of HFP in both species (rats: LFB:49.38±5.37%; HFP:13.90±2.34%; primates: LFB:72.64±4.94%; HFP:10.36±1.61%; main effect, ANOVAN; $p<0.001$; Fig. 3F). In addition, the mean burst frequency of LFB neurons was 124.9±82.9/min and 238.4±14.9 bursts/min in rats and primates, respectively. LFB neurons were burstier than HFP neurons; consequently their CV was higher than that of the HFPs in both species (rats: LFB: 1.65±0.12; HFP: 0.98±0.08; and primates: LFB: 1.92±0.09; HFP: 1.42±0.10, main effect, cell type, ANOVAN; $p<0.001$; Fig. 3G). Considering the overlap in firing rate between the HFP and LFB subgroups in rats, we carefully tested whether GPe neurons could make a transition from one mode of operation to the other. None of the recorded

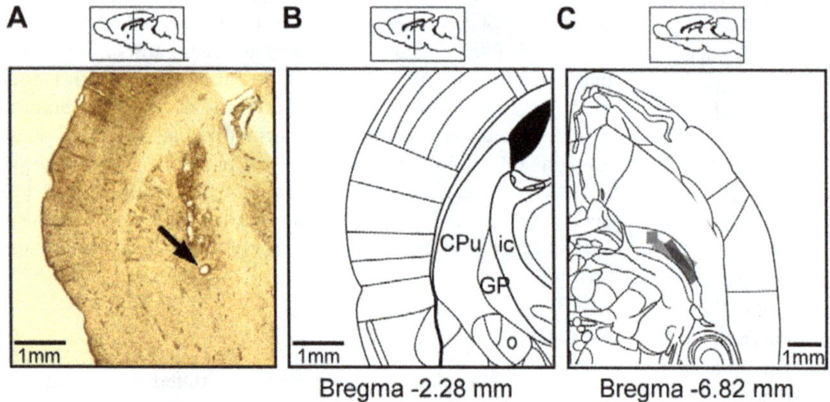

Figure 1. Verification of electrode placement in the Globus Pallidus of rats. A: a 60 micron slice showing electrode placement in a rat GPe following electrolytic lesion. B: Appropriate coronal section from atlas (Bregma: −2.28 mm; [47]). C: Recording sites marked (grey rectangle) for all animals on a planar rat atlas slice (Bregma: −6.82 mm; [47]).

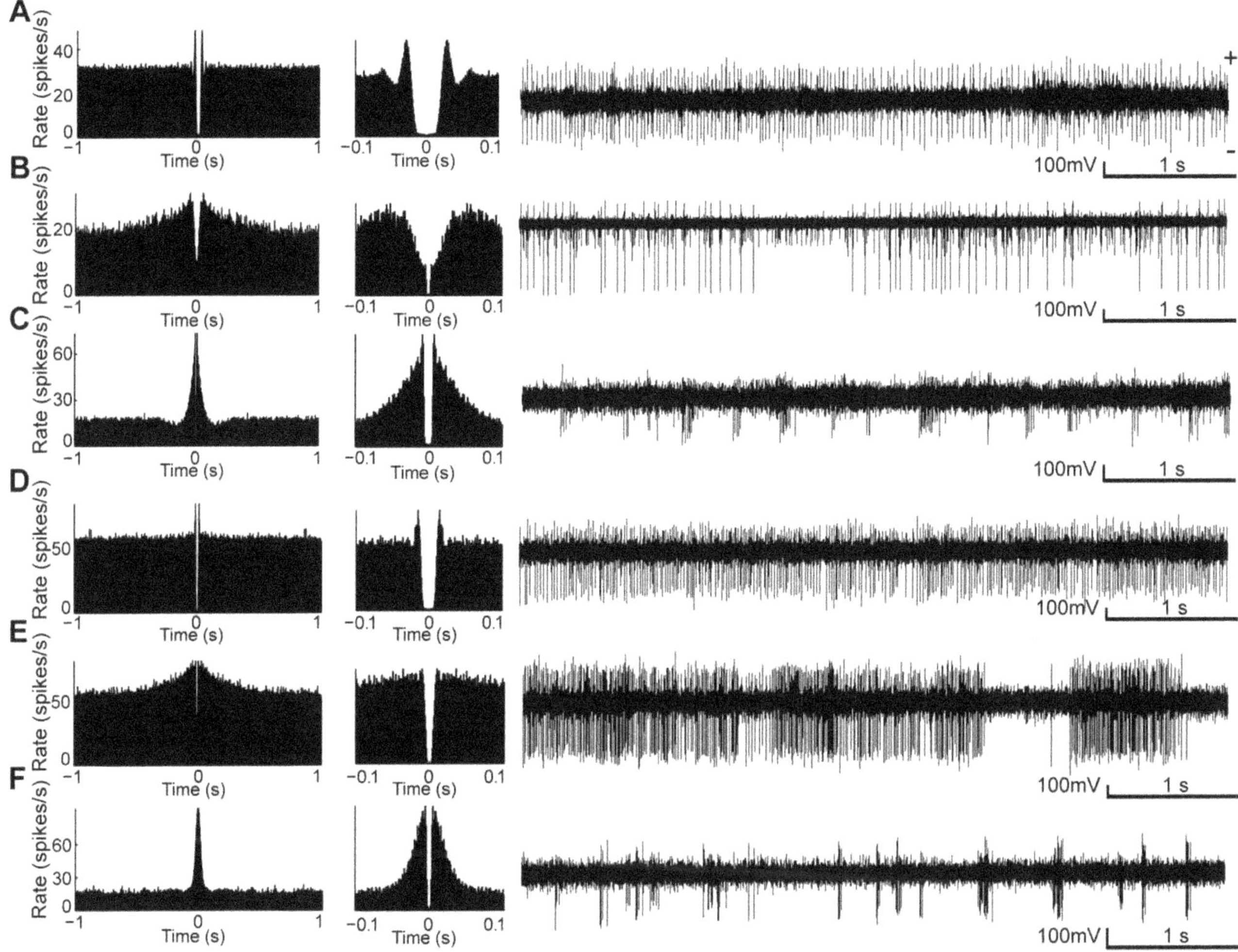

Figure 2. Typical firing patterns observed in rats (A–C) and primates (D–F). Left panel: autocorrelation using a time window of ±1 s, middle panel: autocorrelation with x-axis expanded to ±0.1 s, right panel: spike train of the example neuron. A: example of HFP neuron exhibiting tonic Poisson firing without pauses. B: HFP neuron displaying pauses (pauser). C: LFB neuron (burster). D–F: same type of neurons as in A–C but in primates.

neurons displayed a transition between firing pattern typical of HFPs and that typical of LFBs.

As mentioned previously, similar percentages of tonically firing neurons in both rats and primates presented periods of pauses (rats: 28% - 10 out of 36; and primates: 29% - 16 out of 56). The mean pause frequency in the HFP subpopulation of pausers was not significantly different in rats (11.5±4.2 pauses/min) compared to primates (17.0±4.8 pauses/min). Overall, both species exhibited similar fractions of time spent in pauses (rats: 29.9±3.6%, primates: 27.9±2.3%; $p>0.9$). As expected from bursters, the mode ISI of LFB neurons was significantly shorter than HFP neurons both in rats and in primates (rats: LFB: 8.4±1.5 ms, HFP: 36.7±7.9 ms; $p<0.001$; primates: LFB: 4.1±1.0 ms, HFP: 8.0±0.7 ms, $p<0.01$; post-hoc Mann-Whitney U-test; Fig. 3H). In addition, the peri-modal width was significantly smaller in LFB than in HFP neurons (rats: LFB: 15.9±3.5 ms, HFP: 31.4±4.5 ms; $p<0.005$; primates: LFB: 5.9±1.5 ms, HFP: 10.2±0.5 ms; $p<0.05$, post-hoc Mann-Whitney U-test). Therefore, we can assume that the mode ISI approximated the intra-burst ISI in LFB neurons, whereas in HFP neurons it represented the most frequent ISI value observed. Conversely, the median ISI was not significantly different between groups (rats: LFB: 52.5±16.1 ms, HFP: 73.3±11.7 ms; primates: LFB: 8.1±1.5 ms, HFP: 10.5±0.9 ms) suggesting that the ISI distribution location itself does not differ between neuronal groups, but they have different forms. Overall, all the firing patterns parameters we looked at exhibited similar group differences among GPe neurons in rats and primates.

We then addressed the similarities and differences observed in various waveform parameters within each species. Unlike neuronal classification in other basal ganglia structures such as the striatum, we were unable to reliably classify the neurons into two distinct populations using rat or primate waveform parameters. However, following the firing pattern based classification, we tested whether the HFPs and the LFBs exhibited distinct waveform parameters in primates (Fig. 4A) and in rats (Fig. 4B). In primates, the mean valley to peak duration of LFB neurons (423.2±37.7 μs) was significantly longer than that of HFP neurons (228.0±10.8 μs; $p<0.001$, Mann-Whitney U-test; Fig. 4C). The same was observed for the zero cross parameter (LFB: 389.3±54.5 μs; HFP: 220.9±7.9 μs; $p<0.001$, post-hoc Mann-Whitney U-test; Fig. 4C). In rats, the mean valley to peak duration of LFB neurons (273.1±31.3 μs) was significantly shorter than that of HFP neurons (353.5±21.2 μs; $p<0.05$, Mann-Whitney U-test; Fig. 4D). This tendency was also observed for the zero cross

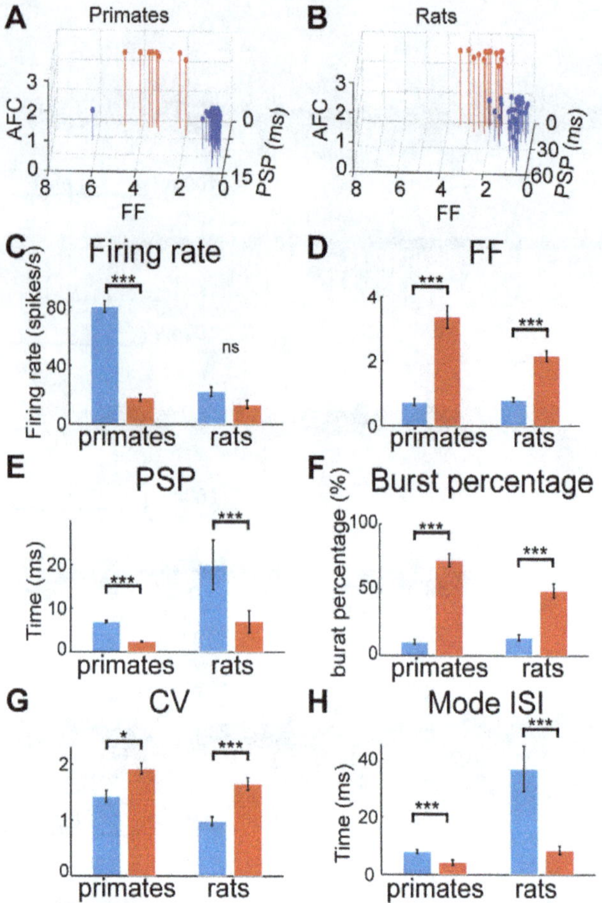

Figure 3. Neuronal classification and firing properties in primates and rats. A and B: 3 dimensional presentation of firing properties leading to the formation of distinct clusters in primates (A) and rats (B). C–H: Bar plots representing parameters of the two groups (HFP - blue, LFB - red) in the two species (left two bars - primates, right two bars - rats).

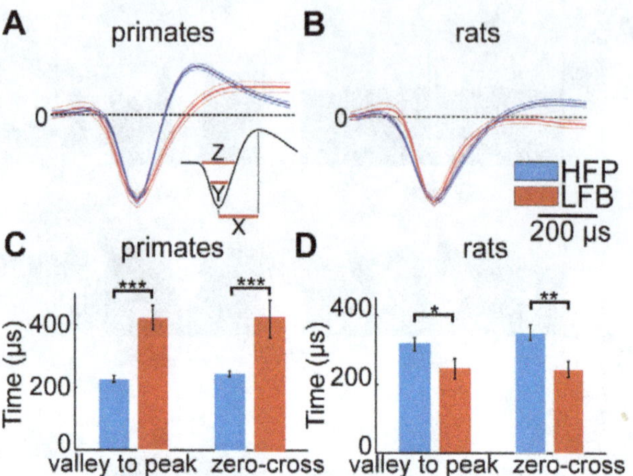

Figure 4. Waveform characteristics. A and B: normalized average waveforms of HFP (blue) and LFB (red) neurons in primates (A) and rats (B). Inset: X represents the valley to peak duration, Y the valley width and Z the zero-cross parameter. C and D Bar plots representing waveform parameters in HFP (blue) and LFB (red) neurons in primates (C) and in rats (D).

parameter (LFB: 244.2±22.0 μs; HFP: 350.0±21.5 μs; $p<0.01$; Mann-Whitney U-test; Fig. 4D).

Last, we examined the temporal interactions between neuronal pairs by calculating their cross-correlograms and testing whether different neuronal pairs were significantly correlated. The vast majority (30 out of 31–97%) of rat neuronal pairs exhibited flat cross-correlograms suggesting a lack of interaction between GPe neurons, which is consistent with the primate neuronal pairs which unanimously exhibited flat cross-correlograms (30 out of 30–100%). In rats, the only pair with a significant correlation (LFB and HFP) exhibited a wide peak centered around time 0, pointing to a probable common input that caused correlated changes in firing rate rather than a direct synaptic connection. Overall, neuronal pairs in both rat and primate GPe neurons displayed very little interaction (Fig. 5).

Discussion

In the present study, we extracellularly recorded GPe neuron activity in rats and primates to compare neuronal activity between the two species and specifically tested whether, as in primates, rat GPe neurons could be categorized as HFPs and LFBs. Our results show that the most striking difference between the two species is the neuronal firing rate, which is extremely high in primate HFPs compared to rats. Most primate studies report high firing rates of about 50 to 80 spikes/s [30,31] within a wide range of individual cell rates [32]. It appears that HFP neurons in rats exhibit a shifted range of activation and consequently a slower maximal firing rate (range of 2 to 74 spikes/s). This has been reported elsewhere [33,34,35,36] and likely reflects interspecies functional differences rather than major differences in GPe information processing strategies and capabilities. Supporting evidence for this view comes from a similar phenomenon observed in cerebellar Purkinje cells, in which rats and mice [37,38] show slower simple spike firing rates than primates [39] (approximately 40 spikes/s vs. 80 spikes/s

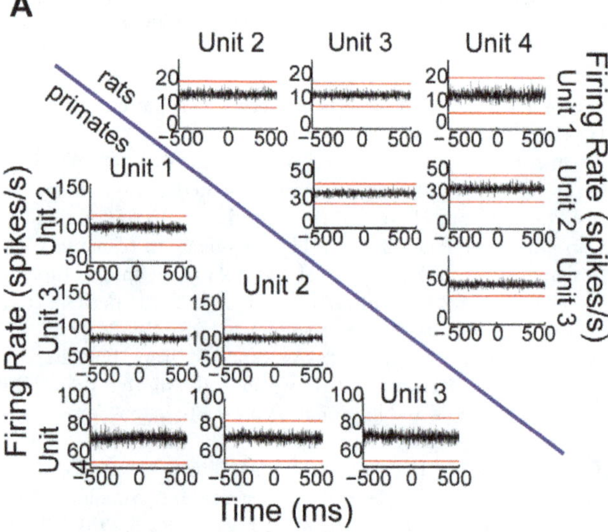

Figure 5. GPe neurons exhibit negligible interactions between pairs of neurons. Cross-correlations in the two species. Below the blue line: cross-correlations during a time window of ±1 s in four units recorded simultaneously in primates. Above the blue line: same in rats. Red lines in every cross-correlogram represent the lower and upper confidence levels (see Methods).

on average, respectively). Waveform parameters in the two species were insufficient to create distinct subpopulations of GPe neurons in both species. Classification of the rat neuronal population based on firing pattern divergence according to the conventional division in primates since the beginning of basal ganglia electrophysiology [8] resulted in the formation of two groups: HFPs and LFBs. These subpopulations represented a proportion of 73.5% and 26.5% respectively in rats, similar to previous intracellular studies [16,18]. Importantly, previous studies in primates have characterized a proportion of 85% of HFP and 15% LFB neurons [8,15,19]. These numbers may be skewed by interspecies differences, the fact that acute experiments entail biased neuronal sampling towards the high-frequency neurons over the more quiescent neurons, or deliberate bias due to lack of scientific interest in the LFB neurons. It remains to be determined whether and how the difference in group fractions influences basal ganglia information processing.

Other diverging parameters observed in this study, such as LFB waveform duration compared to HFP neurons in rats and group fractions are in line with previous electrophysiological studies in rats [18,20]. Of special interest, previous *in-vitro* studies in rats obtained slight inter-population differences [18,19]. Our *in-vivo* results reveal that the same parameters (waveform and firing rate) could not be used to categorize GPe neurons into distinct subgroups and may not be conserved in the two species. In contrast, firing patterns led to a similar classification compared to primates; thus firing patterns *in-vivo* differ from those observed *in-vitro* and were the main basis of GPe neuron differentiation into subpopulations. In contrast to the observed firing rates, waveform characteristics and group fractions that differed between rats and primates, all of the firing pattern characteristics measured in the rat HFPs and LFBs showed similar properties typical of primate HFPs and LFBs. These characteristics reflect firing pattern differentiators indicative of different modes of operation employed by the two cell types. We believe that their similarity in rats and primates likely emphasizes conservation of GPe processing properties which are fundamental to normal basal ganglia function. Moreover, measuring the interactions between pairs of GPe neurons in rats revealed negligible correlations between neurons in this structure. Similarly, negligible interactions of less than 5% have previously been reported between primate GPe neurons [40,41] regardless of inter-neuronal distance [11]. This lack of interaction between GPe neurons supports the idea of functionally independent processing pathways within the GPe that has been preserved over the two species [42,43,44]. This fascinating property, along with the anatomical connectivity features of the basal ganglia, give rise to many questions about the processing properties (input/output organization) of the GPe and the basal ganglia in general [45].

Given the similarities and differences found in this study between and within rat and primate GPe neurons, we suggest that as in primates, rat GPe neurons can be reliably divided into two subgroups of cell types: HFPs and LFBs. This conclusion is based on the neuronal firing patterns which capture the differences between the two cell types to a greater extent than other parameters such as waveform characteristics and firing rates which do not support such a categorization. Interestingly, all the parameters affording a clear separation of rat GPe neurons into two cell types are conserved between primates and rats, thus supporting the notion that they are important for normal GPe processing. In contrast, parameters that did not allow for a clear distinction between the two cell types are not conserved between the two species. Specifically, waveform shapes and percentages in the population could arise from technical differences in the recording device and, in any case, are unlikely to directly influence the GPe mode of operation. Nonetheless, the substantial difference in the firing rates between primate and rat HFPs calls for further investigation to determine whether and how the firing rate influences GPe function during behavior.

From an evolutionary perspective, it was claimed that basal ganglia circuitry has been conserved as an action selection mechanism in vertebrates [46] that evolved through reuse of existing ancestral structures. Thus we could expect to encounter similar neuronal groups in vertebrate basal ganglia. Indeed we found similar neuronal firing patterns in the rat GPe neurons as in primates. Given the known similarity between the same neuronal groups in humans and nonhuman primates and the well-known evolutionary conservation of the basal ganglia it seems likely that human, primate and rat studies could play a complementary role in our understanding of the basal ganglia circuitry. Knowledge of the basal ganglia has increased over the past decades; however, its function remains to be elucidated. Parallel recording of basal ganglia nuclei activity in behaving animals will help determine how the firing patterns and interactions observed during rest are altered during behavior and thus could lead to a better understanding of the basal ganglia network function and organization.

Acknowledgments

We thank Mr. Yuval Baumel for the interesting discussions and Dr. Katya Belelovsky for technical assistance.

Author Contributions

Conceived and designed the experiments: IBG DC. Performed the experiments: LB MB. Analyzed the data: LB. Wrote the paper: LB MB IBG DC.

References

1. Haber SN (2003) The primate basal ganglia: parallel and integrative networks. J Chem Neuroanat 26: 317–330.
2. Alexander GE, DeLong MR, Strick PL (1986) Parallel organization of functionally segregated circuits linking basal ganglia and cortex. Annu Rev Neurosci 9: 357–381.
3. Alexander GE, Crutcher MD (1990) Functional architecture of basal ganglia circuits: neural substrates of parallel processing. Trends Neurosci 13: 266–271.
4. Albin RL, Young AB, Penney JB (1989) The functional anatomy of basal ganglia disorders. Trends Neurosci 12: 366–375.
5. Kita H, Kitai ST (1994) The morphology of globus pallidus projection neurons in the rat: an intracellular staining study. Brain Res 636: 308–319.
6. Levesque M, Parent A (2005) The striatofugal fiber system in primates: a reevaluation of its organization based on single-axon tracing studies. Proc Natl Acad Sci U S A 102: 11888–11893.
7. Turner RS, Anderson ME (2005) Context-dependent modulation of movement-related discharge in the primate globus pallidus. J Neurosci 25: 2965–2976.
8. DeLong MR (1971) Activity of pallidal neurons during movement. J Neurophysiol 34: 414–427.
9. Richardson RT, DeLong MR (1986) Nucleus basalis of Meynert neuronal activity during a delayed response task in monkey. Brain Res 399: 364–368.
10. Hutchison WD, Lozano AM, Davis KD, Saint-Cyr JA, Lang AE, et al. (1994) Differential neuronal activity in segments of globus pallidus in Parkinson's disease patients. Neuroreport 5: 1533–1537.
11. Bar-Gad I, Heimer G, Ritov Y, Bergman H (2003) Functional correlations between neighboring neurons in the primate globus pallidus are weak or nonexistent. J Neurosci 23: 4012–4016.
12. Kita H, Nambu A, Kaneda K, Tachibana Y, Takada M (2004) Role of ionotropic glutamatergic and GABAergic inputs on the firing activity of neurons in the external pallidum in awake monkeys. J Neurophysiol 92: 3069–3084.
13. Elias S, Joshua M, Goldberg JA, Heimer G, Arkadir D, et al. (2007) Statistical properties of pauses of the high-frequency discharge neurons in the external segment of the globus pallidus. J Neurosci 27: 2525–2538.

14. Joshua M, Adler A, Rosin B, Vaadia E, Bergman H (2009) Encoding of probabilistic rewarding and aversive events by pallidal and nigral neurons. J Neurophysiol 101: 758–772.
15. Bronfeld M, Belelovsky K, Bar-Gad I (2011) Spatial and temporal properties of tic-related neuronal activity in the cortico-basal ganglia loop. J Neurosci 31: 8713–8721.
16. Kita H, Kitai ST (1991) Intracellular study of rat globus pallidus neurons: membrane properties and responses to neostriatal, subthalamic and nigral stimulation. Brain Res 564: 296–305.
17. Nambu A, Llinas R (1994) Electrophysiology of globus pallidus neurons in vitro. J Neurophysiol 72: 1127–1139.
18. Cooper AJ, Stanford IM (2000) Electrophysiological and morphological characteristics of three subtypes of rat globus pallidus neurone in vitro. J Physiol 527 Pt 2: 291–304.
19. Bugaysen J, Bronfeld M, Tischler H, Bar-Gad I, Korngreen A (2010) Electrophysiological characteristics of globus pallidus neurons. PLoS One 5: e12001.
20. Millhouse OE (1986) Pallidal neurons in the rat. J Comp Neurol 254: 209–227.
21. Nambu A, Llinas R (1997) Morphology of globus pallidus neurons: its correlation with electrophysiology in guinea pig brain slices. J Comp Neurol 377: 85–94.
22. Gunay C, Edgerton JR, Jaeger D (2008) Channel density distributions explain spiking variability in the globus pallidus: a combined physiology and computer simulation database approach. J Neurosci 28: 7476–7491.
23. Nicolelis MA, Ghazanfar AA, Faggin BM, Votaw S, Oliveira LM (1997) Reconstructing the engram: simultaneous, multisite, many single neuron recordings. Neuron 18: 529–537.
24. Jacobson GA, Lev I, Yarom Y, Cohen D (2009) Invariant phase structure of olivo-cerebellar oscillations and its putative role in temporal pattern generation. Proc Natl Acad Sci U S A 106: 3579–3584.
25. Erez Y, Czitron H, McCairn K, Belelovsky K, Bar-Gad I (2009) Short-term depression of synaptic transmission during stimulation in the globus pallidus of 1-methyl-4-phenyl-1,2,3,6-tetrahydropyridine-treated primates. J Neurosci 29: 7797–7802.
26. Schmitzer-Torbert NC, Redish AD (2008) Task-dependent encoding of space and events by striatal neurons is dependent on neural subtype. Neuroscience 153: 349–360.
27. Legendy CR, Salcman M (1985) Bursts and recurrences of bursts in the spike trains of spontaneously active striate cortex neurons. J Neurophysiol 53: 926–939.
28. Cocatre-Zilgien JH, Delcomyn F (1992) Identification of bursts in spike trains. J Neurosci Methods 41: 19–30.
29. Bronfeld M, Belelovsky K, Erez Y, Bugaysen J, Korngreen A, et al. (2010) Bicuculline-induced chorea manifests in focal rather than globalized abnormalities in the activation of the external and internal globus pallidus. J Neurophysiol 104: 3261–3275.
30. Hashimoto T, Elder CM, Okun MS, Patrick SK, Vitek JL (2003) Stimulation of the subthalamic nucleus changes the firing pattern of pallidal neurons. J Neurosci 23: 1916–1923.
31. Goldberg JA, Bergman H (2011) Computational physiology of the neural networks of the primate globus pallidus: function and dysfunction. Neuroscience 198: 171–192.
32. Adler A, Katabi S, Finkes I, Israel Z, Prut Y, et al. (2012) Temporal convergence of dynamic cell assemblies in the striato-pallidal network. J Neurosci 32: 2473–2484.
33. Kita H, Kita T (2011) Role of Striatum in the Pause and Burst Generation in the Globus Pallidus of 6-OHDA-Treated Rats. Front Syst Neurosci 5: 42.
34. Gardiner TW, Kitai ST (1992) Single-unit activity in the globus pallidus and neostriatum of the rat during performance of a trained head movement. Exp Brain Res 88: 517–530.
35. Gage GJ, Stoetzner CR, Wiltschko AB, Berke JD (2010) Selective activation of striatal fast-spiking interneurons during choice execution. Neuron 67: 466–479.
36. Chang JY, Shi LH, Luo F, Woodward DJ (2006) Neural responses in multiple basal ganglia regions following unilateral dopamine depletion in behaving rats performing a treadmill locomotion task. Exp Brain Res 172: 193–207.
37. de Solages C, Szapiro G, Brunel N, Hakim V, Isope P, et al. (2008) High-frequency organization and synchrony of activity in the purkinje cell layer of the cerebellum. Neuron 58: 775–788.
38. Shin SL, Hoebeek FE, Schonewille M, De Zeeuw CI, Aertsen A, et al. (2007) Regular patterns in cerebellar Purkinje cell simple spike trains. PLoS One 2: e485.
39. Lisberger SG, Fuchs AF (1978) Role of primate flocculus during rapid behavioral modification of vestibuloocular reflex. I. Purkinje cell activity during visually guided horizontal smooth-pursuit eye movements and passive head rotation. J Neurophysiol 41: 733–763.
40. Nini A, Feingold A, Slovin H, Bergman H (1995) Neurons in the globus pallidus do not show correlated activity in the normal monkey, but phase-locked oscillations appear in the MPTP model of parkinsonism. J Neurophysiol 74: 1800–1805.
41. Raz A, Vaadia E, Bergman H (2000) Firing patterns and correlations of spontaneous discharge of pallidal neurons in the normal and the tremulous 1-methyl-4-phenyl-1,2,3,6-tetrahydropyridine vervet model of parkinsonism. J Neurosci 20: 8559–8571.
42. Francois C, Yelnik J, Percheron G, Fenelon G (1994) Topographic distribution of the axonal endings from the sensorimotor and associative striatum in the macaque pallidum and substantia nigra. Exp Brain Res 102: 305–318.
43. Groenewegen HJ, Galis-de Graaf Y, Smeets WJ (1999) Integration and segregation of limbic cortico-striatal loops at the thalamic level: an experimental tracing study in rats. J Chem Neuroanat 16: 167–185.
44. Percheron G, Filion M (1991) Parallel processing in the basal ganglia: up to a point. Trends Neurosci 14: 55–59.
45. Bar-Gad I, Morris G, Bergman H (2003) Information processing, dimensionality reduction and reinforcement learning in the basal ganglia. Prog Neurobiol 71: 439–473.
46. Redgrave P, Prescott TJ, Gurney K (1999) The basal ganglia: a vertebrate solution to the selection problem? Neuroscience 89: 1009–1023.
47. Paxinos G, Watson C (2007) The Rat Brain in Stereotaxic Coordinates. 6th ed., New York: Elsevier.

15

Development of the Horse Grimace Scale (HGS) as a Pain Assessment Tool in Horses Undergoing Routine Castration

Emanuela Dalla Costa[1]*, Michela Minero[1], Dirk Lebelt[2], Diana Stucke[2], Elisabetta Canali[1], Matthew C. Leach[3]

1 Università degli Studi di Milano, Dipartimento di Scienze Veterinarie e Sanità Pubblica, Milan, Italy, **2** Pferdeklinik Havelland / Havelland Equine Hospital, Beetzsee-Brielow, Germany, **3** Newcastle University, School of Agriculture, Food & Rural Development, Newcastle upon Tyne, United Kingdom

Abstract

Background: The assessment of pain is critical for the welfare of horses, in particular when pain is induced by common management procedures such as castration. Existing pain assessment methods have several limitations, which reduce the applicability in everyday life. Assessment of facial expression changes, as a novel means of pain scoring, may offer numerous advantages and overcome some of these limitations. The objective of this study was to develop and validate a standardised pain scale based on facial expressions in horses (Horse Grimace Scale [HGS]).

Methodology/Principal Findings: Forty stallions were assigned to one of two treatments and all animals underwent routine surgical castration under general anaesthesia. Group A (n = 19) received a single injection of Flunixin immediately before anaesthesia. Group B (n = 21) received Flunixin immediately before anaesthesia and then again, as an oral administration, six hours after the surgery. In addition, six horses were used as anaesthesia controls (C). These animals underwent non-invasive, indolent procedures, received the same treatment as group A, but did not undergo surgical procedures that could be accompanied with surgical pain. Changes in behaviour, composite pain scale (CPS) scores and horse grimace scale (HGS) scores were assessed before and 8-hours post-procedure. Only horses undergoing castration (Groups A and B) showed significantly greater HGS and CPS scores at 8-hours post compared to pre operatively. Further, maintenance behaviours such as explorative behaviour and alertness were also reduced. No difference was observed between the two analgesic treatment groups.

Conclusions: The Horse Grimace Scale potentially offers an effective and reliable method of assessing pain following routine castration in horses. However, auxiliary studies are required to evaluate different painful conditions and analgesic schedules.

Editor: Edna Hillman, ETH Zurich, Switzerland

Funding: The authors would like to thank the EU VII Framework program (FP7-KBBE-2010-4) for financing the Animal Welfare Indicators (AWIN) project. The funders had no role in study design, data collection and analysis, decision to publish, or preparation of the manuscript.

Competing Interests: The authors have declared that no competing interests exist.

* E-mail: emanuela.dallacosta@unimi.it

Introduction

The recognition and alleviation of pain is critical for the welfare of horses. Although considerable progress has been made in understanding physiology and treatment of pain in animals over the past 20 years, the assessment of pain in horses undergoing management procedures, such as branding, pin firing and castration, remains difficult and frequently suboptimal [1–4]. Equine castration is a husbandry practice routinely performed to: avoid undesired mating, facilitate handling, and reduce aggression and other undesirable behaviours. Annually, it is estimated that 240,000 horses are castrated in Europe [5]. Studies in other species demonstrate that animals experience pain and discomfort both acutely and chronically following castration [6,7]. Despite the limited research in horses, castration has been shown to be associated with some degree of pain that can persist for several days and, therefore, requires adequate analgesic treatment [2–4,8]. Price et al. [1] reported that only 36.9% of horses received analgesics for post operative pain, with one perioperative administration of Flunixin appearing to be one of the most common analgesic procedure provided following castration [9]: one possible explanation for this is the difficulty in assessing and quantifying pain in this species [2,10]. For example, even though castration of horses is a common procedure, no gold standard for pain assessment is available to date. As in other animal species, pain in horses is difficult to assess because of their inability to communicate with humans in a meaningful manner. This could be further compounded by horses potentially suppressing the exhibition of obvious signs of pain in the presence of possible predators (i.e. humans) as is suggested with other prey species. Several behaviour-based assessments of pain in horses already exist [11–17]. The Post Abdominal Surgery Pain Assessment Scale (PASPAS) is a multidimensional scale that can be used to quantify pain after laparotomy [14]. The Composite Pain Scale (CPS)

Table 1. Breed and mean age of the stallions of the two treatment groups.

Group (N)	Breed (N)	Age (Mean)
Treatment A (19)	Arabian horse (1)	2
	German Warmblood (3)	2.6
	Friesian (3)	1.7
	Iceland pony (5)	2.6
	Irish draught horse (1)	2
	Polo horse (1)	2
	Quarter horse (3)	2
	Mini-Shetland pony (1)	2
	Tennessee Walker horse (1)	2
Treatment B (21)	German Warmblood (4)	2.5
	Edles Warmblood (1)	1
	Friesian (3)	1.7
	Iceland pony (6)	2.5
	Irish draught horse (1)	1
	Polo horse (2)	1.5
	Quarter horse (2)	2
	Mini-Shetland pony (1)	4
	Trakehner (1)	5

Table 2. Details of the horses of the control group.

Sex	Breed	Age	Procedure
Mare	Polo horse	7	control X-ray pelvis
Mare	German warmblood	14	control X-ray cervical
Gelding	Haflinger	3	hoof correction
Gelding	Haflinger	3	hoof correction
Gelding	Haflinger	4	teeth rasping
Gelding	Haflinger	2	hoof correction

focuses on the presence of pain-related behaviours and the change in the frequency of normal behaviour patterns and physiological parameters [16]and has been successfully applied following both surgery (e.g. castration), injury and disease (e.g. laminitis, colic) [16,17]. However, behaviour-based assessments of pain are not without limitations that constrain their routine application. These include the need for trained and experienced observers [8,16,17], prolonged observation periods [18], particularly in conditions inducing only mild pain, and the palpation of the painful area in some cases [14,16,17]. Furthermore, many of the pain related behaviours described so far have been identified in response to what are perceived to be severely painful conditions (e.g. colic, laminitis [14,16]), rather than those that are perceived to be mildly to moderately painful conditions (e.g. identification procedures [19]). Recently, a new approach to pain assessment has been developed in rodents and rabbits utilising the assessment of facial expressions [20–23]. Facial expressions are commonly used to assess pain and other emotional states in humans, particularly in those who are unable to communicate coherently with their clinicians (e.g. those with cognitive impairment and neonates [24,25]). In humans, facial expressions are routinely scored both manually [25] and automatically [26] using the Facial Action Coding System (FACS), which is considered as an accurate and reliable method that describes the changes to the surface appearance of the face resulting from individual or combinations of muscle actions, referred to as 'action units' [27]. Action units relating to pain have been identified in rodents and rabbits and incorporated into species-specific "grimace scales" [20–23]. These grimace scales are considered to give a number of advantages over other routinely used methods of assessing pain in animals. Firstly, grimace scales are less time consuming to carry out [20–23]. Secondly, observers can easily and rapidly be trained to use them [20–23]. Thirdly, grimace scales may utilise our potential tendency to focus on the face when scoring pain [28,29]. Fourthly, they can be used to effectively assess a range of painful conditions, from mild to severe pain [20]. Finally, it can increase the safety of the observer when assessing pain in large animals, as grimace scales do not require the observer to approach the subject and palpate the painful area for the assessment. Therefore the Horse Grimace Scale (HGS) may offer an effective and practical method of identifying painful conditions and the efficacy of the methods we use to ameliorate pain in horses (i.e. analgesia administration). Furthermore, it can be applied in association with other behaviour-based methods to enhance the assessment of pain in horses and could be implemented in practice by owners and stable managers as an effective on farm early warning system.

The objectives of this study were to develop and validate a standardised pain scale based on facial expressions in horses (Horse Grimace Scale) using routine castration, and to investigate whether the HGS could be successfully implemented with minimal training, enabling the development of an on-farm pain assessment tool. Castration was considered a suitable model for the development of HGS because it is amongst the most common management procedures carried out in veterinary practice. In addition, utilising animals that are undergoing routine castration for husbandry reasons allows the researchers to avoid carrying out a surgical procedure solely for the evaluation of a method of assessing post-procedural pain.

Materials and Methods

Ethics statement

Castration is a routinely conducted husbandry procedure that was carried out in compliance with the European Communities Council Directive of 24 November 1986 (No. 86/609/EEC). This study was registered as an animal experiment at the Brandenburg State Veterinary Authority (V3-2347-A-42-1-2012). Horses involved in this study underwent routine veterinary procedures for health or husbandry purposes at the request of their owner on a voluntary basis. Consequently, no animals underwent anaesthesia or surgery or were directly used in order to record data for the purposes of this study. Verbal informed consent was gained from each participant prior to taking part in this research. Written consent was deemed unnecessary as no personal details of the participants were recorded. No animals received less than the standard analgesic regimen for the purposes of the study. This study employed a strict "rescue" analgesia policy: if any animal was deemed to be in greater than mild pain (assessed live by an independent veterinarian), then additional, pain relieving medication would immediately be administered and the animal removed from the study. The choice of medication and dosage would be based on the severity of pain identified thorough the clinical examination of the individual horse.

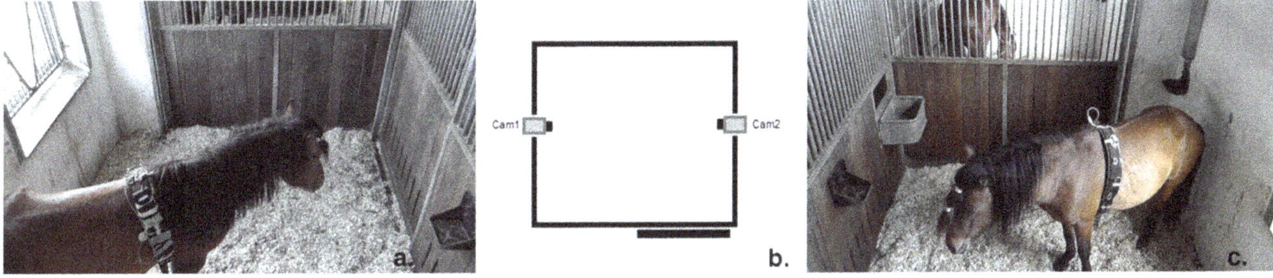

Figure 1. Video cameras position. The drawing in the middle (b) shows the position of the two HD cameras. Pictures on the left (a) and on the right (c) show frames grabbed from Cam1 and Cam2 respectively.

Animals and Husbandry

Forty stallions of different breeds, coat colour and aged between 1 and 5 years (mean age 2.3 years) underwent routine castration (see Table 1 for details). In addition, six horses of mixed age and gender that were undergoing general anaesthesia for different non-invasive and indolent procedures were used as a control group (see Table 2 for details). All animals were recruited from the hospital's clinical cases. In order to be included in this study, all the subjects had to be deemed healthy and without signs of cryptorchidism by an equine veterinarian after physical examination and behavioural evaluation. All horses were hospitalised in a veterinary clinic for 5 days to undergo castration or anaesthesia alone. In order to control for any possible effect of stress related to being in a novel environment and separated from their peers, all the subjects were allowed to acclimatise to their new environment, clinicians and video cameras for 2 days prior to the beginning of the study. In order to control for any possible differences in behaviour between stallions, geldings and mares, the acclimation period before starting with data collection was the same for all the horses. All subjects were kept in the same housing and management conditions: they were housed in standard single horse boxes (4×3 m with an outside window, see Figure 1) on wood shavings (German Horse Span Classic, German Horse Pellets, Wismar, Germany), and in visual contact with other conspecifics. They were fed twice a day with hay (approx. 3 kg/100 kg body weight per day) and water was provided ad libitum by automatic drinkers. Food was withheld from all horses for 8-hours before and 5 hours after anaesthesia (standard protocol for general anaesthesia [30]). In order to collect videos and images without disturbing the behaviour of the horses, two digital video cameras (Panasonic, HDC-SD99, Panasonic, Japan) were positioned on the top of the grate section on opposite sides of the box (see Figure 1).

Surgery and Analgesic Treatment Groups

Horses undergoing castration were divided into two breed-matched treatment groups using a blocked randomization process. Group A (N = 19) received a single perioperative injection of Flunixin (1.1 mg/Kg i.v., Flunixin 5%, medistar, Aschberg, Germany) approximately 5 minutes prior to anaesthesia immediately after administration of sedative drug. Group B (N = 21) received a perioperative injection of Flunixin (1.1 mg/Kg i.v.) as for group A and a subsequent oral application of Flunixin (Flunidol 5%, cp-pharma, Burgdorf, Germany, 1.1 mg/Kg p.o.) 6 hours after castration. All the medications were administered by a veterinary nurse who was aware of group allocation; the veterinarians responsible for pain assessment were blinded to treatment group. Horses underwent routine surgery castration with closed technique through a scrotal approach without primary closure of the wound in dorsal recumbency under general anaesthesia [9], as recommended by the National Equine Welfare Council (NEWC) and the Canadian Veterinary Medical Association [31,32]. The surgeries were all carried out by one of two equally experienced veterinary surgeons. To investigate the impact of general anaesthesia on the HGS, a control group (C) of horses was recruited. The control horses (N = 6) underwent the same general anaesthesia protocol as horses in groups A and B and received a single perioperative injection of Flunixin (1.1 mg/Kg i.v.) 5 minutes prior to anaesthesia. All castrated horses also received antibiotic treatment for three days starting at the morning before surgery (Synutrim 72% Pulver, Vétoquinol, Ravensburg, Germany), 2–4 mg Trimethoprim and 12 mg Sulfadiazin /Kg p.os every 12 h. Prior to the first drug application the weight of each horse was estimated with a weight tape in order for the correct drug doses to be administrated. The anaesthesia protocol was the same for all the subjects: pre-medication with Romifidine (Sedivet, Boehriger Ingelheim Vetmedica, Ingelheim, Germany, 80 micrograms Romifidinehydrochloride/Kg), induction with Diazepam (Diazepam-ratiopharm, Ratiopharm, Ulm, Germany, 0.1 mg/Kg) and Ketamine (Ketamin 10%, medistar, Ascheberg, Germany, 2.2 mg/Kg) intravenously via a jugular catheter. When necessary, general anaesthesia was maintained by another injection of Ketamine (1.1 mg/Kg). Twenty-six out of 40 castrated horses (65%) and 2 out of 6 control horses (33.3%) needed a second injection of Ketamine to maintain an appropriate level of anaesthesia in order to complete the surgery or the non-invasive procedure; the duration of anaesthesia was comparable long all the subjects. Surgery lasted 10–15 min, following which horses were moved to a recovery box; then, as soon as they were able to walk (20–60 minutes after anaesthesia), returned to their home box. Recovery from anaesthesia is the time that a horse need to stand up; it strongly depends on individual differences and it does not necessarily reflect the duration of previous anaesthesia. Horses recovered from anaesthesia without assistance inside the recovery box under visual supervision of a veterinary nurse. No intra-operative complications were reported and all horses recovered from anaesthesia fully and uneventfully prior to the first data collection post-procedure. All surgeries/general anaesthesia were carried out between 9 and 11am.

Pain Assessment

At each time interval an overall pain assessment was conducted by two trained veterinarians blinded to treatment group using a Composite Pain Scale (CPS) (see Table S1) based on the one developed by Bussieres and colleagues [16,17] and adapted according to Søndergaard and Halekoh [33].

Video Recording

Thirty-minute video sequences were recorded using 2 High Definition Cameras with a 28 mm wide angle objective lens (Panasonic, HDC-SD99, Panasonic, Japan), the videos were recorded one day before procedure in the evening (baseline observation, pre-procedure) and at similar time 8-hours following procedure (8 h post-procedure). The cameras were positioned at opposite sides of the box, on the top of the grate section. This arrangement gave the highest probability of capturing the behaviour and face of the horse during filming without interfering with their normal behaviour (see Figure 1).

Behavioural Recording

Behaviour of horses undergoing castration was evaluated. For each video, the last 15 minutes were analysed. A focal animal continuous recording method [34] was used to describe the horse's activity. The frequency and duration of thirty categories of behaviour (see Table S2) was continuously recorded using Solomon Coder (beta 12.09.04, copyright 2006–2008 by András Péter) by two trained treatment and session blind observers. Behaviours recorded as states (movement, licking and chewing, alertness, agitation, investigative behaviour, drinking, eating, lowered head carriage, head orientation, grooming) were reported as durations, and those recorded as events (weight-shifting, pawing, kicking, flank watching, rolling, yawning, masturbating, vocalization, urinating, defecating, tail swishing, flehmen) were reported as frequency of occurrence. Duration of maintenance behaviours showing the same pattern were added to form the composite maintenance behaviour score, comprising exploration, alertness and grooming.

Horse Grimace Scale (HGS) Recording

The HGS was created following the methods developed by Langford et al. [20] and Sotocinal et al. [21] for rodents and Keating et al. [23] for rabbits. Changes in horse behaviour and facial expressions were identified using a pilot study [8] following eight stallions undergoing surgical castration with the same anaesthetic and analgesic protocol as used in the main study. According to the published literature [2,4] and pilot study results [8], 8-hours post-castration was deemed the appropriate time interval between observations as this was when the most of the pain related behaviours were observed. Furthermore, the estimated duration of sedation from pre-medication drugs and anaesthetics used in this study should have subsided at 8-hours post-intervention [35–37]. Still images were extracted from each video sequences whenever the horse was found in a position with the head and face clearly visible. This enabled a number of clear and high quality images to be extracted. Each image was then cropped so that only the head of the horse was visible to prevent observers from being biased by the body of the animal when looking at each image. Images of each subject before and 8-hours after surgery were compared to identify changes in facial expressions associated with these procedures by a trained treatment blind observer experienced in assessing facial expressions in other species (MCL). Based on these comparisons, the Horse Grimace Scale (HGS) was developed, and comprises six facial action units (FAUs): stiffly backwards ears, orbital tightening, tension above the eye area, prominent strained chewing muscles, mouth strained and pronounced chin, strained nostrils and flattening of the profile (see Figure 2). One hundred and twenty six images were randomly selected by a non-participating assistant with no experience of assessing pain in horses for further scoring (63 pre and 63 post procedure images). In order to maintain a balanced design for the statistical analysis, the image set comprised 1 or 2 pictures of each horse pre and 8-hours post procedure (e.g. lateral images pre and post and frontal images pre and post). The 126 images were then scored in a random order using the Horse Grimace Scale by five treatment and session (pre or post-surgery) blind observers. A detailed hand out with the description of the six identified FAUs and the scoring system was distributed to the observers (see Figure 2). Briefly, for each image each observer was asked to give a score for each of FAU using a 3-point scale (0 = not present, 1 = moderately present, 2 = obviously present). If the participant was unable to score a particular FAU clearly, they were asked to score it as 'I don't know'. The Horse Grimace Scale (HGS) score was determined by adding the individual scores for each of the six action units identified (stiffly backwards ears, orbital tightening, tension above the eye area, prominent strained chewing muscles, mouth strained and pronounced chin and strained nostrils and flattening of the profile) in each image. Consequently, the maximum possible HGS score was 12 (i.e. a score of 2 for each of the 6 FAUs). In addition, the observers were asked to make a global pain judgment for each picture (no pain vs. pain) based upon their own clinical experience. If they deemed the individual to be in pain, then they were asked to score the intensity of that pain (mild, moderate or severe). In order to explore the effect of time (pre vs. post-procedure) and treatment (analgesia and surgery), the mean HGS scores were calculated for each image across all participants.

Observer Selection

Five observers were selected as they had expertise either with horses or scoring facial expressions. The observers had diverse backgrounds including horse welfare researchers, veterinary surgeons, research scientists and veterinary students.

Statistical Analysis

All statistical analyses were conducted using SPSS 19 (SPSS Inc., Chicago, USA). Differences were considered to be statistically significant if $P \leq 0.05$. The data were tested for normality and homogeneity of variance using Kolmogorov-Smirnov and Levene test, respectively. CPS and HGS scores were not normally distributed and therefore the scores were transformed using square root transformation. Repeated Measures General Linear Model (RGLM) was used to analyse the data with the time points (pre and 8-hours post-procedure) as the *within-subjects* factor and the treatment group as the *between-subjects* factor. Any treatment effects were further investigated using analysis of variance (ANOVA) with data from the separate time periods forming the dependent variables and treatment as the fixed effect. Post-hoc analysis of treatment group effects was conducted using Bonferroni post-hoc test. The reliability of HGS scale was determined using inter-class correlation coefficient (ICC) to compare mean scores for each of the facial action units across all the participants. Accuracy was determined by comparing the global pain and no pain judgement made by the treatment and period blind observers with actual pain state of the horse in each photograph. The reliability of the Composite Pain Scale scores were analysed using an inter-class correlation coefficient (ICC). Reliability of the manual behaviour analysis was assessed by means of independent parallel coding of a random sample of videotaped sessions (5 clips) using percentage agreement. Wilcoxon test was conducted to determine differences in behaviour shown before and 8 hour after procedure. Spearman correlation coefficients were calculated to investigate the relationship between the CPS, HGS and behaviour.

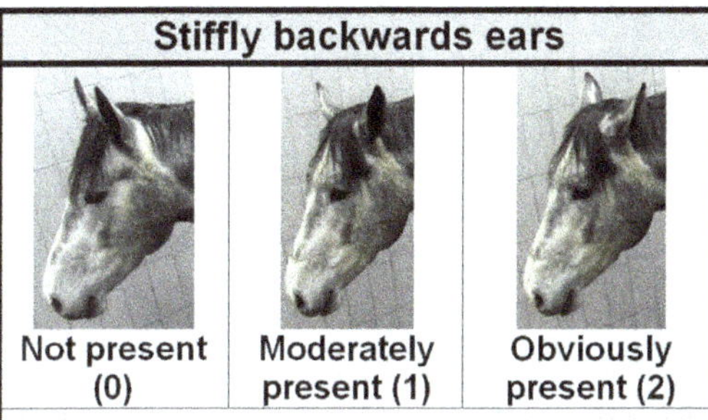

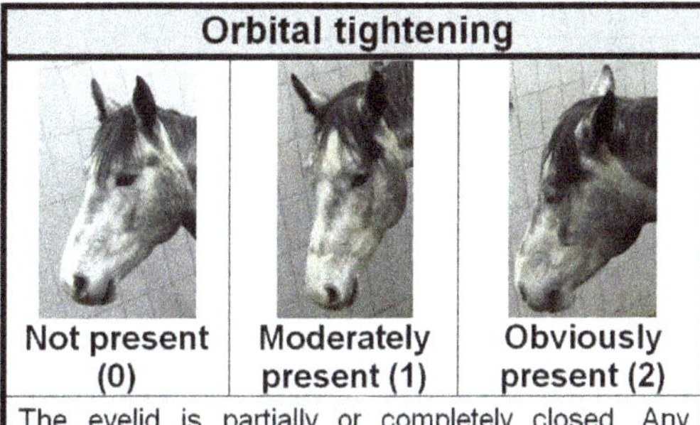

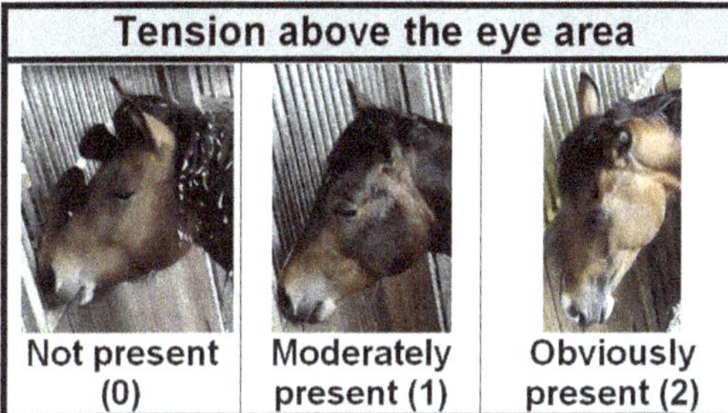

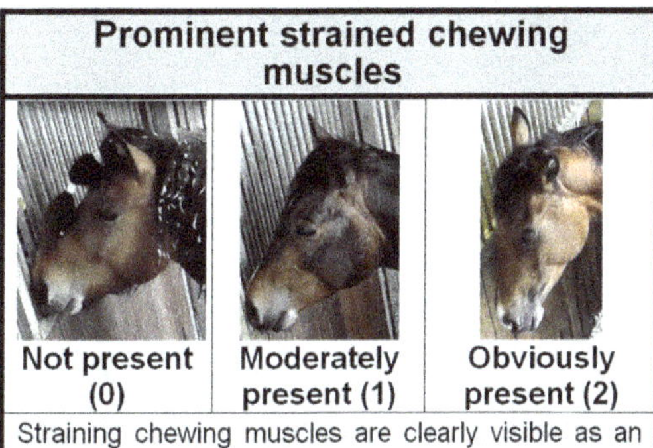

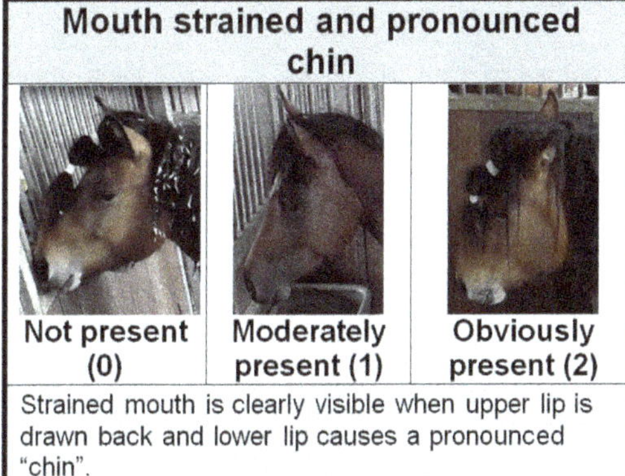

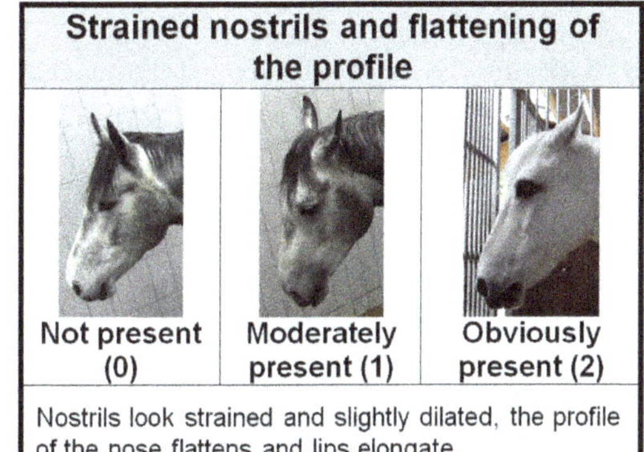

Figure 2. Horse Grimace Pain Scale (HGS). The Horse Grimace Pain Scale with images and explanations for each of the 6 facial action units (FAUs). Each FAU is scored according to whether it is not present (score of 0), moderately present (score of 1) and obliviously present (score of 2).

Results

During this study, no horses required the administration of rescue analgesia or had to be removed from the study due to adverse events.

Horse Grimace Scale (HGS)

Time, treatment and time*treatment interaction had significant effects on HGS score (RGLM, P = 0.000, P = 0.007 and P = 0.000, respectively; $\eta^2 = 0.03$). In the pre-procedure period there was no significant difference between the three treatments (ANOVA, P = 0.84; $\eta^2 = 0.00$). At eight-hours post-procedure the HGS score was significantly different between the three treatments (ANOVA, P = 0.000; $\eta^2 = 0.11$), with the HGS score being significantly higher in horses undergoing routine castration (Groups A and B) compared to the control group (Group C) (Bonferroni post-hoc, P = 0.000 for both comparisons). No significant differences were found between groups with the single (A) or multiple (B) Flunixin administration (Bonferroni post-hoc, P = 1.000) (see Figure 3). Example images and associated HGS scores of horses in groups undergoing castration compared to control are shown in Figure 4.

Total observation time was approximately 40 minutes for scoring all the pictures. The average accuracy of global pain judgement was 73.3%, with false positives being slightly more prevalent (17.0%) than misses (false negatives) (9.8%). Individual accuracy of participants varied from 67.5% to 77.8%. The Horse Grimace Scale demonstrated high inter observer reliability with an overall Intraclass Correlation Coefficient (ICC) value of 0.92. The individual action units comprising the HGS also showed high ICC

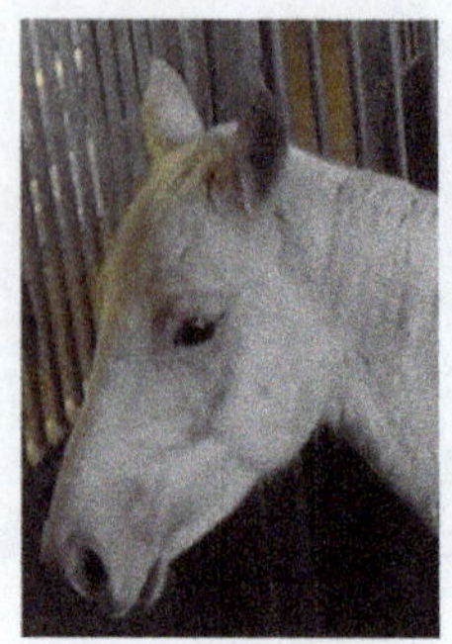

Facial Coding Unit	Score
Ears stiffly backwards	1
Orbital tightening	0
Tension above eye area	0
Prominent strained chewing muscles	0
Mouth strained and pronounced chin	0
Strained nostrils and flattening of the profile	0
Total pain score	1

a.

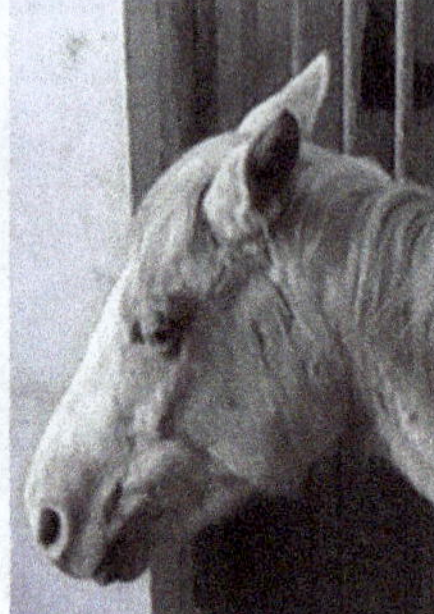

Facial Coding Unit	Score
Ears stiffly backwards	2
Orbital tightening	2
Tension above eye area	0
Prominent strained chewing muscles	2
Mouth strained and pronounced chin	1
Strained nostrils and flattening of the profile	1
Total pain score	8

b.

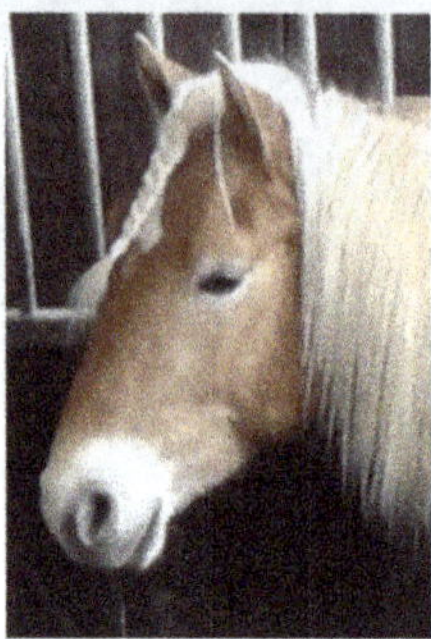

Facial Coding Unit	Score
Ears stiffly backwards	0
Orbital tightening	0
Tension above eye area	1
Prominent strained chewing muscles	0
Mouth strained and pronounced chin	0
Strained nostrils and flattening of the profile	0
Total pain score	1

c.

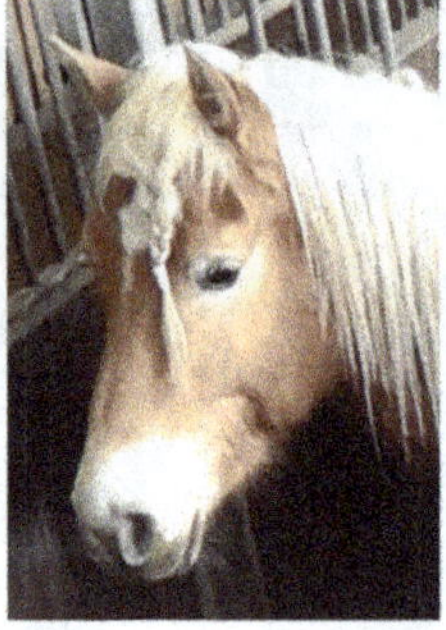

Facial Coding Unit	Score
Ears stiffly backwards	0
Orbital tightening	0
Tension above eye area	1
Prominent strained chewing muscles	0
Mouth strained and pronounced chin	0
Strained nostrils and flattening of the profile	0
Total pain score	1

d.

Figure 3. Mean Horse Grimace Scale (HGS) scores pre and 8-hours post-procedure. HGS scores are presented on the y-axis (±1 SE) for horses undergoing routine castration (A and B), and anaesthesia control group (C) with the pre and 8-hours post-procedure recordings on the x-axis (** P = 0.000).

values of: 0.97 for stiffly backwards ears, 0.83 for orbital tightening, 0.86 for tension above the eye area, 0.88 for prominent strained chewing muscles, and 0.72 for mouth strained and pronounced chin. The only exception was for strained nostrils and flattening of the profile (ICC = 0.58). On average, all the six facial action units (FAUs) were assessed easily by all the participants, as shown by the percentage of "not able to score" ranging from 0% for ear position to 21% for the tension above eye and strained mouth and pronounced chin (see Table 3). Front-view images were more difficult to score than profile view images, in particular for the evaluation of prominent strained chewing muscles and mouth strained and pronounced chin (46% and 81% respectively of "not able to score"). In profile view images, horses with dark-brown or black coats were more difficult to score than grey and light brown coat, especially for the orbital tightening and prominent strained chewing muscles (12% and 16% respectively).

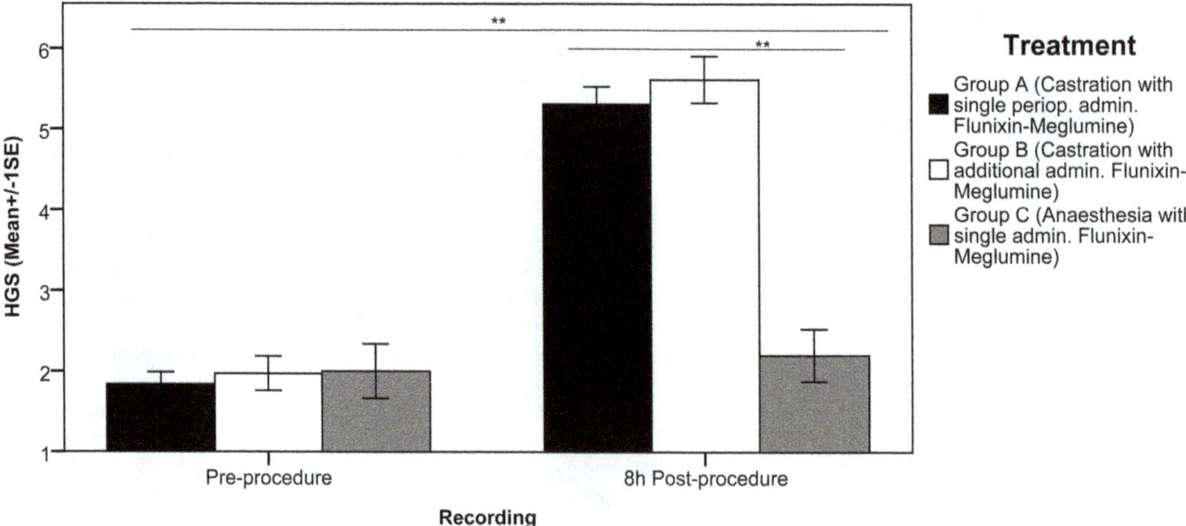

Figure 4. Example images and HGS scores. Example images and associated HGS scores of the same horse pre (a; c) and 8-hours post-procedure (b; d). Images a and b underwent castration; c and d were control animals.

Table 3. The percentage of "not able to score" for each Facial Action Unit identified.

Facial Action Units (FAUs)	Not able to score (%)
Stiffly backwards ears	0
Orbital tightening	9
Tension above the eye area	21
Prominent strained chewing muscles	15
Mouth strained and pronounced chin	21
Strained nostrils and flattening of the profile	8

Composite Pain Scale (CPS)

Time, treatment and time*treatment interaction had significant effects on CPS score (RGLM, P = 0.002, P = 0.002 and P = 0.050, respectively; $\eta^2 = 0.28$). In the pre-procedure period there was no significant difference between the treatments (ANOVA, P = 0.65; $\eta^2 = 0.02$). At eight-hours post-procedure the CPS score was significantly different between the three treatments (ANOVA, P = 0.000; $\eta^2 = 0.41$), with the CPS score being significantly higher in horses undergoing routine castration (Groups A and B) compared to the control group (Group C) (Bonferroni post-hoc, P = 0.000 for both comparisons). No significant differences were found between groups with the single (A) or multiple (B) Flunixin administration (Bonferroni post-hoc, P = 1.000) (see Figure 5).

The CPS demonstrated good inter observer reliability between the two analgesic treatment blind observers with an overall ICC of 0.79.

Behaviour analysis

Percentage agreement between the 2 observers was more than 80% for all the behaviours. Many of the pain related behaviours were observed too infrequently to be meaningfully analysed. Low head carriage showed a tendency to increase in duration at 8-hours after castration (Wilcoxon, P = 0.068) compared to baseline. Duration of exploration and alertness significantly decreased at 8-hours post-castration (Wilcoxon, P = 0.000 and P = 0.008, respectively) compared to baseline. The composite maintenance behaviour score (comprising the sum of the duration of exploration, alertness and grooming) significantly decreased at 8-hours post-surgery (148.1±21.7 sec) compared to pre (363.5±36.4 sec) (Wilcoxon, P = 0.000). There was no significant effect of treatment A or B on either maintenance or pain related behaviours. Total observation time needed to analyse all the videos was approximately 20 hours.

Relationship between behaviour, CPS and HGS

The HGS score was correlated positively with the CPS score (Spearman correlation, r = 0.580, P = 0.000) and negatively with duration of explorative behaviour (Spearman correlation,

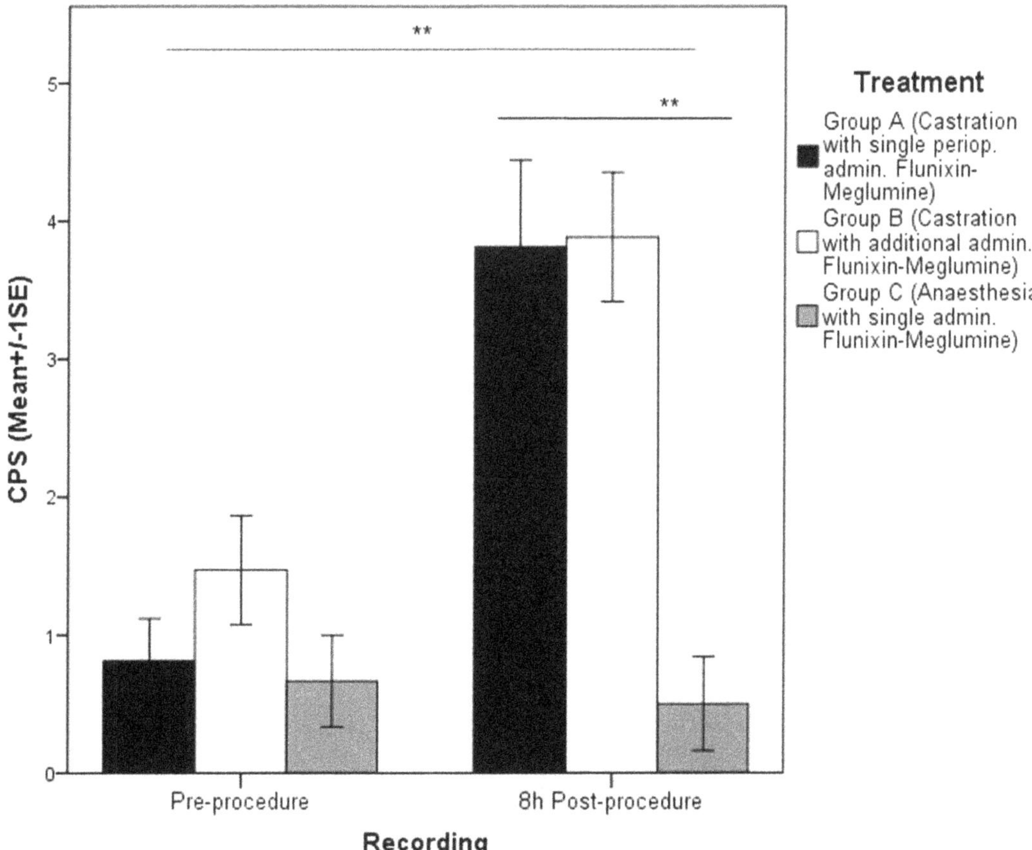

Figure 5. Mean Composite Pain Scale (CPS) scores pre and 8-hours post-procedure. CPS scores are presented on the y-axis (±1 SE) for horses undergoing routine castration (A and B), and anaesthesia control group (C) with the pre and 8-hours post-procedure recordings on the x-axis (** P = 0.000).

r = −0.461, P = 0.002). The HGS score was negatively correlated with the composite maintenance behaviour score (Spearman correlation, r = 0.508, P = 0.001).

Discussion

Despite the severity of pain associated with routine castration in horses being contentious [10,38,39], the findings of previous studies [2–4,40] have demonstrated that this procedure is associated with some degree of pain. An untreated control group undergoing castration without any analgesic treatment was not included in this study for both ethical and welfare reasons, as pain can cause a long lasting welfare issue in horses [40]. Although better balanced control group would be preferable, the control group used in this study to evaluate the effect of general anaesthesia on HGS was similar (in size, age, sex, and clinical conditions) to control groups presented in other scientific studies on the assessment of pain in horses [14,17]. As general anaesthesia for horses is not without risks for health and welfare [41], recruit more horses or healthy stallions to have a more homogenous control group would be questionable for both ethical and welfare reasons. This study has identified changes in facial expressions in horses undergoing surgical castration that appear to be similar to those previously described in other species [20–23], with some subtle variation due to differences in the species subjected to a variety of painful conditions. Changes in ear position, orbital tightening and some tension in the chewing muscles are largely similar to those described in other "grimace scales" [20–23]. In this study, differences in Horse Grimace Scale scores were observed following a routine surgical castration, with an increase in scores from pre to 8-hours post-procedure. Importantly, no differences in the HGS scores were found in control horses, undergoing general anaesthesia for non-invasive procedures, demonstrating that general anaesthesia has no effect on the HGS. Pain related behaviours and physiological parameters assessed using the Composite Pain Scale [16,17] showed a similar pattern to that of the HGS, with only horses undergoing routine castration exhibiting differences in score between the pre and 8-hours post-surgery periods. Low mean CPS scores in relation to the maximum possible score were likely due to the fact that an analgesic treatment was administrated to all the castrated horses and that the CPS was originally developed for a broad spectrum of pain intensities (e.g. orthopaedic pain). Our results confirm the findings of other authors [4] that duration of exploration and alertness decreased in horses between pre and 8-hours post-surgical procedure. The horses showing high HGS scores also exhibited high Composite Pain Scale scores and low duration of explorative behaviour, alertness and grooming 8-hours post-surgery. Differently from other species (e.g. dogs, mice), grooming in horses was never reported to be linked to stress or suffering; whilst several authors reported that, in healthy horses, a considerable portion of the daily time budget can be consumed with grooming [42,43]. It has been clearly demonstrated previously that pain in horses can be expressed through the exhibition of general non-specific indicators such as decrease in normal activity, lowered head carriage, fixed stare, rigid stance and reluctance to move [4,15]. In a preliminary study on castration pain in horses, Eager and colleagues also found that grooming decreased six hours post-operatively[44]. In the present study horses undergoing routine castration showed the tendency to keep their head in a lower position 8-hours post-surgery. Although non-specific behavioural indicators of pain in equids are considered not to correlate strictly with severity of pain [15], the tendency to carry the head below the withers is of relevance because several authors reported that lower head carriage is shown in case of chronic or severe pain [18,45]. The results of this study demonstrate that the HGS is a potentially effective method of assessing castration related pain in horses. Horse Grimace Scale scores significantly increased from pre to post castration and were unaffected by anaesthesia alone indicating that the action units relate directly to post procedure pain and/or distress. As there was no difference in the HGS between the two analgesic treatment groups, we are unable to fully differentiate between post-procedure pain and distress in this study. However, the significant difference between control and treatment groups and correlation between HGS, CPS and some non-specific behavioural indicators of pain suggest that the action units comprising the HGS are likely to change in response to pain. There are two potential explanations for lack of difference in HGS scores between those horses receiving a single pre-operative administration (Group A) and those receiving a pre and post-operative administrations (Group B) of Flunixin. It is possible that both the HGS and CPS were insufficiently sensitive to discriminate between effects of the analgesic schedules used. Alternatively, the two administrations of 1.1 mg/kg of Flunixin 6 hours apart (i.e. pre and post operatively) may not provide greater pain relief than a single pre-operative administration. Duration of pain relief of Flunixin is contradictory, Johnson et al. [46] found that additional Flunixin was needed 12,8±4,3 h after surgery, for this reason we decided to give a second dose of Flunixin before the 8-hour measurement (12,8–4,3 = 8,5 h minus time for oral absorption of Flunixin). As we did not include untreated control group undergoing castration without any analgesic treatment in this study for ethical and welfare reasons we are unable to provide insight into which explanation is correct. Therefore, further studies investigating the HGS, CPS and behavioural indicators of pain as well as the efficacy of 1.1 mg/kg of Flunixin and other analgesics with routine castration are needed to answer the above question.

The overall accuracy of the HGS (73.3%) was slightly lower than that of the other "grimace scales" (97% for the mouse grimace scale [20], 82% for the rat grimace scale [21], and 84% for the rabbit grimace scale [23]). The most likely explanation for this, is a combination of a slightly lower quality for some of the images used compared to those scored in other grimace scales and considerable variation in coat colour of the horses observed. Coat colour of the horse combined with the quality of some of the images meant that dark horses were often more difficult to score than those with lighter coats, especially if the background was dark. This issue has already been observed in mice [20,47] where the higher the quality of the images and a contrasting background allowed the observers to more accurately score the images. Four out of six control horses had a light coat which allowed easier scoring meaning that the finding that the control horses did not present any differences in HGS before and after anaesthesia is highly reliable.

The inter observer reliability (as measured by inter-class correlation coefficients [ICC]) of the overall HGS and its component action units was similar to those of the mouse grimace scale (0.90) [20], rat grimace scale (0.90) [21] and rabbit grimace scale (0.91) [23]. As with other grimace scales applied to animals (e.g. rodents & rabbits), the observers in this study gave images of the horses in a non-painful state (e.g. pre-procedure) low but not zero scores which is inevitable when using a scale that is a composite of six individual action units. In a non-painful state these action units can be observed occasionally in isolation at a low intensity (score of 1 rather than 2), for example if an image is taken of a horse as it 'blinks,' then an observer may give orbital tightening a score of 1 or 2 but it is likely that they will score 0 for all the other action units. It is unlikely that HGS scores lower than two were due to stress related to being in a novel environment as all the horses were acclimated to the new environment. Using the Horse Grimace Scale to score horses 'live' rather than from images will help to solve this issue. The use of Horse Grimace Scale for scoring post-operative pain has distinct advantages over that of manual behaviour analysis, which can be complex due to the a greater number of behaviours that potentially need to be scored. Behaviour-based assessments appear to be more time-consuming to conduct (analysis time was 20 hours for behavioural based assessment compared to 40 minutes for the HGS). Furthermore, changes in facial expressions in the horses were detectable, without the need of approaching the subject, and by observers with differing expertise with only the HGS manual for guidance.

The HGS requires some further validation for assessing post castration pain (for instance in horse with administration of flunixin compared to horses with flunixin associated with an opioid post-surgery, considering longer follow up intervals) and could be further developed for other potentially painful procedures before it can be considered fully validated. Further studies could also be conducted to identify facial action units associated with other states such as fear and anxiety so that we are able to differentiate pain from these other states. Among the limitations of other routinely used methods of assessing pain in horses, there is considerable concern that prey species have evolved the ability to mask obvious signs of pain under specific circumstances (i.e. the presence of a predator such as humans). In humans it has been demonstrated pain related facial expressions cannot be completely suppressed by voluntary control [28] and in another prey species, for example the rabbit, it has been demonstrated that facial expressions are an easy and reliable cage-side method of assessing acute pain associated with ear tattooing in the presence of an observer [23]. It has been shown that humans tend to focus on head and face when assessing pain in humans [28] and rabbits [29] therefore this method could represent a reliable and feasible method that utilises the natural human instinct. Furthermore, HGS could be used as an animal-based indicator of spontaneously emitted pain, and it may provide insights into the experience of pain in horses in their own environment, and so be a useful tool in the assessment of horse welfare on-farm. Even though further evaluation of the HGS is required, the present results suggests that HGS may offer a reliable tool for assessing post-castration pain than other routinely used methods.

Acknowledgments

The authors would like to thank Dr Dario Polli, Dr Alessandra Torraco and Dr Giulia Borino for assistance with video analysis, the 5 observers for their help and assistance in scoring the pictures, and Miss Mareile Groβe Ruse, University of Lund, Sweden, for her assistance in statistical analysis.

The authors also would like to thank horse owners, the colleagues and the personnel of the clinics who patiently helped us with horses during the experiments.

Author Contributions

Conceived and designed the experiments: EDC MM DS DL EC MCL. Performed the experiments: ECD MM DS DL. Analyzed the data: EDC MM. Contributed reagents/materials/analysis tools: EDC MM DS DL EC MCL. Wrote the paper: EDC MM DS DL EC MCL. Development of HGS and technical support by: EDC MCL.

References

1. Price J, Eager RA, Welsh EM, Waran NK (2005) Current practice relating to equine castration in the UK. Research in Veterinary Science 78: 277–280.
2. Love EJ, Taylor PM, Clark C, Whay HR, Murrell J (2009) Analgesic effect of butorphanol in ponies following castration. Equine Veterinary Journal 41: 552–556.
3. Maassen E, Gerhards H (2009) Equine castration: comparison of treatment with phenylbutazon, Traumeel and control group. Pferdeheilkunde 25: 451–460.
4. Sanz MG, Sellon DC, Cary JA, Hines MT, Farnsworth KD (2009) Analgesic effects of butorphanol tartrate and phenylbutazone administred alone and in combination in young horses undergoing routine castration. JAVMA 235: 1194–1203.
5. European Horse Network (2010) Key Figures. Available: http://www.europeanhorsenetwork.eu/index.php?page = horse-industry-in-europe.
6. Molony V, Kent J (1997) Assessment of acute pain in farm animals using behavioral and physiological measurements. Journal of animal science: 266–272. Available: http://www.journalofanimalscience.org/content/75/1/266.short. Accessed 30 January 2013.
7. Llamas Moya S, Boyle LA, Lynch PB, Arkins S (2008) Effect of surgical castration on the behavioural and acute phase responses of 5-day-old piglets. Applied Animal Behaviour Science 111: 133–145. doi:10.1016/j.applanim.2007.05.019.
8. Dalla Costa E, Rabolini A, Scelsa A, Ravasio G, Pecile A, et al. (2010) Behavioural indicators of pain in horses undergoing surgical castration. Proceedings of the 46th Congress of the International Society for Applied Ethology. Vienna, Austria. p. 235.
9. Searle D, Dart AJ, Dart CM, Hodgson DR (1999) Equine castration: review of anatomy, approaches, techniques and complications in normal, cryptorchid and monorchid horses. Australian Veterinary Journal 77: 428–434.
10. Flecknell P, Raptopoulous D, Gasthuys F, Clarke K, Johnston G, et al. (2001) Castration of horses and analgesia. Veterinary Record 149: 252.
11. Viñuela-Fernández I, Jones E, Chase-Topping ME, Price J (2011) Comparison of subjective scoring systems used to evaluate equine laminitis. Veterinary Journal 188: 171–177.
12. Pritchett L, Ulibarri C (2003) Identification of potential physiological and behavioral indicators of postoperative pain in horses after exploratory celiotomy for colic. Applied Animal Behaviour Science 80: 31–43.
13. Love EJ (2009) Assessment and management of pain in horses. Equine Veterinary Education 21: 46–48.
14. Graubner C, Gerber V, Doherr M, Spadavecchia C (2011) Clinical application and reliability of a post abdominal surgery pain assessment scale (PASPAS) in horses. Veterinary Journal 188: 178–183.
15. Ashley FH, Waterman-Pearson AE, Whay HR (2005) Behavioural assessment of pain in horses and donkeys: application to clinical practice and future studies. Equine Veterinary Journal 37: 565–575.
16. Bussières G, Jacques C, Lainay O, Beauchamp G, Leblond A, et al. (2008) Development of a composite orthopaedic pain scale in horses. Research in veterinary science 85: 294–306.
17. Van Loon J, Back W, Hellebrekers LJ, van Weeren PR, Loon JPAM Van, et al. (2010) Application of a Composite Pain Scale to Objectively Monitor Horses with Somatic and Visceral Pain under Hospital Conditions. Journal of Equine Veterinary Science 30: 641–649.
18. Price J, Catriona S, Welsh EM, Waran NK (2003) Preliminary evaluation of a behaviour-based system for assessment of post-operative pain in horses following arthroscopic surgery. Veterinary anaesthesia and analgesia 30: 124–137.
19. Erber R, Wulf M, Becker-Birck M, Kaps S, Aurich JE, et al. (2012) Physiological and behavioural responses of young horses to hot iron branding and microchip implantation. Veterinary Journal 191: 171–175.
20. Langford DJ, Bailey AL, Chanda ML, Clarke SE, Drummond TE, et al. (2010) Coding of facial expressions of pain in the laboratory mouse. Nature methods 7: 447–449.
21. Sotocinal SG, Sorge RE, Zaloum A, Tuttle AH, Martin LJ, et al. (2011) The Rat Grimace Scale: a partially automated method for quantifying pain in the laboratory rat via facial expressions. Molecular Pain 7: 55. Available: http://www.molecularpain.com/content/7/1/55. Accessed 7 November 2012.
22. Leach MC, Klaus K, Miller AL, Scotto di Perrotolo M, Sotocinal SG, et al. (2012) The assessment of post-vasectomy pain in mice using behaviour and the Mouse Grimace Scale. PloS one 7: e35656. Available: http://www.plosone.org/

article/info%3Adoi%2F10.1371%2Fjournal.pone.0035656. Accessed 31 January 2013.

23. Keating SCJ, Thomas A a, Flecknell P a, Leach MC (2012) Evaluation of EMLA cream for preventing pain during tattooing of rabbits: changes in physiological, behavioural and facial expression responses. PloS one 7: e44437. Available: http://www.plosone.org/article/info%3Adoi%2F10.1371%2Fjournal.pone.0044437. Accessed 31 January 2013.
24. Grunau R, Craig K (1987) Pain expression in neonates: facial action and cry. Pain 28: 395–410.
25. Jordan A, Hughes J, Pakresi M, Hepburn S, O'Brien JT (2011) The utility of PAINAD in assessing pain in a UK population with severe dementia. International journal of geriatric psychiatry 26: 118–126.
26. Ashraf AB, Lucey S, Cohn JF, Chen T, Ambadar Z, et al. (2009) The Painful Face - Pain Expression Recognition Using Active Appearance Models. Image and vision computing 27: 1788–1796.
27. Ekman P, Friesen W (1978) Facial action coding system: a tecnique for the measurament of facial action. Consulting. Palo Alto.
28. Williams ACDC (2002) Facial expression of pain: an evolutionary account. The Behavioral and brain sciences 25: 439–488.
29. Leach MC, Coulter CA, Richardson CA, Flecknell PA (2011) Are we looking in the wrong place? Implications for behavioural-based pain assessment in rabbits (Oryctolagus cuniculi) and beyond? PloS one 6: e13347. Available: http://www.plosone.org/article/info%3Adoi%2F10.1371%2Fjournal.pone.0013347. Accessed 4 July 2013.
30. Hall CW, Clarke KW (1983) Veterinary anesthesia, 8th edition.
31. Canadian Veterinary Medical Association (2006) Castration of horses, donkeys, and mules - Position statement. Available: http://www.canadianveterinarians.net/documents/castration-of-horses-donkeys-and-mules#.UdGrTflM9Zs.
32. National Equine Welfare Council, (NEWC) (2009) Equine Industry Welfare Guidelines Compendium for Horses, Ponies and Donkeys. Available: http://www.newc.co.uk/wp-content/uploads/2011/10/Equine-Brochure-09.pdf.
33. Søndergaard E, Halekoh U (2003) Young horses' reactions to humans in relation to handling and social environment. Applied Animal Behaviour Science 84: 265–280. doi:10.1016/j.applanim.2003.08.011.
34. Martin P, Bateson P (2007) Measuring Behaviour: An Introductory Guide. 3rd ed. Cambridge University Press, Cambridge, Massachusetts, USA.
35. England GCW, Clarke KW (1996) Alpha2 adrenoceptor agonists in the horse A review. British Veterinary Journal 152: 641–657.
36. Figueiredo J, Muir W (2005) Sedative and analgesic effects of romifidine in horses. International Journal of Applied Research in Veterinary Medicine 3: 249–258.
37. Muir WW, Sams R a, Huffman RH, Noonan JS (1982) Pharmacodynamic and pharmacokinetic properties of diazepam in horses. American journal of veterinary research 43: 1756–1762.
38. Capner C (2001) Castration of horses and analgesia. Veterinary Record 149: 252.
39. Jones R (2001) Castration of horses and analgesia. Veterinary Record 149: 252.
40. Heleski MC, Cinq-Mars D, Merkies K (2012) Code of practice for the care and handling of equines: review of scientific research on priority issues. Available: http://www.nfacc.ca/resources/codes-of-practice/equine/Equine_SCReport_Aug23.pdf. Accessed 29 January 2013.
41. Bidwell L a, Bramlage LR, Rood W a (2007) Equine perioperative fatalities associated with general anaesthesia at a private practice—a retrospective case series. Veterinary anaesthesia and analgesia 34: 23–30. Available: http://www.ncbi.nlm.nih.gov/pubmed/17238959. Accessed 10 February 2014.
42. Mcdonnell SM (2003) A practical field guide to horse behavior. The Equid Ethogram. Eclipse Press.
43. McGreevy P (2004) Equine Behaviour. Saunders, London, UK.
44. Eager R (2002) Preliminary investigations of behavioural and physiological responses to castration in horses University of Edinburgh.
45. Taylor PM, Pascoe PJ, Mama KR (2002) Diagnosing and treating pain in the horse. Where are we today? The Veterinary Clinics of North America Equine Practice 18: 1–19.
46. Johnson C, Taylor P, Young S, Brearley J (1993) Postoperative analgesia using phenylbutazone, flunixin or carprofen in horses. Veterinary Record 133: 336–338. doi:doi:10.1136/vr.133.14.336.
47. Scotto di Perrotolo M, Miller A, Leach M, Flecknell P (2010) Mesure de la fiabilité et de la précision des expressions faciales pour évaluer la douleur chez la souris. Sciences & Techniques de l'Animal de Laboratoire (STAL) 36: 49–58.

16

Spatial Distribution of Bednet Coverage under Routine Distribution through the Public Health Sector in a Rural District in Kenya

Wendy Prudhomme O'Meara[1,2,3,4]*, Nathan Smith[2], Emmanuel Ekal[5], Donald Cole[6], Samson Ndege[3,4]

1 Department of Medicine, Duke University School of Medicine, Durham, North Carolina, United States of America, **2** Duke Global Health Institute, Durham, North Carolina, United States of America, **3** Department of Epidemiology and Nutrition, Moi University School of Public Health, Eldoret, Kenya, **4** United States Agency for International Development-Academic Model Providing Access to Healthcare Partnership, Eldoret, Kenya, **5** Ministry of Public Health and Sanitation, Nairobi, Kenya, **6** Division of Global Health, Dalla Lana School of Public Health, University of Toronto, Toronto, Ontario, Canada

Abstract

Insecticide-treated nets (ITNs) are one of the most important and cost-effective tools for malaria control. Maximizing individual and community benefit from ITNs requires high population-based coverage. Several mechanisms are used to distribute ITNs, including health facility-based targeted distribution to high-risk groups; community-based mass distribution; social marketing with or without private sector subsidies; and integrating ITN delivery with other public health interventions. The objective of this analysis is to describe bednet coverage in a district in western Kenya where the primary mechanism for distribution is to pregnant women and infants who attend antenatal and immunization clinics. We use data from a population-based census to examine the extent of, and factors correlated with, ownership of bednets. We use both multivariable logistic regression and spatial techniques to explore the relationship between household bednet ownership and sociodemographic and geographic variables. We show that only 21% of households own any bednets, far lower than the national average, and that ownership is not significantly higher amongst pregnant women attending antenatal clinic. We also show that coverage is spatially heterogeneous with less than 2% of the population residing in zones with adequate coverage to experience indirect effects of ITN protection.

Editor: Steffen Borrmann, Kenya Medical Research Institute - Wellcome Trust Research Programme, Kenya

Funding: The HCT programme was made possible through grants from Abbott Laboratories, the Purpleville Foundation and the Global Business Coalition. The funders had no role in study design, data collection and analysis, decision to publish, or preparation of the manuscript.

Competing Interests: The HCT program was made possible through funding from commercial sources (Global Business Coalition and Abbott Laboratories). However, the funders had no role in data collection, analysis or manuscript preparation. None of the authors are employed by or have any financial or non-financial relationship with either organization that would constitute a competing interest.

* E-mail: wendypomeara@gmail.com

Introduction

Insecticide treated bednets (ITNs) are one of the most cost-effective and widely used malaria interventions [1,2]. Between 2006–2008, more than 140 million nets were manufactured and delivered for distribution in sub-Saharan Africa [3].

Maximum effectiveness of ITNs is achieved when a high percentage of individuals in a geographic area are using ITNs. It is estimated that substantial protective indirect effects are seen with roughly 50% or greater coverage of entire populations[4,5,6]. Strategies for distributing ITNs differ between countries and between programs and they show a high degree of variability in coverage of households and high-risk groups [7,8]. Generally, unsubsidized ITNs provided through the private retail sector produces the lowest coverage with significant differences between socioeconomics groups. Free, community-based mass distribution campaigns have been shown to sharply increase bednet coverage and reduce inequities in bednet ownership across socioeconomic strata [2,7,8,9,10,11]. Although mass distribution campaigns are effective, they are also expensive and require repeated campaigns to replace old, damaged, or expired nets. Many programs provide free or partially subsidized ITNs to high-risk groups through routine contact with government health services, particularly antenatal clinics (ANC) and immunization clinics. Still other countries have relied on social marketing of ITNs, and have scaled-up distribution through both the health sector and the private retail sector, usually involving a small co-pay [9]. Such cost-sharing schemes with private and public sector subsidies have sustained high coverage [10]. Other studies suggest that a mix of distribution mechanisms can both achieve and maintain high and equitable coverage [9,11,12].

Delivery of ITNs, either free or partially subsidized, through the government health sector remains the most common avenue for ITN distribution in most countries in sub-Saharan Africa. It is the most logistically straightforward, least expensive, and targets those who bear the greatest burden of disease. In Kenya, the main channel for ITN distribution is through the government health facilities, particularly to pregnant women who attend antenatal clinics and infants who are seen in the immunization clinics. In some areas, mass distribution campaigns or social marketing channels have been used, but these approaches have been limited in geographic scope and frequency [13].

The purpose of this analysis was to describe the impact of routine distribution of bednets targeted to high-risk groups through government health facilities on household-level ownership, and explore some determinants of ownership. We present bednet ownership data from a complete census conducted in a rural district in western Kenya. We explore spatial heterogeneity of bednet ownership at the household level and compare coverage in targeted groups. We evaluate whether targeting high-risk groups attending health facilities is achieving the required coverage in the targeted groups as well as the population as a whole.

Methods

The bednet study was conducted from retrospective analysis of data collected during implementation of a large, home-based public health program, augmented with data collected from health facilities in the implementation area. Study site, study population and data collection procedures are described below.

Study site

Bungoma East district is located in Western Province, Kenya about 50 km from the border with Uganda. It is divided into 23 administrative units called sublocations. There is a river that borders the district to the east and another river that transects the northwestern part of the district. Residents are primarily subsistence farmers, although there are two large sugar plantations which employ a large number of day-laborers from the surrounding communities. The major road between Nairobi and Uganda runs through the middle of the district. There is a small town center. The population is estimated to be just over 200,000 people. Malaria transmission is year-round with a seasonal peak following the rains in March to May. Annual EIR is 29 and more than 60% of children were parasitemic in cross sectional surveys during the rainy season [14].

Government-owned health facilities are categorized from level 2–6. Level 2 is used to describe dispensaries, level 3 refers to health centres which typically have laboratory capacity, more staff, and larger formularies than dispensaries. Level 4–6 facilities are hospitals at the district, provincial or national level with in-patient services and increasing capacity at each level. The population in the study area is served by 21 government-owned health facilities, including a level-4 district hospital, 3 health centres and 17 dispensaries. There is also a mission-run hospital in the northern part of the district and three mission-run dispensaries.

Routine facility-based data

Insecticide-treated bednets are distributed to pregnant women attending public health facilities for antenatal care and to children less than one year of age attending immunization or well-child clinics in keeping with Government of Kenya, Ministry of Public Health & Sanitation guidelines. There have been no community-based ITN distribution programs in the district in at least the last five years. The number of ITNs distributed through the public health facilities in the two years preceding data collection was recorded from routine records kept by the District Health Management Team.

Population census data collection

Household data were collected as part of a large public health campaign initiated to identify HIV-infected individuals. This Home-based Counseling and Testing (HCT) campaign was undertaken by the Academic Model Providing Access to Healthcare (AMPATH) in Bungoma East District between July 2009 and April 2010. The program is described in detail elsewhere [15]. Briefly, all households in the district were visited to offer counseling and testing for HIV. Data were collected using Palm T|X PDA devices (Palm Inc®, California, USA). Standardized information was entered into data-collection forms programmed with Pendragon Forms Software (DDH Software, Inc®, Florida, USA). The total number of individuals resident in the household was recorded and all individuals older than 13 years were offered testing. All children less than five years were screened for immunization. Other data collected included individual demographic data, household asset information, HIV testing history and outcome, bednet ownership and GPS coordinates of the household via direct cable link to an external e-Trex GPS device (Garmin®, Kansas, USA). Pregnant women were identified and asked about attendance at the antenatal clinic. Data were collected from 96% of households in the district.

We refer to any nets reported in the household as 'bednets' because information about bednet retreatment and long-lasting insecticide treated nets was not collected. We define bednet 'coverage' as household ownership of at least one bednet.

A database of health facilities in Kenya including GPS coordinates was compiled and provided by researchers at KEMRI-Wellcome Trust-Nairobi [16]. The database was augmented with additional mapping within Bungoma East District using the handheld e-Trex GPS devices. All facilities were categorized according to level of service – dispensaries, health centres, and hospitals. Other geographic features, including major town centers and all roads (both paved and unpaved) that were accessible in a four-wheel drive vehicle were also mapped. GPS coordinates were uploaded and imported into a database of geographic features using DNRGarmin GPS application (Minnesota Department of Natural Resources, Minnesota, USA). Data for administrative boundaries and rivers were obtained from the Data Exchange Platform for the Horn of Africa (DEPHA) (United Nations, URL: http://www.depha.org), Africover (Food and Agricultural Organization [FAO] of the United Nations, URL: http://www.africover.org), and the World Resources Institute (URL: http://www.wri.org/publication/content/9291). All data was imported into ArcInfo v10.0 (Esri, California, USA).

Data analysis

Sublocations were divided into urban and rural by comparison with Africover landmaps and knowledge of the local area. Only one of 23 administrative sublocations was classified as urban (~3,900 households). All non-spatial data analysis was done in Stata v10. Chi-square tests were used for pair-wise comparisons of bednet ownership by household characteristics. Multivariable regression models were stratified into urban and rural sublocations. Logistic regression was used to explore the relationship between bednet coverage in urban populations and sociodemographic and geographic variables. For rural areas, mixed effects logistic regression models were used with a random effect for sublocation to account for unobserved differences between sublocations. The random effects were captured as random intercepts for each sublocation. The model with the random effects term fit significantly better than the model without. Coefficients are reported as odds ratios. An independent variable was considered to have a significant correlation with bednet ownership if the p-value was <0.05.

Descriptive spatial analysis was done using ArcInfo v10.0 (mapping), R GUI v1.4 for Mac OSX (cluster analysis), and ArcView 3.2 with the Nearest Feature (NearFeat) v3.8b extension (Jenness Enterprises). Ripley's K-function, K(d), was used to evaluate clustering of households without nets compared to households owning bednets. K-function values were calculated between 50 m and 1500 m in 50 meter increments and underestimation of unobserved neighbors near the edge of the study boundary was corrected for by using a border correction method. Household point patterns were tested against complete spatial randomness using 19 permutations of random point placement, yielding >90% confidence envelope. To compare patterns of clustering (households without bednets versus households owning bednets), the difference between the calculated K-function values was plotted against distance (d).

The NearFeat extension was used to calculate the Euclidean distance between features, including distance to the nearest health facility, type of nearest facility, and nearest mapped road.

Kernel density estimation was used to calculate the density of features within a defined area. A kernel estimation surface, based on the quadratic kernel function and a defined radius of 800 meters, was used to estimate the density of households around each 50 meter by 50 meter area (cell) across the study area. This was repeated to calculate the density of households with bednets for each 50 by 50 meter cell. The ratio of households with bednets to all households was calculated across all 50 meter by 50 meter areas within the study area. Areas with less than 20 households per 800 sq. meters were excluded to limit edge effects. Using ArcInfo v10.0, a raster image of the study area was generated using the values of the estimated ratio of households with bednets to total households for each 50 meter by 50 meter cell. Changing the kernel radius between 400–1600 meters did not significantly change the estimate of percent of households at each level of coverage. 800 meters was chosen to represent a neighborhood and corresponds with approximate vector ranges.

To estimate the neighborhood bednet coverage at each individual household location, the raster image values were extracted at each household location. Using the resulting bednet coverage values at each household location, the percent of households within certain coverage levels was calculated.

Ethical approval

HCT is a home-based public health initiative. All participants gave voluntary informed consent for HIV testing. Consent was obtained verbally prior to data collection or any test being conducted. In the case of children less than 18, parental/guardian consent was obtained. In the context of a community health initiative, written consent was not considered appropriate. Verbal consent is considered the norm for most clinical care procedures and activities in our region. Documentation of verbal informed consent was collected by recording who had accepted household entry and testing.

Table 1. Numbers of ITNs distributed through public facilities in Bungoma East district, Kenya, 2008 and 2009.

Year	2008	2009
ANC Clinics	3,110	5,499
U1 Immunization Clinics	6,038	6,163
Total	9,148	11,662

The Institutional Review and Ethics Committee at Moi University and Moi Teaching and Referral Hospital in Eldoret, Kenya and Duke University Institutional Review Board approved the use of de-identified data from this program for analysis and publication.

Results

Bednet Distribution through public health facilities

Bednets were distributed through ANC and immunization clinics at all health facilities. According to the Bungoma East District Ministry of Health, no community-based, mass distribution campaigns were conducted in at least the previous five years. In 2008, a total of 9,148 bednets were distributed; in 2009, a total of 11,662 bednets were distributed (Table 1).

Household Bednet Ownership

A total of 44,753 households were visited and household characteristics were collected. Only 21% (n = 9,532) of all households reported owning at least one bednet. Seventy-two percent of households with any bednet reported owning only one net, 18% reported two nets and the rest reported owning between 3–10 bednets. The total number of bednets reported in the census was 13,230, about 64% of the number reported distributed through facilities. Among households with a pregnant woman (n = 2,988), 25% owned at least one bednet (Table 2). Among households with children under 5 years old (n = 23,645), 25% owned at least one bednet. Among all other households (n = 19,950), 17% owned at least one bednet.

Household Characteristics and Univariate Analysis

The average household membership was 4.4 persons and 53% of households had one or more children less than five years of age.

Table 2. Bednet Ownership and Distribution within Bungoma East District.

	n	Percent with at least one bednet	p-value
Households with Pregnant Women	2,988	25%	p = 0.97
Households with Pregnant women attending ANC	1,711	25%	
Households with Children Under 5	23,645	24%	p<0.001
Households without U5 or pregnant women	19,950	17%	
Urban households	3,497	18%	p<0.001
Rural households	41,256	22%	
Total households	**44,753**	**21%**	

Table 3. Factors associated with household possession of at least one bednet in multivariable logistic regression analysis, stratified by broad location.

n = 3,497	OR	OR			
URBAN	**unadjusted**	**adjusted**	**p-value**	**95% CI**	
Children <5	1.09 (0.98, 1.22)	1.17	0.01	1.04	1.31
Pregnant mother	1.60 (1.11, 2.28)	2.01	0.02	1.14	3.55
Pregnant mother attending ANC	1.57 (0.98, 2.52)	0.85	0.67	0.41	1.78
Wealth indicators					
Own any animals	1.48 (1.21, 1.82)	1.47	0.00	1.18	1.84
Own any land	1.30 (1.09, 1.55)	1.39	0.05	1.01	1.92
Total animals	1.07 (1.04, 1.12)	1.03	0.35	0.97	1.08
Distance					
To Dispensary	1.83 (1.50, 2.26)	1.30	0.04	1.01	1.68
To Any facility	0.80 (0.73, 0.87)	1.39	0.33	0.72	2.67
To Health Centre[a]					
To Road	0.33 (0.26, 0.43)	0.38	0.00	0.27	0.53
Proximity[b]					
Nearest facility is hospital	7.55 (4.12, 13.86)	2.90	0.01	1.28	6.56
Nearest facility is Health Centre	(omitted)[a]				
Pseudo R^2	*0.056*				
n = 41,246	**OR**	**OR**			
RURAL	**unadjusted**	**adjusted**	**p-value**	**95% CI**	
Children <5	1.21 (1.18, 1.24)	1.21	0.00	1.18	1.24
Pregnant mother	1.22 (1.12, 1.34)	1.18	0.02	1.03	1.36
Pregnant mother attending ANC	1.22 (1.08, 1.36)	1.03	0.72	0.87	1.23
Wealth indicators					
Own any land	1.43 (1.34, 1.52)	1.26	0.00	1.18	1.35
Own any animals	1.37 (1.30, 1.43)	1.15	0.00	1.08	1.23
Total animals	1.04 (1.04, 1.05)	1.02	0.00	1.01	1.04
Distance					
To Dispensary	1.02 (1.00, 1.03)	1.02	0.32	0.98	1.06
To Any facility	0.96 (0.93, 0.98)	0.87	0.00	0.84	0.90
To Health Centre	0.98 (0.97, 0.99)	1.02	0.04	1.00	1.04
To Road	0.91 (0.90, 0.92)	1.09	0.00	1.06	1.13
Proximity[b]					
Nearest facility is hospital	0.80 (0.75, 0.85)	0.90	0.08	0.80	1.01
Nearest facility is Health Centre	1.66 (1.55, 1.77)	1.20	0.01	1.05	1.37
		Random effects parameters			
		Standard dev. of constant (95% CI)	0.55	(0.40	0.74)
		Standard error	0.086		

Data presented here are the odds ratio (OR), p-value, and 95% confidence intervals (CI) for the multivariable logistic regression stratified by urban versus rural households.

[a]Within Webuye town the health centre and hospital are less than 0.5 km apart. The distance and proximity variables were combined to consider these two facilities equal.

[b]Reference variable is nearest facility is dispensary.

The proportion of households owning land was 76%, with 52% of all households owning animals. The majority of households lived closest to a dispensary (65%), a quarter of households lived nearest to a hospital (24%), and 11% lived closest to a health center. Households owning a bednet lived an average 2.07 km (SD = 1.01) from the nearest health facility, and households with no bednets lived an average 2.12 km away (SD = 1.01).

Amongst households with pregnant women, women attending ANC were not more likely to be in a household with a bednet (Table 1; p = 0.97). Households with children under 5 years were

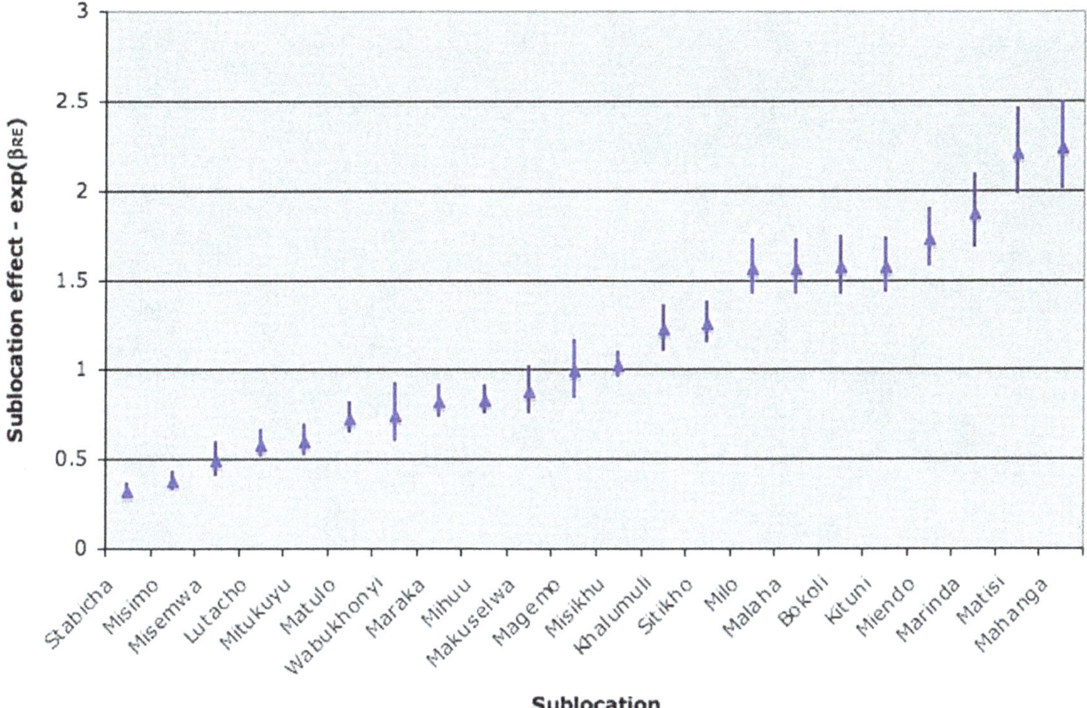

Figure 1. Exponential of the random effects (with 95% CI) for each sublocation for the mixed effects model. This plot shows the effect of sublocation of residence on bednet ownership. The random effects plot is the exponent of the random intercept for each sublocation. The exponent of the random effect can be thought of as the quantity that the exponent of the fixed effects intercept would be multiplied by to account for sublocation. So if exp(RE) = 1.5 then the exp(βo) would be multiplied by 1.5 for households in that sublocation. When exp(RE) = 1, that is the zero effect – location has no effect on the outcome. The plot shows that there is considerable heterogeneity between sublocations due to unobserved factors not captured in the model.

more likely to have a bednet ($p<0.0001$). Among urban and rural areas, households in rural areas were more likely to own a bednet than urban areas ($p<0.0001$).

Multivariate Analysis

To understand the relationship among sociodemographic characteristics and bednet ownership, multivariate regression was performed on household variables. The analysis was stratified by urban and rural households. Table 3 shows the odds ratios of bednet ownership for each independent variable included in the model. In both the rural and urban households, the presence of children under 5 years in the household increased the odds of bednet ownership (OR = 1.17 urban, OR = 1.22 rural, $p<0.01$). The presence of a pregnant woman also significantly increased the odds of bednet ownership, but whether the expectant mother was attending ANC did not affect bednet ownership.

Among urban households, wealth indicators (land ownership OR = 1.39, p = 0.05 and animal ownership OR = 1.47, $p<0.001$) were strongly associated with bednet ownership. Households closest to a hospital were nearly three times as likely to own a bednet (OR = 2.90, p = 0.01). As distance to the nearest road increased, the odds of owning a bednet significantly declined (OR = 0.38, $p<0.001$).

In rural households, the wealth indicators also significantly increased the odds of bednet ownership, but the effect was smaller than for urban households. The largest change in odds of bednet ownership for rural households was related to whether the nearest facility was a health centre (OR = 1.20, p = 0.01) and how far away the household was from any facility (OR = 0.87, $p<0.001$). Although the distance to the nearest health centre (OR = 1.02, p = 0.04) or the nearest road (OR = 1.09, $p<0.001$) were each significant, the effects were very small per kilometer. Nevertheless, the cumulative effects of distance may be substantial; 20% of rural households are located more than 3 km from a facility, giving an odds ratio of 0.66 for bednet ownership in these households.

Significant differences in bednet ownership between sublocations were observed and these differences were not explained by the independent variables reported above. The heterogeneity is captured in the distribution of the random effects by sublocation estimated from the model. The spatial random effects with estimated 95% confidence intervals are plotted in Figure 1.

Spatial Distribution

Bednet coverage varied across the study area but was generally suboptimal; 77% of households lived in areas with 30% coverage or less (Figure 2). No areas were found to have coverage above 70%, and only 2% of households live in areas with greater than 50% coverage. A majority of the areas of higher coverage were seen to be northwest of Webuye town, with other areas to the southwest of the town center.

Computed K-function values showed that the distribution of all households and households owning bednets were significantly more clustered than would be expected from a random distribution of points (data not shown). The difference of the *K*-functions shows that households owning at least one bednet are significantly more clustered than households without bednets over a range of distances. Figure 3 shows the difference curve between the observed K values of households owning a bednet and households without bednets across the study area. Differences greater than zero indicate that households with a bednet are more

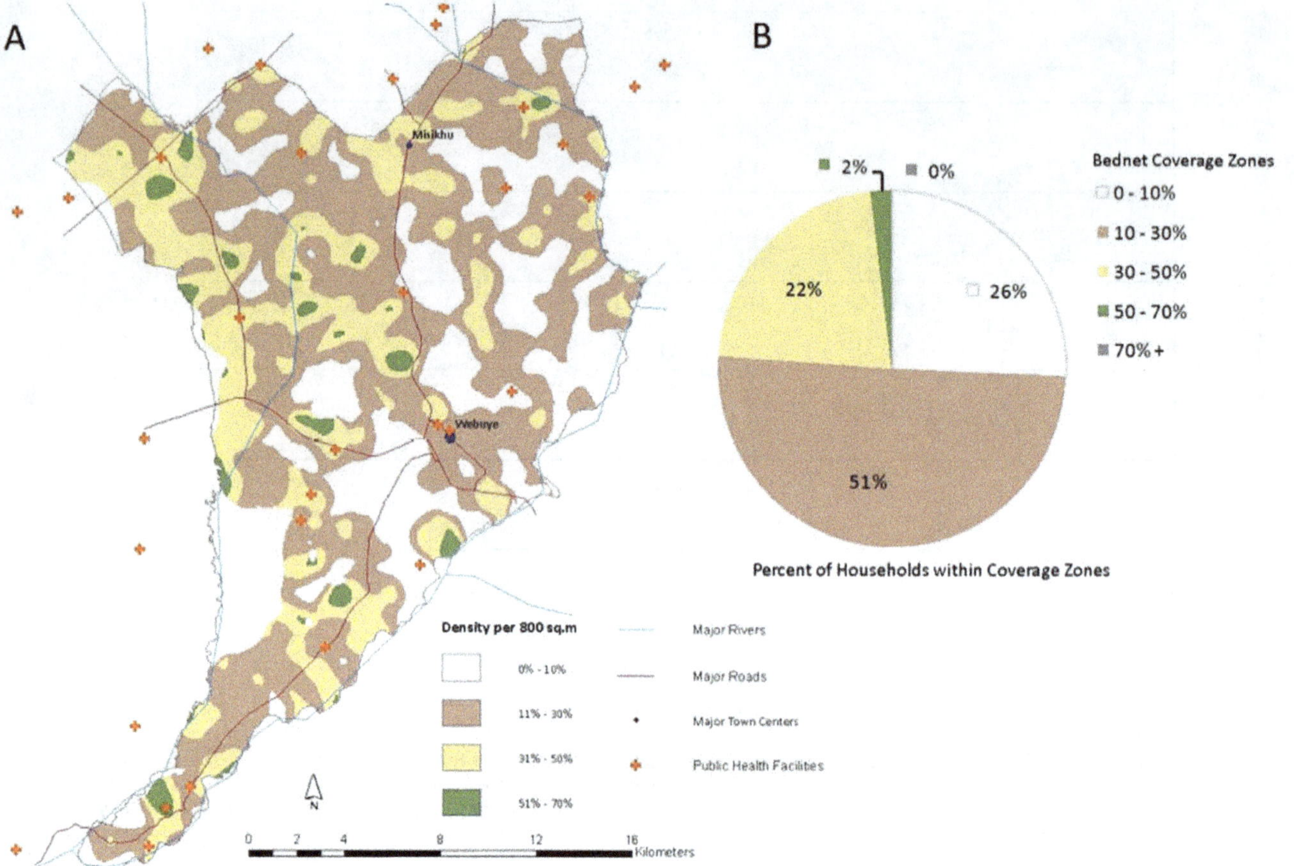

Figure 2. Spatial distribution of bednet coverage. (A) Map of household-level coverage raster. Areas with 0% to 10% community coverage are shown in white; areas with 11%–30% community coverage are shown in brown; areas with 31%–50% community coverage are shown in yellow; and areas with 51% –70% community coverage area shown in green. Major rivers, roads, town centers, and public health facilities are shown. (B) Percent of households within each coverage zones. Colors correspond to map.

clustered, or located near each other more often than households without bednets. Values less than zero would indicate that households with bednets are more dispersed than households without bednets. On average, households with bednets are more clustered than those without within a radius of between 50 m and 1200 m, with the greatest relative clustering seen at about 1000 m. At distances >1200 m, the difference is no longer greater than would be expected under spatial randomness.

Discussion

The Kenya Division of Malaria Control promotes the implementation of insecticide treated bednets as a cornerstone of its malaria control strategy and employs several mechanisms to distribute ITNs. The primary distribution mechanism is through routine visits to government-owned health facilities, although mass distribution campaigns have been used. Countrywide, the percentage of households owning and using any type of bednet is 60%, while ownership of at least one ITN in the house is 56%. In Western Province, where our study area is located, 74% of households owned at least one bednet [17].

Bungoma East district uses targeted distribution of free ITNs through antenatal and immunization clinics. The data presented here show that household bednet ownership in Bungoma East district was far lower than both the national average and the provincial average. Only 21% of households reported owning at least one bednet. District-level data from Kenya shows considerable differences in bednet use between districts, ranging from less than 10% to more than 60% coverage [18]. Previous studies have shown similar population-level coverage in Kenya when ITNs were delivered through health facilities [19] so the low coverage observed here is not entirely unexpected. The low ITN coverage may be responsible for high reported morbidity; there were 49,700 episodes of clinical malaria reported in the district in 2010 (Ministry of Health data, E. Ekal), in a population of approximately 190,000 people.

Fifty-three percent of households in the study area had a child under 5 years and therefore should have recently been eligible for a free ITN, only 24% of these households owned a bednet. Ownership amongst pregnant women attending ANC compared to those not attending ANC was not significantly different despite the fact that women attending ANC were eligible for a free ITN *and* had recently visited the health facility. Recent contact with the ANC clinic should be correlated with high likelihood of bednet ownership and this may be a litmus test for the current availability and effectiveness of the facility-based distribution mechanisms. Our results differ from results seen in Zambia where distribution through ANC was paired with mass distribution[11].

When comparing the number of ITNs reported to be distributed in government health facilities in the two years preceding data collection with the number of households with children less than two years or pregnant women, there should not

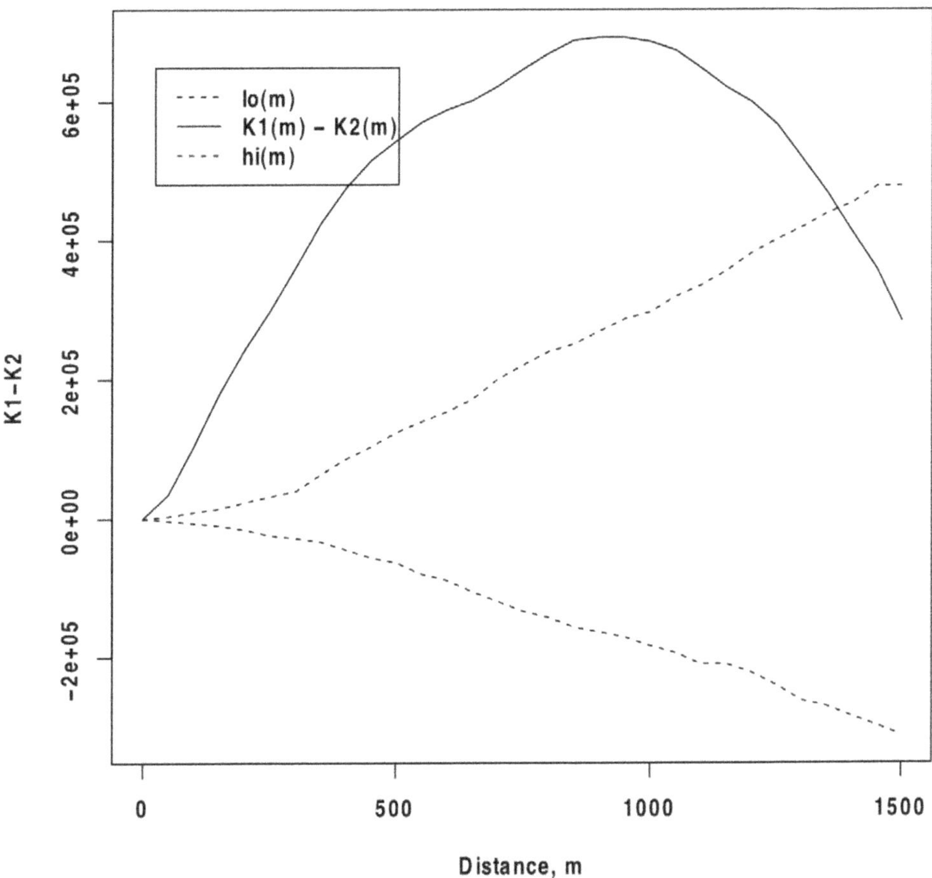

Figure 3. Cluster analysis of bednet coverage. The difference between $K_1(d)$, k-function for pattern of households owning at least one bednet, and $K_2(d)$, k-function for pattern of the underlying household distribution (solid line) and the confidence envelope (dashed lines) around the difference of expected distributions (zero line). Positive values indicate greater clustering of households owning at least one bednet in comparison to the underlying clustering of all households. Negative values indicate households owning at least one bednet have a more dispersed pattern than the underlying household distribution.

have been a shortfall of ITNs. These data suggest appropriate planning for supplies of ITNs but point to other factors limiting distribution. At least one other study has documented misuse of ITN distribution programs at the level of the health facility [20]. We cannot rule out leakage of public-sector ITNs into the retail sector, or informal charges levied by facility staff for ITNs despite Ministry of Health policy to distribute them free of charge. We can also not account for women residing outside the census area attending facilities within the census area, although we do not expect this to be a major factor in the discrepancies noted here. A recent study in Bioko Island of Equatorial Guinea showed a 30% decline in bednet ownership just one year after mass distribution [21]. This indicates that the actual lifespan and retention of bednets may be much lower than their predicted lifespan. This could partially account for the difference between the number of nets distributed and the number identified in the community. Another possible explanation is that new ITNs replace older ones rather than being added to the total number of nets in use.

Wealth indices correlate with bednet ownership even though bednets are provided for free in ANC and immunization clinics. This indicates that many of the bednets may have been purchased in the retail sector. Although wealth indicators may also reflect whether a family can afford to meet the costs of travel to a health facility and time away from daily activities, the observation that those who recently visited a facility (i.e. pregnant women attending ANC) were no more likely to have a bednet suggests that this was probably not a factor in accessing a bednet. Wealth has been shown to be a factor in bednet ownership in a number of other studies [22,23,24] and clear inverse relationships between poverty and uptake of ITNs has been shown [25].

The regression results revealed that distance to a facility is significant in predicting bednet ownership particularly in rural areas but is not as important as the type of facility nearest to each household. This seems to indicate that bednet distribution happens more effectively or more regularly at certain types of facilities (health centres may have a priority) or bednets have been distributed in only select facilities. While few studies have directly looked at bednet ownership and distance to public health facilities, studies elsewhere have looked at distance effects on utilization of health services and malaria morbidity, seeing clear reductions in malaria hospitalization with increasing physical access to primary health facilities [26,27].

Population coverage of bednets is an important determinant of the impact of bednet programs [4,5,6]. Low coverage (less than 50% of individuals) has been shown to be associated with reduced community-level effects [4]. Our study revealed only 21% of households own a bednet, likely resulting in reduced community effects from these bednets. Targeted distribution of ITNs through health facilities generated significant heterogeneity of bednet coverage. Only 16% of households are in zones where the household coverage is at least 35–65% – a range estimated to provide both community and individual-level protection [6]. Only 2% of households were in zones with >50% coverage, a range that has been shown to provide protection from infection and anemia to non-ITN users [4]. Here we have only assessed household-level ownership and have not measured the proportion or household members sleeping under a bednet, a parameter that has been shown to be important in other studies [28]. Furthermore, household ownership (as we have defined "coverage") is not equivalent to population coverage (fraction of the population owning or sleeping under a bednet).

The results presented here showing differences among targeted groups and the general population suggest that targeted distribution strategies have not led to high community-level coverage nor adequate coverage among the targeted groups. Spatial analysis has revealed significant clustering of households owning a bednet above the underlying population clustering at distances less than 1200 meters. Spatial variables such as distance to a road or a health facility did not fully explain the spatial structure of the data, as indicated by the distribution of the random intercepts for sublocations, indicating there are other spatial or neighborhood determinants not captured in our analysis. Previous studies have not incorporated a point-pattern analysis such as the one here. This analysis highlights the spatial heterogeneity of household bednet coverage and may indicate an inequality in physical, financial, or social access not captured in the set of variables we were able to explore.

In our study, bednet ownership was self-reported which may result in an underestimate of bednet ownership if reported absence of bednets is thought to be linked to receiving a new or additional bednet. We did not distinguish between treated and untreated bednets, which limits our ability to extrapolate the results of our study to predict protection. We did not assess bednet usage and it has been shown that bednet ownership does not predict use [29,30]. Our analysis of household-level bednet ownership has highlighted variations in ownership and has estimated factors affecting household ownership and population-level coverage. However, the factors explored here explained only a small fraction of the variation in bednet ownership as evidenced by a small R^2 value. Studies estimating factors affecting household and population-level coverage are critical to evaluating the equity and effectiveness of distribution mechanisms. While the current national malaria strategy has planned for mass distributions every three years, a campaign has not taken place in Bungoma East district in the last five years. Bednet useful life studies have shown rapidly decreasing life after three years, with an average bednet survival of 1–3 years [31]. Further investigations into the impact of frequency and geographic scope of supplemental distribution strategies are therefore critical to achieving adequate coverage to realize population-level indirect effects from bednets.

Acknowledgments

We would like to acknowledge A. Noor (KEMRI-Wellcome Trust, Nairobi) for providing us with GPS coordinates for health facilities and R. Anthopolos (Children's Environmental Health Initiative, Duke University) for assistance with the cluster analysis. Special thanks to the communities and community leaders of Bungoma East district, the community mobilizers and counselors, as well as all the staff who support HCT.

Author Contributions

Conceived and designed the experiments: WO. Performed the experiments: SN NS. Analyzed the data: WO NS. Contributed reagents/materials/analysis tools: EE DC. Wrote the paper: WO NS. Interpretation and significant revisions: DC SN EE.

References

1. Lengeler C (2004) Insecticide-treated bed nets and curtains for preventing malaria. Cochrane Database of Systematic Reviews. Chichester, UK: John Wiley & Sons, Ltd.
2. Noor A, Mutheu J, Tatem A, Hay S, Snow R (2009) Insecticide-treated net coverage in Africa: mapping progress in 2000–07. The Lancet 373: 58–67.
3. World Health Organization (2009) World Malaria Report 2009. Geneva: World Health Organization.
4. Hawley WA, Phillips-Howard PA, Ter Kuile FO, Terlouw DJ, Vulule JM, et al. (2003) COMMUNITY-WIDE EFFECTS OF PERMETHRIN-TREATED BED NETS ON CHILD MORTALITY AND MALARIA MORBIDITY IN WESTERN KENYA. Am J Trop Med Hyg 68: 121–127.
5. Howard SC, Omumbo J, Nevill C, Some ES, Donnelly CA, et al. (2000) Evidence for a mass community effect of insecticide-treated bednets on the incidence of malaria on the Kenyan coast. Transactions of the Royal Society of Tropical Medicine and Hygiene 94: 357–360.
6. Killeen GF, Smith TA, Ferguson HM, Mshinda H, Abdulla S, et al. (2007) Preventing Childhood Malaria in Africa by Protecting Adults from Mosquitoes with Insecticide-Treated Nets. PLoS Med 4: e229.
7. Webster J, Hill J, Lines J, Hanson K (2007) Delivery systems for insecticide treated and untreated mosquito nets in Africa: categorization and outcomes achieved. Health Policy and Planning 22: 277–293.
8. Müller O, De Allegri M, Becher H, Tiendrebogo J, Beiersmann C, et al. (2008) Distribution Systems of Insecticide-Treated Bed Nets for Malaria Control in Rural Burkina Faso: Cluster-Randomized Controlled Trial. PLoS ONE 3: e3182.
9. Khatib RA, Killeen GF, Abdulla SMK, Kahigwa E, McElroy PD, et al. (2008) Markets, voucher subsidies and free nets combine to achieve high bed net coverage in rural Tanzania. Malaria Journal 7: 98–98.
10. Killeen GF, Tami A, Kihonda J, Okumu FO, Kotas ME, et al. (2007) Cost-sharing strategies combining targeted public subsidies with private-sector delivery achieve high bednet coverage and reduced malaria transmission in Kilombero Valley, southern Tanzania. BMC Infectious Diseases 7: 121.
11. Larsen DA, Keating J, Miller J, Bennett A, Changufu C, et al. (2010) Barriers to Insecticide-Treated Mosquito Net Possession 2 Years after a Mass Free Distribution Campaign in Luangwa District, Zambia. PLoS ONE 5: e13129.
12. Skarbinski J, Massaga JJ, Rowe AK, Kachur SP (2007) DISTRIBUTION OF FREE UNTREATED BEDNETS BUNDLED WITH INSECTICIDE VIA AN INTEGRATED CHILD HEALTH CAMPAIGN IN LINDI REGION, TANZANIA: LESSONS FOR FUTURE CAMPAIGNS. Am J Trop Med Hyg 76: 1100–1106.
13. Division of Malaria Control, Ministry of Public Health and Sanitation (2009) Kenya National Malaria Strategy 2009–2017. Nairobi.
14. Shililu JI, Maier WA, Seitz HM, Orago AS (1998) Seasonal density, sporozoite rates and entomological inoculation rates of Anopheles gambiae and Anopheles funestus in a high-altitude sugarcane growing zone in Western Kenya. Trop Med Int Health 3: 706–710.
15. Kimaiyo S, Were MC, Shen C, Ndege S, Braitstein P, et al. (2010) HOME-BASED HIV COUNSELING AND TESTING IN WESTERN KENYA. East African Medical Journal 87: 100–108.
16. Noor AM, Alegana VA, Gething PW, Snow RW (2009) A spatial national health facility database for public health sector planning in Kenya in 2008. Int J Health Geogr 8: 13.
17. Kenya National Bureau of Statistics and Macro ICF (2010) Kenya Demographic and Health Survey 2008-2009. CalvertonMaryland: KNBS and ICF Macro.
18. Kenya Open Data http://www.opendata.go.ke/Health/Country-Health-Visualization-1/ew7x-crc3, accessed July 21, 2011.
19. Noor AM, Amin AA, Akhwale WS, Snow RW (2007) Increasing Coverage and Decreasing Inequity in Insecticide-Treated Bed Net Use among Rural Kenyan Children. PLoS Med 4: e255.
20. Tami A, Mbati J, Nathan R, Mponda H, Lengeler C, et al. (2006) Use and misuse of a discount voucher scheme as a subsidy for insecticide-treated nets for malaria control in southern Tanzania. Health Policy Plan 21: 1–9.
21. Garcia-Basteiro AL, Schwabe C, Aragon C, Baltazar G, Rehman AM, et al. (2011) Determinants of bed net use in children under five and household bed net ownership on Bioko Island, Equatorial Guinea. Malar J 10: 179.
22. Macintyre K, Keating J, Sosler S, Kibe L, Mbogo CM, et al. (2002) Examining the determinants of mosquito-avoidance practices in two Kenyan cities. Malaria Journal 1: 14–14.
23. Matovu F, Goodman C, Wiseman V, Mwengee W (2009) How equitable is bed net ownership and utilisation in Tanzania? A practical application of the principles of horizontal and vertical equity. Malaria Journal 8: 109.
24. Wiseman V, McElroy B, Conteh L, Stevens W (2006) Malaria prevention in The Gambia: patterns of expenditure and determinants of demand at the household level. Tropical Medicine and International Health 11: 419–431.

25. Worrall E, Basu S, Hanson K (2005) Is malaria a disease of poverty? A review of the literature. Tropical Medicine and International Health 10: 1047–1059.
26. O'Meara WP, Noor A, Gatakaa H, Tsofa B, McKenzie FE, et al. (2009) The impact of primary health care on malaria morbidity–defining access by disease burden. Tropical Medicine & International Health 14: 29–35.
27. Müller I, Smith T, Mellor S, Rare L, Genton B (1998) The effect of distance from home on attendance at a small rural health centre in Papua New Guinea. International Journal of Epidemiology 27: 878–884.
28. Gosoniu L, Vounatsou P, Tami A, Nathan R, Grundmann H, et al. (2008) Spatial effects of mosquito bednets on child mortality. BMC Public Health 8: 356.
29. Vanden Eng J, Thwing J, Wolkon A, Kulkarni M, Manya A, et al. (2010) Assessing bed net use and non-use after long-lasting insecticidal net distribution: a simple framework to guide programmatic strategies. Malaria Journal 9: 133.
30. Githinji S, Herbst S, Kistemann T, Noor A (2010) Mosquito nets in a rural area of Western Kenya: ownership, use and quality. Malaria Journal 9: 250.
31. Kilian A (2007) Useful life of a mosquito net and its impact on distribution strategies. Forth meeting of the RBM Working Group on Scalable Malaria Vector Control (WIN) 2007 Oct 24-26 http://www.rollbackmalaria.org/partnership/wg/wg_itn/docs/rbmwin4ppt/4-4.pdf. Accessed September 19, 2011.

17

Emerging Infectious Diseases in Free-Ranging Wildlife–Australian Zoo Based Wildlife Hospitals Contribute to National Surveillance

Keren Cox-Witton[1]*, Andrea Reiss[2], Rupert Woods[1], Victoria Grillo[1], Rupert T. Baker[3], David J. Blyde[4], Wayne Boardman[5¤], Stephen Cutter[6], Claude Lacasse[7], Helen McCracken[8], Michael Pyne[9], Ian Smith[5], Simone Vitali[10], Larry Vogelnest[11], Dion Wedd[6], Martin Phillips[2], Chris Bunn[12], Lyndel Post[12]

1 Australian Wildlife Health Network, Mosman, New South Wales, Australia, **2** Zoo and Aquarium Association Australasia, Mosman, New South Wales, Australia, **3** Healesville Sanctuary, Zoos Victoria, Healesville, Victoria, Australia, **4** Sea World, Gold Coast, Queensland, Australia, **5** Adelaide Zoo, Zoos South Australia, Adelaide, South Australia, Australia, **6** Territory Wildlife Park, Berry Springs, Northern Territory, Australia, **7** Australia Zoo Wildlife Hospital, Beerwah, Queensland, Australia, **8** Melbourne Zoo, Zoos Victoria, Parkville, Victoria, Australia, **9** Currumbin Wildlife Sanctuary, Currumbin, Queensland, Australia, **10** Perth Zoo, South Perth, Western Australia, Australia, **11** Taronga Zoo, Taronga Conservation Society Australia, Mosman, New South Wales, Australia, **12** Australian Government Department of Agriculture, Canberra, Australian Capital Territory, Australia

Abstract

Emerging infectious diseases are increasingly originating from wildlife. Many of these diseases have significant impacts on human health, domestic animal health, and biodiversity. Surveillance is the key to early detection of emerging diseases. A zoo based wildlife disease surveillance program developed in Australia incorporates disease information from free-ranging wildlife into the existing national wildlife health information system. This program uses a collaborative approach and provides a strong model for a disease surveillance program for free-ranging wildlife that enhances the national capacity for early detection of emerging diseases.

Editor: Patrick C Y. Woo, The University of Hong Kong, Hong Kong

Funding: The zoo based wildlife disease surveillance program described in this paper was funded by the Australian Government Department of Agriculture and the Australian Centre of Excellence for Risk Analysis. The funders had no role in study design, data collection and analysis, decision to publish, or preparation of the manuscript.

* E-mail: kcox-witton@wildlifehealthaustralia.com.au

¤ Current address: School of Animal and Veterinary Sciences, The University of Adelaide, Adelaide, South Australia, Australia

Introduction

Emerging infectious diseases are increasingly originating from wildlife, due in part to increasing urbanisation, globalised trade, habitat loss and other environmental changes. This is a real trend that cannot be fully explained by an increase in detection through improved surveillance, recognition, diagnosis or reporting [1], [2], [3], [4], [5]. Many of these diseases have significant impacts on human health, domestic animal health, wildlife health and biodiversity.

Zoonoses represent a rising threat to global health [5], [6]. Recent examples of emerging infectious diseases in humans with a wildlife origin include severe acute respiratory syndrome (SARS), Nipah virus and Ebola virus. Wildlife can act as a source and reservoir of diseases of domestic livestock such as bovine tuberculosis and avian influenza, and can result in significant economic losses [7], [8], [9]. Emerging diseases may also directly threaten wildlife health and biodiversity, as demonstrated in recent years by the emergence of white nose syndrome, Tasmanian devil facial tumour disease (DFTD) and chytridiomycosis [10], [11], [12], [13]. In Australia a number of diseases have emerged over the last 15 years with confirmed or suspected involvement of wildlife. Many of these diseases have had significant impacts on biodiversity, human health and domestic animal health, including chytrid fungus, DFTD, Australian bat lyssavirus (ABLV), Menangle virus, Japanese encephalitis and Hendra virus [14], [15], [16].

With the growing understanding of the importance of wildlife as a source or reservoir of emerging diseases, there is increased recognition of the need for disease surveillance in free-ranging wildlife. There are however inherent difficulties in conducting effective wildlife disease surveillance. Many wildlife disease events go unrecognised due to remote locations and a lack of obviously ill individuals or carcasses. Further challenges include a lack of validated diagnostic tests and laboratory capacity for the investigation of wildlife diseases, under-developed surveillance networks, difficulties in determining key parameters such as prevalence for diseases in wildlife populations, and lack of accurate ecological data on population size and density [17], [18]. Collection and validation of wildlife disease data can be challenging due to lack of funding, the 'anecdotal' nature of some reports, and the need to integrate data from disparate sources [16].

Utilising existing systems to establish a coordinated approach is an effective and efficient mechanism to overcome some of these difficulties, where they relate to reporting and data collection. This approach can be strengthened by a functional network that facilitates communication and information flow between those engaged at all levels in surveillance, diagnosis and management of wildlife disease. Surveillance information collected in this way may contribute to the early detection of new or emerging diseases [16], [19]. This paper describes a zoo based wildlife disease surveillance program, as an example of how such a system can assist in managing some of the issues associated with disease surveillance in free-ranging wildlife.

In Australia, the national animal health system is supported by a co-ordinated general wildlife health surveillance system. The primary responsibility for gathering animal health data, including wildlife disease data, rests with state and territory government agencies [20]. The Australian Wildlife Health Network (AWHN) is a national network of government and private stakeholders with an interest in wildlife health that receives core funding from the Australian Government Department of Agriculture. The AWHN is charged with collation and management of national wildlife surveillance data, and works within a 'One Health' framework by encouraging collaboration on wildlife health issues and investigations across human health, animal health and environmental sectors [21]. The AWHN manages wildlife health data through a national web-based database known as eWHIS (the 'electronic Wildlife Health Information System'). A key component of the wildlife health surveillance system are the 'wildlife coordinators', with a government representative in each of Australia's states and territories. Wildlife coordinators manage wildlife disease investigations in their jurisdiction and report data into eWHIS. State, territory and commonwealth agriculture, environment and human health agencies, universities, private veterinary practices and zoos all contribute to Australia's coordinated wildlife health surveillance system. The zoo based wildlife disease surveillance program was developed to formally incorporate disease information from free-ranging wildlife presented to Australian zoos into this existing national wildlife health information system.

Zoos are well suited to participation in surveillance efforts, as many zoos conduct active disease surveillance of collection animals as part of their routine preventative medicine programs, maintain serum and tissue banks and detailed medical records, and have staff with technical expertise in wildlife health [22], [23], [24]. The Zoo Animal Health Network in the USA, for example, is a collaborative program with the United States Department of Agriculture that is involved in early disease detection and outbreak response programs [25], [26], [27], [28]. The value of zoos for surveillance was demonstrated in 1999 when investigation of wild bird mortalities by veterinarians at New York City's Bronx Zoo led to the diagnosis of the first known occurrence of West Nile virus (WNV) in the western hemisphere, a disease with significant human and animal health impacts [22], [23].

Typically, however, zoo surveillance has largely focused on captive animals within zoo collections. In Australia, wildlife hospitals operated by the major zoos also treat a significant caseload of free-ranging and rehabilitation wildlife. A survey in 2008 found that 15 Australian zoos treated over 14,000 wildlife cases each year in their wildlife hospitals [29] and admissions to these hospitals appear to be increasing over time. As well as providing expertise in veterinary care, these hospitals have strong links to a network of wildlife rehabilitation, conservation, research and welfare organisations in their region.

The zoo based wildlife disease surveillance program was developed in recognition of the strong capacity and potential for wildlife hospitals at Australian zoos to contribute to national and international wildlife disease surveillance. The program aimed to integrate zoo based wildlife hospitals into Australia's animal health surveillance system. This paper describes the program and reviews the outcomes in the context of wildlife diseases that impact on human health, livestock health, trade and biodiversity.

Materials and Methods

Planning

In 2009 the Zoo Animal Health Reference Group [30] held a workshop to identify the role that Australian zoos could play in biosecurity, and surveillance was identified as a key area where a contribution could be made. A zoo based wildlife disease surveillance program was proposed and a collaborative project was subsequently developed between the AWHN and the Zoo and Aquarium Association Australasia (ZAA). The ZAA, with over 80 institutional members, is the peak body representing the zoo and aquarium industry in Australia and New Zealand. The AWHN and the ZAA worked with the Zoo Animal Health Reference Group and the senior veterinarians from the participating zoos to develop the scope and methodology for a pilot project to evaluate the potential of a zoo based surveillance program. The aim of the pilot project was to trial the integration of free-ranging wildlife disease information from zoo based wildlife hospitals into the national wildlife health information system. An additional objective was to strengthen and improve communication and the flow of information between zoo veterinarians and relevant government agencies.

Six major Australian zoos were selected to participate in the pilot project, each with a well-established and resourced on-site veterinary hospital treating free-ranging and rehabilitation wildlife and a permanent staff of experienced zoo and wildlife veterinarians. The six participating zoos are located in five Australian states: Adelaide Zoo in South Australia, Australia Zoo Wildlife Hospital in Queensland, Healesville Sanctuary and Melbourne Zoo in Victoria, Perth Zoo in Western Australia and Taronga Zoo in New South Wales (Figure 1). A formal survey of these zoos was conducted to gather baseline information and assist in planning for the pilot project. Data were collected on the number and taxonomic breakdown of wildlife cases seen by each of the zoo veterinary hospitals over a 12-month period during 2009 to 2010 (Table 1).

Operation

The pilot project commenced in November 2010 and finished in October 2011. During this time an agreed data set was collected from free-ranging and rehabilitation wildlife cases seen by the participating zoo veterinary hospitals. The scope of the pilot project did not include data from zoo collection animals and focused on the reporting of existing work, rather than expansion of disease investigations. Reporting into the national wildlife health information system in the pilot project was limited to selected disease event categories (Table 2), which had previously been established as a high priority for wildlife surveillance in Australia and aligned with data being reported from other sources. These categories are designed to collect wildlife disease information of potential importance to human health, livestock health, trade and biodiversity. While the priority for data collection was positive results, reporting of negative results was also encouraged, particularly where a specific disease was excluded that is a locally, nationally, or internationally notifiable or reportable disease. The 'interesting or unusual' category was designed to capture unusual events or findings that could indicate an emerging disease, syndrome or trend. Examples of disease events that could be reported in this category are significant clusters or patterns of disease, unexpected morbidities or mortalities, toxicity events,

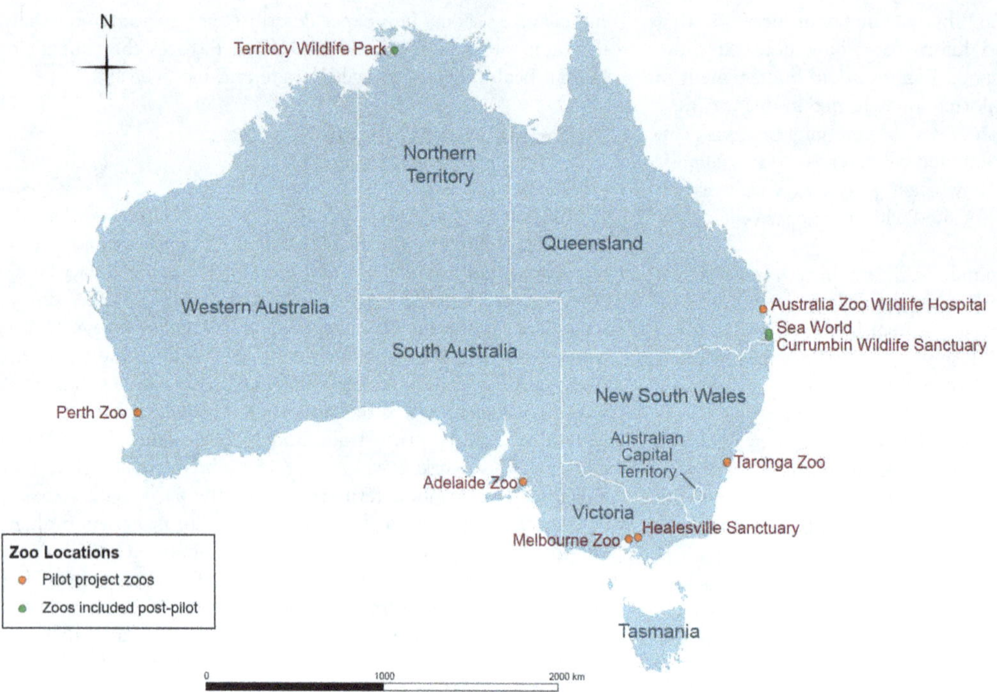

Figure 1. Geographic location of the zoos participating in the surveillance program.

marine wildlife strandings, and cases with possible linkages to international events or drivers. Cases for reporting were not confined to those where a necropsy or laboratory test had been conducted. Participants were encouraged to report a range of cases using different diagnostic tools, including where the diagnosis was based solely on clinical examination.

Cases were reported into the national wildlife health surveillance system via a web-enabled database, the 'electronic Wildlife Health Information System' (eWHIS). After initial training sessions provided by the AWHN, the zoo veterinarians entered data directly into the eWHIS database on a monthly basis for the duration of the pilot project, with ongoing training and support provided as needed. Fields captured included: event dates, event location, event type (e.g. individual, outbreak, monitoring), event category (see Table 2), species, number (affected and dead), state of captivity, presenting syndrome, diagnosis (one or multiple),

Table 2. Categories for selection of wildlife disease events for reporting into eWHIS.

Category
World Organisation for Animal Health (OIE) Listed diseases
Bat viral diseases
Mass mortalities
Arboviral diseases
Salmonella cases
'Interesting or unusual' cases

Table 1. Indicative numbers of free-ranging wildlife cases seen by veterinary hospitals at six major Australian zoos over a 12 month period during 2008/2009.

	Native species*				Feral species*	
ZOO	**Mammals**	**Birds**	**Reptiles**	**Amphibia**	**All taxa**	**TOTAL**
Australia Zoo Wildlife Hospital	2,579 (38%)	2,835 (42%)	1,126 (17%)	49 (0.7%)	197 (3%)	**6,786**
Healesville Sanctuary	567 (37%)	851 (56%)	95 (6%)	14 (0.9%)	*	**1,527**
Taronga Zoo	276 (39%)	341 (48%)	92 (13%)	5 (0.7%)	*	**714**
Perth Zoo	75 (12%)	328 (53%)	188 (31%)	8 (1%)	15 (2%)	**614**
Melbourne Zoo	135 (37%)	135 (37%)	76 (21%)	23 (6%)	*	**369**
Adelaide Zoo	85 (39%)	100 (46%)	8 (4%)	2 (0.9%)	18 (8%)	**213**
TOTAL	**3,717 (36%)**	**4,590 (45%)**	**1,585 (16%)**	**101 (1%)**	**230 (2%)**	**10,229**

*Data from three zoos did not differentiate feral from native species; for these zoos, feral animal cases are included with native species numbers.

laboratory test details and confidentiality level. The data entered into eWHIS were reviewed and moderated by the AWHN.

Participating zoo veterinarians were given the opportunity to discuss interesting disease events and operational aspects of the pilot project at regular teleconferences. All zoo participants were encouraged to engage with their state or territory agriculture agency via the wildlife coordinator, however this did not replace or bypass the legislated reporting of notifiable animal diseases through appropriate channels.

Evaluation

An independent review was conducted at the end of the pilot project by an internationally-recognised consulting company with expertise and experience in epidemiology and wildlife disease surveillance. Their evaluation of the project included an assessment of the value of the surveillance data and the potential for the project to deliver benefits to stakeholders, including the Australian commonwealth, state and territory governments. The sustainability of the system was also assessed. The evaluation process included an online stakeholder survey, interviews with the project coordinators and analysis of collected data.

Results

The preliminary survey indicated that the six zoos treated over 10,000 wildlife cases in a year (Table 1). All six selected zoos agreed to participate in the pilot project and the zoo veterinarians commenced entering data directly into the eWHIS database from November 2010. Sixteen zoo veterinarians participated for some or all of the pilot project period. A total of 211 events that occurred during the 12-month pilot project were reported into eWHIS by the participating zoos. This represented almost a third of all cases submitted to eWHIS during that period from all sources including state and territory departments of agriculture and human health, university researchers and private veterinary practitioners. A small subset of the cases presented to the zoo veterinary hospitals met the agreed criteria for data entry into eWHIS (Table 2). This subset was between 1 and 8% of all cases for individual zoos and approximately 2% for the six zoos overall. Examples of disease events reported for each of the categories are provided in Table 3.

A wide range of wildlife species was represented by the data collected during the pilot project. Accurate taxonomic identification of the animals under investigation was possible due to the expertise of the participating zoo veterinarians. The 211 disease events reported for the period from November 2010 to October 2011 covered 52 different species from 31 families and included birds (12 orders), turtles, marsupials, monotremes, marine mammals and bats (Table 4). The pilot project increased the overall species coverage of the data collected in eWHIS, with 18 species (9 bird, 7 mammal and 2 reptile species) reported through the pilot project that were not reported from other sources during the same period. A number of events reported through the pilot project came from geographic areas not represented by other sources.

The project captured data on diseases with potential human health implications, including confirmed or highly suspicious cases of salmonellosis, avian chlamydiosis (*Chlamydophila psittaci*), Australian bat lyssavirus in bats, mycobacteriosis (unspeciated) in a koala (*Phascolarctos cinereus*), and cryptosporidiosis in a hand-raised macropod. The cases of salmonellosis occurred in a variety of birds, marsupials and reptiles, and typing of these isolates contributed to the National Enteric Pathogens Surveillance Scheme [31]. Multiple cases of neurological signs in tawny frogmouths (*Podargus strigoides*) in urban areas of Sydney were of interest as this species has been suggested as a sentinel for the emerging zoonosis angiostrongylosis [32], [33].

Of the records entered in eWHIS through the pilot project, 73% were categorised by the submitter as 'interesting or unusual', a grouping designed to capture information on possible emerging syndromes and trends. As an example, 14 cases of neoplasia were reported. Cancers have been recognised as emerging diseases of wildlife with potentially serious impacts, including Tasmanian devil facial tumour disease [11] and fibropapillomatosis of green turtles (*Chelonia mydas*) [34]. Additionally, cancer clusters in wildlife due to environmental causes such as chemical contamination can act as sentinels for risk to human health [35], [36]. Cases were also reported of recognised syndromes where the cause has not been fully identified, such as non-suppurative encephalitis in corvids and paralysis in rainbow lorikeets (*Trichoglossus haematodus*). This information could contribute to a better understanding of syndromes with unknown aetiology.

Cases in threatened species were reported, including the endangered Carnaby's black-cockatoo (*Calyptorhynchus latirostris*) and loggerhead turtle (*Caretta caretta*) and a number of vulnerable species (Table 5) [37], some of which were not represented in data captured from other sources for the same period. Data were collected on cases of psittacine circoviral (beak and feather) disease, which is listed as a key threatening process in endangered psittacine species under the *Environment Protection and Biodiversity Conservation (EPBC) Act 1999* [38]. Also reported was a diabetes syndrome affecting koalas in care that could impact on the rehabilitation success of koalas in Queensland, a species now listed as vulnerable under the *EPBC Act 1999* [37]. The first two confirmed clinical cases of chlamydiosis in koalas in South Australia were reported to the AWHN through the pilot project [39]. The South Australian koala population was thought to be free of *Chlamydia* [40], so these reports may be an indicator of an emerging disease in the South Australian koala population.

The project provided a framework for improved data capture for monitoring programs. For example, the AWHN holds responsibility for collating, moderating and maintaining a national dataset of bats tested for ABLV, and the pilot project resulted in the capture of more detailed information on the history and clinical signs of bats for this dataset.

The project framework assisted the management of a disease outbreak in 2011. A strain of avian paramyxovirus 1 (APMV1) not previously reported in Australia was detected in hobby pigeons in the Melbourne area in Victoria, and the virus was subsequently detected in free-living feral rock doves (*Columba livia*) and a spotted turtle dove (*Streptopelia chinensis*), and in a native collared sparrow hawk (*Accipiter cirrocephalus*) [41], [42]. The project provided a mechanism to update zoo veterinarians about the outbreak, highlighted the possible involvement of native pigeons and raptors, and most likely resulted in increased submission of free-ranging sick and dead birds to the Victorian Department of Primary Industries for testing. A number of notifications of other disease events and outbreaks of relevance to wildlife were disseminated through the project, including a cluster of Hendra virus cases in horses in New South Wales and Queensland [43], and neurological disease in horses due to arboviruses in New South Wales [44] in 2011.

Information reported into eWHIS by the participants contributed to Australia's reports to the World Organisation for Animal Health (OIE). Australia, as a contributor to the OIE, regularly reports on the country's animal health status, which is important to ensure that Australia's health status for animals and animal products is well recognised internationally [45].

Table 3. Examples of disease events captured for each reporting category (see Table 2).

Reporting Category	Examples
OIE Listed diseases*	• Avian chlamydiosis (*Chlamydophila psittaci*)
	• Botulism
	• Psittacine circoviral (beak and feather) disease
	• Toxoplasmosis
	• Trichomoniasis
Bat viral diseases	• Australian bat lyssavirus
Mass mortalities	• Six Carnaby's black-cockatoos (*Calyptorhynchus latirostris*) found dead in a similar location over a two-week period
	• Twenty-one rainbow lorikeets (*Trichoglossus haematodus*) and scaly-breasted lorikeets (*Trichoglossus chlorolepidotus*) with neurological signs over a period of a month
Arboviral diseases	• None reported
Salmonella cases	Salmonella cultured from:
	• Green turtle (*Chelonia mydas*) – corneal abscess
	• Australian Raven (*Corvus coronoides*) with neurological signs – muscle
	• Two hand-raised eastern grey kangaroos (*Macropus giganteus giganteus*) with diarrhoea and anorexia – faeces
	• Hand-raised koala (*Phascolarctos cinereus*) joey with neurological signs and septicaemia - caecum, blood and liver
'Interesting or unusual' cases	• Fourteen cases of neoplasia in a variety of species including yellow-bellied glider (*Petaurus australis*), New Zealand fur seal (*Arctocephalus forsteri*), koala (*Phascolarctos cinereus*), wedge-tailed eagle (*Aquila audax*), laughing kookaburra (*Dacelo novaeguineae*)
	• Australian fur seal (*Arctocephalus pusillus doriferus*) with acute suppurative meningitis; heavy growth of *Arcanobacterium*
	• Multisystemic lymphoproliferative disease in a wedge-tailed eagle (*Aquila audax*)
	• Green turtle (*Chelonia mydas*) with fibropapillomatous lesions on flippers
	• Australian raven (*Corvus coronoides*) with non-suppurative encephalitis; flavivirus, avian influenza and Newcastle disease excluded

*Includes 'non-listed' pathogens and agents of wildlife [49].

Evaluation

The independent review found that the pilot project increased the volume of cases and expanded the sources of data being entered into the national database [46]. According to the review, the project resulted in increased geographic and taxonomic coverage of the wildlife population, with data collected from additional 'catchment' areas and an increased species distribution, as well as a wider range of presenting syndromes and reporting reasons. The review concluded from these outcomes that the pilot project enhanced the capacity of the national wildlife health information system for early detection of disease and improved the sensitivity for demonstration of freedom from disease.

The survey of zoo participants found that most considered their institution had benefited from the pilot project. Participants

Table 4. Cases* for November 2010– October 2011 reported through the pilot project, by taxonomic group.

Taxonomic group	
A. ALL CASES	**No. of cases (%)**
Birds	109 (52%)
Mammals	79 (37%)
Reptiles	23 (11%)
Total	**211**
B. MAMMALS	**No. of cases (% of mammal cases)**
Non-macropod marsupial	34 (43%)
Bat⁺	28 (35%)
Macropod	10 (13%)
Marine mammal	4 (5%)
Monotreme	2 (3%)
Other mammal	1 (1%)
Total	**79**

*A case may involve single or multiple animals.
⁺The majority of bat cases were submitted for exclusion testing for Australian bat lyssavirus (ABLV).

Table 5. Threatened species for which data was captured through the pilot project.

Species	EPBC Act Listing Status
Carnaby's black-cockatoo (*Calyptorhynchus latirostris*)	Endangered
Loggerhead turtle (*Caretta caretta*)	Endangered
Chuditch or Western quoll (*Dasyurus geoffroii*)	Vulnerable
Flatback turtle (*Natator depressus*)	Vulnerable
Green turtle (*Chelonia mydas*)	Vulnerable
Grey-headed flying fox (*Pteropus poliocephalus*)	Vulnerable
Hawksbill turtle (*Eretmochelys imbricata*)	Vulnerable
Koala (*Phascolarctos cinereus*)*	Vulnerable
Quokka (*Setonix brachyurus*)	Vulnerable
Sub-Antarctic fur seal (*Arctocephalus tropicalis*)	Vulnerable

*The koala (combined populations of Queensland, New South Wales and the Australian Capital Territory) was listed as vulnerable in May 2012.

reported that the project provided additional focus for the zoos to investigate wildlife diseases; resulted in better recognition of their contribution to wildlife health; and improved collaboration, connection and communication with other institutions and organisations. It also contributed to a better understanding of the wider context of wildlife disease events, and assisted in identifying patterns in these events by providing a forum to share information on similar syndromes from different locations. The majority of participants agreed that participation in the project increased their awareness and understanding of diseases of national concern. The review identified some limitations of the program, including the clustering of cases around major population centres, and the collection of only a small proportion of the total caseload of the participating zoo wildlife hospitals.

The reviewers concluded that there was value in the project to both the stakeholders and the participants, and that it was sustainable. They recommended the program be continued and expanded to include more zoos in order to increase the coverage and volume of data collected and to build on the improved capacity for early detection of wildlife disease. Factors recommended for consideration in the selection of additional zoos included geographic location and the 'catchment' area of wildlife covered by the zoo, veterinary presence, caseload, nature of cases, and availability of resources for data entry.

Outcomes

Based on the success of the pilot project and the recommendations of the independent review, the zoo based wildlife disease surveillance program has continued. Each of the participating zoos has remained with the program, which has expanded to incorporate three additional zoos with the aim of increasing both the geographic and species range. These zoos are Currumbin Wildlife Sanctuary and Sea World in Queensland, and Territory Wildlife Park in the Northern Territory (Figure 1). This brings the total number of free-ranging wildlife cases seen by the nine participating zoos to around 17,000 cases each year. A total of 25 zoo wildlife hospital staff have directly participated in the program since its inception.

Discussion

Animal health surveillance is the key to early detection and management of emerging diseases. The need to include free-ranging wildlife populations in animal health surveillance programs is increasingly recognised in Australia and globally [1], [5], [14], however effective disease surveillance in free-ranging wildlife populations presents many challenges. In Australia, as in many countries, there is an established system for investigating wildlife disease events and reporting them into the national system, however a considerable number of wildlife cases are inevitably seen outside of this system. A significant caseload of free-ranging wildlife is presented for treatment to Australian zoo based veterinary hospitals by members of the public, wildlife carers and park rangers, or are referred by state and territory government agencies, and the cost of providing this service is mostly covered by the zoos' operating budgets [29].

Australian zoo based hospitals are recognised as one of the chief sources of information on wildlife health and are well placed to participate in wildlife disease surveillance as these zoos have veterinary staff with expertise in wildlife health, are well organised and represented by their peak body, the Zoo and Aquarium Association, and have an existing framework of communication and collaboration. Zoos also have strong linkages with a broad network of wildlife rehabilitators, wildlife researchers, conservation organisations and environmental officers in their districts. For these reasons, the existing framework for the national reporting of wildlife disease information was expanded to include zoo veterinarians working with free-ranging wildlife. A pilot project demonstrated that a zoo based surveillance program was able to capture useful information on disease in free-ranging wildlife that might otherwise not have been reported into the national system, or was reported earlier than would otherwise have occurred. The program has the ability to capture valuable information on diseases of humans and domestic animals originating from wildlife, diseases in threatened species and recognised syndromes of unknown aetiology.

Some limitations of the zoo surveillance pilot project were identified by the independent review and the authors. Geographic coverage of cases reported through the project was, as expected, clustered around the physical locations of the participating zoos, which are primarily in or near the major population centres in coastal areas of Australia. This reflects the inherent bias of general surveillance systems. Although primarily in coastal locations, the zoos are situated in a variety of geographic and climatic zones, and in both urban and rural settings. This source of surveillance information does not stand alone, but complements other sources of data. The program also allows clear identification of geographic areas where general surveillance is of lower intensity, which is valuable for planning and assessment of risk.

As described, the scope of the project resulted in the collection of only a small proportion of the total caseload of the zoo wildlife hospitals into the eWHIS database (1–8%). The majority of cases presenting to zoo wildlife hospitals involve orphaned animals and cases involving dog, cat or vehicular trauma. Most of these do not align with the categories for reporting, which are selected on the basis of nationally-agreed priorities for wildlife disease surveillance in Australia. Nonetheless a large volume of potentially valuable data is not captured through the program, and this aspect of data collection will be further investigated by the authors. There may also be cases that meet the selection criteria but are not being reported into eWHIS, as the decision on what to report rests with the submitter, however the AWHN provides training and ongoing guidance on case selection to minimise the loss of eligible data.

This program focuses on wildlife hospitals at zoos, however the caseload varies significantly between participating institutions and in some instances there are other organisations in the same region with a higher caseload, such as private veterinary clinics, and not-for-profit wildlife hospitals and rehabilitation centres, which are not yet formally integrated into the surveillance system. This program may be used as a model in future to integrate other types of organisations into the national wildlife health surveillance system.

The Australian zoo based wildlife disease surveillance program provides a model for an effective, low cost system that utilises existing capacity and routine activities to contribute to national and international surveillance efforts. The program generates information with the potential to assist earlier detection of emerging diseases and trends, as well as strengthening networks, improving communication and information flow, and building capacity in wildlife health professionals. These elements form the basis of a successful surveillance program. This program acknowledges the value of data where a range of diagnostic tools, including clinical assessment has been used. As a model, it demonstrates that meaningful surveillance can be conducted in a variety of circumstances, including those where laboratory capacity and financial resources are limited.

There is a recognition that successful surveillance relies on communication between stakeholders, including private practitioners and public officers [47]. There is a need for greater integration and linkage of animal - both wild and domestic - and human pathogen surveillance systems at the international and national level [48]. The need for a systematic approach to communication between the human and animal disease surveillance systems in Australia has been outlined [19]. A 'One Health' approach can result in increased interaction between professionals working in the veterinary, medical, wildlife and environmental spheres [14]. In an evaluation of the WNV surveillance program in the USA, an association was found between submission of samples by zoos for WNV testing and the level of communication between the zoos and the public health agency [24]. The authors concluded that a greater awareness of the importance of surveillance by zoos could result in better collaboration and detection of possible human health threats from animal disease events.

The AWHN maintains a 'first alert' framework based on a national network of wildlife health professionals that can be used to coordinate and disseminate information in an emergency or a significant disease event. This network receives regular notifications of disease alerts, requests for information and samples, and publication of significant articles, guidelines and policy documents. The pilot project demonstrated the potential of the program to widen this network and raise the level of awareness of emerging diseases and diseases of potential national importance. The collaborative framework of the program also encourages discussion on new and interesting events and patterns of disease across multiple locations, and facilitates sharing of samples for testing and research.

The program has resulted in improved communication and flow of information, and strengthened relationships between the zoo industry and government agencies, in particular the state and territory departments of agriculture. Linking with zoos provides an avenue for information gathering and dissemination, and an opportunity to utilise the expertise and resources within their extensive networks. The program has the potential to build the capacity of zoos to play a rapid and effective role in a disease emergency by integrating zoo veterinarians into the national biosecurity surveillance network.

Conclusion

The science of understanding emerging infectious diseases with wildlife as part of their ecology has gained much attention over recent years, but it is often difficult to conduct meaningful surveillance in this area. The Australian zoo based wildlife disease surveillance program uses a collaborative approach involving government and the zoo industry, with a focus on collecting and reporting of wildlife disease events with potential impact on human health, livestock health and biodiversity. It provides a strong model for a disease surveillance program for free-ranging wildlife that could be adapted and utilised in other contexts. There is potential for expansion of the program to groups outside of zoo hospitals such as private veterinary practitioners from 'sentinel' hospitals with a high wildlife caseload, veterinary hospitals run by animal welfare organisations and universities involved in clinical wildlife work and research. Integration of these groups into the national wildlife health surveillance system has the potential to assist in the early detection of emerging diseases in Australia's free-ranging wildlife population.

Acknowledgments

Australia's states and territories, the zoos mentioned in the paper and the Zoo and Aquarium Association Australasia provided significant in-kind resources to enable the work to proceed. We thank Angus Cameron and Jenny Hutchison from AusVet Animal Health Services for their independent review of the pilot project, Susan Hester from ACERA for her interest and support, and the state and territory wildlife coordinators for their support and participation. We acknowledge the contribution of Helen Crabb, Bonnie McMeekin, Cree Monaghan, Tim Portas, Kimberley Vinette Herrin and Sam Young to the planning of the project. A particular thank you to the participating zoo veterinarians and staff, without whom the program could not run: Paul Eden, Sarah Frith, Leesa Haynes, Peter Holz, Robert Johnson, Trine Kruse, Anna Le Souef, Jenna McKenzie, David McLelland, Phillipa Mason, Jade Patterson, Karen Payne, Franciscus Scheelings, Tania Theuma, Gabrielle Tobias and Rebecca Vaughan-Higgins.

Author Contributions

Conceived and designed the experiments: KCW AR RW VG RTB DJB WB SC CL HMcC M. Pyne IS SV LV DW M. Phillips CB LP. Performed the experiments: KCW AR RW VG RTB DJB WB SC CL HMcC M. Pyne IS SV LV DW. Analyzed the data: KCW AR. Wrote the paper: KCW AR.

References

1. Kruse H, Kirkemo AM, Handeland K (2004) Wildlife as source of zoonotic infections. Emerg Infect Dis 10: 2067–2072.
2. Daszak P, Cunningham AA, Hyatt AD (2001) Anthropogenic environmental change and the emergence of infectious diseases in wildlife. Acta Trop 78: 103–116.
3. Daszak P, Cunningham AA, Hyatt AD (2000) Emerging infectious diseases of wildlife – threats to biodiversity and human health. Science 287: 443–449.
4. Cook RA, Karesh WB (2008) Chapter 6 - Emerging Diseases at the Interface of People, Domestic Animals, and Wildlife. In: Fowler ME, Miller RE, editors. Zoo and Wild Animal Medicine (Sixth Edition). Saint Louis: W.B. Saunders. pp. 55–65.
5. Jones KE, Patel NG, Levy MA, Storeygard A, Balk D, et al. (2008) Global trends in emerging infectious diseases. Nature 451: 990–993.
6. McFarlane R, Sleigh A, McMichael T (2012) Synanthropy of wild mammals as a determinant of emerging infectious diseases in the Asian-Australasian region. Ecohealth 9: 24–35.
7. O'Neil BD, Pharo HJ (1995) The control of bovine tuberculosis in New Zealand. N Z Vet J 43: 249–255.
8. Nolan A, Wilesmith JW (1994) Tuberculosis in badgers (Meles meles). Vet Microbiol 40: 179–191.
9. Alexander DJ (2007) An overview of the epidemiology of avian influenza. Vaccine 25: 5637–5644.
10. Frick WF, Pollock JF, Hicks AC, Langwig KE, Reynolds DS, et al. (2010) An emerging disease causes regional population collapse of a common North American bat species. Science 329: 679–682.
11. McCallum H (2008) Tasmanian devil facial tumour disease: lessons for conservation biology. Trends Ecol Evol 23: 631–637.
12. Skerratt L, Berger L, Speare R, Cashins S, McDonald K, et al. (2007) Spread of chytridiomycosis has caused the rapid global decline and extinction of frogs. EcoHealth 4: 125–134.
13. Berger L, Speare R, Daszak P, Green DE, Cunningham AA, et al. (1998) Chytridiomycosis causes amphibian mortality associated with population declines in the rain forests of Australia and Central America. Proceedings of the National Academy of Sciences 95: 9031–9036.
14. Black PF, Murray JG, Nunn MJ (2008) Managing animal disease risk in Australia: the impact of climate change. Rev Sci Tech 27: 563–580.
15. Bunn C, Woods R (2005) Emerging wildlife diseases – impact on trade, human health and the environment. Microbiology Australia 26: 53–55.
16. Prowse SJ, Perkins N, Field H (2009) Strategies for enhancing Australia's capacity to respond to emerging infectious diseases. Vet Ital 45: 67–78.
17. Sleeman J, Brand C, Wright S (2012) Strategies for wildlife disease surveillance. In: Aguirre A, Ostfeld R, Daszak P, editors. New Directions in Conservation Medicine. New York, NY: Oxford University Press. pp. 539–551.
18. Mathews F (2009) Zoonoses in wildlife integrating ecology into management. Adv Parasitol 68: 185–209.
19. Murray KA, Skerratt LF, Speare R, Ritchie S, Smout F, et al. (2012) Cooling off health security hot spots: getting on top of it down under. Environ Int 48: 56–64.
20. Animal Health Australia (2013) Animal Health in Australia 2012. Canberra, Australia.
21. Australian Wildlife Health Network (2014) *About AWHN.* Available: http://wildlifehealthaustralia.com.au/AboutUs.aspx. Accessed 2014 Mar 10.
22. McNamara T (2007) The role of zoos in biosurveillance. International Zoo Yearbook 41: 12–15.
23. Ludwig GV, Calle PP, Mangiafico JA, Raphael BL, Danner DK, et al. (2002) An outbreak of West Nile virus in a New York City captive wildlife population. Am J Trop Med Hyg 67: 67–75.
24. Pultorak E, Nadler Y, Travis D, Glaser A, McNamara T, et al. (2011) Zoological institution participation in a West Nile Virus surveillance system: implications for public health. Public Health 125: 592–599.
25. McNamara T, Travis D, Nadler Y (2011) A bird in hand: the power of zoo sentinels. Ecohealth 7: S21–22.
26. Watanabe M (2003) Zoos act as sentinels for infectious diseases. BioScience 53: 792.
27. Zoo Animal Health Network (2012) *Flu At The Zoo Tabletop Exercise.* Available: http://www.zooanimalhealthnetwork.org/FluAtTheZoo.aspx. Accessed 2013 Nov 20.
28. USDA/AZA Avian Influenza Surveillance System for Zoological Institutions (2012) Available: http://www.zooanimalhealthnetwork.org/ai/Home.aspx.Accessed 2013 Nov 20.
29. Beri V, Tranent A, Abelson P (2010) The economic and social contribution of the zoological industry in Australia. International Zoo Yearbook 44: 192–200.
30. Australian Wildlife Health Network (nd) *Zoo Animal Health Reference Group.* Available: http://wildlifehealthaustralia.com.au/ProgramsProjects/ZooAnimalHealthReferenceGroup.aspx. Accessed 2014 Mar 10.
31. Powling J (2012) Quarterly Statistics – Surveillance Activities – *Salmonella* Surveillance. Animal Health Surveillance Quarterly Report 17: 27.
32. Spratt D (2005) Neuroangiostrongyliasis: disease in wildlife and humans. Microbiology Australia 26: 63–64.
33. Ma G, Dennis M, Rose K, Spratt D, Spielman D (2013) Tawny frogmouths and brushtail possums as sentinels for *Angiostrongylus cantonensis*, the rat lungworm. Vet Parasitol 192: 158–165.
34. Herbst LH, Klein PA (1995) Green turtle fibropapillomatosis: challenges to assessing the role of environmental cofactors. Environ Health Perspect 103 Suppl 4: 27–30.
35. McAloose D, Newton AL (2009) Wildlife cancer: a conservation perspective. Nat Rev Cancer 9: 517–526.
36. Newman SJ, Smith SA (2006) Marine mammal neoplasia: a review. Vet Pathol 43: 865–880.
37. Australian Government Department of the Environment (2009) *EPBC Act List of Threatened Fauna.* Available: http://www.environment.gov.au/cgi-bin/sprat/public/publicthreatenedlist.pl?wanted=fauna. Accessed 2013 Nov 20.
38. Australian Government Department of the Environment (2009) *Listed Key Threatening Processes.* Available: http://www.environment.gov.au/cgi-bin/sprat/public/publicgetkeythreats.pl. Accessed 2013 Nov 20.
39. Funnell O, Johnson L, Woolford L, Boardman W, Polkinghorne A, et al. (2013) Conjunctivitis Associated with *Chlamydia pecorum* in Three Koalas (*Phascolarctos cinereus*) in the Mount Lofty Ranges, South Australia. Journal of Wildlife Diseases 49: 1066–1069.
40. Australian Government Department of the Environment (2013) *Species Profile and Threats Database 2012:* Phascolarctos cinereus *(combined populations of Qld, NSW and the ACT) – Koala (combined populations of Queensland, New South Wales and the Australian Capital Territory).* Available: http://www.environment.gov.au/cgi-bin/sprat/public/publicspecies.pl?taxon_id=85104. Accessed 2013 Nov 20.
41. Paskin R (2011) Avian paramyxovirus in pigeons. Animal Health Surveillance Quarterly Report 16: 3–5.
42. Grillo T, Post L (2012) Australian Wildlife Health Network. Animal Health Surveillance Quarterly Report 17: 6–8.
43. Field H, Crameri G, Kung NY, Wang LF (2012) Ecological aspects of Hendra virus. Curr Top Microbiol Immunol 359: 11–23.
44. Arthur R (2011) State and Territory Reports – New South Wales. Animal Health Surveillance Quarterly Report 16: 10–13.
45. Australian Government Department of Agriculture (2011) *Australia and the World Organization for Animal Health.* Available: http://www.daff.gov.au/animal-plant-health/animal/oie. Accessed 2013 Nov 20.
46. Cameron A, Hutchison J (2011) Review of the Zoo Based Wildlife Disease Surveillance Pilot Project. Unpublished report to the Australian Wildlife Health Network.
47. Halliday J, Daborn C, Auty H, Mtema Z, Lembo T, et al. (2012) Bringing together emerging and endemic zoonoses surveillance: shared challenges and a common solution. Philos Trans R Soc Lond B Biol Sci 367: 2872–2880.
48. Kuiken T, Leighton FA, Fouchier RA, LeDuc JW, Peiris JS, et al. (2005) Public health. Pathogen surveillance in animals. Science 309: 1680–1681.
49. World Organisation for Animal Health (OIE) (2012) Report of the Meeting of the OIE Working Group on Wildlife Diseases, Paris, 12–15 November 2012. Available: http://www.oie.int/fileadmin/Home/eng/Internationa_Standard_Setting/docs/pdf/WGWildlife/A_WGW_Nov2012.pdf. Accessed 2013 Nov 20.

Association of Veterinary Third-Generation Cephalosporin Use with the Risk of Emergence of Extended-Spectrum-Cephalosporin Resistance in *Escherichia coli* from Dairy Cattle in Japan

Toyotaka Sato[1¤], Torahiko Okubo[1], Masaru Usui[1], Shin-ichi Yokota[2], Satoshi Izumiyama[3], Yutaka Tamura[1*]

1 Laboratory of Food Microbiology and Food Safety, Department of Health and Environmental Sciences, School of Veterinary Medicine, Rakuno Gakuen University, Ebetsu, Japan, **2** Department of Microbiology, Sapporo Medical University School of Medicine, Sapporo, Japan, **3** Nemuro District Agriculture Mutual Aid Association, Nakashibetsu, Japan

Abstract

The use of extended-spectrum cephalosporins in food animals has been suggested to increase the risk of spread of *Enterobacteriaceae* carrying extended-spectrum β-lactamases to humans. However, evidence that selection of extended-spectrum cephalosporin–resistant bacteria owing to the actual veterinary use of these drugs according to criteria established in cattle has not been demonstrated. In this study, we investigated the natural occurrence of cephalosporin-resistant *Escherichia coli* in dairy cattle following clinical application of ceftiofur. *E. coli* isolates were obtained from rectal samples of treated and untreated cattle (n = 20/group) cultured on deoxycholate-hydrogen sulfide-lactose agar in the presence or absence of ceftiofur. Eleven cefazoline-resistant isolates were obtained from two of the ceftiofur-treated cattle; no cefazoline-resistant isolates were found in untreated cattle. The cefazoline-resistant isolates had mutations in the chromosomal *ampC* promoter region and remained susceptible to ceftiofur. Eighteen extended-spectrum cephalosporin–resistant isolates from two ceftiofur-treated cows were obtained on ceftiofur-supplemented agar; no extended-spectrum cephalosporin–resistant isolates were obtained from untreated cattle. These extended-spectrum cephalosporin–resistant isolates possessed plasmid-mediated β-lactamase genes, including $bla_{CTX\text{-}M\text{-}2}$ (9 isolates), $bla_{CTX\text{-}M\text{-}14}$ (8 isolates), or $bla_{CMY\text{-}2}$ (1 isolate); isolates possessing $bla_{CTX\text{-}M\text{-}2}$ and $bla_{CTX\text{-}M\text{-}14}$ were clonally related. These genes were located on self-transmissible plasmids. Our results suggest that appropriate veterinary use of ceftiofur did not trigger growth extended-spectrum cephalosporin–resistant *E. coli* in the bovine rectal flora; however, ceftiofur selection *in vitro* suggested that additional ceftiofur exposure enhanced selection for specific extended-spectrum cephalosporin–resistant β-lactamase-expressing *E. coli* clones

Editor: Axel Cloeckaert, Institut National de la Recherche Agronomique, France

Funding: This study was supported in part by a Grant-in-Aid from the Japanese Ministry of Agriculture, Forestry, and Fisheries and a grant from the Program for Developing the Supporting System for Upgrading Education and Research from the Japan Ministry of Education, Culture, Sports, Science, and Technology. The funders had no role in study design, data collection and analysis, decision to publish, or preparation of the manuscript.

Competing Interests: The authors have declared that no competing interests exist.

* E-mail: tamuray@rakuno.ac.jp

¤ Current address: Laboratory of Human Retrovirology, Leidos-Frederick, Inc., Frederick National Laboratory for Cancer Research, Frederick, Maryland, United States of America

Introduction

β-Lactam antimicrobials are used worldwide in clinical settings. Extended-spectrum cephalosporins (ESCs; third- and fourth-generation cephalosporins such as cefpodoxime [CPD], ceftazidime [CAZ], and cefepime [FEP]) are broad-spectrum antimicrobials that have been listed by the World Health Organization (WHO) as critically important for human health [1]. However, the clinical occurrence of ESC-resistant *Enterobacteriaceae* has increased [3,4]. Numerous bacterial infections in food-producing animals and humans are treated with first- or second-generation cephalosporins such as cefazoline (CFZ), cefalexin (LEX), and cefuroxime (CXM), and ESCs such as ceftiofur (CTF) and CPD. In the WHO ranking of antimicrobials according to their importance in human medicine, the ESCs that are also used in veterinary medicine are listed at the highest rank (critically important antimicrobial agents) on the basis of 2 criteria: (1) the agent or class is the sole therapeutic option or one of few alternatives available to treat serious human disease; and (2) the antimicrobial agent or class is used to treat diseases caused by organisms that may be transmitted via nonhuman sources or diseases caused by organisms that may acquire resistance genes from nonhuman sources [5]. ESCs used in humans and animals are of the same general class and share the same mode of action, even if they differ chemically [6]. Thus, the appearance of ESC-resistant bacteria can be attributable to mechanisms common between humans and animals (mainly by the acquisition of extended-spectrum β-lactamase genes and AmpC-type β-lactamase genes such as bla_{CTX-M} and bla_{CMY}), and interspecies transmission of ESC-resistant bacteria can occur [7,8]. ESC-resistant *Enterobacteriaceae* are found in food animals and their products [7,9–12]. Therefore, discussing issues related to the use of ESCs in veterinary medicine necessitates scientific evidence regarding the joint role played by ESCs in human and veterinary medicine.

CTF is a third-generation cephalosporin that is commonly used in veterinary medicine worldwide [13–15]. In Japan, CTF has been approved for use in cattle as a second-line drug for the treatment of pneumonia and as a first-line drug in serious infectious diseases in dairy cattle. *E. coli* is a commensal bacterial species in cattle feces [16]; some *E. coli* strains act as enteric pathogens in humans and/or are resistant to antimicrobials. [17]. Therefore, it is essential to characterize the *E. coli* with naturally occurring ESC resistance in bovine rectal flora because of the veterinary use of CTF, which may select for antimicrobial resistance. Previous studies have suggested an association between CTF use and the occurrence of ESC-resistant *E. coli* in cattle [2,13–15]. However, it is not known if *E. coli* with naturally occurring ESC resistance is selected for by appropriate veterinary ECS use because many studies have involved artificial intragastric inoculation with extended-spectrum β-lactamase–producing *E. coli* mutants and most do not record antimicrobial use or clinical criteria, such as, detail methods for ECS use, dose, or washout for every cow. All of these factors are important to consider when evaluating for a causal relationship between ECS use and naturally occurring ECS resistance.

In this study, to evaluate the risk of selection of ESC-resistant bacteria related to veterinary treatment with a suitable third-generation cephalosporin, we tried to isolate *E. coli* with naturally occurring ESC resistance from the rectal flora of CTF-treated or untreated dairy cattle after the washout period.

Materials and Methods

Bacterial Samples

We collected 20 dairy bovine rectal feces samples from dairy cattle treated with Excenel (cows 1–20; CTF sodium injection; Pfizer, New York City, USA). Ethical authority was not required according to the Epidemiological and Animal Ethical Research Committee of Rakuno Gakuen University because CTF treatment in this case was performed as part of general clinical treatment, compliant with the Veterinarians Acts and the Pharmaceutical Affairs Law defined by the Ministry of Agriculture, Forestry, and Fisheries in Japan. Briefly, cattle received intramuscular injections of 1–2 $mg{\cdot}kg^{-1}{\cdot}day^{-1}$ CTF for 3 days for serious infectious diseases such as refractory pneumonia, puerperal fever, and hoof disease. This represented the first CTF treatment for these animals, and none had received any other antimicrobials for at least 3 months before sampling. Rectal feces samples were collected after the 8-day washout period, at which point the remaining CTF concentration in the organs and products have no effect on human health, according to the Pharmaceutical Affairs Law defined by the Ministry of Agriculture, Forestry, and Fisheries. The untreated controls included 20 dairy cattle (numbers 21–40) that did not receive any other antimicrobials for at least 3 months and no CTF use for at least 1.5 years before sampling. We did not sample non-treated cattle from herds that contain CTF-treated cattle. All samples were collected from independent farms in Betsukai (Hokkaido, Japan), the most productive dairying area in Japan (at least 100 cattle per farm). We had permission from the farms to collect fecal matter from their private property and CTF use in this study.

Table 1. β-lactam antimicrobial susceptibilities and detection of β-lactamase genes in AMP-resistant isolates in non-supplemented agar.

Cow number	Number of strains/tested colonies	CTF treatment	MIC (μg/mL)						β-lactamase gene
			AMP (≥32)[a]	AMP /CVA	CFZ (≥32)	CXM (≥32)	CTF (≥8)	CTF/CVA	
5	10/10	+	>128	64/32	64–128	32	1	1/0.5	−1(CtoT)/−18(GtoA)/−42(CtoT)/−82(AtoG)*
7	1/10	+	>128	64/32	128	32	2	2/1	−1(CtoT)/−18(GtoA)/−42(CtoT)/−82(AtoG)*

[a]Breakpoint; *Mutations in the chromosomal *ampC* promoter region.

Table 2. β-Lactam susceptibilities and detection of β-lactamase genes in cephalosporin-resistant isolates in CTF-supplemented agar.

Cow number	Number of strains	CTF treatment	MIC (μg/mL) AMP (≥32)[a]	AMP/CVA	CFZ (≥32)	LEX (≥32)	CXM (≥32)	CTF (≥8)	CTF/CVA	CPD (≥8)	CAZ (≥16)	FEP (≥32)	Inc. type	β-lactamase gene
7	9	+	>128	8/4	>128	>128	>128	>32	1/0.5	>128	2	16	N, FIA, FIB	$bla_{CTX\text{-}M\text{-}2}$
7	1	+	128	64/32	>128	32	32	8	8/4	>128	32	≤0.125	I1-Iγ, FIB	$bla_{CMY\text{-}2}$
13	8	+	>128	8/4	>128	>128	>128	>32	1/0.5	>128	1–2	4–8	I1-Iγ	$bla_{CTX\text{-}M\text{-}14}$

[a]Break point.

Isolation of *E. coli*

Fecal samples (1 g) were dissolved in 9 mL of 0.85% sterile saline solution; 100 μL was immediately spread on deoxycholate-hydrogen sulfide-lactose (DHL) agar (Nissui, Tokyo, Japan) supplemented with 4 μg/mL CTF and incubated for 24 h at 37°C. CTF-free DHL plates served as controls. Samples were subcultured on nutrient agar (Nissui) at a maximum of 10 colonies per agar plate. The biochemical properties of these colonies were examined using triple sugar iron medium (Nissui), lysine indole motility medium (Nissui), and oxidase tests. Final identification of *E. coli* was performed by API20E (bioMérieux, Tokyo, Japan).

Susceptibility Testing

β-Lactam resistance was screened using CFZ KB-disks (Eiken, Tokyo, Japan) according to the manufacturer's instructions. Isolates showing resistance to CFZ in the KB-disk method were assessed to determine the minimum inhibitory concentration (MIC) by using the microdilution method according to the recommendations of the Clinical and Laboratory Standards Institute (CLSI; 2008) [18]. MICs were determined for eight β-lactam antimicrobials: AMP, CFZ, LEX, CXM, CTF, CPD, CAZ, FEP, and two mixtures of clavulanic acid (CVA) (CVA/AMP and CVA/CTF). Breakpoint values were defined according to 2008 CLSI recommendations, except in the case of LEX, CXM, CAZ, and FEP, which were defined according to 2011 CLSI recommendations [19], because the break points for these agents have not been defined for veterinary pathogens. Antimicrobial plates for microdilution testing were purchased from Eiken.

Detection of β-lactamase Genes

β-Lactamase genes were identified by PCR and direct DNA sequencing. $bla_{CTX\text{-}M}$ was detected as described by Xu et al. [20], and plasmid-mediated *ampC* was detected as described by Pérez-Pérez et al. [21]. The presence of bla_{TEM}, bla_{SHV}, and mutations in the chromosomal *ampC* promoter region was detected according to Kojima et al. [11]. Nucleotide sequences were determined with a BigDye Terminator v3.1 Cycle Sequencing Kit and a 3130 Genetic Analyzer (Applied Biosystems, Foster City, CA).

Pulsed-field Gel Electrophoresis (PFGE)

PFGE was performed according to the method outlined by PulseNet USA [22] by using *Xba*I (Takara-Bio, Tokyo, Japan). The CHEF-DR III system (Bio-Rad Laboratories, Hercules, CA, USA) was used with the following running conditions: 19 h at 11.3°C, voltage of 6 V, ramped with an initial forward time of 2.2 s, and a final forward time of 54.2 s. After electrophoresis, gels were stained with ethidium bromide and photographed. The banding patterns were visually interpreted using published guidelines, and Dice similarity indices were calculated by cluster analysis.

Transferability Test of β-lactamase Genes

Broth-mating experiments were performed using rifampicin-resistant ML4909 (F$^-$ *galK2 galT22 hsdR metB1 relA supE44* rifampicin-resistant) as a recipient strain [21]. Donors and recipients were grown in tryptic soy broth (TSB, Nissui) to the logarithmic phase; they were then mixed in a total volume of 2 mL at a 1:9 (v/v) ratio, and 2 mL fresh TSB was added. The mating cultures were incubated overnight at 37°C. Transconjugants were selected on CTF (final concentration, 4 μg/mL)- and rifampicin (final concentration, 64 μg/mL)-containing MH agar.

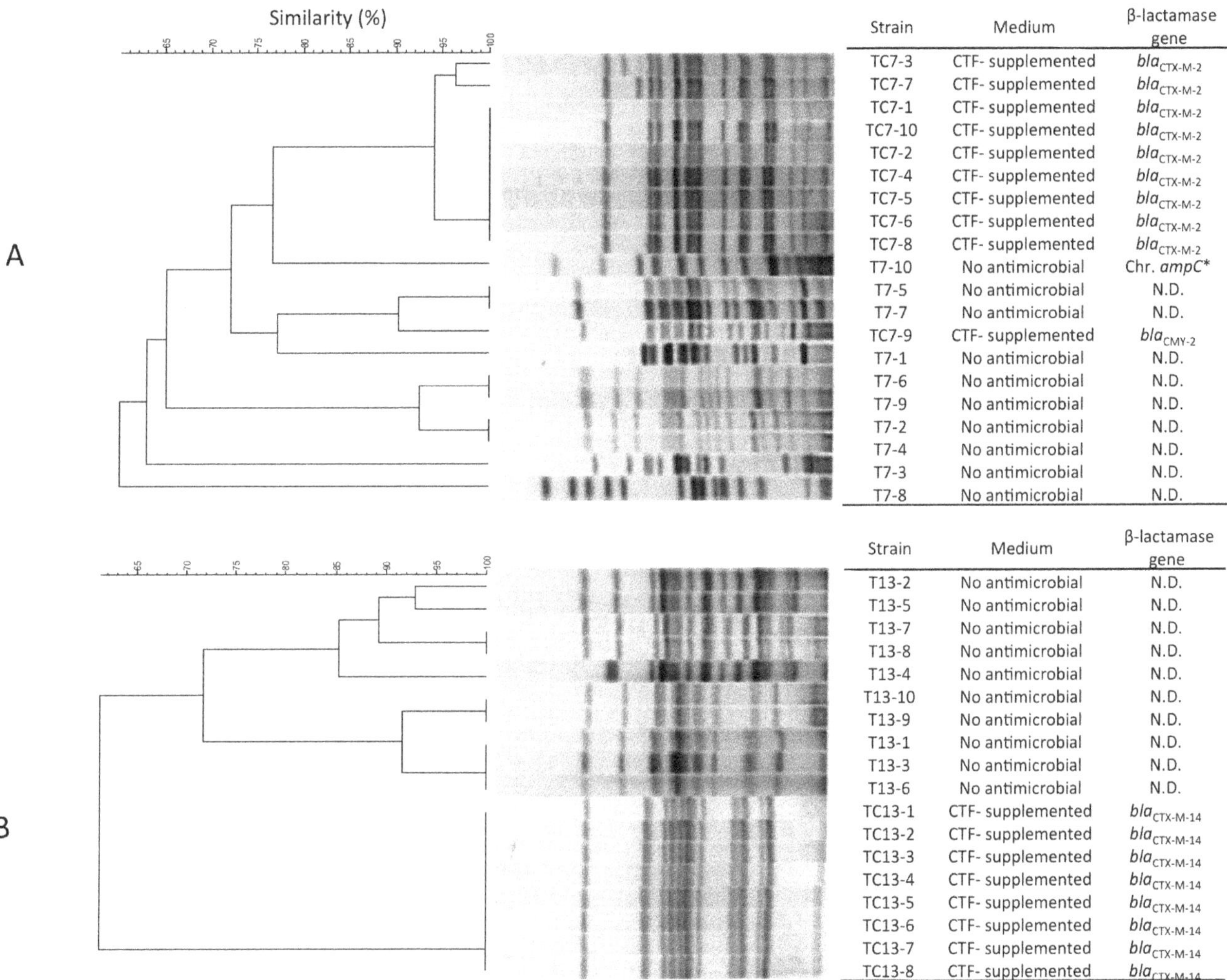

Figure 1. Pulsed-field gel electrophoresis of CTF-resistant *E. coli* isolates from two CTF-treated cattle. A, PFGE analysis of 20 isolates obtained from cow No. 7. Strains T7 and TC7 were isolated in the absence or presence of CTF, respectively. B, PFGE analysis of 18 isolates obtained from cow No. 13. Strains T13 and TC13 were isolated in the absence or presence of CTF, respectively.

Plasmid Profiling and Southern Hybridization Analysis

Plasmid profiling was performed according to previously described methods [24]. Plasmid incompatibility (Inc) groups were determined by PCR with the following primers: HI1, HI2, I1-Iγ, X, L/M, N, FIA, FIB, W, Y, P, FIC, A/C, T, FIIAs, F, K, and B/O [25].

Southern hybridization was performed as follows. Probes were prepared by PCR. Probes for $bla_{CTX-M-2}$ and $bla_{CTX-M-14}$ were prepared using a CTX-M consensus primer set [26]. The probe for bla_{CMY-2} was prepared using primers described by Pérez-Pérez and Hanson [21]. These PCR products were labeled using a PCR DIG Labeling Mix (Roche Diagnostic, Tokyo, Japan) according to the manufacturer's instructions. Plasmid DNA was separated by 0.8% (w/v) agarose gel electrophoresis at 100 V for 70 min. The DNA in the gel was transferred to a positive membrane (Roche Diagnostics) by the capillary method. Pre-hybridization (>30 min) and hybridization (>16 h) were performed using Easy Hyb solution (Roche Diagnostics) under high-stringency conditions, and digoxigenin (DIG) in the hybrids was detected using a DIG Luminescent Detection Kit (Roche Diagnostics) according to the manufacturer's instructions. A hyper MP film (GE Healthcare Japan, Tokyo, Japan) was exposed to the membranes for 2 min at room temperature and developed in a Kodak X-Omat processor.

Statistical Analysis

Statistical significance was determined using chi-square test and Fisher's exact tests. Significance was set at $p<0.05$.

Results

Isolation and Antimicrobial Resistance of *E. coli*

Using non-supplemented agar. In this study, 193 and 182 *E. coli* isolates were obtained from CTF-treated and untreated cattle, respectively. We screened for CFZ resistance by the disk diffusion method. From the 193 strains isolated from CTF-treated cattle, 11 isolates resistant to CFZ were obtained; however, no CFZ-resistant *E. coli* was obtained from untreated cattle ($p<0.05$). The 11 CFZ-resistant isolates (from cow No. 5 [10 strains] and cow No. 7 [1 strain]) were also resistant to AMP and CXM, but not CTF; CVA did not affect the MICs of AMP or CTF (Table 1). All 11 isolates carried mutations in the chromosomal *ampC* promoter region.

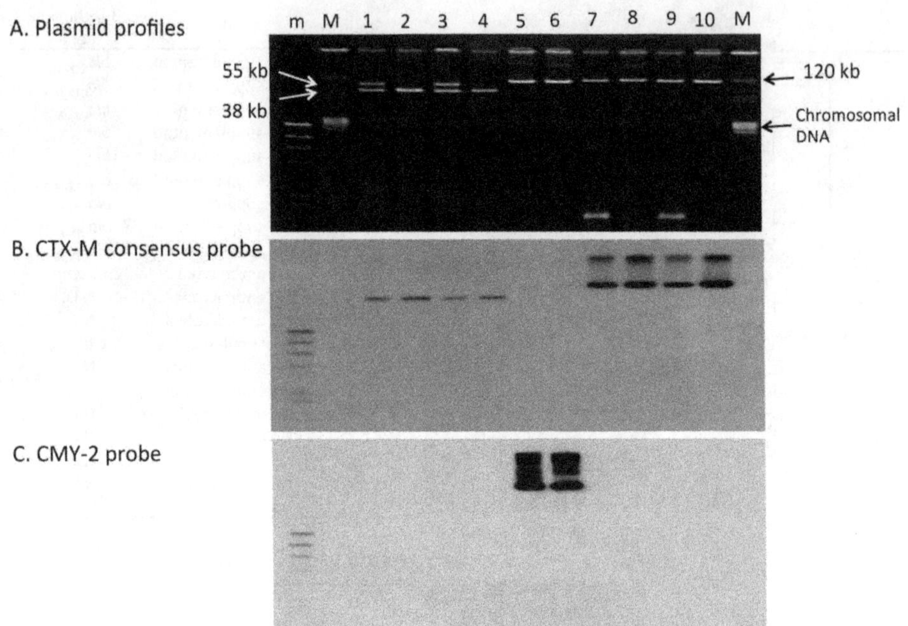

Figure 2. Plasmid profiling and Southern hybridization of β-lactamase genes in *E. coli* isolates from CTF-treated cattle. A, Plasmid profiling. B, Southern hybridization of the bla_{CTX-M} consensus probe. C, Southern hybridization of the bla_{CMY-2} probe. Lane1, ML4909 (recipient); lane 2, TC7-1 (possesses $bla_{CTX-M-2}$); lane 3, TcTC7-1; lane 4, TC7-2 (possesses $bla_{CTX-M-2}$); lane 5, TcTC7-2; lane 6, TC7-9 (possesses bla_{CMY-2}); lane 7, TcTC7-9; lane 8, TC13-1 (possesses $bla_{CTX-M-14}$); lane 9, TcTC13-1; lane 10, TC13-2 (possesses $bla_{CTX-M-14}$); lane 11, TcTC13-2; m, DNA Molecular Weight Marker II, DIG-labeled; M, BAC-Tracker Supercoiled DNA Ladder. $bla_{CTX-M-2}$ and $bla_{CTX-M-14}$ were detected using a CTX-M consensus probe.

Using CTF-supplemented agar. Eighteen *E. coli* isolates were obtained on CTF-supplemented agar (from CTF-treated cow No. 7 [10 strains] and cow No. 13 [8 strains]); no resistant strains were isolated from the untreated group ($p<0.05$). Seventeen isolates were resistant to AMP, CFZ, LEX, CXM, CPD, and CTF, and CVA influenced the MICs of AMP and CTF (Table 2). The *E. coli* isolates showed CTF resistance from cow nos. 7 and 13 possessed $bla_{CTX-M-2}$ and $bla_{CTX-M-14}$, respectively. The last strain from CTF-treated cow No. 7 showed resistance to AMP, CFZ, LEX, CXM, CPD, CAZ, and CTF; however, CVA did not affect the MICs of AMP and CTF in this isolate. This strain possessed bla_{CMY-2}. None of the isolates exceeded the breakpoint of FEP (Tables 1 and 2).

PFGE Analysis and Plasmid Analysis

To determine the clonal relationship of isolates exhibiting differential CTF selection properties, we performed PFGE of isolates derived from non-supplemented and CTF-supplemented agar after collection from two CTF-treated cattle (Nos. 7 and 13; Figure 1). The PFGE pattern showed that these isolates were clearly different clones. Isolates harboring $bla_{CTX-M-2}$ and $bla_{CTX-M-14}$, which were isolated from CTF-supplemented agar, exhibited mostly identical PFGE patterns. Plasmid profiling also showed that strains isolated from CTF-supplemented agar possessed identically sized plasmid(s) harboring their respective β-lactamase gene types (Figure 2). These results indicated that resistant strains carrying $bla_{CTX-M-2}$ from cow No. 7 and those carrying $bla_{CTX-M-14}$ from cow no. 13 originated from a single clone in each cow.

Transferability Test and Southern Hybridization of β-lactamase Genes

We investigated the transferability of β-lactamase genes using recipient ML4909 cells. The donors were TC7-1 and TC7-2, which possessed $bla_{CTX-M-2}$ (isolated from cow No. 7); TC7-9, which possessed bla_{CMY-2} (isolated from cow No. 7); and TC13-1 and TC13-2, which possessed $bla_{CTX-M-14}$ (isolated from cow No. 13). All detected β-lactamase genes could be transferred to the recipient, and the MICs of the transconjugants increased at a level similar to that of the donor (Table 3). Replicon typing and Southern hybridization showed that $bla_{CTX-M-2}$ was located in an IncN plasmid (about 40 kb), bla_{CMY-2} was located in I1-Iγ and/or FIB plasmids (more than 100 kb), and $bla_{CTX-M-14}$ was located in an I1-Iγ plasmid (more than 100 kb; Table 3 and Figure 2).

Discussion

The occurrence of antimicrobial-resistant bacteria, including cephalosporin-resistant bacteria, is thought to be related to selection pressures resulting from antimicrobial consumption [27–29]. Previous studies have suggested an association between CTF use and the occurrence of ESC-resistant *E. coli* in cattle [2,13–15]. Although it has not reported an association between CTF use and the occurrence of ESC-resistant *E. coli* in cattle in Japan, a previous study showed that 6 (1.5%) of 396 *E. coli* isolates obtained from bovine fecal samples in Japan showed ESC resistance [30]. These data indicate an association between the isolation of ESC-resistant *E. coli* and ESC use in Japan. However, evidence supporting this association is lacking because the histories of clinical CTF use and compliance with clinical criteria were unknown and a cohort study on veterinary CTF use has never been performed. Thus, the estimation of emergence of ESC-resistant *E. coli* due to suitable clinical ESC use could help re-evaluate antimicrobial therapy to avoid the spread of ESC-resistant bacteria.

CTF was used to treat refractory pneumonia and other serious infectious diseases such as puerperal fever and hoof disease in dairy cattle, according to our inquiry survey. In this study, cephalospo-

Table 3. β-Lactam susceptibilities and detection of β-lactamase genes in transconjugants from CTF-resistant isolates.

Strain	Characteristic	MIC (μg/mL)						Inc. group	β-lactamase gene
		AMP	AMP/CVA	CFZ	CXM	CTF	CTF/CVA		
ML4909	Recipient	4	2/1	2	<1	<0.5	<0.5/0.25	ND	ND[a)]
TC7-1	Donor	>128	8/4	>128	>128	>32	1/0.5	N, FIA, FIB	$bla_{\text{CTX-M-2}}$
TcTC7-1	Transconjugant	>128	8/4	>128	>128	>32	1/0.5	N	$bla_{\text{CTX-M-2}}$
TC7-2	Donor	>128	8/4	>128	>128	>32	1/0.5	N, FIA, FIB	$bla_{\text{CTX-M-2}}$
TcTC7-2	Transconjugant	>128	8/4	>128	>128	>32	1/0.5	N	$bla_{\text{CTX-M-2}}$
TC7-9	Donor	128	64/32	>128	32	8	8/4	I1-Iγ, FIB	$bla_{\text{CMY-2}}$
TcTC7-9	Transconjugant	64	64/32	128	8	8	4/2	I1-Iγ, FIB	$bla_{\text{CMY-2}}$
TC13-1	Donor	>128	8/4	>128	>128	>32	1/0.5	I1-Iγ	$bla_{\text{CTX-M-14}}$
TcTC13-1	Transconjugant	>128	8/4	>128	>128	>32	<0.5/0.25	I1-Iγ	$bla_{\text{CTX-M-14}}$
TC13-2	Donor	>128	8/4	>128	>128	>32	1/0.5	I1-Iγ	$bla_{\text{CTX-M-14}}$
TcTC13-2	Transconjugant	>128	4/2	>128	>128	>32	<0.5/0.25	I1-Iγ	$bla_{\text{CTX-M-14}}$

[a]ND, not detected.

rin-resistant isolates were found only in CTF-treated animals. All of these isolates possessed mutations in chromosomal *ampC* and were resistant to AMP and first- and second-generation cephalosporins (CFZ and CXM), but not CTF. Thus, we conclude that if CTF is used appropriately (1–2 $mg{\cdot}kg^{-1}{\cdot}day^{-1}$ for 3 days) in Japanese veterinary practice, washout periods will increase the frequency of naturally occurring first- and second-generation cephalosporin resistance in *E. coli*, but will not influence the natural occurrence of ESC-resistant *E. coli* in dairy cattle.

A previous study reported the isolation of ESC-resistant *E. coli* (possessing $bla_{\text{CMY-2}}$) from fecal samples of calves on 8 μg/mL CTF-supplemented agar, but not on non-supplemented agar [14]. This finding suggests that ESC-resistant *E. coli* are present in the bovine rectal flora at low frequency, and additional CTF exposure selects for these ESC-resistant *E. coli*. However, the applicability of this result to real-world CTF treatment in dairying is unknown, because the histories of clinical CTF use (or other β-lactams) in these calves were unknown. In this study, all CTF-resistant isolates were obtained from treated cattle and after culture on CTF-supplemented agar; these isolates possessed a plasmid-encoded β-lactamase gene, $bla_{\text{CTX-M-2}}$, $bla_{\text{CTX-M-14}}$, or $bla_{\text{CMY-2}}$. Importantly, PFGE analysis showed that although ESC-resistant clones were not yet predominant in the rectal flora at the end of the washout period after CTF treatment, *in vitro* CTF exposure led to the selection of specific ESC-resistant clones in CTF-treated cattle. However, we could not determine which CTF dose (1 or 2 mg/kg of CTF) was high risk in terms of selection of ECS-resistant *E. coli* by *in vitro* testing because these dose were scattered regardless of whether ECS-resistant *E. coli* were isolated or not. Therefore, these results suggest that although appropriate CTF use (1–2 $mg{\cdot}kg^{-1}{\cdot}day^{-1}$ for 3 days) in Japanese veterinary practice dose not influence the natural occurrence of ESC-resistant *E. coli* in cattle, if CTF is used inappropriately, such as by overuse and/or subcutaneous use, it might encourage the selection and spread of broad-spectrum cephalosporin-resistant *E. coli* clones in bovine flora as suggested by *in vitro* CTF selection.

β-Lactamase genes in ESC-resistant isolates were located on Inc-type plasmids, i.e., $bla_{\text{CTX-M-2}}$ (Inc-N), $bla_{\text{CTX-M-14}}$ (Inc-I1-Iγ), and $bla_{\text{CMY-2}}$ (Inc.I1-Iγ and/or FIB), and all were capable of self-transmission. $bla_{\text{CTX-M2}}$ was found in *E. coli* from cattle in Japan from 2000 to 2001 [30]. $bla_{\text{CMY-2}}$ was found in I1-Iγ and A/C plasmids in *Salmonella enterica* serovar Typhimurium isolated from cattle in Japan in 2007 [31]. $bla_{\text{CTX-M-14}}$ was found in *S. enterica* serovar Enteritidis from chicken meat imported from China and sold by a retailer in Japan in 2004 [32]. The presence of these genes suggests β-lactamase genes producing ESC resistance are already widespread in Japanese livestock and their products. Although these data do not show an association between veterinary ESC use and the presence of β-lactamase genes in ESC-resistant *E. coli*, the presence of these genes might be selected for by cephalosporin use or co-selected by other antimicrobials used in veterinary medicine.

Furthermore, the ESC-resistant *E. coli* isolated in current study showed resistance to both ESCs used in veterinary medicine and to ESCs used in human medicine, and their transferable β-lactamase genes have been detected in humans in a variety of clinical settings worldwide [33]. Remarkably, $bla_{\text{CTX-M-2}}$ and $bla_{\text{CTX-M-14}}$ have also been found in *E. coli* isolates from humans in Japan ($bla_{\text{CTX-M-2}}$ in Inc-N and $bla_{\text{CTX-M-14}}$ in Inc-Il plasmids [4,34], similar to the pattern observed in our study). In particular, *E. coli* O25 (undetermined H-antigen)-ST131, which frequently possesses $bla_{\text{CTX-M-14}}$, is the most common strain that spreads to humans [34]. Our study and other studies suggest that human health may be at increased risk from the overuse of cephalosporins in livestock and that further genetic and epidemiological investigations are required to determine whether there is direct transmission of ESC-resistant *E. coli* and their β-lactamase genes from livestock to humans.

In conclusion, although appropriate veterinary use of a third-generation cephalosporin, CTF, increased the occurrence of first- and second-generation cephalosporin-resistant *E. coli*, it did not influence the natural occurrence of ECS-resistant *E. coli* in dairy cattle. However, *in vitro* CTF selection suggested that inappropriate CTF use in veterinary practice might increase the risk of selection of ESC-resistant *E. coli* possessing $bla_{CTX\text{-}M\text{-}2}$, $bla_{CMY\text{-}2}$, or $bla_{CTX\text{-}M\text{-}14}$. Therefore, veterinary use of ESCs should be carefully monitored and used appropriately as described by the Joint FAO/WHO/OIE Expert Meeting on Critically Important Antimicrobials [6] to prevent the spread of ESC-resistant bacteria in veterinary medicine.

Author Contributions

Performed the experiments: TS TO. Analyzed the data: TS TO. Contributed reagents/materials/analysis tools: TS TO MU SY SI YT. Wrote the paper: TS. Contributed to, prepared and approved the manuscript: MU SY YT.

References

1. World Health Organization (WHO): Critically Important Antimicrobials for Human Medicine: Categorization for the Development of Risk Management Strategies to contain Antimicrobial Resistance due to Non-Human Antimicrobial Use Report of the Second WHO Expert Meeting, Copenhagen, 2007, 29–31.
2. Chantziaras I, Boyen F, Callens B, Dewulf J (2014) Correlation between veterinary antimicrobial use and antimicrobial resistance in food-producing animals: a report on seven countries J Antimicrob Chemother 69: 827–834.
3. Chong Y, Yakushiji H, Ito Y, Kamimura T (2011) Clinical and molecular epidemiology of extended-spectrum β-lactamase-producing Escherichia coli and Klebsiella pneumoniae in a long-term study from Japan. European Eur J Clin Microbiol Infect Dis 30: 83–87.
4. Suzuki S, Shibata N, Yamane K, Wachino J, Ito K, et al (2009) Change in the prevalence of extended-spectrum-beta-lactamase-producing *Escherichia coli* in Japan by clonal spread. J Antimicrob Chemother 63: 72–79.
5. Collignon P, Powers JH, Chiller TM, Aidara-Kane A, Aarestrup FM (2009) World Health Organization ranking of antimicrobials according to their importance in human medicine: A critical step for developing risk management strategies for the use of antimicrobials in food production animals. Clin Infect Dis 49: 132–141.
6. FAO/WHO/OIE: Report of the Joint FAO/WHO/OIE Expert Meeting on Critically Important Antimicrobials (2007) FAO, Rome, Italy.
7. Bertrand S, Weill FX, Cloeckaert A, Vrints M, Mairiaux E, et al. (2006) Clonal emergence of extended-spectrum β-lactamase (CTX-M-2)-producing *Salmonella enterica* serovar Virchow isolates with reduced susceptibilities to ciprofloxacin among poultry and humans in Belgium and France (2000 to 2003). J Clin Microbiol 44: 2897–2903.
8. Winokur PL, Vonstein DL, Hoffman LJ, Uhlenhopp EK, Doern GV (2001) Evidence for transfer of CMY-2 AmpC beta-lactamase plasmids between *Escherichia coli* and *Salmonella* isolates from food animals and humans. Antimicrob Agents Chemother 45: 2716–2722.
9. Cavaco LM, Abatih E, Aarestrup FM, Guardabassi L (2008) Selection and persistence of CTX-M-producing *Escherichia coli* in the intestinal flora of pigs treated with amoxicillin, ceftiofur, or cefquinome. Antimicrob Agents and Chemother 52: 3612–3616.
10. Jouini A, Vinue L, Ben Slama K, Saenz Y, Klibi N, et al. (2007) Characterization of CTX-M and SHV extended-spectrum beta-lactamases and associated resistance genes in *Escherichia coli* strains of food samples in Tunisia. J Antimicrob Chemother 60: 1137–1141.
11. Kojima A, Ishii Y, Ishihara K, Esaki H, Asai T, et al. (2005) Extended-spectrum-beta-lactamase-producing *Escherichia coli* strains isolated from farm animals from 1999 to 2002: Report from the Japanese Veterinary Antimicrobial Resistance Monitoring program. Antimicrob Agents Chemother 49: 3533–3537.
12. Liebana E, Batchelor M, Hopkins KL, Clifton-Hadley FA, Teale CJ, et al. (2006) Longitudinal farm study of extended-spectrum β-lactamase-mediated resistance. J Clin Microbiol 44: 1630–1634.
13. Daniels JB, Call DR, Hancock D, Sischo WM, Baker K, et al. (2009) Role of ceftiofur in selection and dissemination of *bla(CMY-2)*-mediated cephalosporin resistance in *Salmonella enterica* and commensal *Escherichia coli* isolates from cattle. Appl Environ Microbiol 2009, 75: 3648–3655.
14. Donaldson SC, Straley BA, Hegde NV, Sawant AA, DebRoy C, et al. (2006) Molecular epidemiology of ceftiofur-resistant *Escherichia coli* isolates from dairy calves. Appl Environ Microbiol 72: 3940–3948.
15. Singer RS, Patterson SK, Wallace RL (2008) Effects of therapeutic ceftiofur administration to dairy cattle on *Escherichia coli* dynamics in the intestinal tract. Appl Environ Microbiol 74: 6956–6962.
16. Nuru S, Osbaldiston GW, Stowe EC, Walker D (1972) Fecal microflora of healthy cattle and pigs. Cornell Vet 62: 242–253.
17. Clermont O, Olier M, Hoede C, Diancourt L, Brisse S, et al. (2011) Animal and human pathogenic *Escherichia coli* strains share common genetic backgrounds. Infect Genet Evol 11: 654–662.
18. Clinical and Laboratory Standards Institute: Performance standards for antimicrobial disk and dilution antimicrobial susceptibility tests for bacteria isolated from animals. Approved standard, 3rd ed. CLSI document 2008, M31-A3. CLSI, Wayne, PA.
19. Clinical and Laboratory Standards Institute: Performance standards for antimicrobial susceptibility testing standards 2011, M100-S21. CLSI, Wayne, PA.
20. Xu L, Ensor V, Gossain S, Nye K, Hawkey P (2005) Rapid and simple detection of bla(CTX-M) genes by multiplex PCR assay. J Med Microbiol 54: 1183–1187.
21. Pérez-Pérez FJ, Hanson ND (2002) Detection of plasmid-mediated AmpC β-lactamase genes in clinical isolates by using multiplex PCR. J Clin Microbiol 40: 2153–2162.
22. The National Molecular Subtyping Network for Foodborne Disease Surveillance: One-day (24–28 h) standardized laboratory protocol for molecular subtyping of *Escherichia coli* O157:H7, non-typhoidal *Salmonella* serotypes, and *Shigella sonnei* by pulsed field gel electrophoresis (PFGE) (2004) MAF, 1–12.
23. Ma L, Ishii Y, Ishiguro M, Matsuzawa H, Yamaguchi K (1998) Cloning and sequencing of the gene encoding Toho-2, a class A beta-lactamase preferentially inhibited by tazobactam. Antimicrob Agents Chemother 42: 1181–1186.
24. Kado CI, Liu ST (1981) Rapid procedure for detection and isolation of large and small plasmids. J Bact 145: 1365–1373.
25. Carattoli A, Bertini A, Villa L, Falbo V, Hopkins KL, et al. (2005) Identification of plasmids by PCR-based replicon typing. J Microbiol Methods 63: 219–228.
26. Saladin M, Cao VT, Lambert T, Donay JL, Herrmann JL, et al. (2002) Diversity of CTX-M beta-lactamases and their promoter regions from Enterobacteriaceae isolated in three Parisian hospitals. FEMS Microbiol Lett 209: 161–168.
27. Alexander TW, Inglis GD, Yanke LJ, Topp E, Read RR, et al. (2010) Farm-to-fork characterization of *Escherichia coli* associated with feedlot cattle with a known history of antimicrobial use. Int J Food Microbiol 137: 40–48.
28. Asai T, Kojima A, Harada K, Ishihara K, Takahashi T, et al. (2005) Correlation between the usage volume of veterinary therapeutic antimicrobials and resistance in *Escherichia coli* isolated from the feces of food-producing animals in Japan. Japan J Infect Dis 58: 369–372.
29. Bergman M, Nyberg ST, Huovinen P, Paakkari P, Hakanen AJ (2009) Association between antimicrobial consumption and resistance in *Escherichia coli*. Antimicrob Agents Chemother 53: 912–917.
30. Shiraki Y, Shibata N, Doi Y, Arakawa Y (2004) *Escherichia coli* producing CTX-M-2 beta-lactamase in cattle, Japan. Emerg Infect Dis 10: 69–75.
31. Sugawara M, Komori J, Kawakami M, Izumiya H, Watanabe H, et al. (2011) Molecular and phenotypic characteristics of CMY-2 beta-lactamase-producing *Salmonella enterica* serovar Typhimurium isolated from cattle in Japan. J Vet Med Sci 73: 345–349.
32. Matsumoto Y, Kitazume H, Yamada M, Ishiguro Y, Muto T, et al. (2007) CTX-M-14 type beta-lactamase producing *Salmonella enterica* serovar Enteritidis isolated from imported chicken meat. Japan J Infectious Dis 60: 236–238.
33. Bonnet R (2004) Growing group of extended-spectrum beta-lactamases: The CTX-M enzymes. Antimicrob Agents Chemother 48: 1–14.
34. Uchida Y, Mochimaru T, Morokuma Y, Kiyosuke M, Fujise M, et al. (2010) Clonal spread in Eastern Asia of ciprofloxacin-resistant *Escherichia coli* serogroup O25 strains, and associated virulence factors. Int J Antimicrob Agents 35: 444–450.

19

Transmission of Methicillin-Resistant *Staphylococcus aureus* CC398 from Livestock Veterinarians to Their Household Members

Erwin Verkade[1,2*], Marjolein Kluytmans-van den Bergh[3], Birgit van Benthem[4], Brigitte van Cleef[1,2,4], Miranda van Rijen[1], Thijs Bosch[4], Leo Schouls[4], Jan Kluytmans[1,2,5]

1 Laboratory for Microbiology and Infection Control, Amphia Hospital, Breda, The Netherlands, **2** Laboratory for Medical Microbiology and Immunology, St. Elisabeth Hospital, Tilburg, The Netherlands, **3** Amphia Academy Infectious Disease Foundation, Amphia Hospital, Breda, The Netherlands, **4** Centre for Infectious Disease Control Netherlands, National Institute for Public Health and the Environment, Bilthoven, The Netherlands, **5** Department of Medical Microbiology, VU University medical centre, Amsterdam, The Netherlands

Abstract

There are indications that livestock-associated MRSA CC398 has a reduced human-to-human transmissibility, limiting its impact on public health and justifying modified control measures. This study determined the transmissibility of MRSA CC398 from livestock veterinarians to their household members in the community as compared to MRSA non-CC398 strains. A one-year prospective cohort study was performed to determine the presence of MRSA CC398 in four-monthly nasal and oropharyngeal samples of livestock veterinarians (n = 137) and their household members (n = 389). In addition, a cross-sectional survey was performed to detect the presence of MRSA non-CC398 in hospital derived control patients (n = 20) and their household members (n = 41). *Staphylococcus aureus* isolates were genotyped by staphylococcal protein A (*spa*) typing and multiple-locus variable-number tandem repeat analysis (MLVA). Mean MRSA CC398 prevalence over the study period was 44% (range 41.6–46.0%) in veterinarians and 4.0% (range 2.8–4.7%) in their household members. The MRSA CC398 prevalence in household members of veterinarians was significantly lower than the MRSA non-CC398 prevalence in household members of control patients (PRR 6.0; 95% CI 2.4–15.5), indicating the reduced transmissibility of MRSA CC398. The impact of MRSA CC398 appears to be low at the moment. However, careful monitoring of the human-to-human transmissibility of MRSA CC398 remains important.

Editor: Alex Friedrich, University Medical Center Groningen, Netherlands

Funding: This work was supported by The Netherlands Organization for Health Research and Development (ZonMw) [grant number 125010003]. The funding authority did not interfere with data collection, data analysis, or writing the manuscript, nor did it have the right to approve or disapprove the manuscript.

Competing Interests: The authors have declared that no competing interests exist.

* Email: erwinverkade@gmail.com

Introduction

Infections with methicillin-resistant *Staphylococcus aureus* (MRSA) are associated with increased morbidity, mortality, and (healthcare) costs [1–2]. Traditionally, MRSA has been considered as a hospital-associated pathogen [3–4]. Since approximately 15–20 years, MRSA has expanded its territory to the community causing severe infections in previously healthy persons all over the world [5]. In 2003, a new clade of MRSA emerged in the Netherlands which was related to an extensive reservoir in pigs and cattle [6–7]. This so-called livestock-associated MRSA (LA-MRSA) mostly belongs to clonal complex 398 (MRSA CC398). National Dutch guidelines were adapted in June 2006, recommending persons in contact with live pigs or cattle to be screened upon hospital admission [8]. Since then the number of MRSA CC398 found in the Netherlands has dramatically increased. In 2010, 38% of all newly identified MRSA strains in humans in the Netherlands were of this type, up from 16% by the end of 2006 [9].

Several studies have reported the transmission of healthcare-associated MRSA (HA-MRSA) strains between patients and their household members, with transmission rates varying from below 10% up to 36% [10–14]. Recent surveys showed that MRSA CC398 was 4 to 6-fold less transmissible than other MRSA strains in a hospital-setting [15–17]. At present, the human-to-human transmissibility of MRSA CC398 in a community setting is still unclear. Considering the extensive reservoir in animals and people who work with livestock, the occurrence of MRSA CC398 in people who are not directly involved in farming is strikingly low. So far, there are no indications that MRSA CC398 has spread extensively into the general population. A cross-sectional survey in a livestock-dense region found that only 0.2% of adult individuals without livestock contact were positive for MRSA CC398 [18]. On the other hand, there are observations that proximity of farms is a potential risk factor, even in absence of direct contact between humans and animals [19–21]. In addition, a recent study suggest that incomplete cooking of contaminated meat can cause transmission [22].

Studying the human-to-human transmissibility of MRSA CC398 is hampered by the fact that the reservoir of MRSA CC398 is limited to the livestock agriculture setting, and that the majority of individuals working in this sector live on the farms

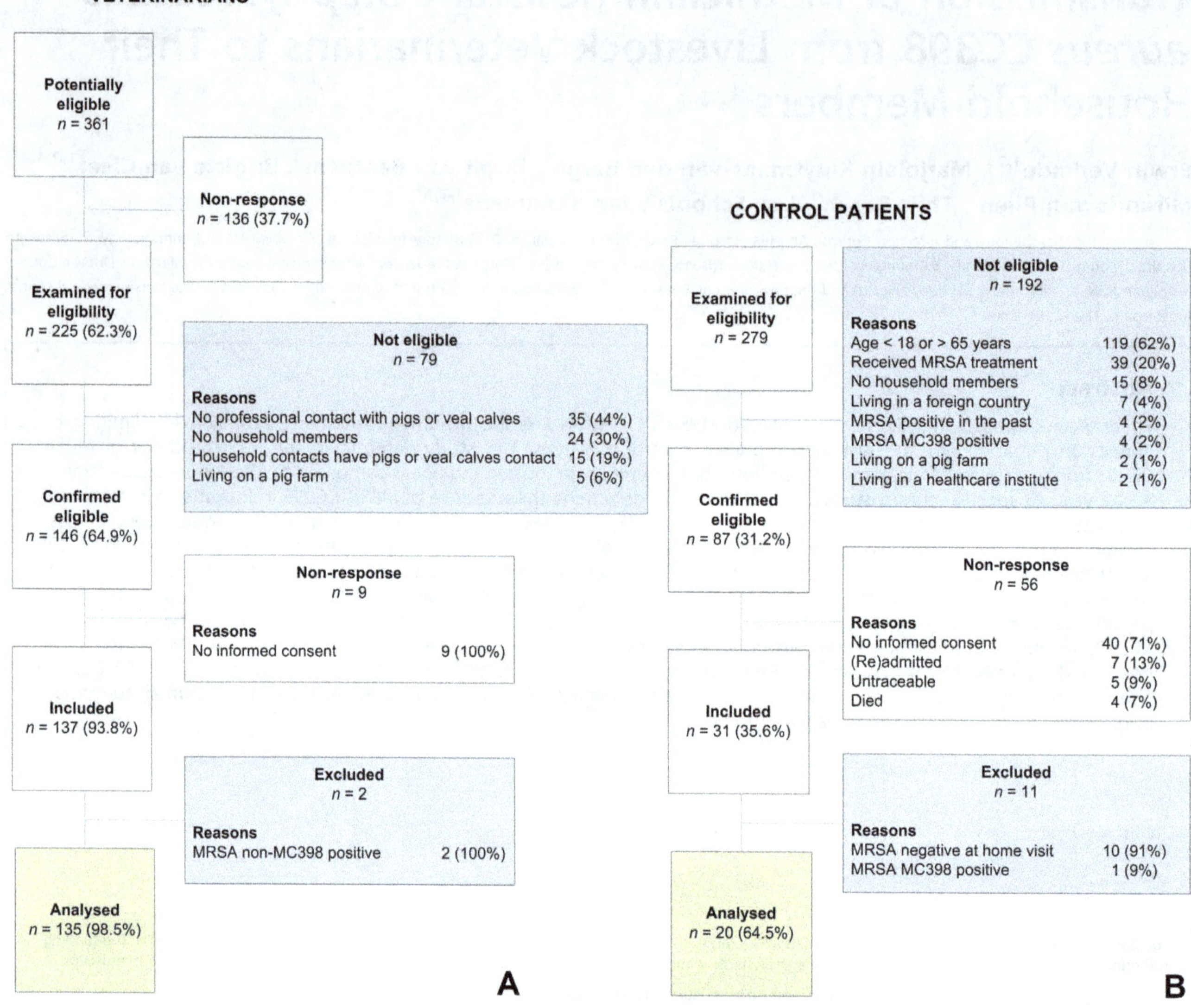

Figure 1. Flow chart of the recruitment of livestock veterinarians (A) and control patients (B).

together with their families, who mostly have direct animal contact themselves. Therefore, livestock veterinarians are an excellent group for studying human-to-human transmissibility of MRSA CC398 since their household members do not have direct contact with pigs or veal calves themselves.

The aim of this study was to determine the transmissibility of MRSA CC398 from livestock veterinarians to their household members compared to other MRSA strains in a community setting.

Materials and Methods

Study design and setting

A one-year prospective cohort study was conducted in Dutch livestock veterinarians and their household members. Individuals were sampled for the presence of MRSA and methicillin-susceptible *S. aureus* (MSSA) in the anterior nares and oropharynx every four months (total study period July 2008 through December 2009). In addition, to compare transmissibility of MRSA CC398 strains with MRSA non-CC398 isolates, a cross-sectional survey was performed in MRSA-positive hospital-based patients and their household members.

Study population

Veterinarians associated with the Dutch Pig Health Department (VGV) were asked to participate in the study in April 2008. Control patients, defined as newly identified carriers of MRSA non-CC398, and their household members were recruited from a network of 16 hospitals and their affiliated microbiological laboratories between July 2009 and May 2011. Veterinarians and control patients were asked to take a nasal and oropharynx swab and to complete a questionnaire, which was used to determine the eligibility for the study. Subjects were eligible for participation if they (1) were aged between 18 and 65 years, (2) had one or more household members who were willing to participate, (3) did not live on a farm with pigs or veal calves, (4) did not have household members with professional pigs or veal calf contact, (5) were not treated for colonisation with MRSA in the previous three months, and (6) had provided written informed consent.

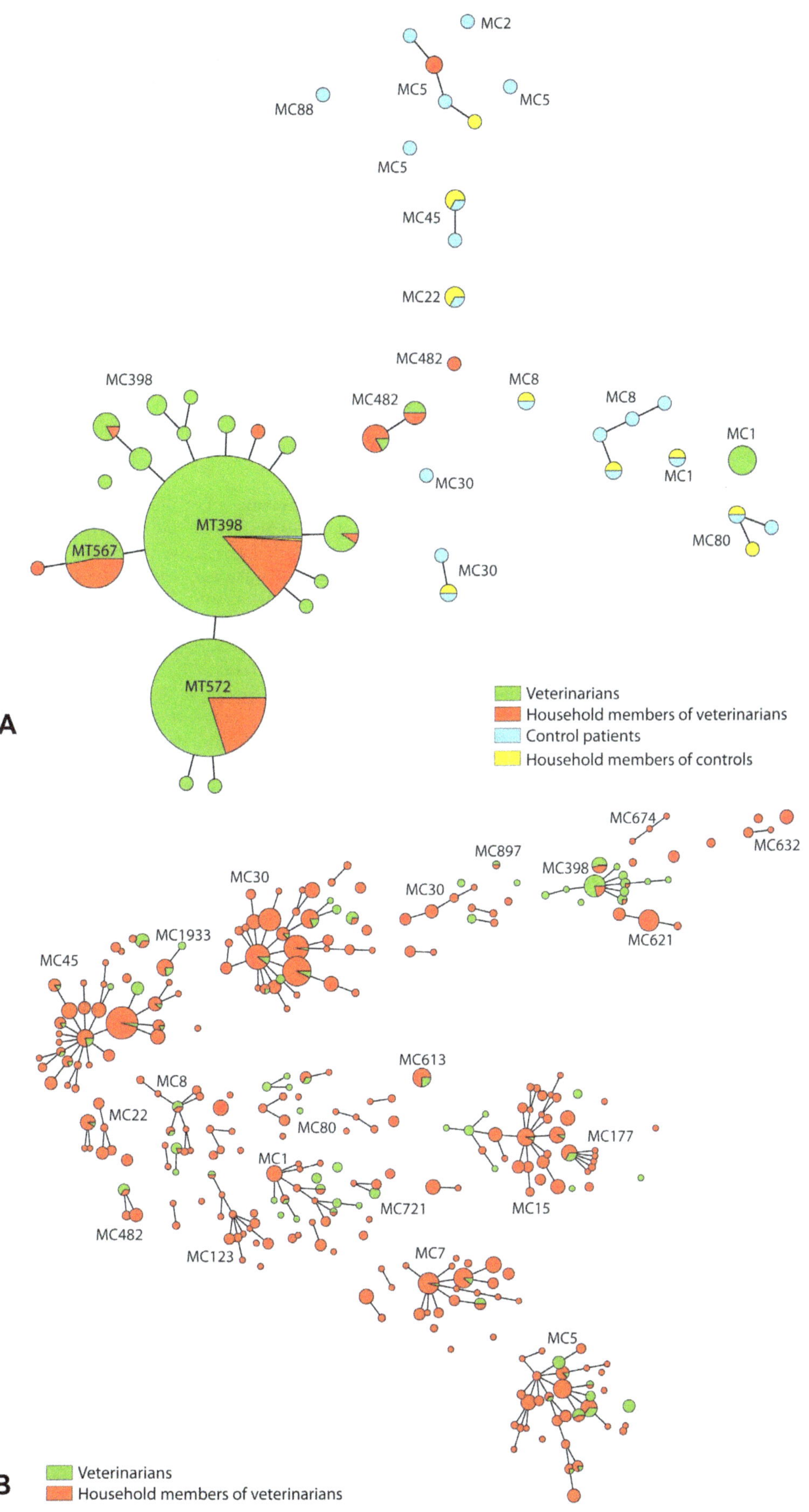
MC2
MC5
MC88
MC5
MC5
MC45
MC22
MC482
MC398
MC482
MC8
MC8
MC1
MC1
MC30
MT398
MT567
MC80
MC30
MT572
A
Veterinarians
Household members of veterinarians
Control patients
Household members of controls
MC674
MC632
MC897
MC398
MC30
MC30
MC621
MC1933
MC45
MC613
MC8
MC22
MC80
MC177
MC1
MC721
MC15
MC482
MC123
MC7
MC5
B
Veterinarians
Household members of veterinarians

Figure 2. Genotypic relatedness of 482 MRSA (A) and 1308 MSSA (B) isolates derived from livestock veterinarians (green), household members of veterinarians (red), control patients (blue) and household members of control patients (yellow), represented as a minimum spanning tree based on MLVA types (MT), which are displayed as circles. The size of each circle indicates the number of isolates with this particular type. MLVA complexes are indicated in characters e.g. MC398 denotes MLVA complex 398.

At baseline, veterinarians and control patients were visited at home and cultures were taken from the anterior nares and the oropharynx. Additional data were collected using a questionnaire that comprised information on age, gender, smoking, composition of the household, exposure to livestock, antibiotic treatment 4 months prior to sampling, and infections. Subsequently, veterinarians and their household members were asked to take nasal and oropharyngeal samples and complete a short questionnaire on the presence of active infections and antibiotic usage at 4, 8, and 12 months and return these by mail to the investigator. Appropriate transport material with Amies medium (Transwab, Medical Wire & Equipment), instructions for sampling and questionnaires were provided during the baseline home visit.

Microbiological procedures

Nasal and oropharyngeal samples were separately plated on chromID *S. aureus* and chromID MRSA agar plates (bioMérieux, La Balme, France), and subsequently placed in two Mueller–Hinton (MH) broth supplemented with 6.5% NaCl. The overnight MH broth were separately subcultured onto both chromID *S. aureus* and chromID MRSA agar plates. All agar plates were read after 18–24 h incubation at 35–37°C according to manufacturer's instructions [23]. All cefoxitin resistant isolates were tested using a PCR for the presence of the *mec*A and *nuc* gene [24–25]. All *S. aureus* strains were genotyped by staphylococcal protein A (*spa*) typing [26] and multiple-locus variable-number tandem repeat analysis (MLVA) as described previously [27]. MLVA types (MTs) were clustered using a categorical clustering coefficient and a minimum spanning tree was constructed to display the relationships between the various MTs. MLVA complexes (MC) were assigned if two neighbouring MTs did not differ in more than one variable number tandem repeat (VNTR) locus and if at least five neighbouring MTs fulfilled this criterion.

Definitions

Subjects were considered positive when either a nasal or an oropharynx swab harboured MRSA or MSSA. Subjects that were MRSA MC398 positive at all four sampling moments were defined as persistent MRSA MC398 carriers. Subjects that yielded MRSA MC398 in one to three samples out of all samples were defined as intermittent MRSA MC398 carriers and subjects that did not have any positive sample during the one-year study were defined as MRSA MC398 non-carriers.

A transmission event was confirmed when MRSA isolates of the same MLVA type were detected in veterinarians and in their household members on a specific sampling moment. A dyad was defined as a set of two household members, which could be MRSA positive or negative.

Statistical analyses

All analyses were performed using SPSS 19.0 for Windows (SPSS Inc. Chicago, IL, USA). Differences in continuous variables between groups were tested with Student's t-test or Mann-Whitney U test when applicable and differences in categorical variables between groups were tested with the Pearson Chi-square test. Univariate backwards analysis for MRSA carriage were performed in a generalized estimated equations (GEE) model using a Poisson distribution with robust covariance estimators to calculate prevalence risk ratios (PRR) [28] with 95% confidence interval (95% CI).

Ethics Statement

This study was approved by the medical ethics committee of the St. Elisabeth Hospital in Tilburg, the Netherlands (protocol number 0749). All participants had provided written informed consent and the reviewing medical ethics committee approved this consent procedure.

Results

Enrolment

Veterinarians. Two hundred and twenty-five of 361 (62%) veterinarians responded and were examined for their eligibility. One-hundred forty-six veterinarians were eligible and after telephonic consultation, 137 veterinarians were included in the one-year follow-up study (Figure 1A). These veterinarians had a total of 389 household members (mean number of household members per veterinarian 2.8 persons).

Control patients. A total of 279 newly identified MRSA patients were reported to the central laboratory. After assessment of the inclusion – and exclusion criteria, 87 (31%) eligible patients were available (Figure 1B). After consultation by the investigator, 31 (36%) control patients were included and visited at home. Ten control patients that were visited at home were found to be MRSA-negative, and one control patient carried MRSA MC398. These eleven control patients were excluded from the analysis. A total of 20 (65%) control patients harboured MRSA non-MC398 and these subjects were included for the analysis. These patients had a total of 41 household members (mean number of household members per patient 2.1 persons).

Results of MLVA and *spa*-typing

In total, 4246 samples were analysed in this study with the following distribution: 1086 samples from a total of 137 veterinarians and 3036 cultures originating from 389 household members. In addition, there were 42 samples from 21 control patients and 82 cultures originating from their household members. Throughout the study, only 5 out of 548 (response rate 99.1%) sampling moments from veterinarians and 38 out of 1556 (response rate 97.6%) of their household members were not received. Sensitivity analysis on the effect of missing samples had no relevant consequences on the conclusions (data not shown).

A total of 1790 isolates were genotyped by *spa*-typing and MLVA: 365 MRSA and 211 MSSA strains from veterinarians, 84 MRSA and 1097 MSSA strains from household members of a veterinarian, 21 MRSA strains from control patients and 12 MRSA strains from household members of a control patient. In total, 341 different MTs belonging to 24 different MLVA complexes (MC) were found among the *S. aureus* isolates (Figure 2). Thirteen isolates (39%) from control patients and their household members had MCs that belonged to hospital-associated MRSA (HA-MRSA) strains. Two isolates (6%) were placed into MRSA MC398 and 18 isolates (45%) clustered into community-acquired MRSA (CA-MRSA). Eleven of these strains (33%) were

Table 1. Distribution of *spa*-types of MRSA MC398 isolates (n = 430) and MSSA MC398 (n = 54) derived from livestock veterinarians and household members during the one-year study period.

	No. of MRSA MC398 isolates (%)			No. of MSSA MC398 isolates (%)			
Spa-type	**Total**	**Veterinarians**	**Household members**	**Total**	**Veterinarians**	**Household members**	**P-value[a]**
t011	241 (56.0%)	210	31	4 (7.4%)	3	1	<0.001
t108	121 (28.1%)	99	22	3 (5.6%)	3	none	<0.001
t567	17 (4.0%)	12	5	none	none	none	0.24
t1184	14 (3.3%)	3	11	none	none	none	0.38
t081	none	none	none	11 (20.4%)	6	5	<0.001
t034	9 (2.1%)	8	1	31 (57.4%)	25	6	<0.001
t1456	9 (2.1%)	8	1	none			0.61
t571	5 (1.2%)	5	none	2 (3.7%)	2	none	0.18
t1451	3 (0.7%)	2	1	none	none	none	1.00
t8333	3 (0.7%)	0	3	none	none	none	1.00
t899	2 (0.5%)	2	none	none	none	none	1.00
t3479	2 (0.5%)	2	none	none	none	none	1.00
t4652	none	none	none	2 (3.7%)	2	none	0.01
t1606, t2287, t4628, t6606	1 each (0.2%)	1 each	none	none	none	none	1.00
t5902	none	none	none	1 (1.9%)	1	0	0.11
Total	430 (100%)	355	75	54 (100%)	42	12	

[a]proportions of MRSA MC398 isolates vs proportions of MSSA MC398 isolates. A p-value ≤0.05 was considered statistically significant.

Table 2. Assignment to MLVA complex 398 (MC398), non-MC398 or no complex of MRSA and MSSA isolates derived from livestock veterinarians during the one-year study period.

Veterinarians (n = 137)	Mean prevalence % (range)	MC398 n (%)	non-MC398 n (%)	no complex n (%)	Total
MRSA isolates	44.6 (43.1–47.1)	355 (97.3) (97%)	10 (2.7)	0 (0)	365
MSSA isolates	26.3 (22.1–29.2)	42 (19.9)	125 (59.2)	44 (20.9)	211
All *S. aureus* isolates	70.9 (69.1–73.0)	397 (68.9) (68.(69%)	135 (23.4)	44 (7.6)	576

Panton–Valentine leukocidin (PVL) positive. In contrast, none of the *S. aureus* MC398 strains originated from veterinarians and their household members were PVL-positive. Two-hundred twenty-two (12.4%) isolates did not belong to a known MLVA complex. The distribution of the different *spa*-types found in *S. aureus* MC398 isolates among veterinarians and their household members are summarized in Table 1. Two dominant *spa*-types, t011 and t108, accounted for 84% of all MRSA MC398 isolates and 4 *spa*-types were found only once. There were 54 MSSA isolates that belong to MC398; 42 isolates were derived from veterinarians (78%) and 12 isolates were recovered from household members (22%). Most of the MSSA strains had *spa*-type t034 (57%) or t081 (20%), which is in large contrast to the MRSA strains, where 9/430 (2.1%) MRSA MC398 isolates had *spa*-type t034 and none had *spa*-type t081.

Carriage of MRSA MC398 among veterinarians and their household members

Table 2 and 3 depict the distribution of all MRSA and MSSA isolates that belong to MLVA complex 398 or non-MC398 isolates found in nasal and oropharynx samples derived from veterinarians and their household members. From the 576 *S. aureus* isolates derived from veterinarians 365 isolates were MRSA (63%), while the 1181 *S. aureus* strains isolated from household members only 84 strains (7.1%) were methicillin-resistant. The vast majority of MRSA strains recovered from veterinarians (97%) and household members (89%) belonged to MC398. The mean prevalence of MRSA MC398 carriage among veterinarians was 44% (range 41.6–46.0%) and that of their household members was 4.0% (range 2.8–4.7%).

Table 4 shows the carrier state of veterinarians and their household members during the one-year study period. Two veterinarians had samples positive with MRSA non-MC398 strains and were excluded for further analysis. Forty veterinarians had four MRSA-positive test results (30%) and were defined as persistent MRSA MC398 carriers. Furthermore, 41 (30%) veterinarians were intermittent MRSA MC398 carriers and 54 (40%) veterinarians never carried MRSA. Altogether 36 from 386 non-exposed household members (9.3%), originating from 28 families (20.4%) carried MRSA MC398 intermittently. The prevalence of MRSA MC398 carriage in household members was statistically significantly higher for veterinarians with persistent MRSA MC398 carriage as compared to veterinarians with MRSA MC398 non-carriage (PRR 9.3; 95% CI 2.8–38.5) as well as veterinarians with intermittent MRSA MC398 carriage (PRR 2.1; 95% CI 1.0–4.6). MLVA genotyping data were not taken into account here. Results of confirmed transmission events are depicted in Table 4.

Transmissibility of MRSA MC398 compared to other MRSA strains

The prevalence of MRSA carriage among household members of livestock veterinarians and control patients was measured. The baseline characteristics of veterinarians and control patients are depicted in Table 5. There were significant differences between the two groups: gender, educational level, ethnicity, age, number of household members, and number of companion animals. The 59 veterinarians that were found MRSA MC398 positive at the initial sampling moment had a total of 180 household members. During the home visit 8 household members (4.4%) harboured MRSA MC398 with the same MLVA type as the index veterinarian, i.e. 4 partners and 4 children. This result was compared with the prevalence of MRSA non-MC398 in household members of 20 control patients, which had a total of 41 household members. Eleven household members (26.8%) carried MRSA non-MC398 with the same MTs as the control patients during the home visit. The MRSA MC398 prevalence in household members of veterinarians was significantly lower than the MRSA non-MC398 prevalence in household members of control patients (8/180 *vs.* 11/41, $p<0.001$). Hence, the transmission rate of MRSA non-MC398 strains is significantly higher than that of MRSA MC398 strains (PRR 6.0; 95% CI 2.4–15.5).

The MRSA MC398 prevalence per family was 13.6% for veterinarians and 45% for control patients (8/59 *vs.* 9/20, $p = 0.009$). At family level, the transmission rate of MRSA non-MC398 strains to other household members is significantly higher in comparison with MRSA MC398 (PRR 3.3; 95% CI 1.3–8.0). In addition, household member pairs (dyads) colonised with the same MLVA complex were identified to estimate the spread of different

Table 3. Assignment to MLVA complex 398 (MC398), non-MC398 or no complex of MRSA and MSSA isolates derived from household members during the one-year study period.

Household members (n = 389)	Mean prevalence % (range)	MC398 n (%)	non-MC398 n (%)	no complex n (%)	Total
MRSA isolates	4.4 (3.1–5.0)	75 (89.3)	9 (10.7)	0 (0)	84
MSSA isolates	48.6 (45.9–50.3)	12 (1.1)	912 (83.1)	173 (15.8)	1097
All *S. aureus* isolates	53.0 (50.9–54.8)	87 (7.4)	921 (78.0)	173 (14.6)	1181

Table 4. Carriage of MRSA MC398 and transmission events among livestock veterinarians and their household members during the one-year study period.

	Total n (%)	Persistent MRSA MC398 carriage n (%)	Intermittent MRSA MC398 carriagen (%)	Non-carriersn (%)
Veterinarians	135 (100)	40 (29.6)	41 (30.4)	54 (40.0)
Household members	386	123	114	149
MRSA carriers among household members	36 (9.3)	23 (18.7)	10 (8.8)	3 (2.0)
Families with a transmission events	28 (20.7)	16 (40.0)	9 (22.0)	3 (5.6)
Confirmed transmission events to household members[a]	31 (8.0)	22 (17.9)	9 (7.9)	0 (0.0)

[a]A confirmed transmission events was defined as that veterinarian and household members were both MRSA-positive during one sampling moment with the same MLVA type.

MRSA clades. In 59 families with MRSA MC398 colonisation, 8 MRSA MC398-positive member dyads out of 422 possible dyads (1.9%) were detected. By comparison, there were significant more concordant dyads among MRSA non-MC398 carriers (13/78 [16.7%], PRR 8.8; 95% CI 3.5–22.6).

Discussion

Our prospective cohort study demonstrates that the mean prevalence of MRSA MC398 colonisation among household members of livestock veterinarians is relatively high (4.0%). None of these families were living on a farm or raising livestock. In total, 36 household members (9.3%), originating from 28 families (20.4%), harboured MRSA MC398 at least once during the one-year study period. These data confirm the results from a previous study performed in Germany in which an MRSA CC398 prevalence of 9.0% among household members of veterinarians was reported [29]. In our study, the prevalence of MRSA MC398 carriage among household members was shown to be highly dependent on the carrier state of the veterinarian. In addition, the prevalence of MRSA among household members was significantly higher for control patients carrying MRSA non-MC398 strains than for veterinarians carrying MRSA MC398 (PRR 6.0; 95% CI 2.4–15.5). These data suggest that MRSA MC398 spread less easily from humans with professional livestock contact to their household members than other MRSA non-MC398 isolates in a community setting. A possible explanation for this reduced transmissibility is that MRSA CC398 originates in humans as MSSA [30], and then spread to livestock, where it subsequently acquired the SCC*mec* cassette and methicillin-resistance. The jump of CC398 was also accompanied by the loss of phage-carried human virulence genes, making this clade less adapted to humans. In a hospital setting, Wassenberg and colleagues found that MRSA CC398 was 5.0 times less transmissible than other healthcare-associated MRSA (HA-MRSA) strains [15]. In general, transmission of MRSA within families seems to be common [10–14]. Several other studies showed high prevalences of MRSA among household members of individuals with HA-MRSA strains [11,14,31–34].

Guidelines underlying the Search & Destroy policy have been adapted in the Netherlands since 2006 based on conclusions from a case-control study [8]. Humans that work with live pigs and veal calves were defined as new risk populations for MRSA carriage and are now actively screened when admitted to a hospital. These guidelines were revised in December 2012, and all household members of confirmed MRSA patients have to be screened for MRSA on hospital admission. At present, household members of livestock veterinarians are not screened upon admission to a hospital. However, this study showed that they have a relatively high MRSA carriage in comparison to the Dutch general population [35]. Consequently, we advocate that household

Table 5. Characteristics of livestock veterinarians with MRSA MC398 carriage and control patients with MRSA non-MC398 carriage at the initial sampling moment.

Characteristics	Veterinarians (n = 59)	Control patients (n = 20)	P-value
Age – median (IQR)	47.0 (41.0–52.0)	39.0 (24.3–57.8)	0.295
Male sex – no. (%)	55/59 (93.2)	7/20 (35.0)	<0.001
Smoking – no. (%)	10/58 (17.2)	4/15 (26.7)	0.467
Educational level[a] – median (IQR)	6.9 (7.0–7.0)	3.6 (2.0–5.0)	<0.001
Born in the Netherlands – no. (%)	55/59 (93.2)	15/20 (75.0)	0.023
Age of household members – median (IQR)	16.0 (8.3–39.0)	34.0 (15.0–52.0)	<0.001
Number of household members – median (IQR)	3.0 (2.0–4.0)	1.5 (1.0–3.0)	0.006
Number of companion animals[b] – median (IQR)	1.0 (0.8–2.0)	0.0 (0.0–1.0)	0.023

IQR: interquartile range (p25–p75); no.: number.
A P-value ≤0.05 was considered statistically significant.
[a]Highest educational level is a bachelor or master title and was valued with a maximum of 7.
[b]Total amount of cats and dogs in the household.

members of MRSA-positive veterinarians should also be screened for the presence of MRSA carriage upon hospital admission.

Despite the reduced human-to-human transmissibility of MRSA CC398, there are a few recent studies indicating that MRSA CC398 might have spread into the general population. A recent study found that MRSA with no link to established risk factors for acquisition, so-called MRSA of unknown origin (MUO), has now emerged [36]. Two distinct genotypic MUO groups were distinguished: MUO CC398 (26%) and MUO non-CC398 (74%), which suggests spread of MUO CC398, not by direct contact with livestock (pigs, veal calves), but through human-to-human transmission or by incomplete cooking of meat, but also by consumption of simultaneously prepared food products, such as salads, using contaminated kitchen equipment [22]. Furthermore, there are observations that proximity of farms is a potential risk factor, even in absence of direct contact between humans and animals [19–21].

To our knowledge, this study is the largest detailed survey among household members of livestock veterinarians. Unlike previous studies on transmissibility of MRSA CC398 [15,29,37], we performed this survey among veterinarians and their household members in a community setting for a prolonged period. Moreover, household members of veterinarians did not have livestock contact themselves during the study period. Therefore, we could estimate the human-to-human transmissibility of MRSA CC398 in detail. Thus the finding of 4.0% of household members carrying MRSA MC398 very likely represents the frequency of intrafamilial transmission. There are, of course, other possibilities of acquisition such as from pets and/or from horses. In addition, a cross-sectional survey to determine the transmissibility of MRSA CC398 in comparison with MRSA non-CC398 in the community was conducted. Here, the same inclusion - and exclusion criteria were used for control patients and veterinarians. Finally, we performed genotyping of all recovered *S. aureus* isolates, confirming the similarity between MRSA strains isolated from the veterinarians or control patients and their household members.

There are some limitations to our study. First, there was a large difference between response rate of veterinarians compared to control patients which may have caused selection bias. In addition, there were significant differences between gender, educational level and ethnicity, age and number of household members, and number of companion animals between control patients and veterinarians. However, to which extent these differences have influenced transmission rates remains unclear. Second, this study does not provide data on the exact transmission route to the household members (e.g. via direct physical contact or via contaminated household, i.e. doorknob, remote control, chairs, etc.). Third, MRSA CC398 isolates are hard to discriminate when using current molecular typing techniques, such as *spa*-typing and MLVA. This hampers studies that investigate possible transmission events and outbreaks caused by this MRSA clade. Finally, a minor limitation is that the results are somewhat outdated because data collection started in August 2008. However, we believe that human-to-human transmissibility of MRSA CC398 has not changed much in 5 years. Since this was a prospective cohort study with one-year follow-up it was inevitable to report the results after several years.

In summary, MRSA CC398 colonisation was common among household members of livestock veterinarians and this was shown to be highly dependent on the carrier state of the veterinarian. Moreover, the transmissibility of MRSA CC398 in the community setting was found to be substantially lower than that of MRSA non-CC398 strains. Therefore, we believe that screening of household members of MRSA-positive veterinarians upon hospital admission is justified and that the current Dutch MRSA guidelines can be maintained. The present situation is a widespread resistant bacterium with an enormous reservoir in livestock. The impact of MRSA CC398 appears to be low at the moment. However, when MRSA CC398 acquires genetic elements harbouring virulence factors it may pose a significant public health problem in the future. Careful monitoring of the human-to-human transmissibility of MRSA CC398 is therefore important.

Acknowledgments

The investigators are indebted to all participating veterinarians, control patients and their household members. The investigators also thank the Pig Health Department (VGV) of the Royal Dutch Veterinary Society for their support. Finally, the authors acknowledge Marianne Ferket, Renée Ladestein and all the laboratory site staff from the Laboratory for Microbiology and Infection Control of the Amphia Hospital for their efforts.

Author Contributions

Conceived and designed the experiments: EV MK BvB JK. Performed the experiments: EV TB. Analyzed the data: EV MK BvB JK. Contributed reagents/materials/analysis tools: EV TB LS. Wrote the paper: EV MK BvB BvC MvR TB LS JK.

References

1. Klevens RM, Morrison MA, Nadle J, Petit S, Gershman K, et al. (2007) Invasive methicillin-resistant *Staphylococcus aureus* infections in the United States. JAMA 298: 1763–1771.
2. van Rijen MM, Kluytmans JA (2009) Costs and benefits of the MRSA Search and Destroy policy in a Dutch hospital. Eur J Clin Microbiol Infect 28: 1245–1252.
3. Archer GL (1998) *Staphylococcus aureus*: a well-armed pathogen. Clin Infect Dis 26: 1179–1181.
4. Noskin GA, Rubin RJ, Schentag JJ, Kluytmans J, Hedblom EC, et al. (2007) National trends in *Staphylococcus aureus* infection rates: impact on economic burden and mortality over a 6-year period (1998-2003). Clin Infect Dis 45: 1132–1140.
5. Kluytmans-Vandenbergh MF, Kluytmans JA (2006) Community-acquired methicillin-resistant *Staphylococcus aureus*: current perspectives. Clin Microbiol Infect (Suppl. 1): 9–15.
6. Voss A, Loeffen F, Bakker J, Klaassen C, Wulf M (2005) Methicillin-resistant *Staphylococcus aureus* in pig farming. Emerg Infect Dis 11: 1965–1966.
7. de Neeling AJ, van den Broek MJ, Spalburg EC, van Santen-Verheuvel MG, Dam-Deisz WD, et al. (2007) High prevalence of methicillin resistant *Staphylococcus aureus* in pigs. Vet Microbiol 122: 366–372.
8. van Loo I, Huijsdens X, Tiemersma E, de Neeling A, van de Sande-Bruinsma N, et al. (2007) Emergence of methicillin-resistant *Staphylococcus aureus* of animal origin in humans. Emerg Infect Dis 13: 1834–1839.
9. Haenen APJ, Huijsdens XWH, Pluister GN, van Luit M, Bosch T, et al. (2011) Surveillance van meticilline-resistente *Staphylococcus aureus* in Nederland in 2010 (in Dutch). Infectieziekten bulletin 22: 250–255.
10. Mollema FP, Richardus JH, Behrendt M, Vaessen N, Lodder W, et al. (2010) Transmission of methicillin-resistant *Staphylococcus aureus* to household members. J Clin Microbiol 48: 202–207.
11. Johansson PJ, Gustafsson EB, Ringberg H (2007) High prevalence of MRSA in household members. Scand J Infect Dis 39: 764–768.
12. Nerby JM, Gorwitz R, Lesher L, Juni B, Jawahir S, et al. (2011) Risk factors for household transmission of community-associated methicillin-resistant *Staphylococcus aureus*. Pediatr Infect Dis J 30: 927–932.
13. Fritz SA, Hogan PG, Hayek G, Eisenstein KA, Rodriguez M, et al. (2012) *Staphylococcus aureus* colonization in children with community-associated Staphylococcus aureus skin infections and their household contacts. Arch Pediatr Adolesc Med 166: 551–557.
14. Lucet JC, Paoletti X, Demontpion C, Degrave M, Vanjak D, et al. (2009) Carriage of methicillin-resistant *Staphylococcus aureus* in home care settings: prevalence, duration, and transmission to household members. Arch Intern Med 169: 1372–1378.
15. Wassenberg MW, Bootsma MC, Troelstra A, Kluytmans JA, Bonten MJ (2011) Transmissibility of livestock-associated methicillin-resistant *Staphylococcus aureus* (ST398) in Dutch hospitals. Clin Microbiol Infect 17: 316–319.

16. van Rijen MM, van Keulen PH, Kluytmans JA (2008) Increase in a Dutch hospital of methicillin-resistant *Staphylococcus aureus* related to animal farming. Clin Inf Dis 46: 261–263.
17. Bootsma MC, Wassenberg MW, Trapman P, Bonten M (2011) The nosocomial transmission rate of animal-associated ST398 meticillin-resistant *Staphylococcus aureus*. J C Soc Interface 57: 578–584.
18. van Cleef BA, Verkade EJ, Wulf MW, Buiting AG, Voss A, et al. (2010) Prevalence of livestock-associated MRSA in communities with high pig-densities in The Netherlands. PLoS ONE 5:e9385.
19. Feingold BJ, Silbergeld EK, Curriero FC, van Cleef BA, Heck ME, et al. (2012) Livestock density as risk factor for livestock-associated methicillin-resistant *Staphylococcus aureus*, the Netherlands. Emerg Infect Dis 18: 1841–1849.
20. van Cleef BA, Monnet DL, Voss A, Krziwanek K, Allerberger F, et al. (2011) Livestock-associated methicillin-resistant *Staphylococcus aureus* in humans, Europe. Emerg Infect Dis 17: 502–505.
21. Schulz J, Friese A, Klees S, Tenhagen BA, Fetsch A, et al. (2012) Longitudinal study of the contamination of air and of soil surfaces in the vicinity of pig barns by livestock-associated methicillin-resistant *Staphylococcus aureus*. Appl Environ Microbiol 78: 5666–5667.
22. van Rijen MML, Kluytmans-Van den Bergh MFQ, Verkade EJM, ten Ham PB, Feingold BJ, on behalf of the CAM Study Group (2013) Lifestyle-associated risk factors for community-acquired methicillin-resistant *Staphylococcus aureus* carriage in the Netherlands: an exploratory hospital-based case-control study. PloS ONE 8(6):e65594.
23. Verkade E, Ferket M, Kluytmans J (2011) Clinical evaluation of Oxoid Brilliance MRSA Agar in comparison with bioMerieux MRSA ID medium for detection of livestock-associated meticillin-resistant *Staphylococcus aureus*. J Med Microbiol 60: 905–908.
24. Kluytmans JA, van Griethuysen A, Willemse P, van Keulen P (2002) Performance of CHROMagar selective medium and oxacillin resistance screening agar base for identifying *Staphylococcus aureus* and detecting methicillin resistance. J Clin Microbiol 40: 2480–2482.
25. van Griethuysen AJ, Pouw M, van Leeuwen N, Heck M, Willemse P, et al. (1997) Rapid slide latex agglutination test for detection of methicillin resistance in *Staphylococcus aureus*. J Clin Microbiol 37: 2789–2792.
26. Harmsen D, Claus H, Witte W, Rothgänger J, Claus H, et al. (2003) Typing of methicillin-resistant *Staphylococcus aureus* in a university hospital setting by using novel software for spa repeat determination and database management. J Clin Microbiol 41: 5442–5448.
27. Schouls LM, Spalburg EC, van Luit M, Huijsdens XW, Pluister GN, et al. (2009) Multiple-locus variable number tandem repeat analysis of *Staphylococcus aureus*: comparison with pulsed-field gel electrophoresis and spa-typing. PLoS ONE 4(4):e5082.
28. Knol MJ, Le Cessie S, Algra A, Vandenbroucke JP, Groenwold RH (2012) Overestimation of risk ratios by odds ratios in trials and cohort studies: alternatives to logistic regression. CMAJ 184: 895–899.
29. Cuny C, Nathaus R, Layer F, Strommenger B, Altmann D, et al. (2009).Nasal colonization of humans with methicillin-resistant *Staphylococcus aureus* (MRSA) CC398 with and without exposure to pigs. PLoS ONE 4(8):e6800.
30. Price LB, Stegger M, Hasman H, Aziz M, Larsen J, et al. (2012) *Staphylococcus aureus* CC398: host adaptation and emergence of methicillin resistance in livestock. MBio 3:e00305–11.
31. Calfee DP, Durbin LJ, Germanson TP, Toney DM, Smith EB, et al. (2003) Spread of methicillin-resistant *Staphylococcus aureus* (MRSA) among household members of individuals with nosocomially acquired MRSA. Infect Control Hosp Epidemiol 24: 422–426.
32. Miller LG, Eels SJ, Taylor AR, David MZ, Ortiz N, et al. (2012) *Staphylococcus aureus* colonization among household members of patients with skin infections: risk factors, strain discordance, and complex ecology. Clin Inf Dis 54: 1523–1535.
33. Zafar U, Johnson LB, Hanna M, Riederer K, Sharma M, et al. (2007) Prevalence of nasal colonization among patients with community-associated methicillin-resistant *Staphylococcus aureus* infection and their household contacts. Infect Control Hosp Epidemiol 28: 966–969.
34. Davis MF, Iverson SA, Baron P, Vasse A, Silbergeld EK, et al. (2012) Household transmission of meticillin-resistant *Staphylococcus aureus* and other staphylococci. Lancet Infect Dis 12(9): 703–716.
35. Bode LG, Wertheim HF, Kluytmans JA, Bogaers-Hofman D, Vandenbroucke-Grauls CM, et al. (2011) Sustained low prevalence of *Staphylococcus aureus* upon admission to hospital in The Netherlands. J Hosp Infect 79: 198–201.
36. Lekkerkerk WS, van de Sande-Bruinsma N, van der Sande MA, Tjon-A-Tsien A, Groenheide A, et al. (2012) Emergence of MRSA of unknown origin in the Netherlands. Clin Microbiol Infect 18: 656–661.
37. Graveland H, Wagenaar JA, Bergs K, Heesterbeek H, Heederik D (2011) Persistence of livestock associated MRSA CC398 in humans is dependent on intensity of animal contact. PLoS ONE 6(2):e16830.

20

Rat Experimental Model of Myocardial Ischemia/ Reperfusion Injury: An Ethical Approach to Set up the Analgesic Management of Acute Post-Surgical Pain

Maria Chiara Ciuffreda[1,2], Valerio Tolva[3], Renato Casana[3], Massimiliano Gnecchi[1,2,4,5], Emilio Vanoli[6], Carla Spazzolini[7], John Roughan[8], Laura Calvillo[9]*

1 Department of Cardiothoracic and Vascular Sciences - Coronary Care Unit and Laboratory of Clinical and Experimental Cardiology, Fondazione IRCCS (IRCCS: Institute for Treatment and Research) Policlinico San Matteo, Pavia, Italy, **2** Laboratory of Experimental Cardiology for Cell and Molecular Therapy, Fondazione IRCCS Policlinico San Matteo, Pavia, Italy, **3** Surgical Department, IRCCS Istituto Auxologico Italiano, Milan, Italy, **4** Department of Molecular Medicine, Unit of Cardiology, University of Pavia, Pavia, Italy, **5** Department of Medicine, Cape Town University, Cape Town, South Africa, **6** Department of Cardiology, IRCCS Multimedica, Sesto San Giovanni, Milan, Italy, **7** Center for Cardiac Arrhythmias of Genetic Base, IRCCS Istituto Auxologico Italiano, Milan, Italy, **8** Institute of Neuroscience, Comparative Biology Centre, University of Newcastle, Newcastle upon Tyne, United Kingdom, **9** Laboratory of Cardiac Arrhythmias of Genetic Base, IRCCS Istituto Auxologico Italiano, Milan, Italy

Abstract

Rationale: During the past 30 years, myocardial ischemia/reperfusion injury in rodents became one of the most commonly used model in cardiovascular research. Appropriate pain-prevention appears critical since it may influence the outcome and the results obtained with this model. However, there are no proper guidelines for pain management in rats undergoing thoracic surgery. Accordingly, we evaluated three analgesic regimens in cardiac ischemia/reperfusion injury. This study was strongly focused on 3R's ethic principles, in particular the principle of Reduction.

Methods: Rats undergoing surgery were treated with pre-surgical tramadol (45 mg/kg intra-peritoneal), or carprofen (5 mg/ kg sub-cutaneous), or with pre-surgical administration of carprofen followed by 2 post-surgery tramadol injections (multi-modal group). We assessed behavioral signs of pain and made a subjective evaluation of stress and suffering one and two hours after surgery.

Results: Multi-modal treatment significantly reduced the number of signs of pain compared to carprofen alone at both the first hour (61 ± 42 *vs* 123 ± 47; $p<0.05$) and the second hour (43 ± 21 *vs* 74 ± 24; $p<0.05$) post-surgery. Tramadol alone appeared as effective as multi-modal treatment during the first hour, but signs of pain significantly increased one hour later (from 66 ± 72 to 151 ± 86, $p<0.05$). Carprofen alone was more effective at the second hour post-surgery when signs of pain reduced to 74 ± 24 from 113 ± 40 in the first hour ($p<0.05$). Stress behaviors during the second hour were observed in only 20% of rats in the multimodal group compared to 75% and 86% in the carprofen and tramadol groups, respectively ($p<0.05$).

Conclusions: Multi-modal treatment with carprofen and tramadol was more effective in preventing pain during the second hour after surgery compared with both tramadol or carprofen. Our results suggest that the combination of carprofen and tramadol represent the best therapy to prevent animal pain after myocardial ischemia/reperfusion. We obtained our results accordingly with the ethical principle of Reduction.

Editor: Yulia Komarova, University of Illinois at Chicago, United States of America

Funding: Dr. Roughan is funded by the UK NC3Rs (http://www.nc3rs.org.uk/). This work was supported by the Ministero Italiano della Sanità (GR-2008-1142871; GR-2010-2320533)(http://www.salute.gov.it/), the Fondazione Cariplo (2007–5984)(http://www.fondazionecariplo.it/it/index.html) and the Ministero Italiano degli Affari Esteri (ZA11GR2)(http://www.esteri.it/MAE/IT). The funders had no role in study design, data collection and analysis, decision to publish, or preparation of the manuscript.

Competing Interests: The authors have declared that no competing interests exist.

* E-mail: l.calvillo@auxologico.it

Introduction

Experimental microsurgery on rodents has become a fundamental tool for translational research over the last 20 years. The quality of surgical procedures is a crucial factor especially when the level of technological sophistication, currently required by laboratory investigations, is taken into account. Molecular biology, proteomics, microarrays and biochemistry need a high standard of *in-vivo* methodologies to assure the highest quality of results. Moreover, ethics in animal care is of primary relevance as the surgical procedures in small rodents can result in a high risk of infections and inflammation leading to suffering, equally or probably more than in other experimental preparations. Small rodents do not vocalize nor communicate in the same way as primates or other common pet species, leading to unsubstantiated beliefs that they are comparatively more robust to infections or suffering. Recently, scientists have begun to observe rodent behaviour more closely, and this has led to a greater acceptance that they may experience suffering; perhaps just as intensely as in many other species. Methods developed to quantify pain and suffering in laboratory animals, including rodents, have already provided greater understanding of the need to refine analgesic and anaesthetic protocols in order to minimise suffering [1]. Rodent use has increased considerably in the last 30 years and they are now one of the most commonly used species in the cardiovascular research field [2].

The ability to apply in rats diagnostic techniques similar to those used in humans renders rat models of myocardial disease very useful for preclinical studies [3,4]. Catheterisation, hemodynamic measurements, echocardiography, histological examinations and biochemical procedures are common tools in cardiac pathophysiology research. The need to conduct such research, not only in an ethically acceptable manner, but also with the greatest translational relevance is accepted as an essential aspect in the success of this work. Advances in pre- and post-surgical care of animals, including the use of anaesthetic and analgesic protocols and aseptic techniques are also considered to be likely factors in further improving the scientific reliability of results. However, despite this, not much has been done so far to develop clearly and appropriate guidelines for use of animals subjected to myocardial infarction. The rationale of this study was to verify if the methods developed to quantify surgical pain and distress during laparotomy [1] could be applied in experimental myocardial infarction and to verify if carprofen and tramadol, published as effective analgesic drugs in laboratory rodents, could provide pain relief after cardiac surgery. Thus our goal was to determine the best practice, in terms of rat's care, in this particular model. We than compared different analgesic approaches in myocardial ischemia/reperfusion (I/R) injury: pre-surgical tramadol or carprofen or a combination of the two drugs (multi-modal group). Carprofen is a non-steroidal anti-inflammatory drug, which veterinarians prescribe as a supportive analgesic for various painful conditions, including surgery [1]. Tramadol is an opioid-like analgesic with a potent analgesic effects [5]. The goal was to establish which of the three approaches may reduce post-surgical pain and to apply the principle of Reduction to our experimental protocol.

Materials and Methods

Ethics

All procedures were approved by the Italian Institute of Health (Ministero della Sanità Italiano) (Permit Number 89/2009-B) according to 116/92 Italian Law and performed in accordance with the DIRECTIVE 2010/63/EU OF THE EUROPEAN PARLIAMENT AND OF THE COUNCIL on the protection of animals used for scientific purposes. The manuscript was prepared according to the ARRIVE (Animal Research: Reporting of In Vivo Experiments) guidelines [6].

Refinement and Reduction

In compliance with the 3Rs principle of reduction, the work used rats already scheduled for studies on myocardial infarction, and the monitoring methods were designed to have no impact on the primary study outcomes. The present study focused on the first two hours after surgery as they were considered as the critical period when appropriate use of analgesia would have maximum positive impact on welfare.

Materials

All surgical equipment was provided by 2Biological Instruments, VA, Italy. Drugs were provided by veterinary pharmacies: Contramal® (tramadol, Formenti, Italy), Rimadyl® (carprofen, Pfizer, Italy) and Amplital® (ampicillin, Pfizer, Italy).

Husbandry

Male Sprague Dawley rats (n = 29) weighing between 250 and 295 g were supplied by Charles River (Calco, LC, Italy) and kept in cages with wood-shaving bedding (each cage (530 cm^2) housed two rats). All cages were open to the room environment (no micro-isolation or ventilated caging) and rats were regularly handled by the staff involved in the experimental protocol. Room temperature was maintained at 21°±1°C with 50%±20% relative humidity and ventilated at 15 filtered air changes per hour. Animals were kept on a 12:12 light:dark cycle and were provided *ad libitum* access to water and rodent feed. (Standard diet, Purina 5L79; Charles River, Calco, LC, Italy). Regular blood screenings on sentinel rats certified the absence of endoparasites and ectoparasites.

Pre-surgical Preparation

Each researcher wore disposable clothes, gloves, footwear and a hair cover. An extractor fan was suspended above the surgical workspace as a barrier to extraneous airborne infectious particles.

The operating table, needle electrodes, heating pad and rat skin were disinfected with didecil-dimetilammonium chloride 0.175% (Farmasept, Nuova Farmec s.r.l., Italy) before surgery. The surgical tools were also sterilized with hot glass dry bead sterilizer.

Animals were placed on a rat/mouse rigid thermostatic pad and body temperature was continuously monitored using a rectal temperature probe (1 mm tip).

Ampicillin 100 mg/kg [7], was injected intra-muscularly, 2 minutes before surgery.

Anaesthesia

Anaesthesia was induced with 4% isoflurane in 1.5 litres/min oxygen using a Perspex chamber and maintained with 2% isoflurane in 0.5 litres/min oxygen. We used isoflurane because this provides rapid induction and safe recovery from anaesthesia with relatively minimal effects on cardiovascular parameters or respiratory rate [4].

Analgesia Experimental Protocol

Three different analgesic groups were compared (**Table 1, Figure 1**):

- Group 1 (C): pre-surgery carprofen, 5 mg/kg subcutaneously (s.c.), 30 min before surgery [1] (n = 9).
- Group 2 (T): pre-surgery tramadol, 45 mg/kg intraperitoneally (i.p.) 15 min before surgery [8] (n = 9).
- Group 3 (CT): combination of carprofen (30 min pre-surgery; 5 mg/kg s.c.) and two tramadol injection post-surgery (first injection (45 mg/kg i.p.) after recovery of mobility; second injection (45 mg/kg i.p.) 1 hour later) (n = 11).

The tramadol dose was selected on the basis of several published reports of its effective use in several invasive surgical models in rats [5,9]. Considering that thoracic pain is one of the most acute among several surgical insults, we chose 45 mg/kg, the highest dose published [8].

All groups underwent I/R injury. For ethical reasons we did not consider conducting surgery in untreated animals or exposing rats

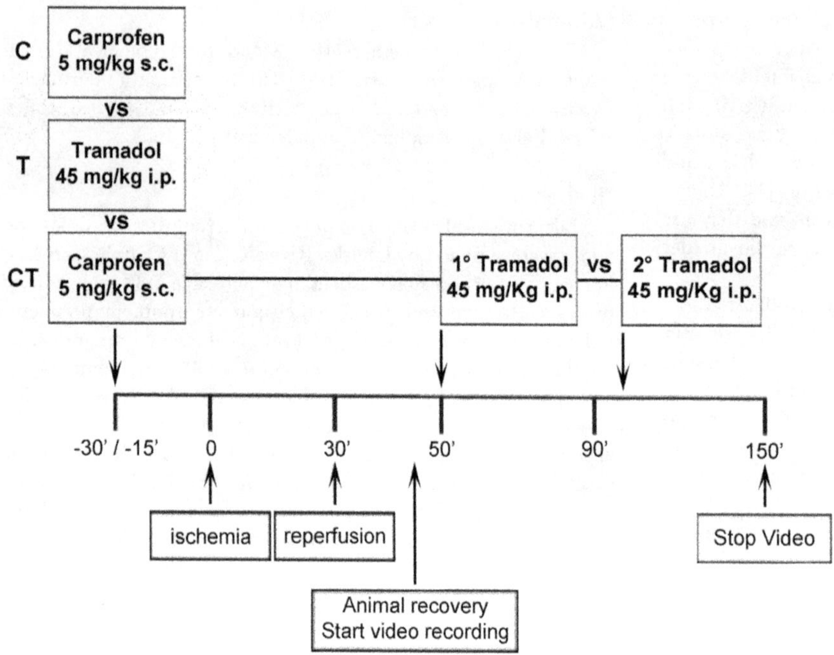

Figure 1. Experimental design. Three different analgesic treatments were compared: (C) 5 mg/kg carprofen (s.c. injection 30 min before surgery), (T) 45 mg/kg tramadol i.p. injection 15 min before surgery). (CT) Pre-treatment with 5 mg/kg of carprofen (30 min before surgery) and 2 i.p. injections of tramadol 45 mg/kg each (immediately after recovery of post-surgical mobility, then 1 hour later).

to anesthesia unnecessarily, thus a saline control group was not used.

Endotracheal Intubation

Under sedation rats were placed supine and a loop of 10 cm length of 3-0 silk-suture was placed around the upper incisors to fix the head. A fiber-optic light source was positioned about 1 cm above the anterior neck for the trans-illumination of the oropharingeal cavity.

The tongue was gently extended to bring the larynx into view. The intubation tube was made from an 18-gauge non-traumatic feeding needle connected to a Y-shaped connector attached to a rat ventilator. Respiration rate was 107 breaths/min; tidal volume 0.6 ml.

Ischemia and Reperfusion

Five−lead ECGs (amplifiers Power Lab-ADInstrument Pty Ltd., UK) were recorded using 4 needle electrodes subcutaneously implanted in each hind/forelimb and 1 electrode placed ventrally on the right side of the chest. A tobacco-pouch suture was implanted through the pectoral muscles to allow rapid closure of the chest at the end of the procedure.

The left coronary artery (LAD) was ligated using a 10 cm length of 4-0 silk suture material (Ethicon, Sommerville, NJ, USA) through a 15 mm opening at the 5th intercostal space. A plain knot was tied and left in-situ for 30 minutes (**Figure 2**). Ischemia was confirmed in all rats by the appearance of discoloration of the heart surface and ST elevation on the ECG recording. Silk suture material was preferred to nylon as this prevented any slippage of the ligature. After 30 minutes the ligature was released [10] and reperfusion was verified by reddening of the previously discoloured area of the heart muscle and by the presence of arrhythmia on ECG recordings. The chest was then closed under negative pressure by gently squeeze of the ribs and pulling the pre-implanted tobacco-pouch suture. Rats were then extubated and observed for approximately 10 minutes under ECG and body temperature monitoring until they were able to move. Following this observational period they were transferred in cages for filming the post-operative behavior.

Table 1. Non-standard Abbreviations.

C	Carprofen
T	Tramadol
CT	Carprofen+Tramadol
I/R	Ischemia/Reperfusion injury
s.c.	Sub-cutaneous
i.p.	Intra-peritoneal
LAD	Left coronary artery

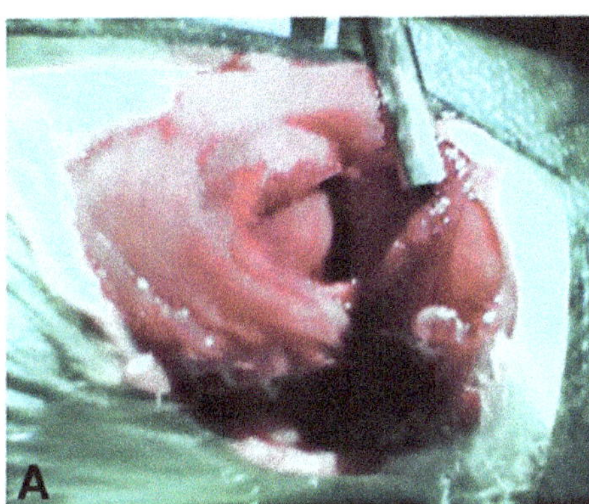
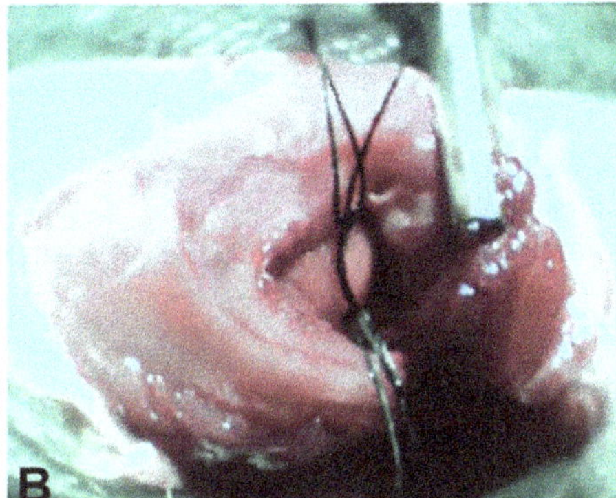

Figure 2. Left coronary artery ligation. (**A**) Heart visualization by the 15 mm opening of the 5th intercostal space. (**B**) LAD was ligated with 4-0 silk suture and the plain knot was tied over two loops of suture. After 30′ ischemia loops were pulled and the knot was released allowing reperfusion.

Post-surgical Pain Assessment

Signs of pain. To assess behaviors indicating post-surgical pain, each rat was filmed for two hours in polycarbonate cages (810 cm^2, Tecniplast S.P.A, Buguggiate, VA, Italy) using a webcam (QuickCam, Logitech). One observer, blind to the treatment, evaluated and counted in each rat predefined pain-specific indicators during the first and second hour after surgery; another researcher repeated the observations and counting for a double blinded check.

There were three main specific indicators previously shown to be effective in describing the presence of post-surgical pain and thought to reflect its severity [1,11]:

1. "Stop" (later named as "Transient Stop"): scored in the absence of all other ongoing activity while rats adopted either a crouched or lying posture.
2. "Twitching": transient involuntary muscular contraction of any body part usually occurring during 'stop'.
3. "Stagger/fall": loss of balance while walking and especially during rapid transition to crouch from high or low rear and/or during grooming.

We hypothesized that signs of pain would increase in response to surgery, but that their relative magnitude would reduce according to the various analgesic treatments tested. This would allow us to determine which treatment regimen afforded maximum pain relief.

Stress behaviors. In addition to pain-specific signs the observer made a subjective welfare assessment to verify whether there was evidence of general distress or suffering. The subjective score was based on whether there were commonly observed abnormal postures namely "Crouch hunch" and "crouch curl" [1,11]. "Crouch hunch" was an abnormal posture during resting or ambulation with the rats head lowered and the back partially arched. "Crouch curl" was an exaggerated version of this with a crouched postured assumed in a hunched position such that the head was lowered between the forelimbs so that the eyes/snout were not visible.

In each case, the presence (yes) or absence (no) of suffering was assessed. A "yes" determination was considered when the animal showed these behavioral signs that the observer thought relevant, and only if lasted several minutes. A "no" evaluation was considered when the rats appeared active, normally responsive, calm, awake and resting normal without appearing agitated (despite the possible presence of signs of pain). The results were expressed as the percentage of rats assessed as 'suffering' in each group at each time point.

Euthanasia

After recordings were completed the rats underwent additional manipulations as part of the investigations for the main study. Depending on that study requirements, rats were either euthanized by exposure to CO_2 at a rate of 6 L/min in their home cages. We decided to use CO_2 to eliminate the animal stress of handling. There is evidence that home-cage euthanasia is at least as acceptable as euthanasia in an induction chamber, as method of human approach, so whenever possible we chose this procedure [12]. In some cases rats were euthanized by induction of anesthesia with isoflurane (as in preparation for surgery) followed by heart explantation.

Statistical Analysis

All analyses used SPSS Statistics version 19 (IBM). Continuous variables are presented as means ± standard deviation (SD). These were compared between groups using one-way ANOVA, followed by post-hoc multiple comparisons using the Tukey's test or the Tamhane method whenever the assumption of homogeneity of variance (evaluated by the Levene test) was violated. Categorical variables were expressed as absolute and relative frequencies and analyzed using chi-squared tests. Within-group comparisons from the first to second assessment period (1 vs. 2 hours following surgery) were made using paired samples t-tests for continuous variables (2-sided). Alpha value was set at 0.05 for all analyses.

Results

Pain Monitoring

Signs of pain during the 1st hour after surgery. Our observations show that the 'stop' behaviour characteristically occurred during rearing and manifested as a transient 'freezing' of all ongoing activity. We hypothesize that this behavior is a transient reaction of few seconds in response to an acute ache. For this reason we named it as "Transient Stop". "Twitching" occurred both during grooming and "Transient Stop", and was the most common behavior that we observed. "Stagger/fall" and "Transient Stop" were less frequent compared to the other signs. ANOVA showed that during the first hour post-surgery the mean frequency of pain-specific behaviors varied significantly according to the treatment group ($p<0.05$); **Table 2**, **Figure 3A**).

Compared to group C, where pain specific signs were most prominent (123±47), group T showed a significant reduction in pain-related behavior (60±67; p<0.05). However, rats treated with tramadol appeared narcotized for most of the assessment period. This effect was absent or considerably less pronounced when the first tramadol injection was administered following recovery (Group CT). The CT combination appeared to be more effective than C alone, with a significantly lower pain score (61±42 *vs* 123±47, p<0.05).

Signs of pain during the 2nd hour after surgery. Animals were completely recovered during the 2nd observation period with the exception of 4 rats who died one hour after the onset of ischemia (one rat in group C, two in group T, and one in group CT). Signs of pain significantly increased in group T from 66±72 during the first hour to 151±86 at the second assessment time (p< 0.05). Group C showed an opposite effect as in the second hour signs of pain significantly reduced compared to the first hour after surgery (from 113±40 to 74±24; p<0.05). In the CT group, the multi-modal treatment caused a small and not significant reduction in the frequency of pain-associated acts from the first and the second hour (65±42 *vs.* 43±21; p = n.s). However, the CT combination confirmed its superior analgesic effectiveness over a prolonged observation time as it resulted in an overall reduction of pain-associated behaviors compared to both the C (43±21 *vs* 74±24; p<0.05) and T (43±21 *vs* 151±86; p<0.05) groups (**Table 2, Figure 3B**).

Stress behaviors during the 1st hour after surgery. As illustrated by **Figure 4A**, a significant (p<0.001) difference in the proportion of rats exhibiting the relevant signs was observed among the three analgesic groups. 'Crouch hunch' and 'crouch curl' were prominent in all rats in group C. In the T group, 8 out of 9 rats (89%) showed distress reactions but, as previously described, these animals were narcotized. It was therefore difficult to determine whether the reduced reactivity was a consequence of suffering or merely sedation. Again, the most effective treatment appeared to be the multi-modal combination of carprofen plus tramadol. Indeed, of the 11 CT treated rats only 3 (27%) showed abnormal behaviour (**Figure 5**).

Stress behaviors during the 2nd hour after surgery. In the second assessment phase, the proportion of rats classed as suffering was relatively unchanged compared to the first hour of the study (**Figure 4B**), and a significant (p<0.05) difference among groups was still observed according to treatment. Indeed, long periods of apparent distress remained relevant in the vast majority of rats in both groups C (6/8, 75%) and T (6/7, 86%). Conversely, only 2 of the 10 (20%) rats injected with the combined drug dose showed the relevant abnormal behavior.

Discussion

The aim of the study was to assess a refined analgesic protocol for rats undergoing experimental thoracotomy and myocardial I/R injury. To accomplish our goal, we applied an effective method to assess pain and distress symptoms and evaluate the effects of different treatments providing pain relief to maximize post-surgical animal care. To test our protocols, we selected a highly traumatic procedure such as open chest I/R myocardial injury. We compared the effects of carprofen or tramadol given alone, with a combination of one dose of carprofen administered pre- and two doses of tramadol given post-operatively (multi-modal treatment). The primary methods of assessment were scoring pain-specific behaviors that accompany pain following other types of surgery (such as laparotomy [1]), and by using a more general (subjective) index of distress: posture and behavioral reactivity changes. Our results show that thoracic surgery caused effects consistent with post-surgical distress and generally poor welfare. Of the 3 groups tested, multi-modal treatment with carprofen and tramadol proved to be the most effective in reducing behavioral abnormalities over a prolonged observation. According to both methods of assessment, carprofen and tramadol given alone showed a relative lack of efficacy during the 2nd hour following surgery.

Pain Scoring

Although combined treatment seemed more effective, it was apparent that pain-specific behaviors and suffering were overall more pronounced than following laparotomy (unpublished observations). This justified our initial belief that surgery to study myocardial I/R may indeed be more painful to rats, as did the fact that none of the treatments completely prevented signs of pain. Also, back-arching, horizontal stretching and abdominal writhing behaviors, activities that can be used effectively to assess the severity of post-laparotomy and the efficacy of its analgesic treatment [1], were presently absent, whereas abnormal postures and twitching behavior were more frequent. This indicates that

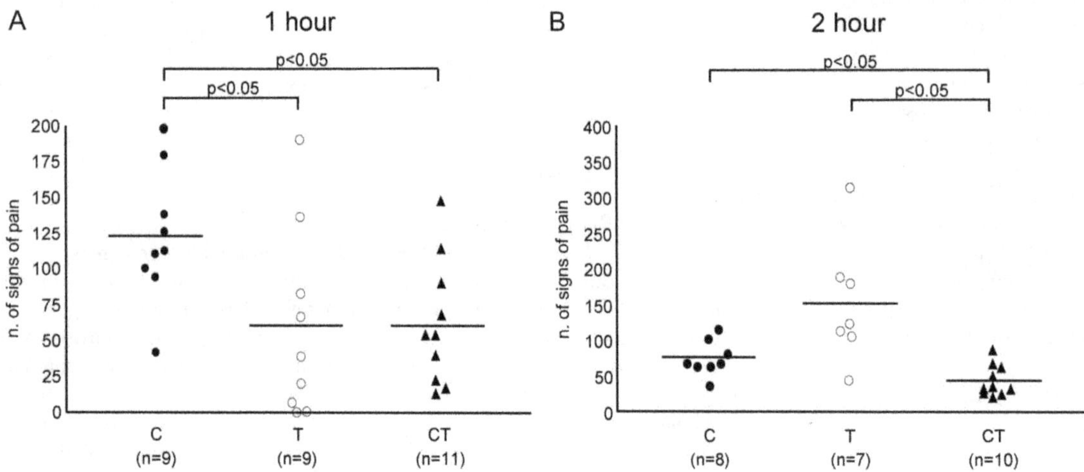

Figure 3. Pain assessment. Number of signs of pain during the first (**A**) and the second hour (**B**) after recovery from surgery. Horizontal lines represent mean values.

Table 2. Signs of pain and analgesic approaches.

Treatment	Time	Twitching	Stagger/Fall	Transient stop	total pains signs
Carprofen	1st hour	112±47	3±3	8±5	123±47*
Tramadol	1st hour	58±67	2±3	1±3	60±67
Carprofen+Tramadol	1st hour	59±42	1±1	2±2	61±42
Carprofen	2nd hour	70±23	0	4±3	74±24
Tramadol	2nd hour	129±87	0	22±33	151±86
Carprofen+Tramadol	2nd hour	42±20	0	1±1	43±21**

*$p<0.05$ *vs* T and CT (1st hour);
**$p<0.05$ *vs* C and T (2nd hour). Data are presented as mean ± SD.

specific signs of pain and stress behaviors largely depend on the type of surgery undertaken. Thus, developing refinements to peri-operative care protocols that improve welfare requires the development of procedure-specific analgesic and pain scoring protocols and probably also refined husbandry practices (e.g. by careful handling and conducting precise surgery). Although our attempt to establish a pain-preventive protocol following myocardial I/R did not completely suppressed animal discomfort, to our knowledge this is the first study describing and evaluating the appropriate signs of pain and suggesting a refined treatment methodology for experimental thoracic surgery in the rat.

Pharmacology and Efficacy

The lack of effectiveness of the pre-surgical treatment with carprofen or tramadol was probably affected by the route of administration and drug pharmacokinetics. Likewise in rats, Roughan and Flecknell concluded that 5 mg/kg carprofen administered subcutaneously had significant analgesic activity lasting between four and five hours following laparotomy [1]. Although, in our study carprofen had more pronounced activity at the 2nd hour compared to the 1st hour following surgery, it was still clearly inadequate as a standalone treatment.

The current observation of tramadol enhanced effectiveness, when given in the form of the combined therapy CT, shows this may be the drug of choice for more severe types of surgery. However, there are two problem issues regarding our use and assessment of the effects of tramadol; post-recovery apnoea and drug-induced narcosis. These effects of tramadol, especially the narcotic effects, may have affected our ability to effectively assess 'suffering'. Those non-specific effects are commonly reported following opioid treatment in rodents, as recently reported in mice undergoing vasectomy following treatment with buprenorphine [13]. Accordingly, from our results it seems that when opioids are used, scoring proven pain-specific signs rather than evaluating generalized appearance provide a more reliable estimate of clinical efficacy. The problem was considerably less when tramadol was given following recovery (Group CT), presumably because the drug reached peak effect after the rat was completely recovered from anesthesia effects. The group treated pre-operatively with carprofen and post-operatively with two doses of tramadol did not appear narcotized, even at the 2nd hour assessment time. This indicated that the timing of treatment could have a significant effect on post-surgical appearance.

The effect of opioids or opioid-like drugs such as tramadol on the immune system presents another possible problem. In a Sprague Dawley rat model of incisional pain, pre-treatment with 1 to 20 mg/kg i.p. of tramadol causes a decrease of IL-6 levels in a dose-dependent manner however, when used in combination with carprofen (CT) had no effect on IL-6 [14]. On the other hand, in Fisher 344 rats 20 to 40 mg/kg tramadol given before laparotomy

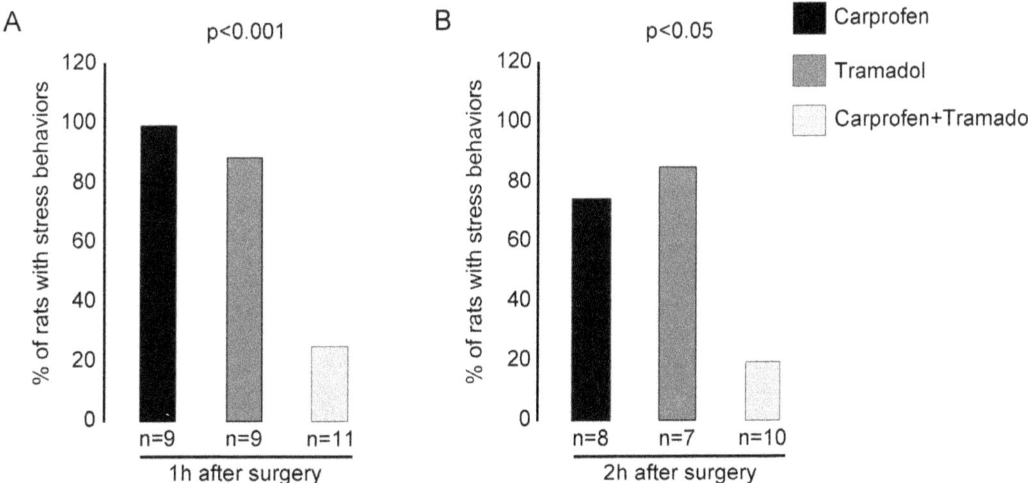

Figure 4. Suffering and distress monitoring. Proportion of rats showing stress behavior during the first (**A**) and the second hour (**B**) after recovery from surgery.

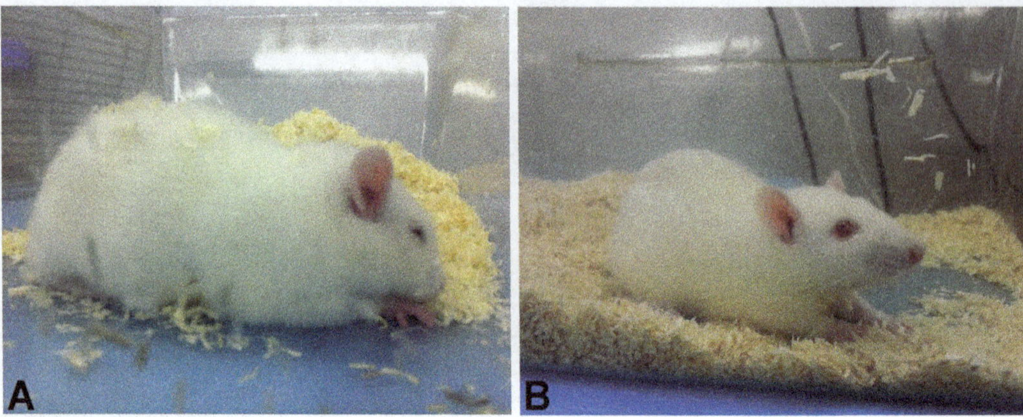

Figure 5. Example of stress behavior. (**A**) Carprofen treated rat exhibiting distress reactions 1 h after surgery. (**B**) Carprofen+Tramadol treated rat showing normal behavior 1 h after surgery.

preserved Natural Killer cells (NK) and IL-2 from the usual depression seen as a consequence of post-surgical stress [15]. Such strain-specific effects are therefore an important consideration in choosing the analgesic combination that is likely to be effective. As a consequence, improving scientific validity may require studies devoted to determining the precise manner of response to surgery for the most widely used rat models (for example Wistar Kyoto, Spontaneous Hypertensive Rats, Fisher, Wistar and Sprague Dawley). Better characterization of the response to analgesics in these is therefore also becoming recognized as essential to progress on refinement, and a basic premise to progress on the 3Rs.

The effect of a chosen analgesic regimen on infarct size is another potential source of variation. When given intravenously at 12.5 mg/kg in male Sprague Dawley rats before the onset of ischemia, tramadol has been shown to have a myocardial protective function against 6 hours of ischemia caused by permanent coronary occlusion, and reduces infarct size by inhibiting NF-kB activation [16]. This mechanism is of primary relevance to studies exploring strategies to modulate infarct expansion, or those concerned with investigating the role of the immune system in cardiac ischemia and failure. In our preliminary studies (data not shown) we verified that tramadol treatment in both groups T and CT did not interfere with infarct expansion. Indeed infarct size did not differ between groups C, T and CT and the calculated infarct size was similar to the necrotic size typically observed in experimental murine models [3,10,17].

Conclusions

The principles of Refinement and Reduction were at the core of our work. This was achieved firstly by performing our experiments in rats already undergoing surgery. Secondly, we identified specific signs of pain and a multi-modal treatment able to reduce post-surgical suffering and improve animal welfare after thoracotomy. We assume that this was obtained by reducing their experience of pain with a development of a new more refined analgesic strategy, for use in this particular surgical model. In the future investigators should aim to further reduce animal suffering. This will require efforts to establish the exact mechanism underlying such multi-modal dosing, and use of the most effective behavioral (or other) methods of pain assessment. Our results indicate such testing should focus on pain-specific outcomes rather than generalized demeanor (due to a relative lack of drug associated non-specific effects).

Study Limitations

The main focus of our study was the 3R's ethic principles, in particular Reduction.

The European Directive *63/2010* recommends that "… the number of animals used in procedures could be reduced by performing procedures on animals more than once, where this does not detract from the scientific objective or result in poor animal welfare…".

Accordingly to this recommendation, our study was planned to test a procedure (the three different analgesic treatments) on animals already undergoing an experimental protocol, thus reducing the number of rats involved and avoiding further suffering. In this context, our protocol guaranteed that animals used to evaluate the post-surgical analgesia were under the same experimental procedure just for the first 2 hours. We were aware that this ethical approach would have caused some limitations which would have prevented some important measurements like corticosterone levels, body weight and food intake and heart rate over the time, being all these procedures further objective parameters to show pain relief [13,18]. Nevertheless, considering the spirit of this manuscript, we feel to have reached the important issue of giving useful observation on analgesia avoiding the use of rats specifically for this aim. Our purpose was to offer a possible alternative way to collect suitable informations without causing further stress to animals.

Acknowledgments

The authors are grateful to Dr. Lidia Cova and Dr. Alice Ghidoni for their very helpful advices and for their professional support.

Author Contributions

Conceived and designed the experiments: LC MC EV MG. Performed the experiments: LC MC EV. Analyzed the data: LC MC CS RC VT JR. Contributed reagents/materials/analysis tools: LC MC MG EV CS. Wrote the paper: LC MC CS JR MG EV.

References

1. Roughan JV, Flecknell PA (2001) Behavioural effects of laparotomy and analgesic effects of ketoprofen and carprofen in rats. Pain 90: 65–74.
2. Selye H, Bajusz E, Grasso S, Mendell P (1960) Simple techniques for the surgical occlusion of coronary vessels in the rat. Angiology 11: 398–407.
3. Calvillo L, Masson S, Salio M, Pollicino L, De Angelis N, et al. (2003) In vivo cardioprotection by N-acetylcysteine and isosorbide 5-mononitrate in a rat model of ischemia-reperfusion. Cardiovasc Drugs Ther 17: 199–208.
4. Calvillo L, Vanoli E, Andreoli E, Besana A, Omodeo E, et al. (2011) Vagal stimulation, through its nicotinic action, limits infarct size and the inflammatory response to myocardial ischemia and reperfusion. J Cardiovasc Pharmacol 58: 500–507.
5. Cannon CZ, Kissling GE, Hoenerhoff MJ, King-Herbert AP, Blankenship-Paris T (2010) Evaluation of dosages and routes of administration of tramadol analgesia in rats using hot-plate and tail-flick tests. Lab Anim (NY) 39: 342–351.
6. Kilkenny C, Browne WJ, Cuthill IC, Emerson M, Altman DG (2010) Improving bioscience research reporting: The ARRIVE guidelines for reporting animal research. PLoS Biol 8: e1000412.
7. Hazir T, Fox LM, Nisar YB, Fox MP, Ashraf YP, et al. (2008) Ambulatory short-course high-dose oral amoxicillin for treatment of severe pneumonia in children: A randomised equivalency trial. Lancet 371: 49–56.
8. Ceyhan A, Ustun H, Altunatmaz K, Ide T, Unal N (2005) Is metoclopramide an alternative to tramadol in management of post-operative pain? an experimental study. J Vet Med A Physiol Pathol Clin Med 52: 249–253.
9. Kongara K, Chambers JP, Johnson CB (2012) Effects of tramadol, morphine or their combination in dogs undergoing ovariohysterectomy on peri-operative electroencephalographic responses and post-operative pain. N Z Vet J 60: 129–135.
10. Michael LH, Ballantyne CM, Zachariah JP, Gould KE, Pocius JS, et al. (1999) Myocardial infarction and remodeling in mice: Effect of reperfusion. Am J Physiol 277: H660–8.
11. Roughan JV, Flecknell PA, Davies BR (2004) Behavioural assessment of the effects of tumour growth in rats and the influence of the analgesics carprofen and meloxicam. Lab Anim 38: 286–296.
12. McIntyre AR, Drummond RA, Riedel ER, Lipman NS (2007) Automated mouse euthanasia in an individually ventilated caging system: System development and assessment. J Am Assoc Lab Anim Sci 46: 65–73.
13. Wright-Williams S, Flecknell PA, Roughan JV (2013) Comparative effects of vasectomy surgery and buprenorphine treatment on faecal corticosterone concentrations and behaviour assessed by manual and automated analysis methods in C57 and C3H mice. PLoS One 8: e75948.
14. Liu YM, Zhu SM, Wang KR, Feng ZY, Chen QL (2008) Effect of tramadol on immune responses and nociceptive thresholds in a rat model of incisional pain. J Zhejiang Univ Sci B 9: 895–902.
15. Gaspani L, Bianchi M, Limiroli E, Panerai AE, Sacerdote P (2002) The analgesic drug tramadol prevents the effect of surgery on natural killer cell activity and metastatic colonization in rats. J Neuroimmunol 129: 18–24.
16. Zhang LZ, Guo Z (2009) Tramadol reduces myocardial infarct size and expression and activation of nuclear factor kappa B in acute myocardial infarction in rats. Eur J Anaesthesiol 26: 1048–1055.
17. Valtchanova-Matchouganska A, Gondwe M, Nadar A (2004) The role of C-reactive protein in ischemia/reperfusion injury and preconditioning in a rat model of myocardial infarction. Life Sci 75: 901–910.
18. Zegre Cannon, Kissling GE, Goulding DR, King-Herbert AP, Blankenship-Paris T (2011) Analgesic effects of tramadol, carprofen or multimodal analgesia in rats undergoing ventral laparotomy. Lab Anim (NY). 40: 85–93.

Estimation of the Use of Antibiotics in the Small Ruminant Industry in the Netherlands in 2011 and 2012

Inge Santman-Berends[1]*, Saskia Luttikholt[2], René Van den Brom[2], Gerdien Van Schaik[1], Maaike Gonggrijp[1], Han Hage[3], Piet Vellema[2]

1 Department of epidemiology, GD Animal Health, Deventer, The Netherlands, **2** Department of small ruminant health, GD Animal Health, Deventer, The Netherlands, **3** Department of cattle health, GD Animal Health, Deventer, The Netherlands

Abstract

The aim of this study was to estimate the quantity of antibiotics and classes of antibiotics used in the small ruminant industry in the Netherlands in 2011 and 2012. Twelve large veterinary practices, located throughout the Netherlands were selected for this study. All small ruminant farms associated with these practices that had complete records on the quantity of antibiotics prescribed were included. The veterinary practices provided data on all antibiotics prescribed, and the estimated animal used daily dose of antibiotics per year (AUDD/Y) was calculated for each farm. The median AUDD/Y in small ruminant farms was zero in both years (mean 0.60 in 2011, and 0.62 in 2012). The largest quantity of antibiotic use was observed in the professional goat industry (herds of ≥32 goats) with a median AUDD/Y of 1.22 in 2011 and 0.73 in 2012. In the professional sheep industry (flocks of ≥32 sheep), the median AUDD/Y was 0 in 2011 and 0.10 in 2012. In the small scale industry (flocks or herds of <32 sheep or goats), the median AUDD/Y never exceeded 0. The most frequently prescribed antibiotics in the small scale industry and professional sheep farms belonged to the penicillin class. In professional goat farms, antibiotics of the aminoglycoside class were most frequently prescribed. This study provides the first assessment on the quantity of antibiotic use in the small ruminant industry. Given a comparable attitude towards antibiotic use, these results might be valid for small ruminant populations in other north-western European countries as well. The antibiotic use in the small ruminant industry appeared to be low, and is expected to play a minor role in the development of antibiotic resistance. Nevertheless, several major zoonotic bacterial pathogens are associated with the small ruminant industry, and it remains important that antibiotics are used in a prudent way.

Editor: Glenn F. Browning, The University of Melbourne, Australia

Funding: This study was funded by the Dutch Ministry of Economic affairs. The funders had no role in study design, data collection and analysis, decision to publish, or preparation of the manuscript.

Competing Interests: The authors have declared that no competing interests exist.

* Email: i.santman@gddiergezondheid.nl

Introduction

In the Netherlands, sheep and goats are generally kept as companion animals. However, there is also a substantial number of professional farms with small ruminants that produce milk and meat for human consumption. In the latter, food safety and food quality are of great importance. To ensure a production of meat and milk by healthy livestock, sick animals need to be treated in a responsible manner. However, the use of antibiotics and other medicines may enhance the development of antimicrobial resistance (AMR) [1–3]. Additionally, the fact that the same classes of antibiotics are used in veterinary and human medicine is a reason for concern [4]. In the last decade, antibiotic resistance in livestock has become a great concern in many European countries because of the association between livestock and the presence of resistant bacteria [5,6]. Nevertheless, the role of small ruminants in this discussion might be of minor importance because earlier research did only find low rates of AMR in sheep [7].

In December 2008, the Dutch Ministry of Agriculture agreed to a covenant entitled "Antibiotic resistance in livestock" for the pig, poultry, cattle and veal industry [8]. The goal of this covenant was to monitor and reduce the use of antibiotics, and therewith achieve a decline in antibiotic resistance in these livestock industries. This resulted in a reduction of the use of antibiotics of over 50% in 2012 relative to the use in 2009 [9]. Because the small ruminant industry did not participate in this covenant, the use of antibiotics in this industry has not been monitored.

From January 1st 2010 onwards, everyone who owns small ruminants in the Netherlands is obliged to register their sheep or goats in the Identification and Registration (I&R) database. The quality of this national database has improved over time, and appears to provide a reasonable and relatively complete representation of the Dutch small ruminant industry in both 2011 and 2012. The combination of improved registration in the central I&R-database and improved registration of prescribed antibiotics in the databases of veterinary practices offered the opportunity to estimate the quantity of antibiotics that were used in the small ruminant industry. Beforehand, the general impression was that the antibiotic use in this industry is fairly low, especially compared to other livestock industries. However, there was no information available on the amount and type of antibiotics used in the small ruminant population. The aim of this study therefore was to estimate the quantity and types of antibiotics that were used in the small ruminant industry in the Netherlands in 2011 and 2012.

Materials and Methods

Ethics Statement

The data that were used for this study belonged to the veterinary practices involved. They gave consent to use the data for this study, given that all data of small ruminant holders and the veterinary practice were anonymised prior to analysis. After combining the different datasets, all identifying information such as names, addresses and unique herd identification (UHI) numbers from both the small ruminant holders and their veterinary practices were either removed or were anonymised. This was done prior to analysis and in this way, it was impossible to trace the data and results to either small ruminant holders or veterinary practices. The Dutch government and the farmers organisation were informed and agreed to this procedure prior to this study.

Study population

For this study, veterinary practices with a minimum of fifty small ruminant holders as client were asked to participate. Eventually twelve large veterinary practices that were located throughout the country were included. The study population consisted of 5,399 holders of small ruminants that were clients of these veterinary practices. The Netherlands had a total of 34,806 registered small ruminant farms in 2012 [10], thus 16% of all registered holdings with small ruminants were covered. Based on species (sheep/goat) and herd size (≤ or > than 32 heads), herds were divided into four different subtypes of small ruminant farms: small scale sheep farms, professional sheep farms, small scale goat farms and professional goat farms. The last group contained both dairy and non-dairy farms. The cut-off value of 32 head was consistent with earlier studies in the Netherlands [11] and was agreed upon by the different stakeholders in the Dutch small ruminant industry.

Available data

The twelve veterinary practices provided data on each delivery of medicines or services to their small ruminant holders. Because four different management systems were used in the veterinary practices that were included in this study, data from the different systems were assigned appropriately before they were combined.

The data from the veterinary practices consisted of names and addresses of clients, services or medicines involved, the species for whom the medicines were provided, date or year of delivery, and delivered amount of prescribed medicines. To be able to calculate quantity of antibiotic delivered to an average animal in the small ruminant industry, data from the veterinary practices were combined with three other data sources, namely:

1. **Animal demographic information** (GD Animal Health) and Ministry of Economic Affairs (EZ)) information on herd level: unique herd identification numbers (UHI), names and addresses of the farms, livestock species present on the farm (sheep/goats/cattle/pigs/poultry). On animal level, this data contained species, birth dates, dates of arrival and removal, reason for arrival (birth, purchase, import), and reason for removal (sale, export, slaughter, death).
2. **Weight information** (Agricultural Economical Institute (LEI)) containing standardized weights for sheep and goats, divided into two and three different age categories respectively.
3. **Pharmacological information** (Faculty of Veterinary Medicine, Utrecht University) containing all relevant information from the manuals of the antibiotics that were approved for use in (small) ruminants. This data included names and registration numbers of products that contain antibiotics, type and concentrate of active substance, and the weight of sheep or goat that could be treated with a certain amount (often mL or g) of active substance.

To be able to combine the different datasets, prior to the start of the validation, the data from the veterinary practices were combined with the demographic information to obtain the UHI numbers for each herd. This was in consent with all stakeholders involved (see also the ethics section). Names and addresses were removed from the data and the UHI numbers were anonymised before the data were analysed.

Data validation

The data from the veterinary practices contained 7,483 records with prescribed antibiotics to be used for small ruminants present on the farms in the years 2011 and 2012.

These data were combined with animal demographics, weight and the pharmacological information in order to calculate the amount of active substances that were delivered to the herds and the total weight of the small ruminants treated. The data in the I&R database were incomplete: for several farms data about the number of animals present was missing. Therefore only 6,297 out of 7,483 antibiotic supply records (84%) were available to calculate the Animal Used Daily Dose of antibiotics per year (AUDD/Y) (Figure 1). The calculated AUDD/Y does not present the truly used daily dose, but presents an estimation of this parameter because 1) the available data contained the amount of antibiotics delivered which may not be completely used by the farmer and 2) for the calculations average weights are used instead of the exact weights of all small ruminants in the herds.

Of those 6,297 prescriptions of antibiotics, 2,970 were delivered to 894 different farms in 2011, and 3,327 were delivered to 1,073 different farms in 2012. Of the remaining 1,186 prescriptions, 584 were delivered to 281 different farms in 2011, and 602 prescriptions were delivered to 276 different farms in 2012. Of 103 and 106 of these herds respectively, a UHI was available, but not registered in the I&R database. Of the remaining 178 and 170 farms respectively, only names and addresses were available that could not be combined with an UHI number to identify individual farms.

The weight (in kilograms) of animals present on the farm was one of the requirements to be able to calculate the AUDD/Y. Since this information was unknown for 281 and 276 farms as described above, it was not possible to include these herds in the calculations of the AUDD/Y. Nevertheless these prescriptions of antibiotics were included for descriptive purposes.

For some antibiotics the prescribed dosage differs between sheep and goats, and in a few cases it was not specified for which species the antibiotics were used. In those cases we decided to include the highest prescribed dose in our calculations.

Finally, farmers use different amounts of ointment to treat eye and skin problems. Therefore it was not possible to determine the animal weight in kilograms that was treated per tube of ointment, resulting in an inaccurate estimation of the AUDD/Y for these applications. For this reason we decided to remove those prescribed antibiotics that are applied locally e.g. ointment in eyes or on the skin. This was in consensus with the calculations of the AUDD/Y in other animal species in the Netherlands [12].

Eventually, 2,785 and 3,113 prescriptions of antibiotics, in 887 and 1,049 farms in 2011 and 2012 respectively, remained for the calculation of the AUDD/Y in small ruminant herds that received antibiotics from their veterinary practice (Figure 1).

Of the 4,231 and 4,074 farms to which veterinary practices had not prescribed antibiotics in 2011 and 2012 respectively, only

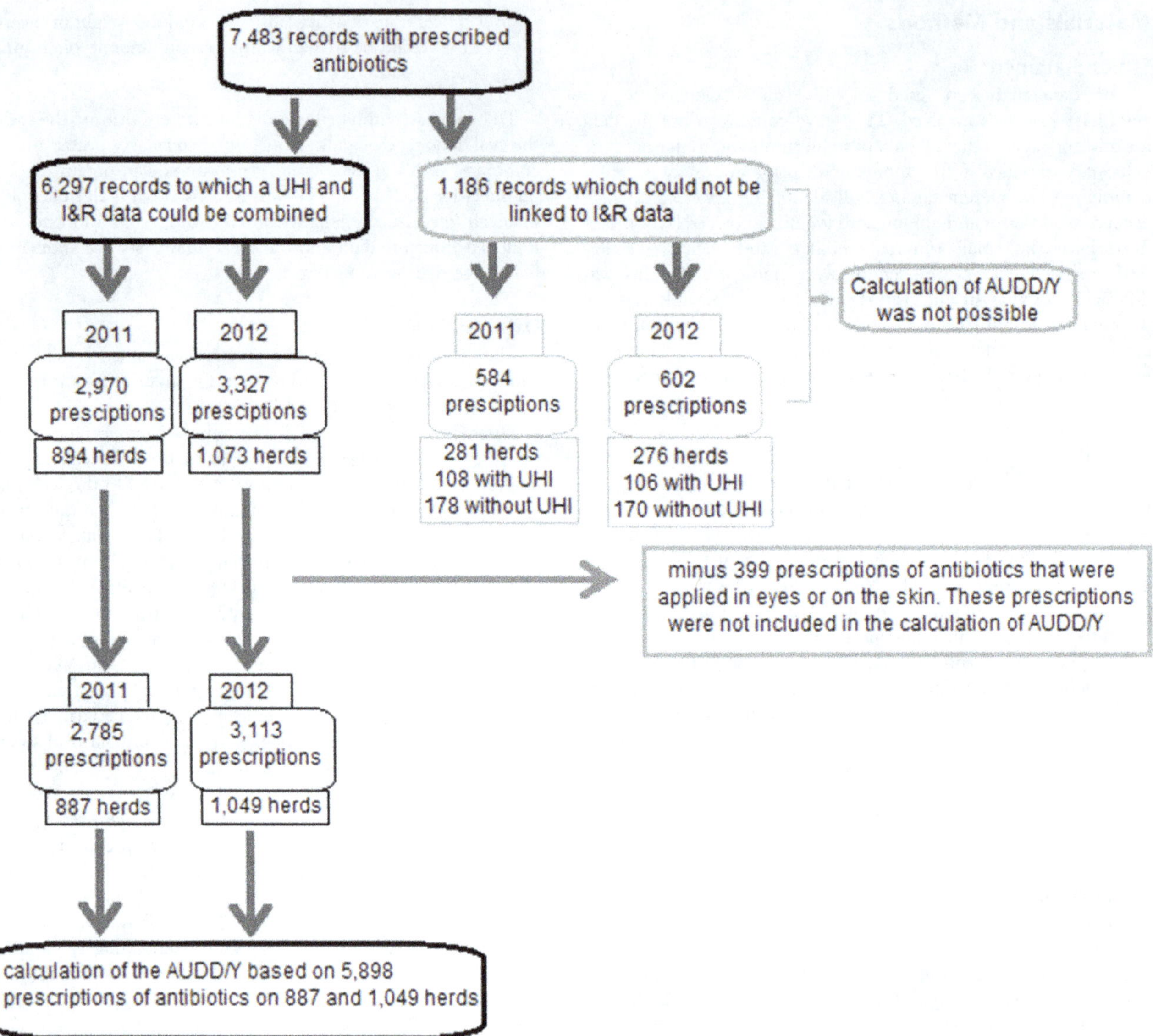

Figure 1. A schematic overview of the validation process of the data of prescribed antibiotics that were provided by the veterinarians for the calculation of the estimated animal used daily dose of antibiotics used per year (AUDD/Y) in farms with small ruminants in 2011 and 2012.

2,989 (71%) and 2,856 (70%) farms had complete I&R data (Figure 2). In accordance with the selection criteria to include only farms with complete data, and analogous to the farms to which antibiotics were prescribed during the analysed period, we decided to include only farms with complete data (2,989 and 2,856 herds in 2011 and 2012, respectively). Lastly, for the calculation of the AUDD/Y in the entire small ruminant industry, data from 3,876 and 3,905 farms with small ruminants respectively, were used for the analyses (Figure 2).

Analyses

All analyses were carried out with STATA version 13 [13]. For each of the 887 and 1,049 farms that had been prescribed antibiotics for their small ruminants in 2011 and 2012 respectively, the total animal weight treated was calculated for each delivery. Weight was used instead of number of animals because antibiotics are prescribed by weight. The total animal treated weight per supply of antibiotics was calculated by multiplying the amount of delivered product (product_i) by the content of active substance ($\text{active substance}_i$) according to the manual of the product. The total amount of active substance divided by the prescribed dose per kg animal (prescribed dose_i per kg) resulted in the total treated animal weight of the small ruminants per herd in kilogram (kg treated) (formula 1).

$$\text{Kg treated} = \frac{\text{product}_i + \text{active substance}_i}{\text{prescribed dose}_i \text{ per kg}} \qquad (1)$$

Where:

Kg treated : the total weight of sheep/goats in kilograms treated with the antibiotics prescribed by the veterinarian per treatment

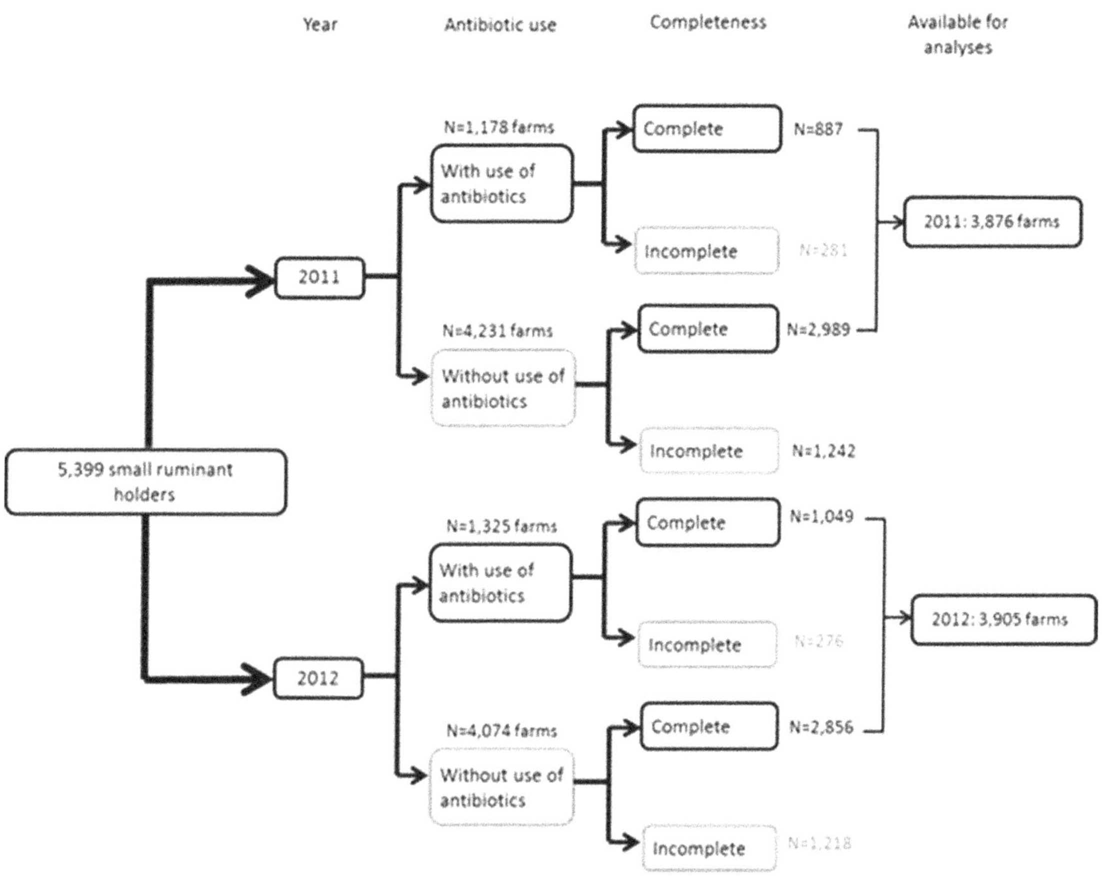

Figure 2. A schematic overview of the number of farms with small ruminants that were clients of the twelve veterinary practices in this study. The figure shows the number of farms with and without antibiotic use and with complete and incomplete data (missing information on the number of animals present in the herd) for both 2011 and 2012.

$Product_i$: the total amount of prescribed antibiotic per unit i

$Active\ substance_i$: the content of active substance per unit i of the antibiotic

$Prescribed\ dose_i$ per kg : the total weight of small ruminant in kilograms treated with a predefined concentration (unit i) of active sub stance

i : mg/gram/mL/piece/pastille etc.

Subsequently, the animal used daily dose of antibiotics (AUD) per prescription was calculated by dividing the total animal weight that was estimated to be treated with antibiotics by the total amount of weight of the sheep/goats in kilograms (kg small ruminant) present in the herd.

Of the 5,989 prescriptions of antibiotics, the exact date of delivery was known for 4,803 deliveries. Of the remaining 1,095 prescriptions only the year of delivery could be provided by the veterinary practices. If the exact date of delivery was known the amount of treated weight was divided by the total amount of weight in kilograms present on that date, otherwise the average weight in the year of delivery was used.

The weight of the small ruminants in the herd was based on the number of sheep and/or goats in each age category, multiplied by the corresponding standard weight. The standard weights differentiate sheep and goats into five categories (Table 1).

The animal used daily dose (AUDD) per prescription was summed to calculate the AUDD/Y for each herd in 2011 and 2012 (Formula 2).

$$AUDD/Y_j = \sum_{ij=1}^{n} \frac{\text{kg treated}_{ij}}{\text{kg small ruminant}_{ij}} \qquad (2)$$

Where:

AUDD/Y : estimated animal used daily dose of antibiotics per year

Kg treated : the total weight of sheep/goat in kilograms treated with the antibiotics prescribed by the veterinarian

Kg small ruminant : the total weight of small ruminant in kilograms present in the herd at the moment the antibiotics are prescribed

i : each of the antibiotic deliveries

j : 2011 or 2012

Herds that did not receive any antibiotics in a year had an AUDD/Y of 0. Descriptive statistics were used to describe the AUDD/Y for the entire small ruminant industry and for each small ruminant subtype. Median tests [14] and proportion tests were used to evaluate differences in proportion of herds with

Table 1. Description of the different weight and age categories that were used by the Agricultural Economical Institute (LEI) to differentiate between species and ages within the small ruminant industry.

Species	Category	Weight in kg	Age in days
Sheep	Ewe	75	>365
Sheep	Lamb	22	0–365
Goat	Milking goat	75	>365
Goat	Rearing kid	37,5	31–365
Goat	Kid	7	0–30

antibiotic use, and to evaluate differences in the AUDD/Y between small ruminant subtypes.

The data that were used for this study are freely available upon request according to the data sharing policies of PLOS ONE. Requests can be directed to the small ruminant department of GD Animal Health in the Netherlands.

Results

Descriptives

The twelve veterinary practices had an average of 423 clients with small ruminants, of which a median of 84 (mean 99) and 120 (mean 113) received antibiotics in 2011 and 2012 respectively. The number of farms for which each veterinary practice prescribed antibiotics varied from 20 to 246 in 2011, and from 26 to 232 in 2012 (Table 2).

In total, the twelve practices prescribed antibiotics to small ruminant holdings 7,483 times during the analysed period. The median number of times each veterinary practice prescribed antibiotics to herds with small ruminants was 261 in 2011, and 299 in 2012. The number of prescriptions of antibiotics ranged from 77 to 841 in 2011, and from 74 to 779 in 2012 (Table 2).

All small ruminant farms with complete data were classified into one of the four small ruminant subtypes (Table 3).

Within the professional goat farms subtype that received antibiotics, 75% and 74% of the farms (46 in 2011, and 51 in 2012) were dairy goat farms. All of the dairy goat farms received antibiotics at least once in both years. The non-dairy professional goat farms were often much smaller than the dairy goat farms and also received antibiotics less often (15 out of 26, and 18 out of 29 non-dairy professional goat farms received antibiotics in 2011 and 2012 respectively). The percentage of farms for which antibiotics had been prescribed ranged from 8% in the small scale goat farms to 85% and 86% in the professional goat farms (Table 3).

The dairy goat farms were the largest herds with a median herd size of 834 and 833 goats in 2011 and 2012, respectively. These herds were part of the professional goat farms subtype, which had a median herd size of 746 and 691 goats in 2011 and 2012. With these herd sizes, the professional goat farms that used antibiotics and were included in this study were somewhat larger compared to the average professional goat herds in the Netherlands (median 658 in 2012). In addition, small scale goat farms that used antibiotics in 2011 and/or 2012 were larger as well, compared to the average small scale goat farm in the Netherlands (median 11 vs. median 3 in both years).

In the professional and small scale sheep farms that used antibiotics in 2011 and/or 2012, there was a median of 64 and 13 sheep in 2011, and 70 and 13 sheep in 2012 respectively. These herd sizes were comparable to the median herd sizes of all professional and small scale sheep farms in the Netherlands (median 65 and 11 in 2012).

Most antibiotics prescribed to small ruminants in this study were applied parentally (78% in 2011 and 81% in 2012) or orally (10% and 7%, respectively). In sporadic cases antibiotics were applied by intramammary or intrauterine routes (Figure 3). The third most used method of application of antibiotics in small ruminants was by means of ointments on the eyes, however, antibiotics that were applied as ointments on the eyes or skin (cutaneous) were excluded for the calculation of the AUDD/Y. (See 2.3 Data validation).

Animal used daily dose of antibiotics per year

For the calculation of AUDD/Y data on antibiotic deliveries and average standard weighs were used. Therefore, the AUDD/Y in this study presents an estimation of the AUDD/Y. The median AUDD/Y in herds with small ruminants that used antibiotics was 0.73 and 0.70 (mean 2.73 and 2.26) in 2011 and 2012 respectively (Table 4). However, there was a large variation in the AUDD/Y between herds, with many farms having an AUDD/Y slightly above 0, and only a small number of farms with a high AUDD/Y (Figure 4). The values of AUDD/Y in farms with small ruminants ranged from 3.7×10^{-4} to 181 in 2011, and from 1.8×10^{-5} to 219 in 2012 (Table 4). The AUDD/Y in the years 2011 and 2012 in

Table 2. Descriptive results of the number of connected small ruminant farmers, the number of farmers that were prescribed antibiotics, and the number of times antibiotics were prescribed by the twelve veterinary practices that cooperated in this study in the Netherlands.

Year	Median [mean] number of farms per veterinary practice	Number of farms for which antibiotics were prescribed		Number of times antibiotics were prescribed by the veterinary practices	
		Median [mean]	Range	Median [mean]	Range
2011	423 [415]	84 [99]	20–246	261 [296]	77–841
2012	423 [415]	120 [113]	26–232	299 [327]	74–779

Table 3. The number of farms included the study with or without the use of antibiotics in 2011 and/or 2012 for each subtype of small ruminant farm in the Netherlands.

Small ruminant farm subtype		With antibiotic use		Without antibiotic use		% with antibiotic use
		dairy	other	dairy	other	
Professional goat farms (≥32 goats)	2011	46	15	0	11	85
	2012	51	18	0	11	86
Professional sheep farms (≥32 sheep)	2011	0	566	0	636	47
	2012	0	686	0	502	58
Small scale goat farms (<32 goats)	2011	0	52	0	566	8
	2012	0	51	0	582	8
Small scale sheep farms (<32 sheep)	2011	0	208	0	1,776	10
	2012	0	243	0	1,761	12

farms with antibiotic use were not significantly different from each other. When farms without antibiotics use in one or both years were included as well, the median AUDD/Y was 0 (mean 0.62 in 2011, and 0.60 in 2012).

In 25 and 27 farms (3%) with small ruminants that used antibiotics in 2011 and 2012 respectively, an AUDD/Y above ten was found. Of the 25 farms with an AUDD/Y above ten in 2011, 18 farms only housed small ruminants, 6 farms also housed cattle, and one farm housed multiple other livestock species besides small ruminants. Of the 27 farms with an AUDD/Y above ten in 2012, 15 only housed small ruminants, ten farms also housed cattle, and two farms housed multiple other livestock species. Out of the seven and eight herds in 2011 and 2012 with the highest AUDD/Y (≥ 50), three and four farms (50%) had a combination of small ruminants and cattle on their farm. This percentage was higher than the percentage of combined farms with small ruminants and cattle in the whole studied population (34%), but this difference was not significant (P-value>0.05).

As stated previously, the percentage of subtypes of farms with small ruminants that used antibiotics ranged from 8% to 85% in 2011 and from 8% to 86% in 2012. Corrected for the percentage of farms with antibiotic use, the median AUDD/Y varied from 0 in both types of small scale holders, and professional sheep farms, to 1.22 in professional goat farms in 2011. In 2012, the median AUDD/Y in all farms that were included ranged from 0 in both types of small scale holders, and 0.10 in professional sheep farms, to 0.73 in professional goat farms (Table 5). Professional sheep and goat farms had a significantly higher AUDD/Y compared to the small scale sheep and goat farmers (P-Chisq<0.001). In addition, professional goat farms also had a significantly higher AUDD/Y than the professional sheep farms in both years (P-Chisq<0.001).

Most antibiotics were prescribed in the first months of the year, with the highest quantity in March. In the Netherlands, these months represent the lambing season [15]. Especially in dairy herds, almost no antibiotics were prescribed in the period when no lambs were born, i.e. between September and January. In the non-

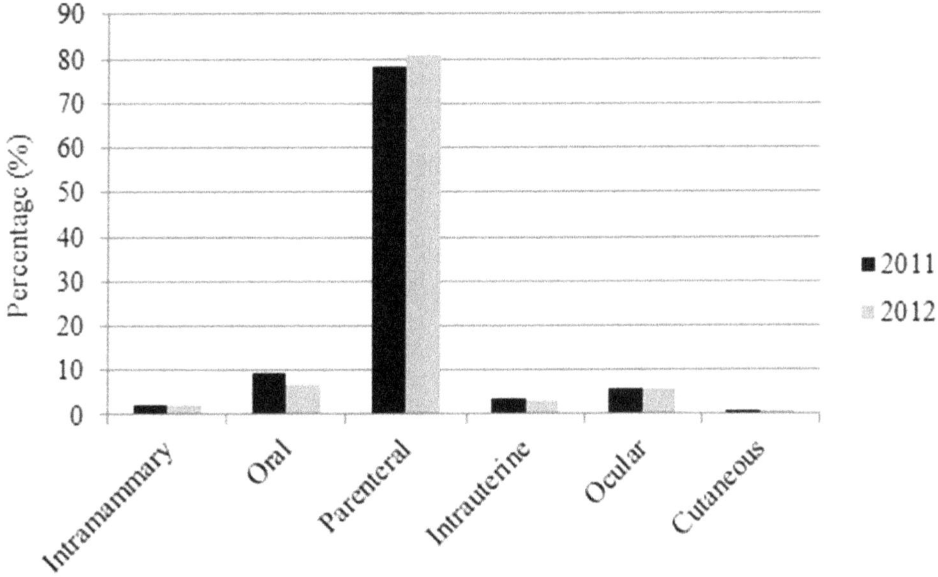

Figure 3. The application methods of antibiotics for small ruminants in 2011 and 2012 in the Netherlands.

Table 4. The percentage of farms for which antibiotics were prescribed, and the estimated animal used daily dose of antibiotics per year (AUDD/Y) in 2011 and 2012 in all farms with small ruminants in the Netherlands, and in farms with antibiotic use only.

	% farms for which antibiotics were prescribed	Median [mean] AUDD/Y in all small ruminant farms	Median [mean] AUDD/Y in farms with antibiotic use	Range in AUDD/Y on farms with antibiotic use
2011	23%	0 [0.62]	0.73 [2,73]	3.7×10^{-4}–181
2012	27%	0 [0.60]	0.70 [2,26]	1.8×10^{-5}–219

dairy herds, besides the prescriptions in the lambing season, antibiotics were prescribed at a low rate throughout the year.

The AUDD/Y per subtype of farms with small ruminants was subdivided into 14 classes based on the active substance of the antibiotic. Penicillin was most commonly used, both in 2011 and in 2012, in small scale sheep and goat farms and in professional sheep farms (Figure 4). In the professional goat farms, antibiotics containing aminoglycosides were the most used class (Figure 5).

Discussion

The median AUDD/Y in farms with small ruminants was 0 in both 2011 and 2012 (mean 0.62 and 0.60). The highest median values of the AUDD/Y were found in the professional goat industry. The small scale farmers had the lowest AUDD/Y values. In this study, all antibiotics that had been prescribed by one of the twelve veterinary practices to clients that kept at least one small ruminant were included. We decided to select veterinary practices rather than individual farmers, because in this way it was possible, within the framework of the study, to include a large number of herds with small ruminants (N = 5,399). The disadvantage of this decision was that the farms included might not be fully representative for the whole small ruminant population in the Netherlands. However, it appeared that parameters such as the ratio of herds between different subtypes, and herd sizes of farms included, were comparable to those of the entire small ruminant population. Therefore it was concluded that the results presented in this study give an accurate representation of antibiotic use in the entire small ruminant population in the Netherlands. Nevertheless, the AUDD/Y calculated in this study might be slightly biased because it was not possible to include farms that 1) did not have an UHI number or 2) did have an UHI number but were not registered in the I&R system. This was the case in 24% and 21% of the farms with antibiotic use in 2011 and 2012 respectively, and in 28% of the farms without antibiotic use. From January 1st 2010 onwards, all farms with small ruminants are obliged to register their animals and animal movements in the I&R database. This database improves every year, but is not yet complete. After some additional research in cooperation with the veterinary practices, it was concluded that the majority of farms with missing I&R data were small herds that only kept a few small ruminants. The descriptive results of small ruminant farms to which antibiotics had been prescribed but for which no AUDD/Y could be calculated, showed that antibiotics were prescribed less frequently to these farms compared to farms with complete data (results not presented). Therefore it was concluded that removal of these farms from the analyses probably has resulted in a slight overestimation of the AUDD/Y in small ruminant farms.

Antibiotics were not prescribed to all farms with small ruminants in 2011 or 2012. According to the participating veterinarians this was as expected, because the likelihood that a farmer with only a few small ruminants would need antibiotics every year was relatively small, especially when these animals are only kept for companion purposes. Nevertheless, prescription of antibiotics to these small scale farms might lead to a theoretical overestimation of the AUDD/Y because veterinarians are obliged to supply a complete bottle of antibiotics while this bottle might not be used completely. This was also apparent in our data on the amount of antibiotic deliveries. If Small scale goat or sheep holders used antibiotics, then the AUDD/Y in their flock was higher than in the professional sheep farms and comparable to the AUDD/Y in professional goat farms.

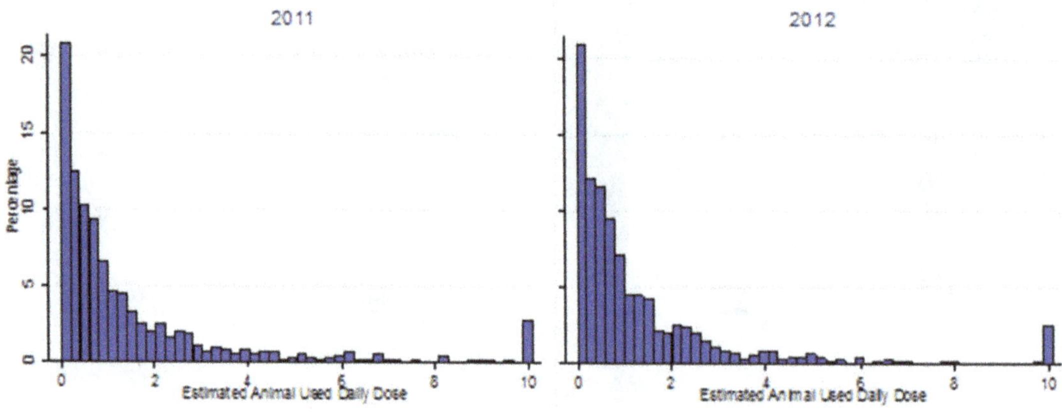

Figure 4. The distribution of the estimated Animal Used Daily Dose of antibiotics per year (AUDD/Y) in farms with small ruminants for which antibiotics were prescribed in 2011 and 2012. Values for AUDD/Y above ten were a rare event and are therefore set at ten for clarity of the figure.

Table 5. The percentage of farms in this study for which antibiotics were prescribed, and the estimated animal used daily dose of antibiotics per year (AUDD/Y) in 2011 and 2012 for farms with antibiotic use and all farms with small ruminants in the Netherlands, per subtype of small ruminant farms.

		% farms for which antibiotics were prescribed	Median [mean] AUDD/Y on farms with antibiotic use	Median [mean] AUDD/Y on all small ruminant farms
Professional goat farms (≥32 goats)	2011	85%	1.57 [16.84]	1.22 [14.27]
	2012	86%	1.27 [8.00]	0.73 [6.81]
Professional sheep farms (≥32 sheep)	2011	47%	0.60 [0.96]	0 [0.45]
	2012	58%	0.59 [1.10]	0.10 [0.63]
Small scale goat farms (<32 goats)	2011	8%	1.52 [2.13]	0 [0.18]
	2012	8%	1.47 [5.48]	0 [0.44]
Small scale sheep farms (<32 sheep)	2011	10%	1.61 [3.55]	0 [0.37]
	2012	12%	1.19 [3.20]	0 [0.39]

We had access to the exact quantity of antibiotics that the participating veterinary practices delivered to small ruminant herds. It was unknown whether these antibiotics were actually used and if they were used at the prescribed dose. Nevertheless, for small ruminant herds in the Netherlands, antibiotics are almost exclusively prescribed to treat clinical signs, which makes it very likely that the prescribed antibiotics were used immediately after delivery. In addition, the possible overestimation in AUDD/Y we assume in small scale farms, is expected to be small in large scale farms. In these herds, in almost all cases complete bottles of antibiotics will be used and if antibiotics remain after treatment, these will be used on a later notice. Although we believe that the obligatory rule of delivering bottles instead of millilitres might have led to a slight overestimation in our calculations, this will only play a minor role because most antibiotics are used by large scale farms in which antibiotic delivery gives a reliable indication of the actual use.

It was remarkable that antibiotics were only prescribed to 47% and 58% of the professional sheep farms in 2011 and 2012 respectively. This percentage did not increase with increasing numbers of animals per farm (>150 sheep; 46% in 2011, and 60% in 2012). This was not as expected, because beforehand it was hypothesized that the large majority of these professional sheep farms would need to use antibiotics every year. This hypothesis was supported by the fact that a Canadian study found that 94% of the sheep herds used antibiotics during a year [16]. Nevertheless, the herds in their study were much larger (average flock size of 197 ewes) compared to the professional sheep farms in this study. The finding that for a part of the professional sheep farms no antibiotics were prescribed in one or both years was discussed with the veterinary practices. The veterinarians indicated that 1) a part of the farms were probably no longer affiliated to the veterinary practice concerned and 2) a part of the farms did receive antibiotics during the analysed years, but that these antibiotics were probably accidentally assigned to the cattle.

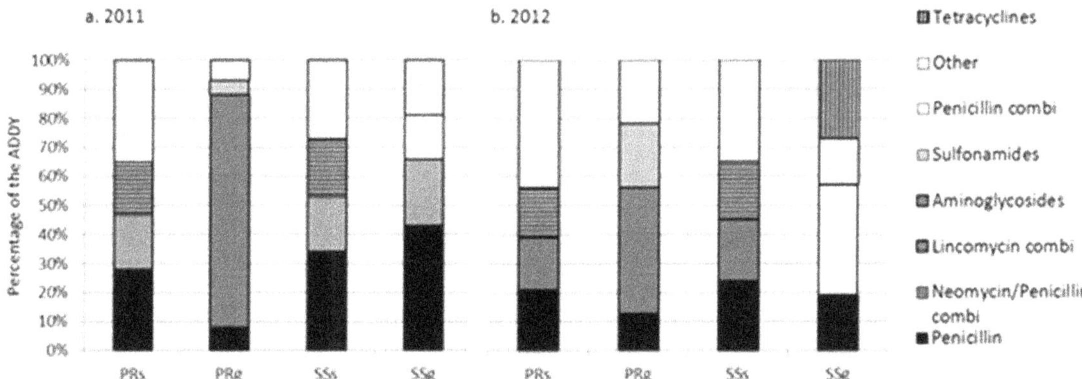

Figure 5. The distribution of the three most frequently used classes of active substances, and the rest summarized in the category "other", presented as percentages of the total estimated animal used daily dose of antibiotics per year (AUDD/Y) in 2011 (a) and 2012 (b) per subtype of small ruminant farms in the Netherlands (PRs: professional sheep farms (≥32 sheep), PRg: professional goat farms (≥32 goats), SSs: small scale sheep farms (<32 sheep), SSg: small scale goat farms (<32 goats). The category "other" can, besides the 7 classes already described in the legend of the figure, also contain TMPS, Polymixins, Macrolides, Lincomycins, Fluoroquinolones, Fenicoles, Cephalosporins.

Nevertheless, all veterinarians stated that they are becoming more and more aware of the importance of a correct registration of prescribed antibiotics, and declared that the registration in 2012 had already been improved compared to 2011. This was also visible in the data that showed an 11% increase in antibiotic use in professional sheep farms in 2012 compared to 2011. There were no indications that the quantity of antibiotics prescribed to herds with small ruminants had increased between 2011 and 2012, and therefore it was assumed that at least a part of this increase was caused by the improved quality of registration. Nevertheless, these flaws in registration might have led to a slight underestimation of the total AUDD/Y in the professional sheep farms.

In the small ruminant industry, a median AUDD/Y of 0 was found both in 2011 and in 2012. This was lower than the median AUDD/Y in veal (27.0 in 2011, and 21.0 in 2012), pigs (5.5 in 2011, and 6.2 in 2012), poultry (20.9 in 2011, and 17.1 in 2012) and cattle (1.5 in 2012) in the Netherlands [12]. The median AUDD/Y of small ruminants was comparable to the median AUDD/Y of suckling and fattening cows that also had a median AUDD/Y of 0. There are a few studies that looked at the number of antibiotic treatments in Canadian sheep, but in these studies the exact amount of prescribed and used antibiotics was unknown [16,17]. To our knowledge, no studies have been published on the quantity of antibiotic use in small ruminants in other European countries, but as in the Dutch situation, antibiotic use in other livestock species appeared to be higher [18–21]. Although no information was available on antibiotic use in small ruminants in other European countries, we have no reasons to believe that there will be large differences, given the fact that the sheep and goat industry in these countries is more or less comparable to the Dutch situation.

Penicillin was most often used in sheep flocks and small scale goat herds, and aminoglycosides were mostly used in the professional goat herds. In Canadian sheep, antibiotics belonging to the penicillin class were also found to be most frequently used [16,17]. In addition, tetracyclines were in the top three of most frequently used antibiotics in Canada, which is in accordance with our study.

In the entire livestock industry, aminoglycosides only play a minor role in the total quantity of prescribed antibiotics. Most antibiotics used in livestock in the Netherlands are tetracyclines or a combination of trimethoprim and sulfonamides. Products with penicillin, or a combination of penicillin and other active substances, were the third most used class of antibiotics in the Netherlands in 2012 [12]. In other countries, the most frequently used class of antibiotics also differs between different livestock species. However, in all species, antibiotics containing penicillin as the active substance were frequently used as well [19–22].

Because there is a relation between the use of antibiotics and development of antibiotic resistance [23], the use of antibiotics should be minimized as much as possible. The quantity of antibiotics used in the small ruminant industry appeared to be low with a median value of 0, which meant that more than 50% of the farms with small ruminants did not use any antibiotic during a whole year. This can partly be explained because a majority of farmers keep small ruminants on a small scale as companion animals. These farms only used antibiotics in sporadic cases. But even in the professional goat industry, median values of the AUDD/Y did not exceed the AUDD/Y of other livestock species that are kept in the Netherlands. Furthermore, in the Dutch small ruminant industry antibiotics appeared to be prescribed mostly to treat illness, while in other livestock industries these products were also used extensively on a prophylactic basis. Although the general use of antibiotics was found to be low, there appeared to be a small number of herds with small ruminants that had a very high AUDD/Y. It is recommended that these herds will be investigated more closely, to determine the reasons for the high rate of antibiotic use and to develop measures to reduce the use in these herds as appropriate.

This study aimed at quantifying the amount of antibiotics used in the small ruminant industry. We did not study the relation between the AUDD/Y and AMR. From a Canadian study it is known that in sheep, most AMR is found to tetracyclines [7]. However, these authors conclude that the overall AMR in Canadian sheep is low. Whether these results are also valid for small ruminants in the Netherlands is unknown and it is recommended to look into the relation of antibiotic use in Dutch small ruminants and AMR in more detail.

Conclusion

In this study, the antibiotic use in the small ruminant industry in the Netherlands was estimated for the years 2011 and 2012. The median AUDD/Y was 0 both in 2011 and in 2012 (mean 0.62 and 0.60). This AUDD/Y is lower than this parameter reported in other livestock industries. Most antibiotics were prescribed to the professional goat industry. Nevertheless, the AUDD/Y in the professional goat industry was also lower compared to the AUDD/Y in other livestock industries. With the low usage of antibiotics in the small ruminant industry, it is likely that this industry might only play a minor role in the development of antibiotic resistance in the entire livestock industry.

Acknowledgments

This study was facilitated by the Dutch Ministry of Economic Affairs. We would like to thank the twelve participating veterinary practices for their data input in this study. In addition, we are very grateful to the pharmacy of the Faculty of Veterinary Medicine, Utrecht University, for providing the dataset that contained all the antibiotic manual information.

Author Contributions

Analyzed the data: ISB. Contributed reagents/materials/analysis tools: ISB SL RvdB PV. Wrote the paper: ISB GvS RvdB PV JH MG SL.

References

1. Ungemach FR, Müller-Bahrdt D, Abraham G (2006) Guidelines for prudent use of antimicrobials and their implications on antibiotic usage in veterinary medicine. Int. J. Med. Mic. 296: 33–38.
2. De Neeling AJ, Van den Broek MJM, Spalburg EC, Van Santen-Verheuvel MG, Dam-Deisz WDC, et al. (2007) High prevalence of methicillin resistant Staphylococcus aureus in pigs. Veterinary Microbiology 122: 366–372.
3. Scott LC, Menzies PI, (2011) Antimicrobial resistance and small ruminant veterinary practice. Vet. Clin. North Am. Food Anim. Pract. 27: 23–32.
4. Silbergeld EK, Graham J, Price LB (2008) Industrial food animal production, antimicrobial resistance, and human health. Annual Review Public Health 29: 151–169.
5. Graveland H, Duim B, van Dijkeren E, Heedrik D, Wagenaar JA (2011) Livestock-associated methicillin-resistant Staphylococcus aureus in animals and humans. Int. J. Med. Microbiol. 301: 630–634.
6. Hendriksen RS, Mevius DJ, Schroeter A, Teale C, Meunier D, et al. (2008) Prevalence of antimicrobial resistance among bacterial pathogens isolated from cattle in different European countries: 2002–2004. Acta Vet. Scand. 50: 28 doi:10.1186/1751-0147-50-28.
7. Scott L, Menzies P, Reid-Smith RJ, Avery BP, McEwen SA, et al. (2012) Antimicrobial resistance in fecal generic Escherichia coli and Salmonella spp. obtained from Ontario sheep flocks and associations between antimicrobial use and resistance. Can. J. Vet. Res. 76: 109–119.

8. LNV (2008) Convenant to reduce antibiotic resistance in livestock farming in the Netherlands (in Dutch). Available: http://www.rijksoverheid.nl/documenten-en-publicaties/kamerstukken/2008/12/08/convenant-antibioticaresistentie-dierhouderij.html. Accessed 15 September 2013.
9. MARAN-2012 (2013) Monitoring of Antimicrobial Resistance and Antibiotic Usage in Animals in the Netherlands in 2012. Available: http://www.wageningenur.nl/nl/Expertises-Dienstverlening/Onderzoeksinstituten/central-veterinary-institute/Publicaties-CVI/MARAN-Rapporten.htm. Accessed 25 September 2013.
10. Santman-Berends IMGA, Van den Brom R, Van Schaik G, Vellema P (2013) Data-analyses of the small ruminant industry in 2013 (in Dutch). GD Animal Health Service, Deventer 2013.
11. Krol DJ (2007) Inventarisation of the small ruminant industry in the Netherlands (in Dutch). GD Animal Health Service, Deventer, 2007.
12. SDA (2013) The use of antibiotics in livestock species in 2012 (in Dutch). Available: http://www.autoriteitdiergeneesmiddelen.nl/. Accessed 15 September 2013.
13. Stata Corporation (2013) Stata Software version 13. Stata Corporation, College Station, Texas, USA.
14. Kruskal WH, Wallis WA (1952) Use of ranks in one-criterion variance analysis. J. Am. Stat. Ass. 47: 583–621.
15. Van den Brom R, Moll L, Van Schaik G, Vellema P (2013) Demography of Q fever seroprevalence in sheep and goats in the Netherlands in 2008. Prev. Vet. Med. 109: 76–82.
16. Avery BP, Rajić A, McFall M, Reid-Smith RJ, Deckert AJ, et al. (2008) Antimicrobial use in the Alberta sheep industry. Can. J. Vet. Res. 72: 137–142.
17. Moon CS, Berke O, Avery BP, McEwen SA, Reid-Smith RJ, et al. (2010) Characteristics of drug use on sheep farms in Ontario, Canada. Can. Vet. J. 51: 1373–1378.
18. Vieira AR, Pires SM, Houe H, Emborg HD (2011) Trends in slaughter pig production and antimicrobial consumption in Danish slaughter pig herds, 2002–2008. Emidemiol. Infect. 139: 1601–1610.
19. Callens B, Persoons D, Maes D, Laanen M, Postma M, et al. (2012) Prophylactic and metaphylactic antimicrobial use in Belgian fattening pig herds. Prev. Vet. Med. 106: 53–62.
20. Pardon B, Catry B, Dewulf J, Persoons D, Hostens M, et al. (2012) Prospective study on quantitative and qualitative antimicrobial and anti-inflammatory drug use in white veal calves. J. Antimicrob. Chemother. 67: 1027–1038.
21. Persoons D, Dewulf J, Smet A, Herman L, Heyndrickx M, et al. (2012) Antimicrobial use in Belgian broiler production. Prev. Vet. Med. 105: 320–325.
22. Sawant AA, Sordillo LM, Jayarao BM (2005) A survey on antibiotic usage in dairy herds in Pennsylvania. J. Dairy Sci. 88: 2991–3000.
23. Tacconelli E (2009) Antimicrobial use: risk driver of multidrug resistant microorganisms in healthcare settings. Current Opinion in Infectious Disease 22: 352–358.

22

Evaluating the Accuracy of Molecular Diagnostic Testing for Canine Visceral Leishmaniasis Using Latent Class Analysis

Manuela da Silva Solcà[1], Leila Andrade Bastos[1], Carlos Eduardo Sampaio Guedes[1], Marcelo Bordoni[1], Lairton Souza Borja[1], Daniela Farias Larangeira[1,2], Pétala Gardênia da Silva Estrela Tuy[3], Leila Denise Alves Ferreira Amorim[3], Eliane Gomes Nascimento[4], Geraldo Gileno de Sá Oliveira[1,5], Washington Luis Conrado dos-Santos[1], Deborah Bittencourt Mothé Fraga[1,2,5], Patrícia Sampaio Tavares Veras[1,5]*

1 Laboratório de Patologia e Biointervenção, Centro de Pesquisa Gonçalo Moniz–Fundação Oswaldo Cruz, Salvador, Bahia, Brazil, 2 Escola de Medicina Veterinária, Universidade Federal da Bahia, Salvador, Bahia, Brazil, 3 Instituto de Matemática –Departamento de Estatística, Universidade Federal da Bahia, Salvador, Bahia, Brazil, 4 Centro de Referência em Doenças Endêmicas Pirajá da Silva (PIEJ), Jequié, Bahia, Brazil, 5 Instituto Nacional de Ciência e Tecnologia em Doenças Tropicais (INCT - DT), Salvador, Bahia, Brazil

Abstract

Host tissues affected by *Leishmania infantum* have differing degrees of parasitism. Previously, the use of different biological tissues to detect *L. infantum* DNA in dogs has provided variable results. The present study was conducted to evaluate the accuracy of molecular diagnostic testing (qPCR) in dogs from an endemic area for canine visceral leishmaniasis (CVL) by determining which tissue type provided the highest rate of parasite DNA detection. Fifty-one symptomatic dogs were tested for CVL using serological, parasitological and molecular methods. Latent class analysis (LCA) was performed for accuracy evaluation of these methods. qPCR detected parasite DNA in 100% of these animals from at least one of the following tissues: splenic and bone marrow aspirates, lymph node and skin fragments, blood and conjunctival swabs. Using latent variable as gold standard, the qPCR achieved a sensitivity of 95.8% (CI 90.4–100) in splenic aspirate; 79.2% (CI 68–90.3) in lymph nodes; 77.3% (CI 64.5–90.1) in skin; 75% (CI 63.1–86.9) in blood; 50% (CI 30–70) in bone marrow; 37.5% (CI 24.2–50.8) in left-eye; and 29.2% (CI 16.7–41.6) in right-eye conjunctival swabs. The accuracy of qPCR using splenic aspirates was further evaluated in a random larger sample (n = 800), collected from dogs during a prevalence study. The specificity achieved by qPCR was 76.7% (CI 73.7–79.6) for splenic aspirates obtained from the greater sample. The sensitivity accomplished by this technique was 95% (CI 93.5–96.5) that was higher than those obtained for the other diagnostic tests and was similar to that observed in the smaller sampling study. This confirms that the splenic aspirate is the most effective type of tissue for detecting *L. infantum* infection. Additionally, we demonstrated that LCA could be used to generate a suitable gold standard for comparative CVL testing.

Editor: Yara M. Traub-Csekö, Instituto Oswaldo Cruz, Fiocruz, Brazil

Funding: This work was supported by grants and fellowships from INCT (Instituto Nacional de Ciência e Tecnologia em Doenças Tropicais - http://inctdt.cebio.org - Grant number: 576269/2008-5) and PPUS - FAPESB (Programa de Pesquisa para o Sistema Único de Saúde - Fundação de Amparo a Pesquisa no Estado da Bahia - http://www.fapesb.ba.gov.br - Grant number: SUS0011/2010). The funders had no role in study design, data collection and analysis, decision to publish, or preparation of the manuscript.

Competing Interests: The authors have declared that no competing interests exist.

* Email: pveras@bahia.fiocruz.br

Introduction

Visceral leishmaniasis (VL) is a disease with both medical and veterinary importance that is endemic in Brazil, and in many other countries throughout Latin America, Asia, and Europe [1]. One of the etiological agents of VL is *Leishmania infantum* (syn. *Leishmania chagasi*), which is transmitted to vertebrate hosts through the bites of female sand flies [2–5].

Dogs are considered the main domestic reservoir for this parasite because of their high rates of infection and the high frequency of parasites found in their skin [6–9]. Once infected with *L. infantum*, dogs have clinical manifestations that range from asymptomatic to systemic, including weight loss or cachexia; hypertrophy of the lymph nodes; and changes to the skin such as onychogryphosis, footpad swelling, localized or generalized alopecia, skin ulcers, and nasal or periocular dermatitis. They can also present with pathological alterations such as anemia or hepatic and renal failure [10,11].

Canine visceral leishmaniasis (CVL) can be diagnosed using parasitological, serological, or molecular methods in conjunction with clinical and epidemiological parameters [12]. Serological tests to diagnose CVL are the most common procedures used worldwide [13], however they lack sensitivity and specificity, which makes diagnosing the disease difficult when animals present with low antibody titers or there is cross-reactivity [14–17]. Hence, additional tests could be advantageous for confirming the diagnosis of inconclusive cases. For use as a confirmatory test, the molecular detection of *Leishmania* spp. provides greater sensitivity and specificity than other diagnostic techniques [8,18].

Numerous studies have described highly sensitive detection of low parasitic loads using quantitative real-time PCR (qPCR) [19–21]. qPCR has also been used to monitor the tissue parasitic load in dogs following anti-*Leishmania* treatment in countries where this procedure is unrestricted [22,23].

Several invasive, and non-invasive, techniques have been used to obtain biological tissue samples to diagnose *Leishmania* infection using conventional PCR and qPCR. The biological samples most widely used for molecular diagnosis of *Leishmania* spp. infection in dogs are the spleen, bone marrow, lymph node, and skin [12,18,24]. However, molecular diagnostic tests in studies using these tissue types have produced variable, and sometimes conflicting results, for identifying *Leishmania*-infected dogs [19,25,26]. This might be because culturing the parasite, which has been used as the gold standard assay [27,28], has a low sensitivity threshold for detecting dogs with a low parasite burden [29,30], which compromises the accuracy evaluation of diagnostic testing.

Therefore, the authors hypothesized that the lack of a reliable gold standard assay could account for the varying accuracy of the molecular diagnostic tests for *Leishmania* infection in different tissues. Latent class analysis (LCA) appraises tests with imperfect reference standards [31–33] using a statistical model to construct the latent class variable. Recently, LCA has been used to accurately evaluate the results of serological tests for diagnosing CVL [34].

The aim of the present study was to determine which type of canine tissue sample in an area with endemic VL provided the highest rate of *Leishmania* DNA detection by qPCR. In addition, qPCR results were compared to parasitological and serological diagnostic tests to determine which test provided the most accurate diagnosis of *L. infantum* infection.

Materials and Methods

1. Ethics Statement

Experimental procedures involving dogs were performed in accordance with Brazilian Federal Law on Animal Experimentation (Law no. 11794), the guidelines for animal research established by the Oswaldo Cruz Foundation [35], and the Brazilian Ministry of Health Manual for the Surveillance and Control of VL [36]. The CPqGM - FIOCRUZ Institutional Review Board for Animal Experimentation approved protocols for both animal euthanasia and sample collection procedures (Permit Number: 015/2009; Permit Number 017/2010).

2. Dogs

As previously described by Lima etal. (2014), over a one week period in July 2010, 51 stray dogs were taken from the streets of Jequié, a municipality located in the State of Bahia, Brazil, which is an area endemic for CVL. These dogs were selected as part of a surveillance and control program for VL that our group conducted in collaboration with the Endemic Diseases Surveillance Program of the State Health Service [37]. A CVL diagnosis was established based on the presence or absence of the following clinical signs: emaciation, alopecia, anemia, conjunctivitis, dehydration, dermatitis, erosion, ulcerations, lymphadenopathy, and onychogryphosis as previously detailed by Lima etal. (2014). Dogs from Jequié were clinically classified as having mild (stage I), moderate (stage II), and severe CVL (stage III) according to Solano-Gallego etal. (2009) [38].

3. Tissue Sampling

Tissue samples were obtained during necropsies as previously described by Lima etal. (2014). Briefly, the dogs were anesthetized and then euthanized by intracardiac injection of a supersaturated solution of potassium chloride (2 mL/kg). Immediately before the lethal injection, 50 mL of blood were collected by intracardiac puncture. Blood samples were preserved in EDTA-2Na tubes (Greiner bio-one, Kremsmünster, Austria) and in blood collection tubes (BD Vacutainer; Becton, Dickinson and Co). During the necropsy, splenic aspirate samples were collected by puncturing the central region of the spleen and bone marrow samples were obtained by puncturing the wing of the ilium, approaching from the dorsal crest. Conjunctival swabs of the right and left eyes were taken by rubbing the swab multiple times against the surface of the lower eyelid. A small fragment of the popliteal lymph node was cut from the whole organ and a skin fragment was collected using a sterile 5 mm punch (Kolplast, Brazil) from the medial portion of the pinna. Tissue samples were collected using sterile needles, swabs, and blades and all of the samples were stored in DNAase- and RNAase-free tubes at $-70°C$ until DNA extraction.

4. Hematological and Biochemical Parameters

Hematological and biochemical parameters were evaluated on the day of the necropsy. Total red blood cell and white blood cell counts were determined using an automated cell counter (Pentra 80 counter, ABX Diagnostics, Montpellier, France). Microhematocrit tubes containing blood samples were centrifuged at 12,000 rpm for 5 min, and then the hematocrit levels were estimated. Serum was collected by centrifuging the Vacutainer tubes, and was used for the biochemical tests including total protein, globulin, albumin, blood urea nitrogen, and creatinine, using an enzymatic colorimetric method with an A15 autoanalyzer (BioSystems, Barcelona, Spain).

5. Serological and Parasitological Tests

The following serological tests were performed to detect anti-*Leishmania* antibodies: the DPP CVL rapid test which detects rk28-specific antibodies and the EIE CVL with crude *L. major* antigen diagnostic test provided by FIOCRUZ (Bio-Manguinhos Unit, Rio de Janeiro, Brazil). These serum tests were performed in accordance with manufacturer instructions. An in-house ELISA, with crude *L. infantum* antigen was also performed as previously described [39,40]. Parasitological evaluation was performed by culturing part of the splenic aspirate collected during necropsy in Novy–MacNeal–Nicolle (NNN) biphasic medium supplemented with 20% Fetal Bovine Serum (FBS – Gibco BRL, New York, USA) and 100 μg/mL gentamicin to avoid contamination (Sigma Chemical Co., St. Louis, MO) for four weeks at 24°C [41]. Parasites were detected using microscopy performed at weekly intervals for no less than four weeks. Each splenic culture was prepared in duplicate. All of the culture labels were double-checked to avoid misidentification.

Parasite isolates were randomly selected from five dogs and sent to the national reference laboratory for *Leishmania* typing at the Oswaldo Cruz Institute (CLIOC, Rio de Janeiro, RJ, Brazil). The isolates were typed using monoclonal antibodies and enzyme electrophoresis analysis in order to determine the *Leishmania* species.

6. Control Samples

Splenic aspirate samples from 20 dogs that had previously been identified as *Leishmania*-positive from an endemic area [18] were used as positive controls. Splenic aspirates of 20 healthy dogs from the municipality of Pelotas, Rio Grande do Sul, Brazil, an area without endemic CVL, were used as negative controls. All of the healthy dogs had no clinical signs of CVL, and tested negative for infection using the in-house ELISA, parasite culturing, and qPCR techniques.

7. Sample Handling and Decontamination Procedures

Due to the high degree of sensitivity inherent in qPCR, exceptional care was taken to avoid cross-contamination during not only the sample collection procedures, but also during DNA extraction and qPCR testing. As previously described [18], all procedures were carried out in an environment that was suitable for sample collection and qPCR procedures. All of the disposable surgical materials were used for a single animal, and the laminar flow hood was decontaminated by UV radiation before each procedure. Filter tips were routinely used throughout all DNA extraction steps and when performing the qPCR [42].

8. DNA Extraction

DNA was obtained from 200 µL of splenic and bone marrow aspirate, 200 µL of blood, 20 mg of lymph node, and 20 mg of a skin fragment using a DNeasy Blood & Tissue Kit (Qiagen, Hilden, Germany) in accordance with the manufacturer's protocols. DNA samples from the conjunctival swabs were purified using a phenol–chloroform method as previously described [42]. The DNA pellets were suspended in 30 µL of Tris–EDTA buffer (10 mmol/L Tris and 1 mmol/L EDTA, pH 8.0). Once extracted, the quality and concentration of each DNA sample were evaluated using a digital spectrophotometer (NanoDrop ND-1000, Thermo Scientific, Wilmington, USA) [43]. All of the DNA samples were adjusted to a final concentration of 30 ng/µL, aliquoted, and kept at −20°C until the qPCR assays were performed.

Parasite DNA was extracted from *L. infantum* (MHOM/BR2000/MERIVALDO), *Leishmania amazonensis* (MHOM/Br88/Ba-125), *Leishmania braziliensis* (MHOM/BR/94/H3456), and *Leishmania major* (MHOM/RI//WR-173) promastigotes cultivated at 24°C. For the DNA extraction, the parasites were counted and centrifuged. DNA was extracted from pellets corresponding to a known number of parasites in accordance with the Qiagen protocols.

9. Quantitative PCR (qPCR)

9.1 Inclusion and exclusion criteria. To assess positivity, DNA samples were only included in the analysis if they met the minimum quality criteria: i) the DNA sample concentration was above 30ng/µl; ii) DNA samples amplified with the same efficiency as the DNA curve; and iii) amplification of the 18s rRNA housekeeping gene was successful. Any samples that did not fulfill one or more of the above inclusion criteria were excluded, only 10 out of 51 for skin fragments and 26 out of 51 for bone marrow aspirate. To compare parasitic load in different tissue types, DNA samples were only included in the analysis if they met the minimum quality criteria for all tissue types (samples from 20 dogs out of 51).

9.2 Quantitative PCR Assay. qPCR was used to determine the amount of parasite DNA in canine tissue samples. qPCR assays were performed following an amplification protocol previously described by Francino etal. (2006). The qPCR technique targeted a conserved region of *L. infantum* kDNA to obtain a 120-bp amplicon. All of the reactions were performed in triplicate. The reaction was in a final volume of 25 µL containing: 5 µL (150 ng) of each DNA sample diluted in deionized water and 20 µL of the PCR mixture. The PCR mixture contained: 12.5 µL of Universal Mastermix (Life Technology Corporation, Carlsbad, CA-USA), the forward primer 5′-AACTTTTCTGGTCCTCCG-GGTAG-3′ (LEISH-1) and the reverse primer 5′-ACCCCCA-GTTTCCCGCC-3′ (LEISH-2) both at a final concentration of 900 nM, and a fluorogenic probe 5′-AAAAATGGGTGCAGAA-AT-3′ with a FAM reporter molecule attached to the 5′ end and an MGB-NFQ quencher (200 nM final concentration) linked to the 3′-end (Life Technology Corporation). In order to overcome limitations caused by endogenous PCR inhibitors in the blood, skin fragment, and conjunctival swab samples, all of the steps leading up to DNA amplification were performed in the presence of bovine serum albumin (5 µg/each reaction) (Sigma Chemical) [44].

9.3 Quantification of *Leishmania* kDNA. Quantification of *Leishmania* kDNA was performed using an absolute method based on comparing the cycle threshold (Ct) values from the samples to a standard curve, which was constructed using serial 10-fold dilutions from 10^5 to 10^{-1} parasites performed in triplicate. Reactions were performed using the Applied Biosystems 7500 Fast Real-Time PCR System (Life Technology Corporation). The reaction was carried out under the following conditions: 1 cycle at 50°C for 2 min, 1 cycle at 95°C for 10 min, and 40 two-step cycles, first at 95°C for 15 s and then at 60°C for 1 min. In order to minimize variability between plates, the values from each plate were normalized using a common fluorescence detection baseline. Each sample's Ct value was calculated by determining the point at which its fluorescence signal was above the established detection baseline. The Ct cut-off value was determined using a Receiver-Operator Characteristic (ROC) curve. The optimal Ct cut-off value for the parasite kDNA qPCR assay was determined by calculating sensitivity and specificity for different Ct cut-off points and the ROC curve derived from the amplification values of *Leishmania*-negative samples and *Leishmania*-positive samples (see item 6). Tissue samples were considered positive when the Ct values were equal to or less than the Ct cut-off point determined using the ROC curve analysis. If the standard deviation between triplicates was >0.38, the sample set was reanalyzed by qPCR [45]. The efficiency of the qPCR protocol was evaluated by calculating the slope value of the standard curve for the parasite kDNA. This value, −3.657 (SD = 0.148), was obtained from the mean slope values of nine independent experiments with a correlation coefficient (R^2) of 0.998.

9.4 Assessment of qPCR Analytical Sensitivity and Specificity. Analytical sensitivity was evaluated by determining whether the presence of host tissue interferes with the amplification profiles when using qPCR to detect *L. infantum* DNA in infected dogs. First, a standard curve was constructed using ten-fold dilutions from reference strain *L. infantum* DNA (see item 9.3). Next, a ten-fold dilutions of reference strain *L. infantum* DNA was mixed with the splenic aspirate DNA from negative control animals (see item 6) and another standard curve was constructed from these dilutions. Finally, the amplification profiles of the two curves were compared. The analytical specificity of the qPCR analysis was assessed by comparing the amplification profiles of DNA samples from the *L. infantum* reference strain to profiles from several other *Leishmania* species, including the New World *L. amazonensis* and *L. braziliensis*, and the Old World *L. major*. As described in item 9.3, standard curves for each species were constructed from ten-fold serial dilutions ranging from 10^5 to 10^{-1} parasites performed in triplicate. Analytical specificity was further assessed by evaluating the amplification profiles of DNA obtained from other canine pathogens, such as *Ehrlichia canis* and *Babesia canis*. Briefly, 150 ng of DNA from each pathogen was amplified and compared to the *L. infantum* amplification profile.

9.5 Quantification of 18S rRNA Gene Expression. The expression of the canine housekeeping gene 18S rRNA was measured in order to normalize the concentration of input DNA for each sample and to obtain a reference amplification value to ensure the use of high-quality DNA samples [46]. TaqMan Pre-Developed Assay Reagents (Life Technology Corporation) were used to detect and quantify 18S rRNA gene expression. All of the reactions were performed at a final volume of 25 μL containing: 5 μL of DNA canine tissue sample diluted in deionized water and 20 μL of PCR mixture. The PCR mixture contained: 12.5 μL of Universal Mastermix (Life Technology Corporation), 1.25 μL of 18S GeneEx Assay primer and probe sets (Life Technology Corporation) at a concentration of 20x, and deionized water to obtain the final volume. The positive and negative controls for the housekeeping genes were plated in triplicate and the samples were plated in duplicate. Reactions were performed on an Applied Biosystems 7500 Fast Real-Time PCR System (Life Technology Corporation) using the following protocol: 1 cycle at 50°C for 2 min; 1 cycle at 95°C for 10 min; and 40 two-step cycles, first at 95°C for 15 s and then 50°C for 1 min. A seven point standard curve was constructed for the housekeeping gene ranging from 450–18.75 ng. The slope of the standard curve for the 18s rRNA gene was −3.399 (SD = 0.296), which represents the mean slope value of 11 independent experiments with the corresponding coefficient of determination (R^2) of 0.990.

9.6 Parasitic Load in DNA Samples. Samples from 20 of the 51 dogs were used to determine which tissue type harbored the highest parasitic load by comparing the splenic and bone marrow aspirates, blood, conjunctival swab of right and left eyes, lymph node and skin fragments. The parasitic load was expressed as the number of parasites normalized to the established reference amplification value for the 18S rRNA gene in 150 ng of DNA from each tissue sample [47]. Then the value obtained was calculated per 100 mg of host tissue DNA.

10. Evaluation of qPCR accuracy using splenic aspirate samples from a prevalence study

The accuracy of the qPCR assay was evaluated using splenic samples obtained from 800 dogs during a random prevalence study performed in Camaçari, BA, an endemic area for CVL in Brazil. All 800 dogs were clinically evaluated and classified as described in item 2. They were also tested using the following CVL diagnostic methods: DPP CVL rapid test, EIE CVL, our in-house ELISA, and parasite cultures from splenic aspirates as described in item 5. qPCR analysis of splenic aspirate samples was performed as described in item 9.

11. Statistical Analysis

In order to prevent bias, serological, parasitological and molecular techniques were performed and their results were judged without knowledge of the outcome of the other tests.

The ROC curve data analysis described in item 9.3 was performed using GraphPad Prism software v.5.0 (GraphPad Prism Inc., San Diego, CA). Differences in the parasitic load between each type of biological sample were assessed using the Friedman test followed by the Dunn's multiple comparison test. The relationship between parasitic load in the spleen and qPCR positivity in each infected tissue was assessed with the Spearman correlation test using log transformed values for the parasitic load ($p<0.05$).

For the 800 dogs evaluated in the cross sectional study, the intensity of the parasitic load in the spleen (item 9.6) was categorized into three ranges: $<10^4$, 10^4–10^6, and $>10^6$. The number of clinical signs in the dogs (item 2) was stratified into four ranges: 0 (no clinical signs), 1–3, 4–6, and >6 clinical signs. Fisher's exact test was used to evaluate the association between the number of clinical signs and the splenic parasitic load ranges.

LCA was performed using a statistical model to define a latent variable that could be used as a gold standard. To define a latent variable that could accurately identify *L. infantum* infection, three indicators representing serologic (DPP CVL), parasitological (culture from splenic samples), and molecular (splenic aspirate qPCR) diagnostic techniques were included. Animals were grouped into two categories, 'infected dogs', and 'not-infected dogs'. The latent classes were estimated and characterized using two parameters: (a) item-response probabilities and (b) class prevalence, which is the probability of belonging to a latent class according to the response pattern. The estimate was performed using the maximum likelihood with expectation-maximization (EM) algorithm. The goodness of fit of the statistical model was evaluated using entropy, which varied between 0 and 1, with the value 1 indicating that the individuals are perfectly classified into the latent classes. Average probabilities for each latent class, which expresses the uncertainty of global classification, were also assessed *a posteriori,* considering a higher *a posteriori* probability to be a better goodness of fit for the statistical model. The Vuong-Lo-Mendell-Rubin likelihood ratio test was used to choose the number of classes in LCA [48]. The Akaike information criterion (AIC) and Bayes information criterion (BIC) were also evaluated for each model. LCA was performed using the software Mplus 5.2, the syntax for fitting LCA in MPlus program is reported in Appendix S1 [49]. Additionally, the conditional independence was checked by evaluation of significant bivariate residuals [50,51].

The sensitivity and 95% confidence interval (CI) were calculated for each diagnostic technique and each tissue type analyzed, using the LCA latent variable as gold standard. The accuracy (sensitivity and specificity) of the qPCR technique using splenic aspirates was further evaluated with the LCA in a random sample of 800 dogs. Sensitivity of each test was measured as the proportion of positive results, only among those identified as such by the gold standard, while specificity was measured as the proportion of negative results, which were correctly identified as such by the gold standard.

Results

1. Sample description

All 51 dogs from the endemic area of Jequié were mixed-breed, their estimated ages varied from 1–10 years old, the animals weighed 5–30 kg, 45% (23/51) were males, and 55% (28/51) were females. All of the dogs exhibited clinical signs that could be related to CVL including splenomegaly (33/51), emaciation (17/51), hypertrophy of the lymph nodes (46/51), alopecia (21/51), cutaneous alterations (41/51), onychogryphosis (29/51), and ocular alterations (10/51). With respect to clinical pathology, 73% of the dogs presented with anemia (35/48), 98% with hypergammaglobulinemia (49/50), and 98% with hypoalbuminemia (49/50). Using the scale published by Solano-Gallego etal. (2009), all of the dogs were classified as having moderate CVL (stage II), except one animal that also exhibited a creatinine value greater than 1.4 mg/dL and was considered to have severe CVL (stage III).

2. Standardization of the qPCR Protocol

The Ct cut-off value for parasite DNA detection was performed using a ROC analysis. This analysis showed an area under the curve of 1.0, indicating a high probability ($p<0.001$) that a randomly chosen positive sample would be correctly classified.

The Ct cut-off value of 37.0 had prediction rates of 100% sensitivity (CI 83.16–100) and 95% specificity (CI 75.13–99.87) with a likelihood ratio of 20. The analytical sensitivity was then determined. We found that the amplification profile of the reference strain *L. infantum* DNA was similar to that of the reference strain mixed with splenic aspirate DNA from negative control animals. The lower limit of detection was then determined and corresponded to 0.016 parasites per reaction.

In terms of the analytical specificity, the Old World *L. major* parasite DNA samples were remarkably similar to those of *L. infantum* at all of the concentrations tested. In contrast, DNA from *L. amazonensis* and *L. braziliensis* could only be successfully amplified at concentrations of 10^4 and 10^5 parasites per reaction. This corresponded to the same number of cycles needed to amplify DNA from 0.02 parasites per reaction of the *L. infantum* reference strain (Figure S1). *E. canis* and *B. canis* DNA did not amplify using this qPCR protocol (data not shown). With respect to the housekeeping gene, attempts to amplify18S rRNA from DNA samples of *Leishmania* spp. resulted in no detectable qPCR amplification using the same primer set that successfully amplified the gene in canine DNA samples (data not shown).

3. Positivity of diagnostic techniques

Using qPCR, 100% of the dogs from Jequié (51/51) tested positive for parasite DNA in at least one of the tissue types analyzed. Among these, 98% (50/51) tested positive in the splenic aspirate samples; 80.4% (41/51) in blood samples; 68.3% (28/41) in skin fragments; 54.9% (28/51) in lymph node fragments; 35% (7/20) in bone marrow aspirate; 37.3% (19/51) in left eye conjunctival swabs, and 33.3% (17/51) in right eye conjunctival swabs.

Parasites were observed in 35.3% (18/51) of the parasite cultures from splenic aspirate and anti-*Leishmania* antibodies were detected in 43.8% (21/48), 47.1% (24/51), and 66.7% (34/51) of the canine serum samples using the EIE CVL, DPP CVL rapid test, and in-house ELISA, respectively.

4. Accuracy of the diagnostic tests

Latent class was used to provide a reliable estimate of sensitivity and specificity in order to select the tissue that provided the greatest accuracy for qPCR DNA detection. Serological, parasitological, and molecular techniques were used to determine prevalence of the latent classes and conditional probabilities in the LCA model for *L. infantum* infection in dogs. The probability that a dog from Jequié would be classified as infected using the LCA model was 47.1%. Among the animals considered infected by the LCA, the probability that a dog would test positive using qPCR of the splenic aspirate was 95.8%. The probability that a dog tested positive using either DPP CVL or by parasite culture from splenic aspirates was 100.0% or 54.2%, respectively (Table 1).

Entropy was then calculated to assess how well the animals were classified *a posteriori* by the model. The entropy of the Jequié samples was 1.0; indicating accuracy in the classification of dogs using LCA. Moreover, *a posteriori* average probabilities that animals were properly classified into the latent classes "Infected" and "Not Infected" were 100% in both cases in the Jequié animals. The Lo-Mendel-Rubin test indicated that the model with 2 classes was a better fit for the data obtained from the Jequié dogs ($p<0.01$) when compared with the model with only 1 class (data not shown). These results are supported by the analysis of the AIC and BIC (data not shown).

The sensitivity of the tests employed in Jequié to diagnose *L. infantum* infection was assessed employing the latent variable obtained by LCA as the gold standard (Figure 1). Splenic aspirates

Table 1. Prevalence of latent classes and conditional probabilities to the LCA model for *L. infantum* infection detection in dogs.

		Dogs from Jequié n = 51			Dogs from Camaçari n = 800		
Technique	**Result**		**Latent Classes**			**Latent Classes**	
			Infected n = 24 (47.1%)	**Not Infected n = 27 (52.9%)**		**Infected n = 120 (14.5%)**	**Not Infected n = 680 (85.5%)**
		Result Frequency (%)	**Conditional Probabilities (%)**		**Result Frequency (%)**	**Conditional Probabilities (%)**	
DPP CVL	**Positive**	47.1	100.0	0.0	16.6	82.9	5.5
	Negative	52.9	0.0	100.0	83.4	17.1	94.5
Splenic Aspirate Culturing	**Positive**	35.3	54.2	18.5	13.2	87.8	0.0
	Negative	64.7	45.8	81.5	86.8	12.2	100.0
Splenic Aspirate qPCR	**Positive**	98.0	95.8	100.0	34.2	93.3	24.1
	Negative	2.0	4.2	0.0	65.8	6.7	75.9

provided the highest sensitivity of the available tissues sampled achieving 95.8% (95%CI 90.4–100) of sensitivity. The sensitivity attained in other tissues ranged from 80% to 30% as follows: lymph node fragments 79.2% (95%CI 68–90.3), skin fragments 77.3% (95%CI 64.5–90.1), blood 75% (95%CI 63.1–86.9), bone marrow aspirates 50% (95%CI 30–70), left eye swab 37.5% (95%CI 24.2–50.8), and right eye swab 29.2% (95%CI 16.7–41.6). It was not possible to calculate splenic qPCR specificity since only one sample tested negative in this method. Specificity of the other tissues achieved 66.7% for lymph node fragments (95%CI 53.7–79.6) as well as for bone marrow aspirates (95%CI 47.8–85.6), 63% (95%CI 49.7–76.2) for right and left eye swabs, 42.1% (95%CI 27–57.2) for skin fragments and 14.8% (95%CI 5.1–24.6) for blood. Considering the other diagnostic tests, the sensitivity of the serological tests was 100% for the DPP CVL, followed by 79.2% (95%CI 68–90.3) for the in-house ELISA, 65.2% (95%CI 51.7–78.7) for EIE CVL, while sensitivity for the splenic aspirate culturing was 54.2% (95%CI 40.5–67.8). The specificity was highest for DPP CVL 100%, followed by splenic parasite cultures 81.5% (95%CI 70.8–92.1), EIE CVL 76% (95%CI 63.9–88.1), in-house ELISA 44.4% (95%CI 30.8–58.1).

5. Parasitic load in different tissue types

To further characterize tissue performance for the molecular diagnostic assay, parasitic loads were determined in the different tissues analyzed. As shown in Table 2 a considerable degree of variation was observed among the samples with values ranging from 120 parasites in a splenic aspirate sample up to 186 million parasites found in a bone marrow aspirate sample. However, the median parasitic load was higher in splenic aspirate samples than in the conjunctival swabs from either eye ($p<0.05$) or bone marrow aspirate ($p<0.05$). No statistically significant differences were observed when comparing parasitic loads in the splenic aspirate to the blood or skin tissue samples.

6. Distribution of parasitic load according to number of clinical signs

The distribution of parasitic load according to the number of clinical signs is displayed in Table 3. We observed a significant positive association between the intensity of parasitic load in the spleen and the number of clinical signs present in the dogs. Animals with no clinical signs ($p<0.01$) or those exhibiting 1–3 clinical signs ($p<0.001$) had lower parasitic loads in splenic tissue

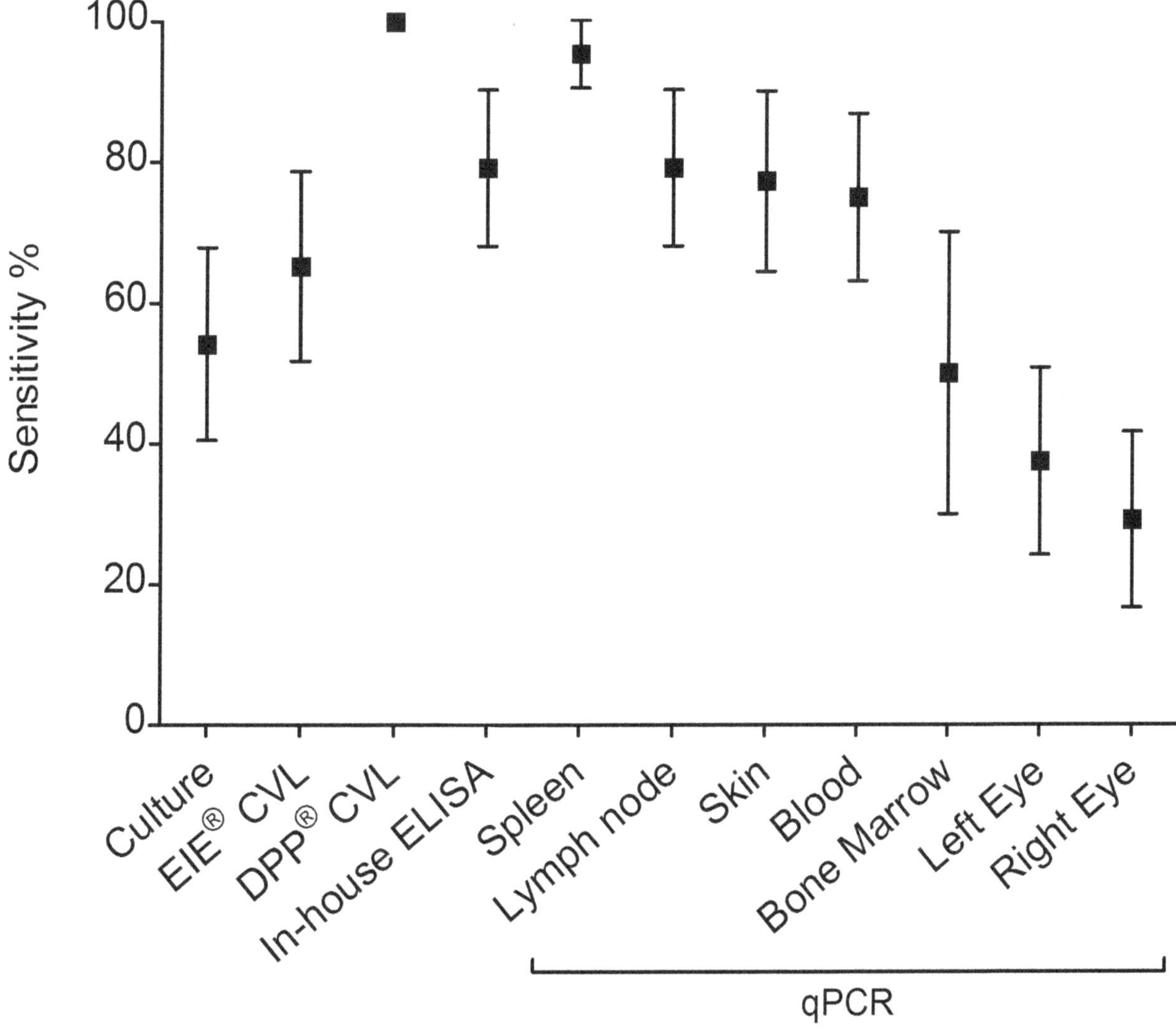

Figure 1. Sensitivity of the different diagnostic techniques employed in the biological samples obtained from Jequié animals (n = 51). Vertical bars represent the 95% confidence intervals. Sensitivity values were obtained using the latent variable as the gold standard.

Table 2. Parasitic loads detected in different canine tissue types from a total of 20 dogs from the endemic area of Jequié.

Tissue type	Positivity	Parasitic loads[a]				
		Minimum	25% Percentile	Median	75% Percentile	Maximum
Splenic Aspirate	100% (20/20)	120	1,088	4,365	14,325	74,000,000
Blood	70% (14/20)	0	0	7,960	19,800	228,000
Skin Fragment	60% (12/20)	0	0	1,870	21,500	32,400,000
Lymph node Fragment	60% (12/20)	0	0	830.5	9,288	7,800,000
Bone Marrow Aspirate	35% (07/20)	0	0	0.0*	28,275	186,000,000
Left Eye Swab	50% (10/20)	0	0	645.0*	2,073	240,000
Right Eye Swab	35% (07/20)	0	0	0.0*	3,141	147,000

[a]number of parasites normalized by the established reference amplification value for the housekeeping gene 18S rRNA in 100 mg of host tissue DNA.
*$p<0.05$ Friedman's together with Dunn's multiple comparisons test of splenic aspirates and swab of right or left eye and splenic aspirates and bone marrow.

($<10^4$). In contrast, animals with >6 clinical signs ($p<0.01$) showed relatively higher loads ($>10^6$). The dogs presenting with 4–6 clinical signs were homogeneously distributed throughout the three ranges.

7. Accuracy of qPCR using splenic aspirate samples from a prevalence study

Splenic aspirate samples collected from a random study conducted in the endemic area of Camaçari were used to evaluate the high sensitivity observed for the qPCR technique developed using convenience sampling from Jequié. Positive diagnoses in the samples from Camaçari varied according to diagnostic test. In this sample, 34.2% were positive using qPCR, 24.4% using EIE CVL, 19.8% using the in-house ELISA, and 16.6% using DPP CVL.

Similar to the samples from Jequié, LCA was used to analyze the results from the Camaçari samples. Reliability of the LCA model was evaluated and the probability of an animal being infected with *L. infantum* was calculated. The response patterns obtained from the latent class model that were used are listed in Table 4. Animals from Camaçari that had at least two positive test results were classified by the LCA model as 'Infected'. However, the presence of a positive result from the splenic aspirate parasite culture implied a 100% probability of being infected with *L. infantum*, regardless of the DPP CVL and splenic aspirate qPCR results. When dogs from this endemic area tested negative by all three diagnostic techniques, the probability that the animal was infected with *L. infantum* was 0%. Furthermore, the probability of animals being infected was still very low when only splenic aspirate qPCR (2.7%) or DPP CVL (1.4%) tested positive according to this LCA model.

The entropy of the Camaçari samples was 0.934, and the *a posteriori* average probabilities of being correctly classified as "Infected" and "Not Infected" were, respectively, 92.4% and 99.3%. Similar to the analysis performed with samples from Jequié, using random samples, the Lo-Mendel-Rubin test indicated that the model with 2 classes was optimal and was supported by the analysis of the AIC and BIC (data not shown).

Using LCA, the sensitivity of the splenic aspirate qPCR (95%; 95%CI 93.5–96.5) was higher than for the other diagnostic tests: DPP CVL (86.4%; 95%CI 84.1–88.8), splenic parasite cultures (83.5%; 95%CI 80.8–86.2), the in-house ELISA (78.3%; 95%CI 75.5–81.2), and EIE CVL (72.5%; 95% CI 69.4–75.6) (Figure 2A). However, the specificity was highest for splenic parasite cultures (100%), followed by DPP CVL (95.6%; 95%CI 94.2–97), the in-house ELISA (90.6%; 95%CI 88.6–92.6), EIE CVL (84.1%; 95%CI 81.6–86.6), and splenic aspirate qPCR (76.7%; 95%CI 73.7–79.6) (Figure 2B).

Discussion

The present study found that a qPCR protocol targeting *Leishmania* kDNA provided the highest diagnostic sensitivity in dogs from Jequié when compared to standard serological and parasitological methods. In this endemic area, the DPP CVL rapid test and EIE CVL were able to detect infection in 47.1% and 43.8%, respectively, of a population of symptomatic dogs. Interestingly, 100% of these dogs tested positive with respect to at least one of the tissue types analyzed using qPCR. Similar results have been obtained by other studies, in which high sensitivity was achieved using molecular techniques [14,16,52]. Together these results reinforce the notion that the number of

Table 3. Distribution of parasitic load according to number of clinical signs in dogs from the prevalence study.

Number of Clinical Signs	Splenic Parasitic Load Ranges			Fisher Exact Test
	$<10^4$	10^4–10^6	$>10^6$	
0	8 (57.1%)	5 (35.7%)	1 (7.1%)	$p<0.01$
1–3	55 (42%)	49 (37.4%)	27 (20.6%)	$p<0.001$
4–6	37 (39.4%)	27 (28.7%)	30 (31.9%)	$p=0.11$
>6	5 (16.1%)	9 (29.0%)	17 (54.8%)	$p<0.01$
Total	105	90	75	

Table 4. Response patterns[a] of Camaçari dogs for LCA model with 2 latent classes for diagnosis of CVL.

Response pattern					
DPP CVL	**Splenic Aspirate Culturing**	**Splenic Aspirate qPCR**	**Frequency Observed % (n)**	**CVL Probability *a posteriori* (%)**	**Result Based on LCA**
N	N	N	60.1 (429)	0.0	Not infected
N	N	P	20.5 (146)	1.4	Not infected
P	N	N	3.6 (26)	2.7	Not infected
N	P	N	0.1 (01)	100.0*	Infected
P	N	P	2.7 (19)	54.7	Infected
N	P	P	2.1 (15)	100.0	Infected
P	P	N	0.7 (05)	100.0	Infected
P	P	P	10.2 (73)	100.0	Infected

[a]Response patterns of all samples tested using the three techniques.
*Estimation based on only one animal sample presenting this pattern.
N: Negative; P: Positive.

infected dogs detected by serological surveys in endemic areas is severely underestimated [53,54].

Several methods have been recently developed for the molecular detection of *Leishmania* spp. [20,21,55], that provide divergent results when used in a variety of clinical canine samples [54]. Among the tissues analyzed, the authors observed that splenic aspirate samples provided the highest detection rate, successfully identifying 98% of the samples that tested positive. This result is supported by the fact that the spleen is a key site for parasite multiplication in naturally infected dogs [24,56]. Interestingly, following splenic aspirate samples, 80.4% of blood samples tested positive using qPCR. In addition, we found that the parasitic loads achieved were similar in the blood and splenic aspirate samples. These are promising results given that drawing blood is a much less invasive sampling technique to detect *Leishmania* infection in dogs than obtaining splenic aspirates. In contrast, several other studies have found that bone marrow and lymph node tissues offered a higher number of positive results than

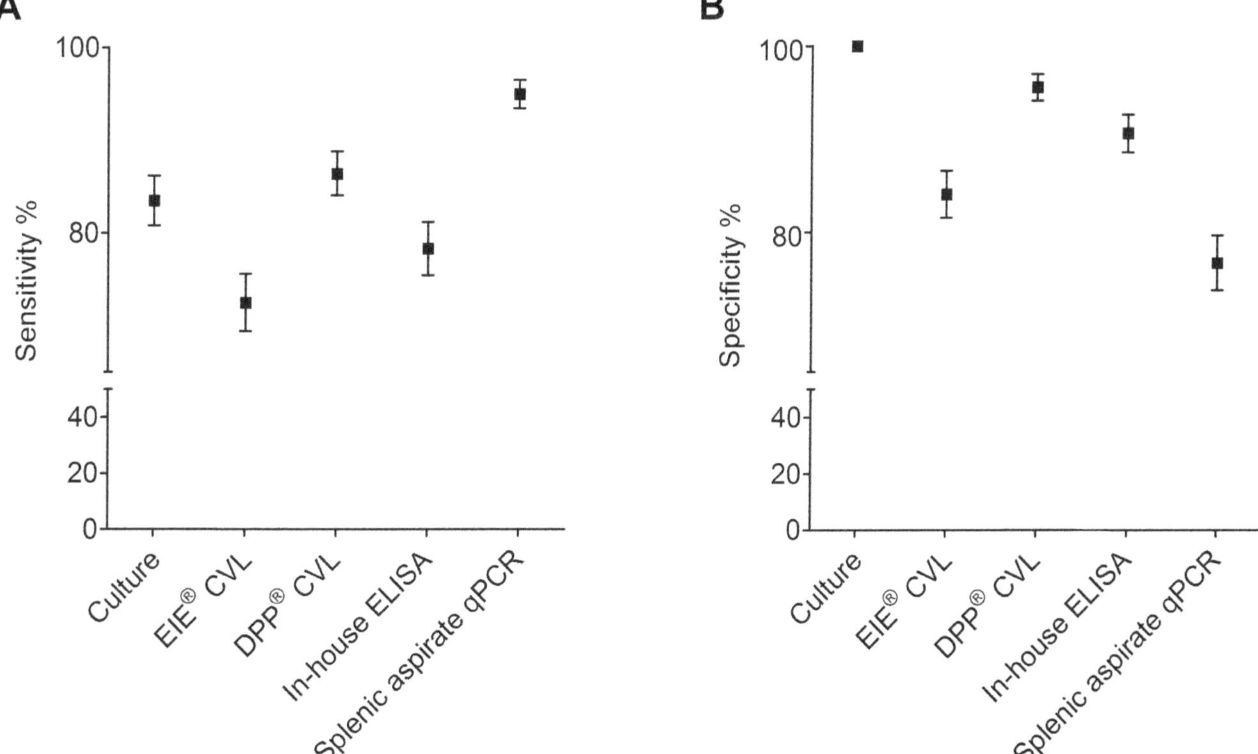

Figure 2. Sensitivity and specificity of the different diagnostic techniques employed in the biological samples obtained from Camaçari animals (n = 800). Vertical bars represent the 95% confidence intervals. **A)** Sensitivity and **B)** Specificity values obtained using the latent variable as the gold standard.

blood [46,55,57,58]. Francino etal. (2006) suggested that using qPCR to detect *Leishmania* parasites in blood samples might be sufficient to diagnose infection given the technique's ability to quantify extremely low parasitemia. However, other authors consider the blood to be a poor source of *Leishmania* DNA [59], mostly because blood samples do not have satisfactory detection rates using conventional PCR. The underlying cause of these poor results may be the high frequency of PCR inhibitors found in blood, in addition to low parasitic loads, which could lead to false negatives especially in asymptomatic dogs [52]. Serum albumin can be added to avoid any potential inhibiting effects in qPCR reaction [44]. In the present study we added serum albumin to blood, skin, and conjunctival swab samples. Our results demonstrate that splenic aspirates or blood can be effectively used to detect parasite DNA using qPCR [18,19].

The analytical specificity of the qPCR technique was also evaluated in the present study by comparing the amplification profiles of *L. infantum* DNA to other Old and New World *Leishmania* species. The amplification profile of the Old World species *L. major* was remarkably similar to that of *L. infantum* (Figure S1). This corroborates other studies that have shown a great deal of similarity between the genomes of these species [60]. To the best of our knowledge, *L. major* is not known to be a causative agent of CVL, nor have any cases linked to this parasite been reported in Latin America [61]. kDNA from New World parasites, such as *L. amazonensis* and *L. braziliensis*, was successfully amplified using this protocol, but only at high concentrations of 10^4 and 10^5 parasites per reaction (Figure S1). Protocols capable of distinguishing between *Leishmania* species are preferable in endemics areas for both cutaneous and visceral forms of the disease [62]. In this study, five *Leishmania* species isolated from the dogs were identified by multilocus enzyme electrophoresis as *L. infantum*. Nonetheless, the use of splenic aspirate samples can avoid misleading diagnostic results since visceralization of *L. braziliensis* has not been reported and visceralization of *L. amazonensis* is a relatively rare event both in humans or dogs [62–64].

Regrettably, an ideal gold standard is still lacking for CVL diagnosis [65]. Historically, parasite culturing and immunofluorescence antibody test (IFAT) have been abundantly used. However, culturing is shown to have low sensitivity, while IFAT low specificity [65]. An alternative to using a single technique as the gold standard is to utilize LCA, once this method defines a latent variable to be used as gold standard, considering all diagnostic tests impartially. Indeed, LCA has been proved to successfully estimate the sensitivities and specificities of different diagnostic tests for several diseases [34,66–69]. LCA has been an useful tool for validating serological diagnostic methods for VL, since this analysis provides more realistic estimates of diagnostic test performance [34,67]. In the scientific community still exist concerns regarding the high sensitivity of qPCR results, especially when this technique is able to detect very low parasitic loads. In addition, some authors state that is impossible for qPCR to differentiate between the DNA of a living parasite and a dead one. Otherwise, Prina etal. (2007) [70] were the only ones that proved that as soon as 1 h after exposure to a substance able to kill the parasites, only less than 1% of the initial *Leishmania* DNA could be detected by qPCR. No other group demonstrated these results, especially using invivo experiments. Thus, in the present study, we have decided not to consider all the dogs as infected, even if they displayed parasite in at least one tissue by the qPCR, and perform the qPCR accuracy evaluation using the latent variable.

Employing the latent class variable as the gold standard, we found that the sensitivity for splenic aspirate qPCR and DPP CVL were 95.8% and 100% respectively, in a population of symptomatic dogs in Jequié. However, these results were limited since it was a small sample size. To address this, the results of the qPCR testing were evaluated using a larger random sampling of dogs that consisted of a population of positive and negative dogs, which are representative of the population of an endemic area for VL. In this random population survey using 800 dogs, the high sensitivity of splenic aspirate qPCR was confirmed achieving 95% of sensitivity, while the DPP CVL sensitivity was corrected to 83.5%. Despite the high sensitivity of the splenic aspirate qPCR, the specificity was relatively low (76.7%). This could be due to the large number of dogs from the randomly sampled population that tested positive only by splenic aspirate qPCR (20.5%) and were considered as 'Not infected' by the LCA. These animals were likely misclassified by LCA as false negatives, since the splenic aspirate qPCR is known to be the most sensitive diagnostic technique for CVL, most likely more sensitive than the variables used to define the variable latent class.

Several studies have demonstrated a positive correlation between clinical manifestations of CVL and parasitic load in the spleen, lymph nodes and skin using several techniques [20,41,56,71]. Using qPCR of splenic aspirate in dogs, we also found a positive association between parasitic load and clinical manifestations of CVL, reinforcing the notion that can be used not only for detection of infection but also to monitor disease severity in dogs.

Although splenic aspirate collection is considered an invasive procedure by many dog owners [27,72], Barrouin-Melo etal. (2006) noted that minor complications were observed in only three out of 257 dogs that underwent splenic aspiration. Complications can be further minimized by visualizing the spleen using an ultrasound device to guide splenic aspiration [72,73]. In our experience, during the prevalence study in the municipality of Camaçari, the splenic aspirate procedure assisted by ultrasonography was well tolerated in all 800 dogs without any reported complication.

In conclusion, the authors found that, the splenic aspirates and blood, provided the greatest sensitivity for detecting *Leishmania* DNA using qPCR. In addition, the results indicated that LCA could be used to create a suitable gold standard for diagnosis, since this technique offers a more comprehensive evaluation of the results obtained using different diagnostic testing methods for CVL.

Supporting Information

Figure S1 Amplification profiles of DNA samples from *Leishmania* spp. A) *L. infantum*; **B)** *L. major*; **C)** *L. amazonensis*; **D)** *L. braziliensis*. DNA samples derived from the *L. infantum* reference strain, and several other *Leishmania* species, including New World *L. amazonensis* and *L. braziliensis*, and Old World *L. major*. Standard curves were constructed using amplification patterns from ten-fold serial dilutions performed in triplicate ranging from 10^5 to 10^{-1} parasites per reaction.

Appendix S1 Syntax for fitting LCA in MPlus program.

Acknowledgments

The authors would like to thank Dr. Flávia W. Cruz McBride for support to obtain negative control samples in Pelotas, Dr. Virgínia Maria G. da Silva and Joselli S. Silva for the help in the endemic area. Additionally, the authors acknowledge Kyoshi Fukutani for help in the qPCR analysis. Finally, we are grateful to Andris K. Walter for providing English revision and consulting services and manuscript edition by native English-speaking experts from BioMed Proofreading LLC.

Author Contributions

Conceived and designed the experiments: MSS CESG DBMF PSTV. Performed the experiments: MSS LAB MB LSB DFL. Analyzed the data: MSS CESG PGSET LDAFA WLCS DBMF PSTV. Contributed reagents/materials/analysis tools: DFL GGSO EGN PGSET LDAFA. Wrote the paper: MSS CESG LDAFA DBMF PSTV.

References

1. Desjeux P (2004) Leishmaniasis. Nat Rev Microbiol 2: 692.
2. Killick-Kendrick R (1999) The biology and control of phlebotomine sand flies. Clin Dermatol 17: 279–289.
3. Kuhls K, Alam MZ, Cupolillo E, Ferreira GE, Mauricio IL, et al. (2011) Comparative microsatellite typing of new world *Leishmania infantum* reveals low heterogeneity among populations and its recent old world origin. PLoS Negl Trop Dis 5: e1155.
4. Lainson R, Shaw JJ (1978) Epidemiology and ecology of leishmaniasis in Latin-America. Nature 273: 595–600.
5. Mauricio IL, Stothard JR, Miles MA (2000) The strange case of *Leishmania chagasi*. Parasitol Today 16: 188–189.
6. Deane LM, Deane MP, Alencar JE (1955) [Control of *Phlebotomus longipalpis* by DDT house spraying endemic foci of kala-azar in Ceara]. Rev Bras Malariol Doencas Trop 7: 131–141.
7. Dye C (1996) The logic of visceral leishmaniasis control. Am J Trop Med Hyg 55: 125–130.
8. Gramiccia M, Gradoni L (2005) The current status of zoonotic leishmaniases and approaches to disease control. Int J Parasitol 35: 1169–1180.
9. Molina R, Amela C, Nieto J, San-Andres M, Gonzalez F, et al. (1994) Infectivity of dogs naturally infected with *Leishmania infantum* to colonized *Phlebotomus perniciosus*. Trans R Soc Trop Med Hyg 88: 491–493.
10. Ciaramella P, Oliva G, Luna RD, Gradoni L, Ambrosio R, et al. (1997) A retrospective clinical study of canine leishmaniasis in 150 dogs naturally infected by *Leishmania infantum*. Vet Rec 141: 539–543.
11. Koutinas AF, Polizopoulou ZS, Saridomichelakis MN, Argyriadis D, Fytianou A, et al. (1999) Clinical considerations on canine visceral leishmaniasis in Greece: a retrospective study of 158 cases (1989–1996). J Am Anim Hosp Assoc 35: 376–383.
12. Miro G, Cardoso L, Pennisi MG, Oliva G, Baneth G (2008) Canine leishmaniosis–new concepts and insights on an expanding zoonosis: part two. Trends Parasitol 24: 371–377.
13. Gomes YM, Paiva Cavalcanti M, Lira RA, Abath FG, Alves LC (2008) Diagnosis of canine visceral leishmaniasis: biotechnological advances. Vet J 175: 45–52.
14. Coura-Vital W, Marques MJ, Veloso VM, Roatt BM, Aguiar-Soares RD, et al. (2011) Prevalence and factors associated with *Leishmania infantum* infection of dogs from an urban area of Brazil as identified by molecular methods. PLoS Negl Trop Dis 5: e1291.
15. Ferreira Ede C, de Lana M, Carneiro M, Reis AB, Paes DV, et al. (2007) Comparison of serological assays for the diagnosis of canine visceral leishmaniasis in animals presenting different clinical manifestations. Vet Parasitol 146: 235–241.
16. Solano-Gallego L, Morell P, Arboix M, Alberola J, Ferrer L (2001) Prevalence of *Leishmania infantum* infection in dogs living in an area of canine leishmaniasis endemicity using PCR on several tissues and serology. J Clin Microbiol 39: 560–563.
17. Troncarelli MZ, Camargo JB, Machado JG, Lucheis SB, Langoni H (2009) *Leishmania* spp. and/or *Trypanosoma cruzi* diagnosis in dogs from endemic and nonendemic areas for canine visceral leishmaniasis. Vet Parasitol 164: 118–123.
18. Solca Mda S, Guedes CE, Nascimento EG, Oliveira GG, dos Santos WL, et al. (2012) Qualitative and quantitative polymerase chain reaction (PCR) for detection of *Leishmania* in spleen samples from naturally infected dogs. Vet Parasitol 184: 133–140.
19. Francino O, Altet L, Sanchez-Robert E, Rodriguez A, Solano-Gallego L, et al. (2006) Advantages of real-time PCR assay for diagnosis and monitoring of canine leishmaniosis. Vet Parasitol 137: 214–221.
20. Manna L, Reale S, Vitale F, Gravino AE (2009) Evidence for a relationship between *Leishmania* load and clinical manifestations. Res Vet Sci 87: 76–78.
21. Mary C, Faraut F, Lascombe L, Dumon H (2004) Quantification of *Leishmania infantum* DNA by a real-time PCR assay with high sensitivity. J Clin Microbiol 42: 5249–5255.
22. Maia C, Campino L (2008) Methods for diagnosis of canine leishmaniasis and immune response to infection. Vet Parasitol 158: 274–287.
23. Martinez V, Quilez J, Sanchez A, Roura X, Francino O, et al. (2011) Canine leishmaniasis: the key points for qPCR result interpretation. Parasit Vectors 4: 57.
24. Maia C, Ramada J, Cristovao JM, Goncalves L, Campino L (2009) Diagnosis of canine leishmaniasis: conventional and molecular techniques using different tissues. Vet J 179: 142–144.
25. Ferreira Sde A, Ituassu LT, de Melo MN, de Andrade AS (2008) Evaluation of the conjunctival swab for canine visceral leishmaniasis diagnosis by PCR-hybridization in Minas Gerais State, Brazil. Vet Parasitol 152: 257–263.
26. Lombardo G, Pennisi MG, Lupo T, Migliazzo A, Capri A, et al. (2012) Detection of *Leishmania infantum* DNA by real-time PCR in canine oral and conjunctival swabs and comparison with other diagnostic techniques. Vet Parasitol 184: 10–17.
27. Carvalho D, Oliveira TMFS, Baldani CD, Machado RZ (2009) An enzyme-linked immunosorbent assay (ELISA) for the detection of IgM antibodies against *Leishmania chagasi* in dogs. Pesquisa Veterinária Brasileira 29: 120–124.
28. Sundar S, Rai M (2002) Laboratory diagnosis of visceral leishmaniasis. Clin Diagn Lab Immunol 9: 951–958.
29. Moreira MA, Luvizotto MC, Garcia JF, Corbett CE, Laurenti MD (2007) Comparison of parasitological, immunological and molecular methods for the diagnosis of leishmaniasis in dogs with different clinical signs. Vet Parasitol 145: 245–252.
30. Ndao M (2009) Diagnosis of parasitic diseases: old and new approaches. Interdiscip Perspect Infect Dis 2009: 278246.
31. Baughman AL, Bisgard KM, Cortese MM, Thompson WW, Sanden GN, et al. (2008) Utility of composite reference standards and latent class analysis in evaluating the clinical accuracy of diagnostic tests for pertussis. Clin Vaccine Immunol 15: 106–114.
32. Butler JC, Bosshardt SC, Phelan M, Moroney SM, Tondella ML, et al. (2003) Classical and latent class analysis evaluation of sputum polymerase chain reaction and urine antigen testing for diagnosis of pneumococcal pneumonia in adults. J Infect Dis 187: 1416–1423.
33. Nascimento MC, de Souza VA, Sumita LM, Freire W, Munoz F, et al. (2007) Comparative study of Kaposi's sarcoma-associated herpesvirus serological assays using clinically and serologically defined reference standards and latent class analysis. J Clin Microbiol 45: 715–720.
34. Machado de Assis TS, Rabello A, Werneck GL (2012) Latent class analysis of diagnostic tests for visceral leishmaniasis in Brazil. Trop Med Int Health 17: 1202–1207.
35. Machado CJ, Filipecki AT, Teixeira MD, Klein HE (2010) Regulation of the use of animals in Brazil in the twentieth century and the process of forming the current regime applied to biomedical research. História, Ciências, Saúde-Manguinhos 17: 87–105.
36. Brasil MdSd (2006) Manual de vigilancia e controle da leishmaniose visceral: Ministerio da Saude - Secretaria de Vigilancia em Saude.
37. Lima IS, Silva JS, Almeida VA, Junior FG, Souza PA, et al. (2014) Severe clinical presentation of visceral leishmaniasis in naturally infected dogs with disruption of the splenic white pulp. PLoS One 9: e87742.
38. Solano-Gallego L, Koutinas A, Miro G, Cardoso L, Pennisi MG, et al. (2009) Directions for the diagnosis, clinical staging, treatment and prevention of canine leishmaniosis. Vet Parasitol 165: 1–18.
39. Baleeiro CO, Paranhos-Silva M, dos Santos JC, Oliveira GG, Nascimento EG, et al. (2006) Montenegro's skin reactions and antibodies against different *Leishmania* species in dogs from a visceral leishmaniosis endemic area. Vet Parasitol 139: 21–28.
40. Paranhos-Silva M, Freitas LA, Santos WC, Grimaldi GJ, Pontes-de-Carvalho LC, et al. (1996) A cross-sectional serodiagnostic survey of canine leishmaniasis due to *Leishmania chagasi*. Am J Trop Med Hyg 55: 39–44.
41. Barrouin-Melo SM, Larangeira DF, Trigo J, Aguiar PH, dos-Santos WL, et al. (2004) Comparison between splenic and lymph node aspirations as sampling methods for the parasitological detection of *Leishmania chagasi* infection in dogs. Mem Inst Oswaldo Cruz 99: 195–197.
42. Batista LF, Segatto M, Guedes CE, Sousa RS, Rodrigues CA, et al. (2012) An assessment of the genetic diversity of *Leishmania infantum* isolates from infected dogs in Brazil. Am J Trop Med Hyg 86: 799–806.
43. dos Santos Marques LH, Gomes LI, da Rocha IC, da Silva TA, Oliveira E, et al. (2012) Low parasite load estimated by qPCR in a cohort of children living in urban area endemic for visceral leishmaniasis in Brazil. PLoS Negl Trop Dis 6: e1955.
44. Giambernardi TA, Rodeck U, Klebe RJ (1998) Bovine serum albumin reverses inhibition of RT-PCR by melanin. Biotechniques 25: 564–566.
45. Naranjo C, Fondevila D, Altet L, Francino O, Rios J, et al. (2012) Evaluation of the presence of *Leishmania* spp. by real-time PCR in the lacrimal glands of dogs with leishmaniosis. Vet J 193: 168–173.
46. Solano-Gallego L, Rodriguez-Cortes A, Trotta M, Zampieron C, Razia L, et al. (2007) Detection of *Leishmania infantum* DNA by fret-based real-time PCR in urine from dogs with natural clinical leishmaniosis. Vet Parasitol 147: 315–319.
47. Manna L, Reale S, Viola E, Vitale F, Foglia Manzillo V, et al. (2006) *Leishmania* DNA load and cytokine expression levels in asymptomatic naturally infected dogs. Vet Parasitol 142: 271–280.
48. Muthen B, Asparouhov T (2012) Bayesian structural equation modeling: a more flexible representation of substantive theory. Psychol Methods 17: 313–335.

49. Muthen LK, Muthen BO (2007) Mplus - Statistical analysis with latent variable. Version 6.
50. Garrett ES, Zeger SL (2000) Latent class model diagnosis. Biometrics 56: 1055–1067.
51. Uebersax J (2009) A Practical Guide to Conditional Dependence in Latent Class Models. John Uebersax Enterprises LLC.
52. Lachaud L, Chabbert E, Dubessay P, Dereure J, Lamothe J, et al. (2002) Value of two PCR methods for the diagnosis of canine visceral leishmaniasis and the detection of asymptomatic carriers. Parasitology 125: 197–207.
53. Alvar J, Canavate C, Molina R, Moreno J, Nieto J (2004) Canine leishmaniasis. Adv Parasitol 57: 1–88.
54. Baneth G, Koutinas AF, Solano-Gallego L, Bourdeau P, Ferrer L (2008) Canine leishmaniosis - new concepts and insights on an expanding zoonosis: part one. Trends Parasitol 24: 324–330.
55. Maia C, Nunes M, Cristovao J, Campino L (2010) Experimental canine leishmaniasis: clinical, parasitological and serological follow-up. Acta Trop 116: 193–199.
56. Reis AB, Martins-Filho OA, Teixeira-Carvalho A, Carvalho MG, Mayrink W, et al. (2006) Parasite density and impaired biochemical/hematological status are associated with severe clinical aspects of canine visceral leishmaniasis. Res Vet Sci 81: 68–75.
57. de Almeida Ferreira S, Leite RS, Ituassu LT, Almeida GG, Souza DM, et al. (2012) Canine skin and conjunctival swab samples for the detection and quantification of *Leishmania infantum* DNA in an endemic urban area in Brazil. PLoS Negl Trop Dis 6: e1596.
58. Manna L, Reale S, Vitale F, Picillo E, Pavone LM, et al. (2008) Real-time PCR assay in *Leishmania*-infected dogs treated with meglumine antimoniate and allopurinol. Vet J 177: 279–282.
59. Reale S, Maxia L, Vitale F, Glorioso NS, Caracappa S, et al. (1999) Detection of *Leishmania infantum* in dogs by PCR with lymph node aspirates and blood. J Clin Microbiol 37: 2931–2935.
60. Peacock CS, Seeger K, Harris D, Murphy L, Ruiz JC, et al. (2007) Comparative genomic analysis of three *Leishmania* species that cause diverse human disease. Nat Genet 39: 839–847.
61. Alvar J, Velez ID, Bern C, Herrero M, Desjeux P, et al. (2012) Leishmaniasis worldwide and global estimates of its incidence. PLoS One 7: e35671.
62. Madeira MF, Schubach A, Schubach TM, Pacheco RS, Oliveira FS, et al. (2006) Mixed infection with *Leishmania (Viannia) braziliensis* and *Leishmania (Leishmania) chagasi* in a naturally infected dog from Rio de Janeiro, Brazil. Trans R Soc Trop Med Hyg 100: 442–445.
63. Barral A, Pedral-Sampaio D, Grimaldi Junior G, Momen H, McMahon-Pratt D, et al. (1991) Leishmaniasis in Bahia, Brazil: evidence that *Leishmania amazonensis* produces a wide spectrum of clinical disease. Am J Trop Med Hyg 44: 536–546.
64. Tolezano JE, Uliana SR, Taniguchi HH, Araujo MF, Barbosa JA, et al. (2007) The first records of *Leishmania (Leishmania) amazonensis* in dogs (*Canis familiaris*) diagnosed clinically as having canine visceral leishmaniasis from Aracatuba County, Sao Paulo State, Brazil. Vet Parasitol 149: 280–284.
65. Rodriguez-Cortes A, Ojeda A, Francino O, Lopez-Fuertes L, Timon M, et al. (2010) *Leishmania* infection: laboratory diagnosing in the absence of a "gold standard". Am J Trop Med Hyg 82: 251–256.
66. Hartnack S, Budke CM, Craig PS, Jiamin Q, Boufana B, et al. (2013) Latent-class methods to evaluate diagnostics tests for Echinococcus infections in dogs. PLoS Negl Trop Dis 7: e2068.
67. Boelaert M, Rijal S, Regmi S, Singh R, Karki B, et al. (2004) A comparative study of the effectiveness of diagnostic tests for visceral leishmaniasis. Am J Trop Med Hyg 70: 72–77.
68. Pan-ngum W, Blacksell SD, Lubell Y, Pukrittayakamee S, Bailey MS, et al. (2013) Estimating the true accuracy of diagnostic tests for dengue infection using bayesian latent class models. PLoS One 8: e50765.
69. Wu X, Berkow K, Frank DN, Li E, Gulati AS, et al. (2013) Comparative analysis of microbiome measurement platforms using latent variable structural equation modeling. BMC Bioinformatics 14: 79.
70. Prina E, Roux E, Mattei D, Milon G (2007) *Leishmania* DNA is rapidly degraded following parasite death: an analysis by microscopy and real-time PCR. Microbes Infect 9: 1307–1315.
71. Sanchez MA, Diaz NL, Zerpa O, Negron E, Convit J, et al. (2004) Organ-specific immunity in canine visceral leishmaniasis: analysis of symptomatic and asymptomatic dogs naturally infected with *Leishmania chagasi*. Am J Trop Med Hyg 70: 618–624.
72. Watson AT, Penninck D, Knoll JS, Keating JH, Sutherland-Smith J (2011) Safety and correlation of test results of combined ultrasound-guided fine-needle aspiration and needle core biopsy of the canine spleen. Vet Radiol Ultrasound 52: 317–322.
73. Barrouin-Melo SM, Larangeira DF, de Andrade Filho FA, Trigo J, Juliao FS, et al. (2006) Can spleen aspirations be safely used for the parasitological diagnosis of canine visceral leishmaniosis? A study on assymptomatic and polysymptomatic animals. Vet J 171: 331–339.

23

Using Informatics and the Electronic Medical Record to Describe Antimicrobial Use in the Clinical Management of Diarrhea Cases at 12 Companion Animal Practices

R. Michele Anholt[1]*, John Berezowski[2], Carl S. Ribble[1,3], Margaret L. Russell[4], Craig Stephen[1,3]

1 Faculty of Veterinary Medicine, University of Calgary, Calgary, Alberta, Canada, **2** Veterinary Public Health Institute, University of Bern, Bern, Switzerland, **3** Centre for Coastal Health, Nanaimo, British Columbia, Canada, **4** Community Health Sciences, University of Calgary, Calgary, Alberta, Canada

Abstract

Antimicrobial drugs may be used to treat diarrheal illness in companion animals. It is important to monitor antimicrobial use to better understand trends and patterns in antimicrobial resistance. There is no monitoring of antimicrobial use in companion animals in Canada. To explore how the use of electronic medical records could contribute to the ongoing, systematic collection of antimicrobial use data in companion animals, anonymized electronic medical records were extracted from 12 participating companion animal practices and warehoused at the University of Calgary. We used the pre-diagnostic, clinical features of diarrhea as the case definition in this study. Using text-mining technologies, cases of diarrhea were described by each of the following variables: diagnostic laboratory tests performed, the etiological diagnosis and antimicrobial therapies. The ability of the text miner to accurately describe the cases for each of the variables was evaluated. It could not reliably classify cases in terms of diagnostic tests or etiological diagnosis; a manual review of a random sample of 500 diarrhea cases determined that 88/500 (17.6%) of the target cases underwent diagnostic testing of which 36/88 (40.9%) had an etiological diagnosis. Text mining, compared to a human reviewer, could accurately identify cases that had been treated with antimicrobials with high sensitivity (92%, 95% confidence interval, 88.1%–95.4%) and specificity (85%, 95% confidence interval, 80.2%–89.1%). Overall, 7400/15,928 (46.5%) of pets presenting with diarrhea were treated with antimicrobials. Some temporal trends and patterns of the antimicrobial use are described. The results from this study suggest that informatics and the electronic medical records could be useful for monitoring trends in antimicrobial use.

Editor: Herman Tse, The University of Hong Kong, Hong Kong

Funding: This research was partially funded by the University of Calgary (www.ucalgary.ca) and The Centre for Coastal Health (www.centreforcoastalhealth.ca). The funders had no role in study design, data collection and analysis, decision to publish, or preparation of the manuscript.

Competing Interests: The authors have declared that no competing interests exist.

* Email: rmanholt@ucalgary.ca

Introduction

Diarrhea is a common clinical presentation in companion animals [1]. The pathophysiology of diarrhea is complex, poorly understood and can involve a wide array of infectious and non-infectious etiologies [2,3]. Clinical evaluation of ill animals directs the selection of diagnostic procedures such as parasite studies, microbiological examinations and/or toxin testing. Clinicians must weigh the cost of diagnostic procedures, the owner's willingness to pay for them and the time spent waiting for a result against the likelihood that the results of a diagnostic test will affect their therapeutic recommendations. This cost-benefit analysis often results in diarrhea in pets being managed by empirical therapy with antihelmintics and antimicrobials [4].

Infectious disease specialists advocate restricting antimicrobial use (AMU) to cases where there is evidence that AMU will result in improved clinical outcomes [3,5,6]. Warnings against indiscriminate AMU in animals are increasing because the consequences of AMU include antimicrobial resistance (AMR) with decreased efficacy of important antimicrobials against significant animal and human pathogens [7,8]. In their closely shared environment, pets may be a source of antimicrobial resistant enteric bacteria or resistance genes for their owners [9–11].

Understanding the clinical management of common veterinary problems and patterns of AMU may provide the necessary exposure information to help interpret AMR trends, identify potential problem areas in prescribing practices and provide evidence-based practice guidelines for practitioners [12–16]. Collecting clinical management and AMU data at the veterinary patient level has not been legislated in Canada and remains a challenge in veterinary medicine in Canada [11,17,18].

The uptake of the electronic medical record (EMR) by companion animal practitioners provides an opportunity for accessing case management and AMU data. Informatics is "the application of information and computer science technology to public health practice, research and learning" [19]. Informatics has been applied elsewhere to text-based clinical records to describe disease-drug associations by physicians [20]. In this paper we used the EMR's from a participating practice network and explored text mining for accessing and analyzing the textual orders for diagnostic testing and AMU in the medical records.

The objectives of this study were to:

1. Apply and evaluate text-mining technology of EMR's to characterize the clinical management of diarrhea cases by companion animal veterinarians in a network of participating veterinary practices.
2. Describe the diagnostic management of diarrhea in companion animals and the proportion of cases for which there was documented evidence of an infectious process.
3. Describe the use of antimicrobials in the management of diarrhea cases.
4. Describe the temporal patterns of the use for each antimicrobial class used in the treatment of diarrhea cases for a 4 year period (January 1, 2007 to December 31, 2010).

Materials and Methods

Study area and data

The study area included 6 communities in the province of Alberta, Canada including: Calgary, Cochrane, Airdrie, Chestermere, Strathmore and Okotoks. A survey of all of the companion animal practices in the study area identified the practices that had completely computerized medical records and the same veterinary practice management software. Twelve of the 20 eligible practices agreed to participate in this project; a sample of convenience. A data sharing agreement was signed by each of the practice's managing partners and the author (Anholt). Approval from the University of Calgary Conjoint Faculties Research Ethics Board did not require permission from the pet owners.

A custom-built data extraction program was used to extract the anonymized electronic medical records (n = 428,783) from the veterinary practice management programs from January 1, 2007 to December 31, 2010. All records were stored in a secure data warehouse at the University of Calgary. The appointment schedule, medical notes (history, clinical exam, interpretations of diagnostic tests, assessment, differential diagnoses, and treatment) and prescription data for each case were combined into one free-text variable named '*Note*', in the data file. Data was stored and managed using Microsoft Office Excel 2007 (Microsoft Corporation, Redmond, Washington) and Konstanz Information Miner 2.2.2 (Knime, http://www.knime.org). The features of the participating practices, data extraction and management of the warehoused data have been described elsewhere [21].

Linguistics-based text-mining software (QDAMiner3.1/WordStat6, Provalis Research, Montreal, QC), was used in this study. Text, in the form of individual words or phrases was organized into categorization dictionaries which were used to identify and retrieve cases. A categorization dictionary was applied to the '*Note*' variable in the warehoused records to identify and retrieve records that met the case definition of any companion animal species (dog, cat, small mammal, bird, reptile) with clinical diarrhea or a description of feces consistent with diarrhea (n = 18,827 records). The case definition and the development, optimization and validation of the text miner to identify and retrieve records of diarrhea is further described in Anholt et al.[22].

Each of the 18,827 records represented a uniquely identified patient classified as having diarrhea, seen at a participating practice on a recorded date. After the initial visit, animals may have been hospitalized, returned for re-examination or there may have been a telephone consultation with the owners for the same complaint. To minimize repeated counts of the same case of diarrhea, all records of veterinary utilization (consultations, hospitalizations, laboratory results) for the same animal within 14 days of the initial visit were combined to represent one diarrhea case. There were 15,928 diarrhea cases in this study.

Development of the categorization dictionary in the text miner

Text mining was used to identify and retrieve cases for which one or more of the following activities were recorded:

- diagnostic testing had been performed.
- an etiological diagnosis had been made.
- treatment with an antimicrobial had been initiated.

Case definitions were developed for diagnostic testing and etiological diagnoses to classify cases using the text miner and also by an external reviewer. For classification purposes a diagnostic test was a laboratory test that could either be performed in the practice by the animal health technologist or sent to an external veterinary laboratory. A case was classified as positive for diagnostic testing if any of the following diagnostic tests were recorded within the variable 'Note':

- Fecal flotations and fecal smears and using light microscopy that provided a morphological diagnosis of helminths, protozoa or bacteria.
- Enzyme-linked immunosorbent (ELISA) assays to identify canine parvovirus or *Giardia* spp. infections from fecal samples.
- Real time PCR tests were performed to screen fecal samples for canine distemper virus, canine coronavirus, canine parvovirus, *Clostridium perfringens* enterotoxin A, *Cryptosporidium* spp. *Giardia* spp., *Salmonella* spp., feline coronavirus, feline panleukopenia, *Toxoplasma gondii*, and *Tritrichomonas foetus*.
- Fecal bacteria culture was performed.

A case was classified as positive for etiologic diagnosis if a positive outcome for any of the diagnostic tests described above was recorded. The positive classification included imprecise morphological diagnoses of bacterial infections such as bacterial overgrowth and *Campylobacter*-type spp. as recorded by a veterinarian or technician.

Positive antimicrobial use cases were defined as those diarrhea cases that were administered, dispensed or prescribed antimicrobials for the management of the diarrhea signs.

To calculate the number of diarrhea cases required to assess the ability of the text miner to accurately classify the cases by each management activity (diagnostic testing, etiological diagnosis and antimicrobial treatment), the assumptions of the precision-based sample size calculation were: i) significance level, 0.05, ii) *a priori* estimate of the proportion, conservatively = 0.5, iii) precision = 0.1. The calculated number of cases positive for each activity required in the sample was 96. To reach the target of 96 positive cases in the sample required an estimate of the proportion of cases that would be positive for each activity. This was unknown and was expected to differ for each activity so a proportion of 0.20 was selected. The number of controls required was calculated using, $N_{controls} = N_{Cases}(1\text{-Prev/Prev})$ = 384 controls +96 cases = 480 [23]. A sample of 500 records was randomly selected from the entire file of 15,928 diarrhea cases.

An experienced veterinarian clinician, blinded to the results of the text miner, reviewed all of the information contained in the extracted EMR's for the sample of 500 cases. The clinician reviewer classified each case as positive or negative for each of: i) laboratory diagnostics performed; ii) etiological diagnosis made; and iii) antimicrobial treatment. This served as the external standard.

We cross-tabulated the dichotomous results from the text miner and the external standard. The results for each case definition were summarized as the sensitivity and the specificity of the text miner's ability to correctly classify cases. The 95% confidence intervals for the sensitivity and specificity were also calculated (Exact method, Stata/IC 10.0, StataCorp, College Station, Tx). The cases that were improperly classified (false positives and false negatives) were reviewed to determine why they had been misclassified and if there were any opportunities to improve the text-mining classifier.

The sample of 500 diarrhea positive cases was categorized into three categories: i) no diagnostic testing performed, ii) diagnostic testing performed with a negative result or no result recorded; and iii) diagnostic testing performed with a positive diagnosis. Within each of the 3 categories the proportion of patients that were managed with antimicrobials was determined. Odds ratios (OR) and their 95% confidence intervals (CI) were used to quantify the difference between the odds of cases within each category receiving antimicrobials.

Antimicrobial use trends

The text miner's categorization dictionary for antimicrobial use (described above) was then applied to all of the 15,928 diarrhea cases to classify cases that had been administered, dispensed or prescribed antimicrobials. Antimicrobial use was described by the class of antimicrobial used and by Health Canada's categorization of antimicrobial drugs based on importance to human medicine [24]. Co-occurrences of antimicrobial use were identified by the text miner and the antimicrobials used in combination were described.

We examined the temporal trends of the Category I (very high importance in human medicine) and Category II (high importance in human medicine) antimicrobials [24] for the 4 years of the study. For each month of the study, we determined the proportion of cases that had been treated with any antimicrobial and the proportions treated with each class of antimicrobial. The temporal trend for all antimicrobials combined and for each antimicrobial was examined by fitting a linear regression model to the data. The number of antimicrobial treated cases, normalized by the total number of diarrhea cases for each month, was the dependent variable and the month/year was the independent variable. If the antimicrobial use data fit the slope estimated by the linear regression ($p<0.05$), the proportions of cases treated with this antimicrobial were plotted as a function of time [25]. Further exploratory data analysis included data smoothing by: i) pooling the number of cases treated with each class of antimicrobial in each quarter of each year; and ii) plotting the results in scatterplots with quadratic overlays (Stata/IC 10.0).

Results

Text mining

Estimates of the text miner's ability to distinguish between cases that had diagnostic testing performed (sensitivity = 70% and specificity = 85.1%) and which had an etiological diagnosis made (sensitivity = 72.4% and specificity = 97.4), were relatively low. There were wide confidence intervals around sensitivity which indicated poor precision of the estimate (Table 1, Table 2). The primary reason the text miner performed poorly when classifying these cases was that the context was relevant to the classification of the case. For example, the word "parvo" was associated with a diagnosis, a differential diagnosis, a past diagnosis, a diagnostic test, a serological titer, a vaccine, and a recommendation or a warning to owners. Despite repeated efforts, it was not possible to improve the performance of the text miner to classify cases by the diagnostic test performed or their etiological diagnosis, so the text miner was not used for these purposes.

In contrast, text mining classified cases that had been treated with an antimicrobial with high sensitivity (92.3%) and specificity (85%) when compared to a human reviewer (Table 3). The text miner misclassified cases if the name of the antimicrobial was not provided or improperly spelled, if the record contained information about past treatment or future considerations for treatment or if the pet was receiving antimicrobials but they were being used to treat a co-morbidity (not dispensed for diarrhea). Given the high sensitivity and specificity of the text miner for classifying cases with respect to antimicrobial use, it was used for the remainder of the analysis.

Diagnostic testing, diagnoses and antimicrobial use

As the text miner did not accurately classify cases that had laboratory testing performed or a diagnosis made, the results presented are from the manual review of the sample of 500 diarrhea positive cases only. The remaining diarrhea cases were not described by their diagnostic testing or etiological diagnosis. There were 88 cases (17.6%) in the sample of 500 diarrhea positive cases tested to identify an etiological diagnosis (Figure 1, Table 4). Fecal examinations (smears and/or floats) were performed in 56 of the 88 (63.6%) cases that underwent diagnostic testing; ELISA assays were run on 58 (65.9%) cases to identify canine parvovirus or *Giardia* spp.; multiple testing using a combination of fecal exams and ELISA tests was documented in 29 (33%) of those tested. Fecal cultures or PCR tests were each ordered in 1 (1.1%) and 3 (3.4%) of the cases respectively; all of which were negative. Thirty-six cases (40.9% of those tested, 7.2% of all cases) had a

Table 1. From a random sample of 500 companion animal cases of diarrhea, the accuracy of the text miner for classifying the cases as positive or negative for *'had diagnostic testing'* when compared to a manual review of the medical records serving as the external standard.

	External standard +	External standard -	Sum
Text miner +	63	61	124
Text miner -	27	349	376
Sum	90	410	500
	Sensitivity = 70.0% (95%CI, 59.4% - 79.2%)	Specificity = 85.1% (95%CI, 81.3% - 88.4%)	

Table 2. From a random sample of 500 companion animal cases of diarrhea, the accuracy of the text miner for classifying the cases as positive or negative for *'had an etiological diagnosis made'* when compared to a manual review of the medical records serving as the external standard.

	External standard +	**External standard -**	**Sum**
Text miner +	21	17	38
Text miner -	8	454	462
Sum	29	466	500
	Sensitivity = 72.4% (95%CI, 52.8%–87.3%)	Specificity = 97.4% (95%CI, 95.5%–98.7%)	

stated etiologic diagnosis in the EMR; all were prescribed an antihelmintic or antimicrobial medication. We inferred that given the management of cases with a positive result, that the veterinarians considered the findings to be relevant.

Patients that had diagnostic procedures performed had more antimicrobials administered, dispensed or prescribed (72.7%) than patients that had no diagnostic testing performed (41%) (OR = 3.8; 95% CI 2.2–6.7). There was little difference in the proportion of patients that were treated with antimicrobials and had a positive diagnostic test and those treated with antimicrobials and a negative diagnostic test (OR = 1.2, 95% CI 0.4–3.6) (Figure 1). Two hundred and thirty-three of the 500 diarrhea cases (46.6%) received antimicrobials; none of the cases receiving antimicrobials were culture positive for bacteria (Figure 1, Table 4).

Text mining of the diarrhea cases (n = 15,928) identified 7400 (46.5%) cases that were administered, dispensed or prescribed antimicrobials. There were 8041 occurrences of AMU in the 7400 cases. The distribution of the antimicrobial classes used in the management of diarrhea positive cases is summarized in Table 5. Category 1 (very high importance to human health) antimicrobials were prescribed in most (87.1%) of the antimicrobial-treated diarrhea cases. Veterinarians prescribed more than one antimicrobial in 641 (8.7%) of all cases treated with an antimicrobial. Nitroimidazole plus a penicillin was the most frequent treatment combination (n = 346) followed by nitroimidazole together with first and second generation cephalosporins (n = 79), penicillins with fluorquinolones (n = 67), and nitroimidazoles in combination with fluorquinolones (n = 66).

Antimicrobial use temporal trends

The linear regression analyses of 'all antimicrobials' (n = 7400), 'nitroimidazole' (n = 5814) and 'penicillin' (n = 808) were significant ($p<0.05$) and these variables were plotted against time (Figure 2). The graph and the slope coefficients (0.0002 to 0.0004) indicate a very small statistically significant, upward trend in the proportions of diarrhea cases treated with any antimicrobial and treated with nitroimidazoles and penicillins. The regression analyses of the remaining antimicrobials were not statistically significant.

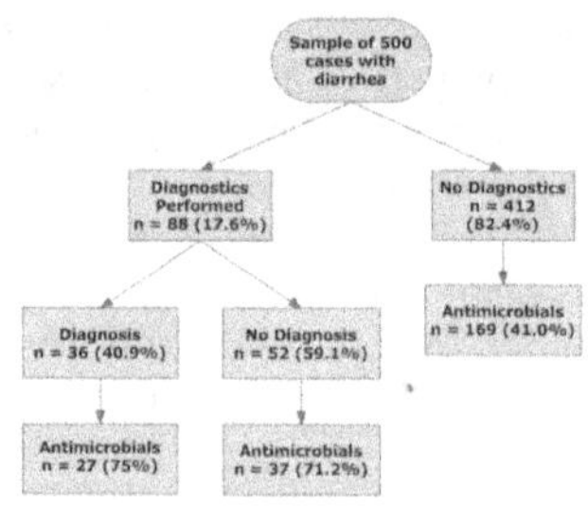

Figure 1. From a random sample of 500 companion animal cases with diarrhea, a flow diagram describing the proportion of cases that had laboratory diagnostics performed, had an etiological diagnosis made, and were administered, prescribed or dispensed antimicrobials.

Smoothed scatterplots of the quarterly counts of cases treated with 3rd/4th generation cephalosporins and the penicillin β-lactamase inhibitor combinations showed patterns of antimicrobial use that were mirror images of each other (Figure 3). Scatterplots of the remaining antimicrobial class combinations did not show any recognizable patterns.

Discussion

Results of the text mining methods used in this study varied depending on the variable of interest. Text mining results for AMU were relatively accurate because the documentation of antimicrobial treatments by veterinarians was usually explicit and unambiguous; the meaning of the words did not depend upon the context in which they were used. However, the language used to

Table 3. From a random sample of 500 companion animal cases of diarrhea, the accuracy of the text miner for classifying the cases as positive or negative for *'had an antimicrobial administered, dispensed or prescribed'* when compared to a manual review of the medical records serving as the external standard.

	External standard +	**External standard -**	**Sum**
Text miner +	215	40	255
Text miner -	18	227	245
Sum	233	267	500
	Sensitivity = 92.3% (95%CI, 88.1%–95.4%)	Specificity = 85.0% (95%CI, 80.2%–89.1%)	

Table 4. Distribution of a sample of companion animal cases with diarrhea by the stated etiological diagnosis (n = 500).

Diagnosis	Number of cases (% of 500 cases)	% of diagnosed cases	Diagnostic test
All	36 (7.2)	-	
Helminths	1 (0.2)	2.7	Morphology
Coccidia	5 (1.0)	13.9	Morphology
Bacterial overgrowth	9 (1.8)	25	Morphology
Campylobacter-type	1 (0.2)	2.8	Morphology
Canine parvovirus	9 (1.8)	25.0	ELISA
Giardia spp.	11 (2.2)	30.6	Morphology or ELISA

record diagnostic procedures and diagnoses was highly context specific and the linguistic-based text mining approach used in this study was unable to discriminate between the various meanings. It is possible that trained or rule-based text-mining software could more accurately distinguish these cases and is an area for future study [26,27].

Most cases of acute (less than 14 days) diarrhea are mild and self-limiting and supportive treatment without a diagnosis is considered appropriate [2]. Therefore, it was not unexpected that less than 18% of the diarrhea cases in our study had diagnostic procedures performed. The recommended initial diagnostic approach to acute diarrhea is a fecal exam [28]. More than half of the diagnostic procedures in our study were fecal flotation and/or fecal smears. In animals with severe disease (febrile, dehydrated, hemorrhagic or persistent diarrhea) further efforts at establishing an etiological diagnosis are warranted [2,28]. Animals in this study that were subjected to diagnostic laboratory testing were more likely to be given antimicrobials than those that were not tested regardless of the test results. This may indicate an assessment of more severe disease by the veterinarian although this judgment was not often explicitly stated in the medical record. Despite efforts to identify an etiological agent, a positive diagnosis was established in less than half of the cases undergoing diagnostic testing.

Giardiasis was the most frequent diagnosis in this study and antimicrobial treatment is usually recommended in *Giardia*-positive diarrheic animals [29]. However, *Giardia* spp. is commonly misdiagnosed in veterinary practice and most cases are self-limiting [30]. Antimicrobials are also recommended in the management of diarrhea in companion animals if there is a positive diagnosis of secondary bacterial overgrowth associated with inflammatory bowel disease or culture-confirmed primary bacterial infections of *Salmonella*, *Campylobacter*, *Clostridium* and enterotoxigenic *E. coli* [2,4,5,29], if there is evidence of a breach in the mucosal integrity of the intestines (hemorrhagic diarrhea), or to manage the immunosuppressive effects of parvovirus [2,4,5,28,29]. Other authors argue that while antimicrobials are commonly used in cases with a confirmed culture or if there is evidence of hematochezia, there is little objective information as to whether they are needed in all cases [3,5].

Our findings indicated that veterinarians commonly prescribed antimicrobials for diarrhea without any documentation that the

Table 5. Distribution of antimicrobials used by the veterinary practices in the treatment of companion animal diarrhea cases (n = 15,928) in 2007, 2008, 2009 and 2010.

Health Canada Category [24]	Antibiotic class	Number of cases (% of 15,928 diarrhea cases)	% antimicrobial treated cases (n = 7400)
Category 1 (Very High Importance)	3rd/4th Generation Cephalosporins	124 (0.8)	1.7
	Fluorquinolones	200 (1.3)	2.7
	Nitroimidazoles	5814 (36.5)	78.6
	Penicillin β – lactam inhibitors	310 (1.9)	4.2
	Total for Category I	**6448 (40.5)**	**87.1**
Category II (High Importance)	1st/2nd Generation Cephalosporins	426 (2.7)	5.8
	Lincosamides	76 (0.5)	1.0
	Macrolides	124 (0.8)	1.7
	Penicillins	808 (5.1)	10.9
	Timethoprim-Sulpha	84 (0.5)	1.1
	Total for Category II	**1518 (9.5)**	**20.5**
Category III (Medium Importance)	Choramphenicol	5 (0.0)	0.1
	Sulphonamides	62 (0.4)	0.8
	Tetracycline	8 (0.1)	0.1
	Total for Category III	**75 (0.5)**	**1.0**

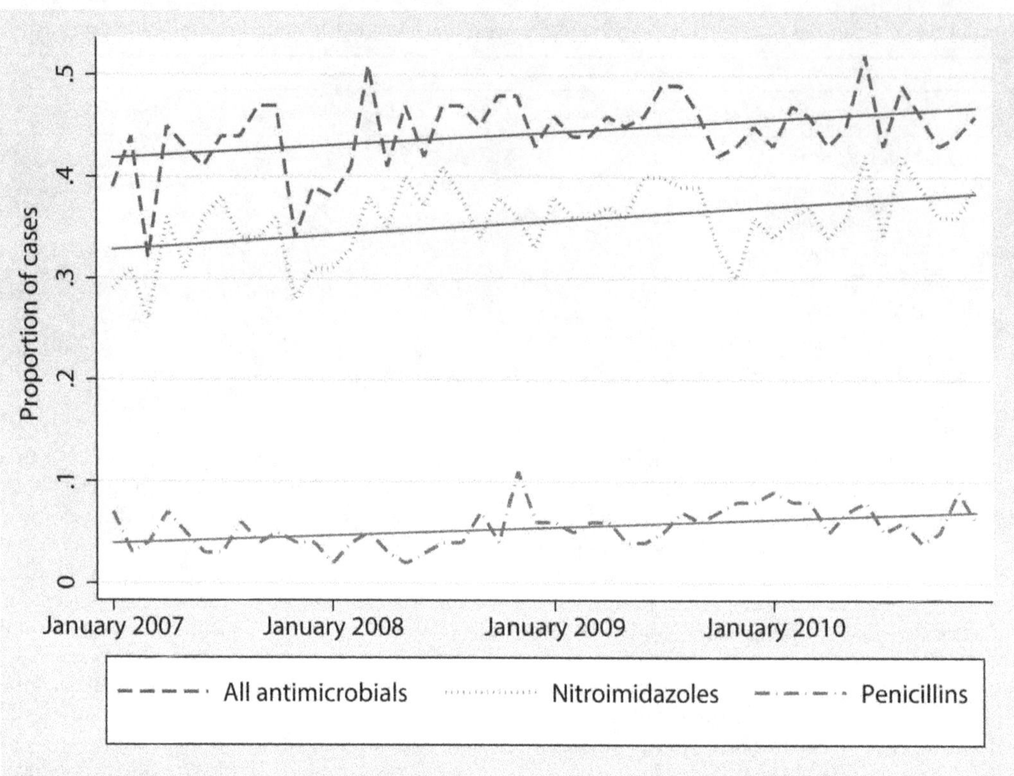

Figure 2. Changes in the proportion of companion animal diarrhea cases (n = 15,928) treated with any antimicrobial, nitroimidazole class and penicillin class from January 1, 2007 to December 31, 2010.

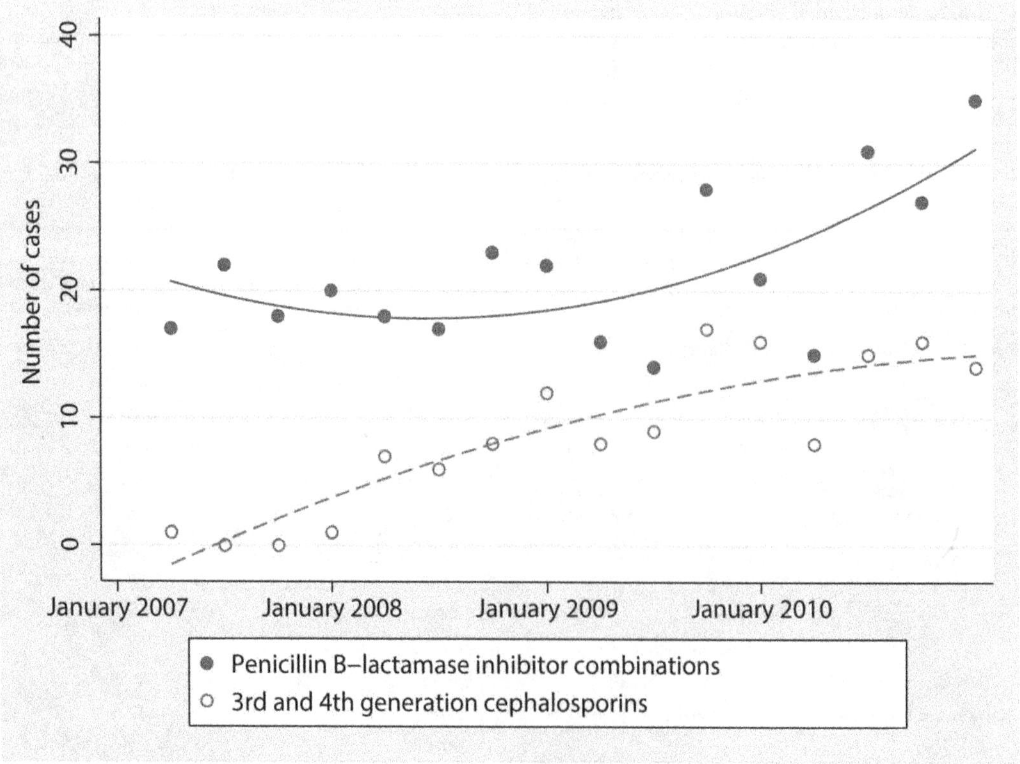

Figure 3. From 15,928 cases of companion animals with diarrhea, scattergrams of the counts of cases treated with B-lactam inhibitors and cephalosporins in each yearly quarter from January 1, 2007 to December 31, 2010.

animal's diarrhea had an infectious etiology. Empirical combinations of antimicrobial treatments was also common. Empirical antimicrobial use may lead to treatment failures and antimicrobial resistance [3,4,28,29]. We found no post-prescription, pharmacoepidemiological studies evaluating empirical antimicrobial management of diarrhea in pets in the refereed literature.

Using the data extracted from medical records it was possible to detect changing trends in AMU. Despite increased AMR concerns [4,6] there was evidence that nitroimidazole and penicillin use for the management of diarrhea in companion animals was increasing. Metronidazole (a drug of the Nitroimidazoles Class) was the most frequently prescribed antimicrobial and its use increased over the 4 years of the study. It is the drug of choice for anaerobic and microaerophilic bacteria (*Bacteroides* and *Clostridia*) and parasites (*Giardia* spp.) in animals [4]. In people it is important in the management of these pathogens and *Helicobacter pylori* [31,32]. There are few therapeutic alternatives for these infections in people and so it is classified as a Category I antimicrobial [24]. Sensitivity testing for anaerobes is not routinely performed but treatment failures have been documented [32,33] and the molecular basis for resistance has been established [31]. We found no papers documenting the transmission of metronidazole-resistant bacteria from pets to people.

The increase in the number of cases treated with 3rd and 4th generation cephalosporins in early 2008 coincided with the Canadian approval on May 30, 2007 and subsequent distribution of Convenia (Pfizer Animal Health, Kirkland, QC) later in 2007 [34]. Convenia is the trade name for cefovecin, a third generation cephalosporin. The increase in cefovecin use corresponded to a decrease in the use of penicillin β-lactamase inhibitor combinations. The indications for use are similar for the 2 classes of drugs so it is possible that one class was being used as an alternative to the other. Starting in the middle of 2009, the relationship appeared to be inverted and this trend continued until the end of 2010, the reason for which is unknown.

The results from this study suggest that informatics and EMR's could be useful for supporting evidence-based practice, and for monitoring trends in AMU and changes in veterinary prescription behavior following interventions to modify their use. Temporal trends and regional differences could prompt further investigations to explore why the observed trends were developing. Interventions such as confidential benchmarking by comparing AMU among veterinarians may serve to help veterinarians recognize problems and reduce AMU [35]. Analytical studies to see if there is an association between AMU in companion animals with diarrhea and the development of AMR in fecal microorganisms are indicated and informatics could provide the exposure data necessary to interpret AMR results.

Author Contributions

Conceived and designed the experiments: RMA JB CS. Performed the experiments: RMA. Analyzed the data: RMA. Contributed reagents/materials/analysis tools: RMA JB CR MR CS. Contributed to the writing of the manuscript: RMA JB CR MR CS.

References

1. Lidbury JA Turpin I, Suchodolski JS (2008) Gastrointestinal disease in a population of insured dogs and cats from the United Kingdome (2006–2007); 18th ECVIM-CA Congress; Ghent, Belgium. pp. 219.
2. Hall EJ, German AJ (2010) Diseases of the small intestine. In: Ettinger SJ, Feldman EC, editors. Textbook of Veterinary Internal Medicine, Diseases of the Dog and Cat. 7th ed. St. Lois, Missouri: Sanders Elsvier. pp. 1527–1572.
3. Weese JS (2011) Bacterial enteritis in dogs and cats: diagnosis, therapy, and zoonotic potential. Vet Clin North Am Small Anim Pract 41: 287.
4. Boothe DM (2012) Principles of antimicrobial therapy. In: Boothe DM, editor. Small Animal Clinical Pharmacology and Therapeutics. 2nd ed. St. Louis, Missouri: Elsevier Saunders.
5. Guerrant RL, Van Gilder T, Steiner TS, Thielman NM, Slutsker L, et al. (2001) Practice guidelines for the management of infectious diarrhea. Clin Infect Dis 32: 331–351.
6. Center for Disease Control Website. Interagency Task Force on Antimicrobial Resistance (2011) A public health action plan to combat antimicrobial resistance. Available: www.cdc.gov/./pdf/public-health-action-plan-combat-antimicrobial-resistance.pdf. Accessed 2013 February 2.
7. Morley PS, Apley MD, Besser TE, Burney DP, Fedorka-Cray PJ, et al. (2005) Antimicrobial drug use in veterinary medicine. J Vet Intern Med 19: 617–629.
8. Coffman JR (Chairman) National National Research Council (1999) The use of drugs in food animals: Benefits and risks. Washington, DC: Institute of Medicine.
9. Weese JS (2008) Antimicrobial resistance in companion animals. Anim Health Res Rev/Conf Res Workers Anim Dis 9: 169–176.
10. Guardabassi L, Schwarz S, Lloyd DH (2004) Pet animals as reservoirs of antimicrobial-resistant bacteria Review. J Antimicrob Chemother 54: 321–332.
11. Prescott JF, Hanna WJ, Reid-Smith R, Drost K (2002) Antimicrobial drug use and resistance in dogs. Can Vet J 43: 107–116.
12. Singer RS, Reid-Smith R, Sischo WM (2006) Stakeholder position paper: epidemiological perspectives on antibiotic use in animals. Prev Vet Med 73: 153–161.
13. Greco PJ, Eisenberg JM (1993) Changing physicians' practices. N Engl J Med 329: 1271–1274.
14. Meyer E, Schwab F, Jonas D, Rueden H, Gastmeier P, et al. (2004) Surveillance of antimicrobial use and antimicrobial resistance in intensive care units (SARI): 1. Antimicrobial use in German intensive care units. Intensive Care Med 30: 1089–1096.
15. Vlahović-Palc???evski V, Dumpis U, Mitt P, Gulbinovic J, Struwe J, et al. (2007) Benchmarking antimicrobial drug use at university hospitals in five European countries. Clin Microbiol Infect 13: 277–283.
16. Goossens H, Ferech M, Vander Stichele R, Elseviers M (2005) Outpatient antibiotic use in Europe and association with resistance: a cross-national database study. Lancet 365: 579–587.
17. Monnet D, López-Lozano JM, Campillos P, Burgos A, Yagüe A, et al. (2001) Making sense of antimicrobial use and resistance surveillance data: application of ARIMA and transfer function models. Clin Microbiol Infect 7: 29–36.
18. Public Health Agency of Canada website. Canadian Integrated Program for Antimicrobial Resistance Surveillance (2008) 2008 Annual Report. Available: http://www.phac-aspc.gc.ca/cipars-picra/2008/index-eng.php. Accessed 2012 November 29.
19. Friede A, Blum HL, McDonald M (1995) Public health informatics: how information-age technology can strengthen public health. Annu Rev Public Health 16: 239–252.
20. Chen ES, Hripcsak G, Xu H, Markatou M, Friedman C (2008) Automated acquisition of disease–drug knowledge from biomedical and clinical documents: an initial study. J Am Med Inform Assoc 15: 87–98.
21. Anholt RM, Berezowski J, MacLean K, Russel M, Jamal I, Stephen C (2014) The application of medical informatics to the veterinary management programs at companion animal practices in Alberta, Canada: A case study. Prev Vet Med 113: 165–174.
22. Anholt R, Berezowski J, Jamal I, Ribble C, Stephen C (2014) Mining free-text medical records for companion animal enteric syndrome surveillance. Prev Vet Med 113: 417–422.
23. Guyatt G SD, Haynes B. (2006) Evaluating diagnostic tests. In: Haynes BSD, Guyatt G., Tugwell P., editor. Clinical Epidemiology; How to do Clinical Practice Research. Third edition. Philadelphia: Lippincott William and Wilkins.
24. Health Canada website. Veterinary Drug Directorate (2009) Categorization of antimicrobial drugs based on importance to human medicine. Available: http://www.hc-sc.gc.ca/dhp-mps/vet/antimicrob/amr_ram_hum-med-rev-eng.php. Accessed 2012 November 29.
25. Jump RLP, Olds DM, Seifi N, Kypriotakis G, Jury LA, et al. (2012) Effective Antimicrobial Stewardship in a Long-Term Care Facility through an Infectious Disease Consultation Service: Keeping a LID on Antibiotic Use. Infect Control Hosp Epidemiol 33: 1185–1192.
26. Mooney RJ, Bunescu R (2005) Mining knowledge from text using information extraction. ACM SIGKDD Explorations newsl 7: 3–10.
27. Meystre SM, Savova GK, Kipper-Schuler KC, Hurdle JF (2008) Extracting information from textual documents in the electronic health record: a review of recent research. Yearbook Med Inform: 128–144.
28. Sherding RG, Johnson SE (2006) Diseases of the intestines. In: Birchard SJ, Sherding, RG, editor. Saunders Manual of Small Animal Practice. 3rd ed. St. Louis, Missouri: Saunders Elsevier.
29. Eddlestone SM (2002) Drug Therapies Used in Gastrointestinal Disease. Compendium: Small animal/exotics 24: 452–468.
30. Payne PA, Artzer M (2009) Biology and control of Giardia spp. and Tritrichomonas foetus. Vet Clin North Am Small Anim Pract 39: 993–1007.

31. Dhand A, Snydman DR (2009) Mechanism of Resistance in Metronidazole. Antimicrob Drug Resist: 223–227.
32. Megraud F, Lamouliatte H (2003) Review article: the treatment of refractory Helicobacter pylori infection. Aliment Pharmacol Ther 17: 1333–1343.
33. Fang H, Edlund C, Hedberg M, Nord CE (2002) New findings in beta-lactam and metronidazole resistant Bacteroides fragilis group. Int J Antimicrob Agents 19: 361.
34. Health Canada website. Veterinary Drug Directorate (2007) Notice of Compliance. Available: http://www.hc-sc.gc.ca/dhp-mps/prodpharma/notices-avis/index-eng.php. Accessed 2012 November 29.
35. Ibrahim OM, Polk RE (2012) Benchmarking antimicrobial drug use in hospitals. Expert Rev Anti Infect Ther 10: 445–457.

24

Controlling Malaria Using Livestock-Based Interventions: A One Health Approach

Ana O. Franco[1,2]*, M. Gabriela M. Gomes[1], Mark Rowland[2], Paul G. Coleman[2], Clive R. Davies[†2]

1 Instituto Gulbenkian de Ciência, Oeiras, Portugal, **2** Faculty of Infectious and Tropical Diseases, London School of Hygiene and Tropical Medicine, London, United Kingdom

Abstract

Where malaria is transmitted by zoophilic vectors, two types of malaria control strategies have been proposed based on animals: using livestock to divert vector biting from people (zooprophylaxis) or as baits to attract vectors to insecticide sources (insecticide-treated livestock). Opposing findings have been obtained on malaria zooprophylaxis, and despite the success of an insecticide-treated livestock trial in Pakistan, where malaria vectors are highly zoophilic, its effectiveness is yet to be formally tested in Africa where vectors are more anthropophilic. This study aims to clarify the different effects of livestock on malaria and to understand under what circumstances livestock-based interventions could play a role in malaria control programmes. This was explored by developing a mathematical model and combining it with data from Pakistan and Ethiopia. Consistent with previous work, a zooprophylactic effect of untreated livestock is predicted in two situations: if vector population density does not increase with livestock introduction, or if livestock numbers and availability to vectors are sufficiently high such that the increase in vector density is counteracted by the diversion of bites from humans to animals. Although, as expected, insecticide-treatment of livestock is predicted to be more beneficial in settings with highly zoophilic vectors, like South Asia, we find that the intervention could also considerably decrease malaria transmission in regions with more anthropophilic vectors, like *Anopheles arabiensis* in Africa, under specific circumstances: high treatment coverage of the livestock population, using a product with stronger or longer lasting insecticidal effect than in the Pakistan trial, and with small (ideally null) repellency effect, or if increasing the attractiveness of treated livestock to malaria vectors. The results suggest these are the most appropriate conditions for field testing insecticide-treated livestock in an Africa region with moderately zoophilic vectors, where this intervention could contribute to the integrated control of malaria and livestock diseases.

Editor: Thomas A. Smith, Swiss Tropical & Public Health Institute, Switzerland

Funding: Ana O. Franco was funded by the Portuguese Fundação para a Ciência e Tecnologia (FCT - SFRH/BD/9605/2002), co-financed by the Programa Operacional Ciência e Inovação 2010 (POCI 2010) and Fundo Social Europeu (FSE), and by EPIWORK - European Commission (Grant Agreement 231807). The publication fees were paid by the London School of Hygiene and Tropical Medicine. The funders had no role in study design, data collection and analysis, decision to publish, or preparation of the manuscript.

Competing Interests: The authors have declared that no competing interests exist.

* Email: afranco@igc.gulbenkian.pt

† Deceased

Introduction

In the last few decades there has been increasing recognition of the need for an integrated public health and veterinary approach, accounting for the surrounding social-ecological system, to face many of the most challenging disease threats: the so-called 'One Health' approach [1]. Broadly speaking, animals play an important role in the epidemiology of several of the most important diseases of man, where they can act as a reservoir source for infectious pathogens, and/or a source of blood-meal to arthropod vectors of human disease. The recognition of this relationship has led to the implementation of human disease control strategies targeted at animal populations. These control opportunities have been investigated both empirically and theoretically. Yet, our knowledge on what determines the public health benefits of many of these veterinary interventions remains limited.

A case study of the 'One Health' concept is human malaria in regions where its mosquito vectors (*Anopheles* spp.) also feed on animals, since the presence of livestock close to the household can affect the rate of vector-human contacts and consequently the risk of disease transmission among people. As the *Plasmodium* malaria parasites that infect humans are not infective to livestock, it has since long been proposed that animals could be used to divert the malaria vector biting from humans, a control intervention known as zooprophylaxis [2,3]. However, despite the large number of studies performed worldwide for over a century to try to assess the value of this strategy in the fight against malaria (reviewed in [4,5,6,7,8,9]), the available evidence is still contradictory and no consensus exists on the prophylactic effect of animals. Indeed, although in several situations the presence of livestock has been referred to as a protective factor for malaria vector-human contact and/or disease, such as in Papua New Guinea [10,11] and Sri Lanka [12], the opposite has been reported in various other studies, where livestock were shown to be a risk factor, such as Pakistan [13,14], Philippines [15,16], and Ethiopia [17,18] (throughout this work the term livestock is used to refer to cattle and other domestic large and small ruminants - buffalos, sheep, goats -, as well as donkeys, horses, and swine).

The apparently contradictory outcomes of the numerous studies conducted result from a combination of several possible effects of livestock on malaria. On one hand, livestock may divert the blood-seeking mosquito vectors from humans, thereby decreasing the biting on people [10,11,19] and, as a result, decreasing the transmission of the malaria parasite [20] and preventing its amplification in people (i.e. the basis for the zooprophylaxis concept). But on the other hand, livestock can provide additional blood-sources and/or larval breeding sites [21,22,23,24,25], which can increase vector survival and/or density [26], consequently increasing the probability of the vector surviving the parasite extrinsic incubation period and becoming infectious, as well as increasing biting on people [2,6,27]. Additionally, livestock may attract more mosquitoes, which, once in the vicinity of the human dwellings, may end up biting humans rather than animals [14,15,16,18]. The resulting net impact of livestock on malaria risk therefore depends on the relative contribution of each of those effects.

In areas where the presence of livestock near people increases malaria transmission, an apparently simple solution could be to change livestock management in order to deploy the animals away from people's houses, between village and vector breeding site [7]. However, in Pakistan as well as in some Ethiopian regions, for instance, this is not likely to be a feasible strategy, given that livestock are such an important source of household income that people prefer to keep the animals near their houses to prevent them from being stolen [13,28,29,30] and to facilitate husbandry practices, such as milking the lactating animals. An alternative solution has therefore been proposed: target the non-human host of the zoophilic mosquito, by treating livestock with insecticides/ acaricides [13] (hereafter referred globally as 'insecticides' for simplicity). This strategy has since long been effectively used to control ectoparasites and the diseases they transmit to animals (and often also to humans), as well as to reduce the direct economic losses they cause due to decrease in productivity (e.g. lower efficiency of feed conversion, weight gain and milk production) [31]. Namely, insecticide treatment of livestock has been applied against tsetse flies transmitted animal and human trypanosomiasis in sub-Saharan Africa [32,33,34,35], tick-borne diseases worldwide (such as anaplasmosis, babesiosis, theileriosis) [33,36], and a variety of other biting and/or nuisance flies [37,38], mosquitoes [38,39], biting midges [40], mites, and lice.

The effectiveness of insecticide-treated livestock (ITL) against malaria was successfully tested by a community-randomised trial in Pakistan [41], where the main vectors, *An. stephensi* and *An. culicifacies*, are highly zoophilic [42]. Notably, following the treatment of virtually all domestic animals (93% of the population of cattle, sheep and goats) with a solution of the pyrethroid deltamethrin applied by sponging, *Plasmodium falciparum* malaria incidence decreased by 56% (95% CI 14%–78%), and prevalence decreased by 54% (95% CI 30–69%). Moreover, efficacy was comparable to that of traditional indoor insecticide spraying but with 80% less costs. Livestock previously infested with ectoparasites also improved in weight and milk yield productivity, enhancing community uptake of the programme [41]. Additional studies have followed to explore whether this strategy could also be applied in sub-Saharan Africa, for integrated control of malaria and animal trypanosomiasis and tick-borne diseases. Notably, bioassays of deltamethrin applied by spot-on and by spray have been conducted in Ethiopia [43], and in Tanzania [44], respectively, to assess the effects of ITL on the mortality and behaviour of malaria vectors. However, despite the encouraging results from these bioassays, the impact of ITL on malaria transmission at the community level is yet to be formally assessed in Africa, where the disease burden is the greatest, but the dynamics and determinants of infection differ from Asia.

A possible concern with ITL is repellency of mosquitoes, which may increase vector feeding on untreated livestock or unprotected humans, and make the intervention detrimental. It is known that certain insecticides exert not only (1) a toxic or direct insecticidal effect, killing mosquitoes that contact with an insecticide-impregnated surface, but also (2) behavioural avoidance responses. These sub-lethal behavioural effects include a) contact-mediated irritancy, inhibiting mosquitoes from remaining on the treated surface, thereby stimulating them to exit prematurely (common with pyrethroid insecticides), and b) non-contact or spatial repellency, which acts from a distance of the treated surface inhibiting mosquitoes from entering treated areas [45,46]. Hereafter, the latter two responses will be referred together as repellency, since any of them could cause mosquitoes diversion to another host, in analogy with the shift in host feeding from humans to domestic animals that has occasionally been associated with the use of pyrethroid-treated nets [47,48,49,50,51]. Additionally, a case-control study in the Pokot territory of Kenya and Uganda [52] found that people with ITL had a higher risk of Visceral Leishmaniasis, suggesting that the insecticide might have repelled sandflies attempting to feed on animals and diverted them to feed on humans. Although, to the best of our knowledge, such behavioural shift has not been reported for ITL and anopheline mosquitoes, the possibility of it occurring should not be disregarded and is therefore important to investigate, particularly because the most promising insecticides tested on livestock to target malaria vectors have been pyrethroids [19,39,43,44,53,54,55]. The popularity of pyrethroids is due to their high insecticidal action associated with low mammalian toxicity [56,57] which makes them safe for both the treated animals and for the consumers of animal products.

An additional concern with using ITL against malaria in Africa is that, even in areas where the moderately zoophilic *An. arabiensis* vector (which can easily feed on humans or livestock, depending on host abundance and accessibility) predominates over more anthropophilic vectors such as *An. gambiae s.s.*, the ITL intervention is still likely to achieve a smaller reduction in malaria transmission than in Pakistan (and other areas of South Asia), where the vectors are highly zoophilic, taking most of their bloodmeals upon livestock. A possible way to overcome this problem could be to artificially increase the attractiveness of insecticide-treated animals to the malaria vector. Although such has not been tested in the field yet, the use of synthetic attractants to lure anopheline vectors towards baits or traps and away from humans is an area of increasing research [58,59].

This work aims to clarify the different effects of livestock on malaria and to understand under what circumstances livestock-based interventions could play a role in malaria control programmes. This was achieved by, firstly, developing a mathematical model that predicts the apparently contradictory outcomes that have been associated with the presence of untreated livestock in different ecological settings, and secondly, by expanding the model to incorporate insecticide treatment of livestock and fitting it to data from Pakistan (where the ITL trial was performed [41]) and from Ethiopia (where a field study was conducted [9]) to investigate the potential and limitations of ITL. We focus on livestock-based interventions, without comparing their effect with other malaria control interventions, such as insecticide-treated bednets and indoor spraying with residual insecticides. The model characterizes situations where livestock by itself can lead to a decrease, increase, or no net impact on malaria transmission to humans, and it further indicates that treating livestock with insecticide can be a useful complementary tool to control malaria, not only in Asia, but also in sub-Saharan Africa.

Materials and Methods

Malaria model

A mathematical model for the transmission dynamics of human malaria was developed based on the Ross and Macdonald models [60,61], where humans are compartmentalized into either susceptible (uninfected and not immune), or infected/infectious (SIS model), and mosquito vectors are divided into susceptible (uninfected and not immune), exposed/latent (have been infected but are not yet infectious) or infectious (SEI model). Here, the Ross-Macdonald model is extended by discriminating the feeding behaviour of the vector on its alternative hosts: livestock and human populations, and by incorporating the treatment of livestock with insecticide as a potential *novel* method to control human malaria. The new model explicitly incorporates the effects of untreated and insecticide treated livestock on the vector population feeding behaviour, mortality and population density, allowing exploration of the impact of livestock-based interventions on malaria transmission dynamics. A diagrammatic flow chart of the model is presented in Figure 1. Throughout the article, the human, vector and livestock populations will be referred to with the subscripts h, v and l, respectively.

The model is formally represented by a system of ordinary differential equations as follows. For the dynamics of infection in the human population, we have

$$\frac{dS_h}{dt} = -\left(aqb\frac{I_v}{N_h}\right)S_h + rI_h, \tag{1}$$

$$\frac{dI_h}{dt} = \left(aqb\frac{I_v}{N_h}\right)S_h - rI_h,$$

where $N_h = S_h + I_h$ (total human population). Transmission of infection from vectors to humans depends on the number of infected vectors per human, I_v/N_h, the vector blood feeding rate on any host, a, (the interval between bloodmeals on any host is $1/a$), the proportion q of feeds taken on humans (so-called human blood index - HBI), the probability b that a human will become infected following the bite of an infectious vector, and the number of susceptible hosts, S_h. Once susceptible humans are infected the parasite undergoes a period of latency before infective gametocytes appear, but as this period is short compared to the duration of infection, it is not represented explicitly in the model [62]. Infected individuals, I_h, recover from infection at a rate r, eventually becoming fully susceptible to re-infection (the average duration of infection is $1/r$). It is therefore assumed that there is no boosting immunity due to repeated infections, as done for simplification in earlier zooprophylaxis models [27,63,64,65,66]. Human natural mortality and reproductive rates are omitted from the model because humans have a long life expectancy relative to other time periods used in the model (such as the latent period, infectious period and vector life span). We also assume no disease-induced death and therefore, the human population size remains constant.

The disease dynamics in the vector population is represented by

$$\frac{dS_v}{dt} = \rho N_v - \left(aqc\frac{I_h}{N_h} + \mu\right)S_v,$$

$$\frac{dL_v}{dt} = \left(aqc\frac{I_h}{N_h}\right)S_v - (\omega + \mu)L_v, \tag{2}$$

$$\frac{dI_v}{dt} = \omega L_v - \mu I_v,$$

where $N_v = S_v + L_v + I_v$ (total vector population). The vector population comprises only adult female anopheline mosquitoes, since males do not blood feed. Transmission of infection from

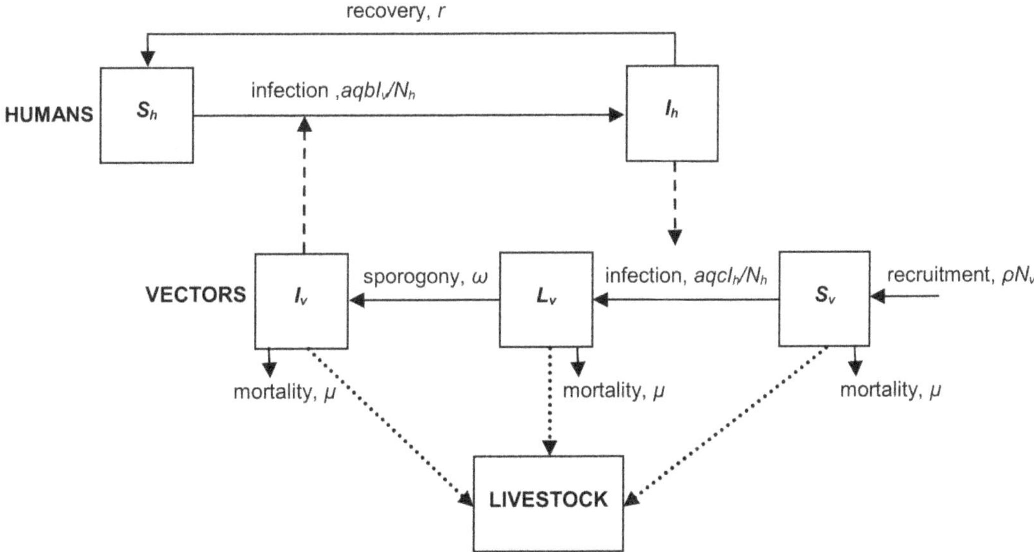

Figure 1. Schematic representation of the malaria model. Horizontal solid lines denote transitions between epidemiological states, and dashed lines represent transmission of infection between human hosts and mosquito vectors. Dotted lines denote vectors feeding on livestock. The vector population consists of adult female anopheline mosquitoes.

humans to vectors depends on the proportion of infectious humans, I_h/N_h, the vector feeding rate on humans, aq, and the probability c that a vector will become infected after feeding upon an infectious human. Infected latent mosquitoes, L_v, become infectious after a sporozoite maturation period (latent period $= 1/\omega$). Anopheline vectors are assumed to remain infectious throughout their life, as usually observed. Infection is assumed to have no impact on vector feeding behaviour, reproduction, nor mortality, as in most malaria models. Although some effects from infection have been described [67], they are not considered in the approximation adopted here.

The vector life expectancy is often about the same order of magnitude as the latent period in the vector. Consequently, only a minority of the infected vector population survives to become infectious, and therefore the model must incorporate the class of latent vectors as well as vector mortality and recruitment. The mortality rate of adult vectors, μ, is assumed to be age independent, such that the average vector life-span is $1/\mu$. We consider two implementations for the recruitment rate. One where the vector population is kept constant by assuming that recruitment and mortality rates are equal $\rho = \mu$.

Another where the density-dependent regulation of the adult vector population due to competition within the larval stages, which depends on the abundance and extent of breeding sites, is explicitly modelled. Following Lord et al. [68] and Kawaguchi et al. [66], the recruitment rate of newly emerged female adults entering the susceptible class is given by

$$\rho = \rho_0 - \rho_s N_v \text{ and } \rho_s = \frac{\rho_0}{K},$$

$$\Leftrightarrow \rho = \rho_0 \left(1 - \frac{N_v}{K}\right),$$

where ρ and ρ_s are the vector recruitment rate in the absence of density-dependence constraints and the strength of the density-dependence in recruitment, respectively, and K is the vector-carrying capacity of the ecosystem. It is assumed that the number and capacity of the breeding sites (and therefore, the vector-carrying capacity) remain the same independently of the hosts' abundance and availability. For instance, the potential increase in breeding sites due to livestock hoof prints is not considered here. While density dependence is essential for the systematic investigation of the zooprophylactic effects of livestock populations with different sizes and characteristics, this is no longer a focus on the investigation of insecticide treatment later on. As such, variable vector population is primarily used in the first part of the Results (Untreated Livestock) and the constant vector population is the implementation of choice throughout the second part (Insecticide Treated Livestock).

As done for simplification in previous malaria models, we assume that vectors take one bloodmeal per gonotrophic cycle, and therefore, the interval between bloodmeals corresponds to the length of the gonotrophic cycle. Similarly, female mosquitoes are assumed to feed homogenously with a fixed preference for humans and/or animals.

Formulation of livestock effects

In the absence of insecticide treatment, the effects of livestock on the human blood index, q, follow what has been proposed by Sota and Mogi [63] and are defined by:

$$q = \frac{N_h A_h}{N_h A_h + N_l A_l},$$

which can be simplified to:

$$q = \frac{1}{1 + \frac{N_l A_l}{N_h A_h}},$$

where A_h and A_l are the proportional availabilities of the human and livestock hosts, respectively, and can take any value between 0 and 1, inclusive. The term availability encompasses all the factors that can influence the likelihood of the vector feeding on a given type of host, when two types of alternative hosts are present in equal numbers. Namely, these factors include the accessibility of each host to the vector (which can vary with distance between vector breeding sites and location of humans/livestock at night, whether located indoors or outdoors, under a bednet or not, or livestock enclosed inside a shed or not), and on the intrinsic propensity to feed upon humans *versus* animals (anthropophily *versus* zoophily), and to feed in the location where the host resides (endophagy *versus* exophagy), which can be modified by vector genetics and learning. In the presence of insecticide treatment, the expression for the human blood index is generalized as

$$q = \frac{1}{1 + \frac{N_l}{N_h} \frac{A_l(1-\varepsilon\alpha)}{A_h}}, \tag{3}$$

where ε is the proportion of livestock population treated with insecticide, hereafter referred as treatment coverage, and α is the diversion probability, defined as the probability that a host-seeking mosquito will be diverted away from ($\alpha > 0$, repellency) or towards ($\alpha < 0$, attractancy) an insecticide-treated animal. Therefore, the insecticide treatment of livestock only affects the human blood index if the intervention has some diversion effect upon the vectors, either repellency or attractancy (see **Text S1.1** for more details).

The baseline mortality rate of the vector is decomposed as being the sum of the minimum mortality rate (μ_m) due to causes other than searching for a bloodmeal host (i.e. mortality due to hazards during the act of feeding on a host, the gestation period, the search for oviposition sites, and the underlying aging process), and the mortality due to searching for a bloodmeal host (μ_s). The search-related mortality is assumed to be proportional to the length of the searching period, which is inversely related to the abundance and availability of potential blood meal hosts. These assumptions follow previous models by Saul [27] and Killeen and Smith [65].

When no livestock are treated with insecticide, the expression for the vector mortality rate therefore becomes

$$\mu = \mu_m + \left(\frac{1}{(N_h A_h + N_l A_l)j}\right) a,$$

where the last term is the search-related mortality, μ_s. Parameter j is a factor to scale the proportional availabilities (A_h, A_l) of hosts to the mosquito vectors into absolute availability values. As in most previous malaria models, it is assumed that the feeding success of malaria vectors is independent of the density of vectors per available host [69].

When livestock are treated with insecticide the mortality rate is generalized as

$$\mu = \mu_m + \mu_s + \mu_k$$
$$= \mu_m + \left(\frac{1}{(N_h A_h + (1-\epsilon\alpha)N_l A_l)j}\right)a + \left(\frac{\epsilon(1-\alpha)N_l A_l}{N_h A_h + N_l A_l}k\right)a. \quad (4)$$

In the μ_s term, as seen for the human blood index, if there is repellency ($\alpha > 0$) it is as if the availability of livestock became reduced by the proportion $\varepsilon\alpha$, which corresponds to the proportion of bites attempted on a given animal that will be diverted to another animal or human host. This will cause an increase in the time it takes for the vector to find a bloodmeal host, with consequent increase in the search-related vector mortality. Conversely, if there is attractancy ($\alpha < 0$), it is as if the availability of livestock became increased by the proportion $\varepsilon\alpha$, which corresponds to the proportion of bites attempted on a given animal that were diverted from another animal or human host. This will decrease the time for the vector to find a bloodmeal host, thereby decreasing the search-related vector mortality. The μ_k term accounts for the direct lethal effect of insecticide applied on livestock, and is a function of the vector biting rate on livestock, the treatment coverage, ε, the diversion probability, α, and the insecticidal probability, k. The daily biting rate, a, needs to be included in the expressions for μ_s and μ_k, since the additional mortalities, either due to searching for a bloodmeal host or due to attempting to feed on insecticide-treated livestock, are only suffered by the vector when it attempts to blood feed (see **Text S1.2** for more details). Our model assumes that the insecticide effects (diversion and insecticidal probabilities) are constant, therefore reflecting average values of what would be observed throughout the year.

Simulations

The system of equations (1)–(2) was analysed symbolically for the derivation of endemic equilibrium solutions (see **Text S2**) and numerically for the simulation of dynamical trajectories over time. Numerical integration was performed using BERKELEY MADONNA v. 8.3.9, with the built-in method *fourth order Runge-Kutta*. The equilibrium solutions were further explored with MATLAB v. R2011a.

We first investigate the effects of untreated livestock in malaria transmission and then move to explore the impact of treating livestock with an insecticide that has lethal and possible diversionary effects (repellency or attractancy) upon malaria vectors. For this purpose, a range of simulations was performed with system (1)–(2), focusing on scenarios of endemic *Plasmodium falciparum* malaria.

Threshold derivation

We also determined the threshold conditions required for persistence of malaria, by analyzing the equilibria of the model represented by system (1)–(2). The average number of secondary cases generated by a single infectious individual introduced in a population of fully susceptible individuals, is known as the basic reproduction number, denoted by R_0 [61,70]. This threshold quantity expresses the transmission potential of an infectious disease and must exceed unity for the infection to be maintained in the population. The expression for R_0 was derived by linearization around the disease-free equilibrium (DFE), based on the next-generation operator approach [71,72]. We then explored the impact of ITL on R_0 for different intervention scenarios. Namely, by setting $R_0 = 1$, we obtained the critical proportion of the livestock population that must be treated with insecticide, and assessed how this critical coverage would be affected by the insecticide diversionary properties.

Parameterization

Parameters values for the untreated livestock model were obtained directly or derived from the literature and are provided in Table 1. The effects of insecticide treatment were explored using parameter values that were either extracted or derived from empirical data from the index studies in the North-West Frontier Province of Pakistan (ITL trial conducted by Rowland et al. [41]) and in the Konso district of South-West Ethiopia (field study by Franco [9]), or from previous studies within or near the area of the index studies, as listed in Table 2. See **Text S3** for details on parameterization.

Results

Untreated livestock

Here we explore the effects that varying the abundance and/or availability untreated livestock could have on different outcome measures of malaria transmission. All the simulations used parameter values as listed in Table 1, unless otherwise specified.

Figure 2 shows the vector population density and prevalence of human infection over time as livestock are introduced in a setting where previously only humans and no livestock were present. Simulations were performed assuming a fix human density ($N_h = 100$) and 1 head of livestock per person ($\theta_{Nl} = 0.25$). The proportional availability of livestock to vectors was the same as that of humans for all plots in this figure ($A_l = 0.5$), illustrating the case of a moderately zoophilic vector, like *An. arabiensis* in Ethiopia. Additional scenarios of host density and availability were also explored.

Firstly, we simulate a modified model with the best case scenario where the vector population is kept constant ($N_v(t) = 1000$) by assuming that recruitment and mortality rates are the same ($\rho = \mu$) (black line), and secondly, the carrying capacity was set to a higher level ($K = 5{,}000$ to $100{,}000$) and the vector population density increased from its initial equilibrium ($N_v(0) = 1000$) towards carrying capacity (coloured lines). As we would expect, in the case of constant vector density, the introduction of livestock leads to consistent reductions in the prevalence of human cases by diverting vector feeds to livestock (black line). Overall, the higher the numbers and/or availability of the introduced livestock, the stronger is the predicted zooprophylactic effect on malaria transmission. When the vector population density is allowed to increase, however, the prevalence of human cases might increase (coloured lines). For a given density and availability of livestock, the higher the carrying capacity is in relation to the initial vector population density, the higher the vector density and consequently malaria transmission levels in the new endemic equilibrium. In all simulated scenarios in **Figure 2** the system reaches a new equilibrium in less than 3 years after the introduction of livestock.

Figure 3 examines various outcome measures of malaria transmission that characterize the new endemic equilibrium that is reached under a range of relative livestock to human density (θ_{Nl} varying from 0 to 1), when the proportional availability of livestock to vectors is either the same ($A_l = 0.5$) or nine times higher ($A_l = 0.9$) as that of humans, the latter resembling a scenario of a highly zoophilic vector, ~ *An. culicifacies* in Pakistan. The outcome measures investigated include the human blood index (HBI, designated as q in our model), daily overall vector mortality (μ), vector density (N_v),daily entomological inoculation rate (EIR),

Table 1. Parameter values for modelling the effects of untreated livestock on malaria.

Symbol	Definition	Value	[Reference]
a	Vector daily biting rate on any host	0.5	[89]
b	Probability that humans become infected from the bite of an infectious vector	0.04	[90]
c	Probability that vectors become infected after biting on an infectious human	0.3	[90]
r	Human daily recovery rate from infection (1/average duration of infection)	0.05	[29,30,90]
ω	Daily rate at which infected mosquitoes become infectious (1/latent period)	0.07	[91]
μ	Overall average vector daily mortality rate ($\mu_m + \mu_s$)	Varied	Derived
μ_h	Vector daily mortality rate in absence of available livestock	0.1	[89]
μ_m	Vector daily minimum mortality rate when there are no hazards due to search for a bloodmeal host	0.05**	[89]
μ_s	Vector daily mortality rate due to searching for a bloodmeal host	Varied**	Derived
ρ	Overall average vector daily recruitment rate	Varied	Derived*
ρ_0	Vector daily recruitment rate in the absence of density-dependence constraints	Varied	Derived*
ρ_s	Strength of the density-dependence in recruitment (/day)	Varied	Derived*
K	Carrying capacity of the vector population (/ha)	10^3 to 10^5	-
$N_v(0)$	Initial vector density, prior to change in livestock abundance and/or availability (/ha)	10^3	-
N_h	Human density (/ha)	100	-
θ_{Nl}	Relative density of livestock:humans (N_l/N_h)	0 to 20	-
A_l	Proportional availability of livestock to vectors	0 to 1	-
A_h	Proportional availability of humans to vectors (= 1-A_l)	0 to 1	-
q	Proportion of vector bloodmeals on humans (Human Blood Index)	0 to 1	Derived
j	Scaling factor to transform proportional availabilities into absolute availabilities	Varied	Derived

*For simulations with constant vector population density: $\rho = \mu$; for variable vector density: $\rho = \rho_0(1 - N_v/K)$ and $\rho_0 = \mu_h K/(K - N_v(0))$.
**The relative magnitudes of μ_s and μ_m were varied in a sensitivity analysis.

and prevalence of infection in humans (I_h). The EIR is the number of infective mosquito bites received by a human per unit time, estimated multiplying the daily human-biting rate (HBR) by the proportion of mosquitoes with sporozoites in their salivary glands (I_v/N_v). The HBR is the total number of mosquito bites received by a human, per day, and is calculated as the product of the number of vectors per human and the number of daily bites on humans per vector (HBR = (N_v/N_h)aHBI).The figure illustrates the effects of livestock on decreasing the human blood index while decreasing vector mortality (**Figure 3A,B**) and increasing vector population density (**Figure 3C,D**). The combination of these effects may lead to situations where the presence of livestock increases, decreases, or has no significant impact on malaria transmission (all other panels in **Figure 3**). The introduction of livestock is predicted to have a zooprophylactic effect, i.e. decrease malaria transmission, in two situations. One is that the vector population density does not increase as a result of livestock introduction. The other is that although the vector population density increases as a result of livestock introduction, the livestock numbers and availability to vectors are sufficiently high, such that the increase in vector density is counteracted by the diversion of bites from humans to animals (**Figure 3**). Otherwise, the introduction of livestock is predicted to increase malaria transmission.

Impact of vector search-related mortality on the effects of untreated livestock. For the purpose of illustrating the model behaviour, the simulations for untreated livestock assume that the vector-search mortality when no livestock are available (i.e. when $N_l = 0$ or $A_l = 0$), has the same value as the vector minimum mortality rate ($\mu_s = \mu_m = \mu_h 0.5 = 0.05$/day). A sensitivity analysis was done to explore the impact of different relative magnitudes of the vector search-related mortality (**Figure S1** in **Text S4.1**). If the vector search-related mortality is already negligible before livestock are introduced, then introducing livestock will have no impact on the vector mortality, and will simply decrease HBI, consequently decreasing malaria transmission. Conversely, if the vector search-related mortality is considerable, introducing livestock can considerably decrease vector mortality, which can increase the proportion of vectors surviving the extrinsic incubation period to become infectious, and thereby counteracting the decrease of the HBI due to diversion of mosquito bites from humans to livestock, consequently increasing malaria transmission. After a certain threshold of livestock density, further increasing their abundance produces negligible reduction on vector mortality.

Insecticide treated livestock

To explore the effects of ITL on malaria the model was fitted to *P. falciparum* malaria transmitted by the highly zoophilic *An. culicifacies* in Pakistan and the more anthropophilic *An. arabiensis* in Ethiopia. Parameter values are listed in Table 2. The main differences in the malaria transmission parameters between the Asian and African settings are as follows. In Ethiopia, livestock were 8.1 times more abundant, although with an estimated 56.8 times lower availability to the main malaria vector, than in Pakistan, resulting in a predicted HBI over 4 times higher in the African than in the Asian setting. Additionally, the estimated duration of the latent period in vectors was slightly shorter, while the vector life expectancy was 75% higher in Ethiopia than in Pakistan. The initial density of vectors per human and the probability of infection in vectors were set to be, respectively, 3.3 and 13.6 times higher in Pakistan than in Ethiopia.

Table 2. Parameter values for modelling the effects of insecticide-treated livestock on malaria.

Symbol	Definition	Value		[Reference]	
		Pakistan	Ethiopia	Pakistan	Ethiopia
a	Vector daily biting rate on any host (1/gonotrophic cycle)	0.4	0.4	[92]	[93,94]
b	Probability that humans become infected from the bite of an infectious vector	0.5	0.5	[95,96]	[95,96]
c	Probability that vectors become infected after biting on an infectious human	0.95	0.07	**	**
r	Human daily recovery rate from infection (1/average duration of infection)	0.05	0.05	***	***
ω	Daily rate at which infected mosquitoes become infectious (1/latent period)	0.057	0.064	Derived from [9,91]	Derived from [9,91]
μ	Overall average vector daily mortality rate ($\mu_m+\mu_s+\mu_k$)	Varied	Varied	Derived	Derived
μ_0	Vector daily natural mortality rate in the absence of ITL (1/natural life expectancy)	0.22	0.12	Derived from [41,92]	Derived from [93,94,97]
μ_m	Vector daily minimum mortality rate when there are no hazards due to search for a bloodmeal host (1/vector maximum life expectancy)	0.11****	0.06****	-	-
μ_s	Vector daily mortality due to searching for a bloodmeal host*	0.11****	0.06****	Derived	Derived
μ_k	Vector daily mortality due to the direct lethal effect of insecticide applied on livestock	Varied	Varied	Derived	Derived
ρ	Overall average vector daily recruitment rate	$=\mu$	$=\mu$	-	-
N_v	Vector density (/ha)	5000	1500	**	**
N_h	Human density (/ha)	100	100	-	-
θ_{Nl}	Relative density of livestock:humans (N_l/N_h)	0.14	1.13	[41]	[9]
θ_{Al}	Relative availability of livestock:humans (A_l/A_h)	53.24	0.938	Derived from [98]	Derived from [99]
A_l	Proportional availability of livestock to vectors ($\theta_{Al}/(1+\theta_{Al})$)	0.982	0.484	Derived	Derived
A_h	Proportional availability of humans to vectors (1-A_l)	0.018	0.516	Derived	Derived
q	Proportion of vector bloodmeals on humans*	0.118	0.485	Derived	Derived
j	Scaling factor to transform proportional availabilities into absolute availabilities	Varied	Varied	Derived	Derived
ε	Treatment coverage: proportion of livestock population that is treated with insecticide	0 to 1	0 to 1	-	-
k	Insecticidal probability	0.1 (0 to 0.9)	0.1 (0 to 0.9)	Derived from [54]	-
α	Diversion probability ($\alpha>0$, repellency; $\alpha<0$, attractancy)	0 to 1	−1 to 1	-	-

Malaria vectors: *An. culicifacies* in Pakistan, *An. arabiensis* in Ethiopia.
*Parameter values pre-intervention that will be affected if livestock are treated with an insecticide with diversion properties.
**Values chosen to produce malaria prevalence similar to the observed in the index study areas.
***M. Rowland unpublished data.
****The relative magnitudes of μ_s and μ_m were varied in a sensitivity analysis.

It was assumed that, prior to the ITL intervention, an endemic equilibrium of malaria transmission had been reached and, as in most previous zooprophylaxis models [27,65,66], vector population density was at its equilibrium level, and remained constant throughout the intervention (i.e. vector recruitment and mortality rates are the same). We therefore consider the scenario where the insecticide has no impact on the overall vector population density. Thus, the beneficial impact of an ITL intervention with a non-diversionary insecticide is assumed to be due only to the decrease on vector survival caused by the toxic insecticidal effect, and consequent reduction in the proportion of vectors that become infectious. When the insecticide additionally has some repellent properties, there is some beneficial effect from increasing the vector search-related mortality, which partially counteracts the increase in vector bloodmeals on humans. Conversely, when there is attractancy, there is the greater benefit of decreasing the bloodmeals in humans, which counteracts the decrease in vector search mortality.

Impact on malaria prevalence. We started by exploring the predicted impact of ITL on the prevalence of human infection. This is represented in terms of the prevalence ratio (PR), which is defined as the ratio between the prevalence under a given coverage of insecticide-treated livestock (ε) and the prevalence pre-intervention. The proportional reduction on the pre-intervention prevalence is given by 1-(prevalence ratio).

Simulations were initially performed to estimate the coverage of treated livestock (ε) and insecticidal probability (k) required to obtain the 54% reduction in *P. falciparum* prevalence observed in the Pakistan ITL trial, for the Pakistan and the Ethiopian simulated scenarios, assuming the use of an insecticide with no diversion properties ($\alpha = 0$, **Figure 4**). For any given intervention effort, ITL is predicted to cause a stronger reduction in malaria prevalence in Pakistan than in Ethiopia. Nevertheless, the same reduction in prevalence could be achieved in Ethiopia, if using higher treatment coverage and/or a product with stronger or longer lasting insecticidal properties. For instance, for the scenario of $k = 0.1$ (estimated value from Pakistan data, as detailed in **Text S3.2**), the predicted treatment coverage required to obtain the observed reduction in prevalence (PR = 0.46) is $\varepsilon = 15\%$ in Pakistan and 25% in Ethiopia (**Figure 4**).

We also investigated whether by increasing the attractiveness of insecticide treated livestock to vectors it would be possible to obtain in Ethiopia the same reduction in prevalence as observed in the Pakistan trial, with the same intervention effort used in the Asian setting (**Figure 5**). To achieve in Ethiopia the same PR = 0.46 with similar coverage as predicted for Pakistan ($\varepsilon = 15\%$, for $k = 0.1$, assuming no repellency) would require an attractancy of 20%, while with attractancy of 10% or 30%, the coverage would be approximately 19% or 13%, respectively.

We then explored how the coverage would be affected if the insecticide had a repellency effect upon vectors, and what might be the repellency probability above which the intervention could become deleterious, by causing prevalence to increase above the pre-intervention level. Not surprisingly, the intervention benefits considerably decrease if the insecticide has repellency properties. Considering again the case of the estimated $k = 0.1$ (**Figure 5**), to achieve the observed reduction in prevalence (PR = 0.46) with the 93% coverage that was actually applied in the Pakistan trial, the model suggests that a repellency probability of ~17% would need to be acting in Pakistan. If that same repellency level was acting in Ethiopia, the required coverage was predicted to be 60%. For repellency above 17% in Pakistan or above 21% in Ethiopia, the achieved reduction in prevalence is expected to be always smaller than the observed (i.e. the prevalence ratio, PR, would always be >0.46), even if all livestock are treated ($\varepsilon = 1$). The intervention would become deleterious (PR >1) for repellency above 20% in Pakistan and above 28% in Ethiopia (**Figure 5**). The smaller the coverage (for a given k), or the greater the k (for a given coverage), the higher is the repellence threshold above which ITL will start becoming detrimental (PR >1) (**Figure S2** in **Text S4.2**).

Threshold phenomena. The derived basic reproduction number for the malaria model is given by:

$$R_0 = \frac{N_v}{N_h} \frac{(aq)^2 bc}{r\mu} \frac{\omega}{(\omega + \mu)} \qquad (5)$$

where q is given by expression (3) and μ is given by expression (4).

By setting $R_0 = 1$ in (5) we see that the critical proportion of the livestock population that must be treated with insecticide in order to interrupt malaria transmission is

$$\varepsilon_c = \frac{\sqrt{r\omega\left(4\frac{N_v}{N_h}(aq')^2 bc + r\omega\right)} - r\left(\omega + 2\left(\mu_m + \frac{a}{(N_h A_h + N_l A_l)j}\right)\right)}{2ra(1-q')k}, \qquad (6)$$

where q' is the HBI in the absence of insecticide treatment: $q' = \dfrac{1}{1 + \frac{N_l}{N_h}\frac{A_l}{A_h}}$.

This expression for ε_c is valid for the best-case scenario regarding repellence and the worst case scenario regarding attractancy, i.e. when using an insecticide without any diversionary effects upon vectors ($\alpha = 0$).

To explore how repellency ($\alpha > 0$) or attractancy ($\alpha < 0$) would impact ε_c numerical simulations were performed (**Figure 6**). The stronger the insecticidal probability (k), the smaller is the critical proportion of treated livestock (ε_c) required to potentially reduce R_0 below unity, for any given α in Ethiopia, and for $\alpha < 0.4$ in Pakistan. In the Asian scenario, for $\alpha \geq 0.4$, above a certain treatment coverage and insecticidal probability, there could be a shift from $R_0 < 1$ to $R_0 > 1$. For instance, for $\alpha = 0.4$ and $k = 0.4$, R_0 becomes less than 1 if coverage is above 36% and below 90%, while for coverage above 90% then R_0 increases to greater than 1. Similarly, for $\alpha = 0.5$ and $k = 0.6$, R_0 is reduced to less than 1 for coverage between 29% and 70%, but for coverage above 70% the R_0 becomes above 1. For any given k, the stronger the repellence, the higher is the critical coverage, while the stronger the attractancy, the lower is the critical coverage. Furthermore, for any given k, with or without repellency, the critical coverage is always higher for Ethiopia than for Pakistan (**Figure 6**).

Impact of vector search-related mortality on the effects of insecticide-treated livestock. The baseline simulations for ITL assume that the background vector search-related mortality (pre-livestock treatment) has the same value as the vector minimum mortality rate ($\mu_s = \mu_m = \mu_0.0.5$). Additional simulations were done to explore the sensitivity of the findings to alternative search-related vector mortality values (**Figure 5** and **Figure 6** can be contrasted with **Figure S3** and **Figure S4** in **Text S4.2.1**, respectively).

Although there is uncertainty about its exact value, the relative magnitude of the background vector search-related mortality will only affect the intervention impact if the insecticide has diversionary properties. Namely, decreases in the background search mortality will counteract the only benefit of repellence (which was an increase on the search-associated vector mortality), and consequently decrease the beneficial impact of an ITL intervention. In general, the smaller the background search-related mortality, the stronger is the detrimental effect of any given repellency probability ($\alpha > 0$) on malaria prevalence or R_0, and consequently, the greater is the coverage required to achieve a given reduction in prevalence or R_0, and the lower is the repellence threshold above which the intervention would become deleterious (and *vice-versa*). For instance, comparing the baseline scenario with the worst-case scenario of null background vector search-related mortality, the repellence threshold would decrease from 20% to 13% in Pakistan and from 28% to 19% in Ethiopia (**Figure S3** in **Text S4**). This relationship becomes however increasingly non-linear with increase in the insecticidal effect (k) of a treatment with repellency, namely in Pakistan (**Figure S4** in **Text S4**). For a given attractancy probability ($\alpha < 0$), the smaller the background vector-search related mortality, the stronger are the intervention benefits, and consequently, the smaller is the coverage required to achieve a given reduction in prevalence or R_0 (**Figure S3** and **Figure S4** in **Text S4**).

Discussion

By combining a mathematical model with field data we have explored the different effects that livestock can have on human malaria in areas where the disease is transmitted by zoophilic vectors, allowing us to understand under which circumstances livestock-based interventions could play a role in malaria control programmes.

Our model predicts that the presence of untreated livestock will have a zooprophylactic effect in two scenarios. One is when vector population density does not increase as a result of livestock introduction. The other is when although the vector population

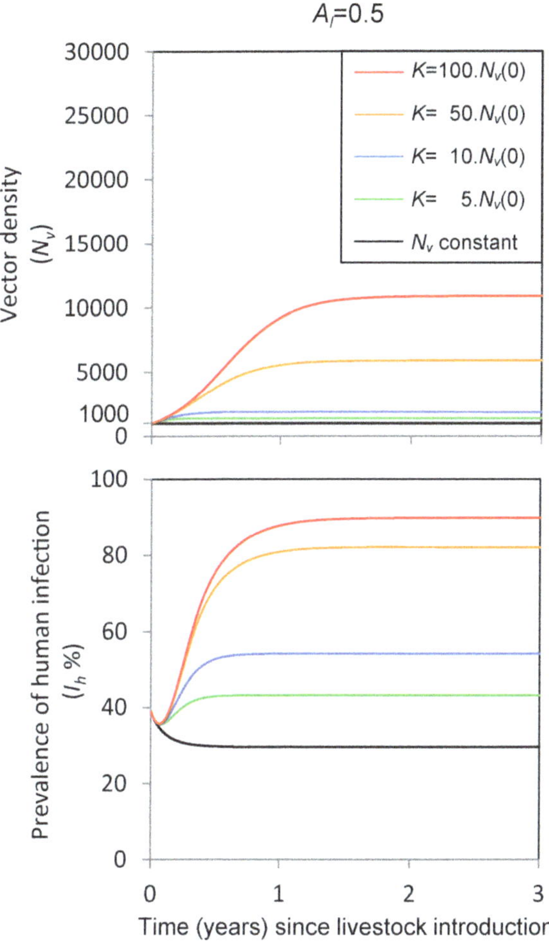

Figure 2. Temporal effect of introducing livestock in a setting with endemic malaria. Effect of introducing livestock in a setting where only humans were present, when: N_v remains constant (black line), and when N_v increases until reaching a maximum, which depends on the carrying capacity, K (increasing from $K=5{,}000$ (green) to 100,000 (red)). $N_v(0)=1000$, $N_h=100$ and $A_l=0.5$: the availability of livestock to vectors is the same as that of humans; $\theta_{Nl}=0.25$ (1 head of livestock per 4 persons). To achieve the same initial equilibrium N_v (and I_h) for various K values, the vector recruitment rate in the absence of density-dependence constraints was set to vary accordingly: $\rho_0=\mu_h K/(K-N_v(0))$. Other parameters are as in Table 1.

density increases, the numbers and availability of livestock to vectors are sufficiently high (such that the resulting diversion of bites from humans to livestock can counteract the increase in vector density), or the vector mortality related with host-search pre-livestock introduction was sufficient low (such that introducing livestock causes no significant decrease on the already small search mortality). Otherwise, the introduction of livestock is predicted to increase malaria transmission.

These results are in agreement with the insights from two previous zooprophylaxis models [27,63]. Namely, Sota & Mogi [63] also identified as key determinants of the beneficial *versus* detrimental effect of untreated livestock on malaria transmission whether the vector population had reached its maximum possible density prior to livestock introduction, and whether the density and/or availability of animal hosts were sufficiently high. It is worthwhile mentioning that these features are captured by both the present model and the Sota & Mogi [63] model although the two works differ in the approach used to model the potential detrimental impact of livestock on malaria transmission. The present work explicitly models the effect of animal or human hosts' abundance and availability on vector mortality, with consequent impact on the dynamics and density of adult vectors. Instead, Sota & Mogi [63] assumed a constant vector mortality rate, and modelled the effect of hosts abundance and availability on the probability of successful blood feeding of the vector, with consequent impact on the number of eggs laid and density of adult vectors in the future generations. Aside from the work by Sota & Mogi [63], two other previous zooprophylaxis models that addressed the effect of untreated livestock on malaria transmission [27,65], have also explicitly modelled the effect of animal or human hosts abundance and availability on vector mortality. Saul [27] also highlighted that the effect of untreated livestock on malaria greatly depended on the magnitude of the search-related vector mortality: when this is significant, increase in livestock density could lead to increased malaria transmission, which is consistent with our results.

Regarding the insecticide-treatment of livestock, when using an insecticide without diversionary properties, any given intervention effort is predicted to achieve a stronger reduction in malaria transmission in a setting with highly zoophilic vectors (exemplified by Pakistan) than with the more anthropophilic *An. arabiensis* (illustrated by Ethiopia), as expected. Yet, the same reduction in malaria prevalence could be achieved in Ethiopia, if treating a high proportion of the livestock population with a product that has stronger and/or lost lasting insecticidal effect than what was used in Pakistan. The predicted intervention effort required to achieve a given reduction in prevalence with a non-repellent insecticide, is however, surprisingly low, and most likely unrealistic. In the Pakistan trial, a 54% reduction in prevalence was obtained, following treatment of 93% of the livestock population in the trial villages (cattle, goats, and sheep) [41]. Our results suggest that, to achieve the observed reduction in prevalence with such high treatment coverage, the insecticidal effect would need to be extremely small.

When accounting for a possible repellency effect of the insecticide, the expected benefits of the intervention decrease considerably in both settings, requiring more realistic parameter values to obtain the results observed in the Pakistan trial. Repellency threshold probabilities were identified above which the intervention could become detrimental, increasing the prevalence of human infection above the pre-intervention levels. For repellency probability below those thresholds any vector diversion to humans was predicted to be overcompensated by the insecticidal (direct lethal) effect and the increased search-related mortality of the mosquitos attempting to blood feed on insecticide-treated animals. Within that range of repellency probability for which ITL is likely to still reduce malaria prevalence, a greater benefit may be observed in Pakistan or in Ethiopia, depending on the repellency and coverage levels.

The results indicate that repellency has a stronger detrimental impact on malaria (prevalence or R_0) in Pakistan than in Ethiopia, and therefore, it would take a smaller level of repellency for ITL to start becoming deleterious in the Asian setting. Above the repellency threshold the intervention becomes always more detrimental in settings with higher availability of livestock to vectors, like in Pakistan and other settings with highly zoophilic vectors.

The repellency level of the insecticide applied to animals can thus have an important effect on the intervention outcome. For a given treatment coverage, the stronger and/or longer lasting the insecticidal effect, the higher is the repellency threshold above

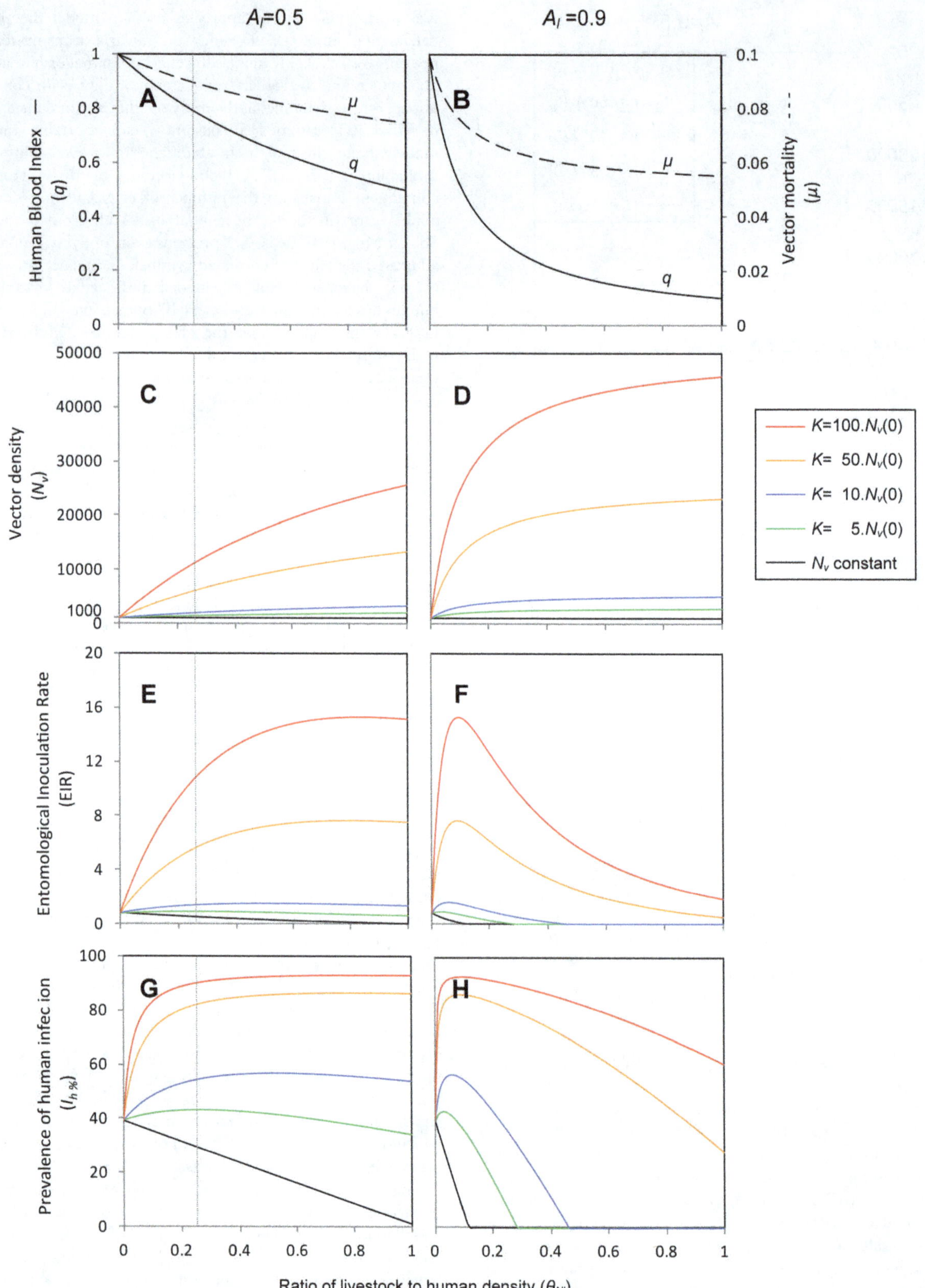

Figure 3. Effect of altering the relative livestock to human density, for different vector density scenarios, at the new endemic equilibrium. Comparing a scenario where the availability of livestock to vectors is the same as that of humans (left, $A_l = 0.5$) *versus* where it is 9 times higher than that of humans (right, $A_l = 0.9$). Along the *x*-axis, representing $\theta_{Nl} = N_l/N_h$, the livestock density N_l is varied relative to a fixed human density $N_h = 100$. $N_v(0) = 1000$. Effect of introducing livestock when: N_v remains constant (black line), and when N_v increases until reaching a maximum, which depends on the carrying capacity, K (coloured lines: K increasing from 5,000 (green line) to 100,000 (red line)). The effects of introducing livestock on the human blood index (HBI) and on the vector mortality rate (μ) are independent from the vector density scenarios (A, B).

The vertical line in the left panels highlights the new endemic equilibrium that is reached after the introduction of 1 head of livestock per 4 persons ($\theta_{NI} = 0.25$), corresponding to the end of the timeline in Figure 2. Other parameters are as in Table 1.

which the intervention starts becoming detrimental. Additionally, when considering doing ITL interventions with high treatment coverage of the livestock population, researchers should be aware that the higher the intervention coverage, the greater the detrimental effect from a given repellency level, and the greater the benefits from reducing repellency. A small decrease in repellency could greatly improve the intervention benefits, with the effect being greater in scenarios with more zoophilic mosquitoes. Interestingly, this is the opposite from the case of insecticide-treated nets (ITNs), where repellency could be beneficial in some circumstances. Namely, the greater the proportion of the human population covered with ITNs the greater are the expected benefits from repellency, and, conversely, the smaller the coverage the greater the likelihood that malaria vectors might be diverted from ITN-protected people to those unprotected (if the density and/or availability of animal hosts to the mosquito vector are small) [65].

In general therefore, the smaller the repellency, the greater the benefits of an ITL intervention. The benefits in settings with moderately zoophilic vectors, such as *An. arabiensis* in sub-Saharan Africa, could be further improved by artificially increasing the attractiveness of livestock to the malaria vector.

If the insecticide has diversionary properties upon the malaria vectors, the magnitude of the vector mortality related with host searching was predicted to considerable affect the model results. Namely, the smaller the vector search-related mortality pre-intervention, the stronger are the insecticide diversionary effects upon malaria prevalence or R_0, be it the detrimental effect of a given repellency probability on transmission, or the reduction in transmission obtained with a given attractancy probability. Given the influential role of the vector search-related mortality upon the effects of untreated and insecticide-treated livestock on malaria transmission, obtaining field estimates for this component of vector mortality is an important challenge that future research should address.

The repellency threshold above which the intervention might become detrimental could be as low as 13% in Pakistan and 19% in Ethiopia, if assuming all livestock population is treated with an average direct insecticidal effect of 10%, under the worst case scenario of null vector search-related mortality. The smaller the treatment coverage, and/or the stronger the insecticidal effect or the search-related mortality, then the higher the repellency level at which ITL can still be safely used.

To our knowledge, this is the first modelling approach that explicitly explores the potential effects of repellency and attractancy in the context of ITL and malaria transmission. The present work is an improvement in relation to previous malaria models of the impact of applying insecticide on animals [27], on animal sheds [66], or on bednets [65]. None of the former two models [27,66], explored a repellent or attractant effect of the insecticide, and although work by Killeen and Smith [65] has looked at repellency and livestock applied to an African setting, it did so in the context of insecticide-treated bednets and diversion of malaria vectors to humans and/or untreated cattle, without referring to insecticide-treatment of cattle.

Considerations on modelling repellency

The present work assumes that when a mosquito tries to bite on an insecticide-treated animal and is repelled, it will be diverted to bite on another host. Nonetheless, it could be that the mosquito is not able to find a successful bloodmeal and does not feed in that night, ending up either feeding only on the following night, or dying earlier. The impact of repellency on vector mortality is

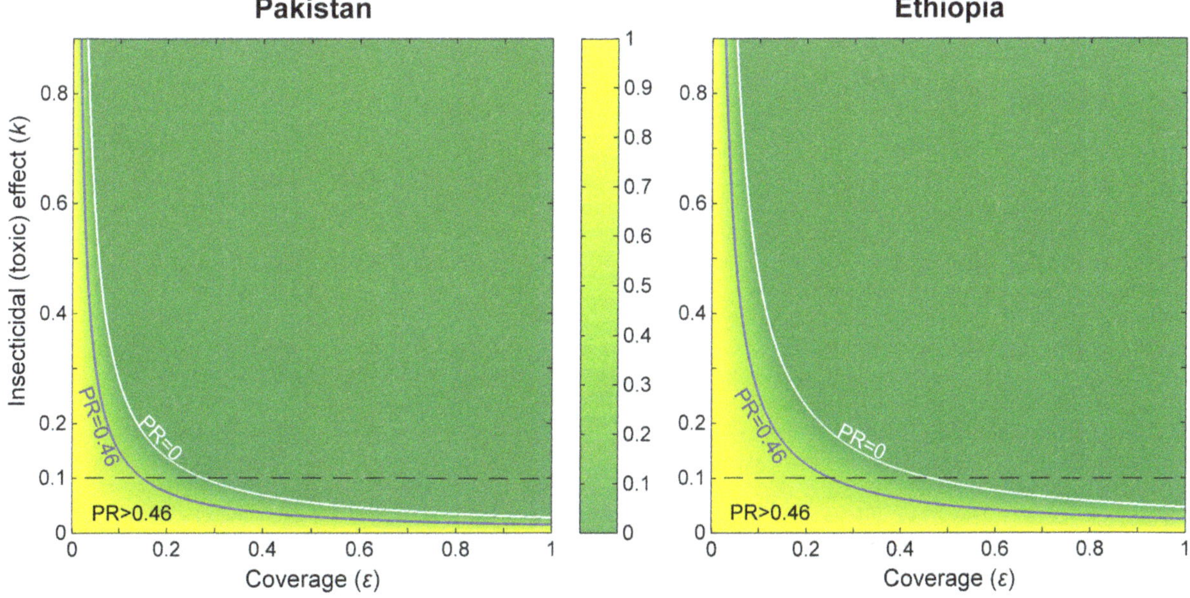

Figure 4. Predicted impact of Insecticide Treatment of Livestock on malaria prevalence, without diversion ($\alpha = 0$)**.** This figure shows the combination of values of coverage and insecticidal probability required to achieve a given prevalence ratio (PR: prevalence with ITL / baseline prevalence). Blue line: PR = 0.46 (like the observed in the Pakistan trial); White line: PR = 0; Dashed line: $k = 0.1$, as estimated for the Pakistan trial. The colour bar shows the scale of PR values, from 0 to 1. Other parameters are as in Table 2.

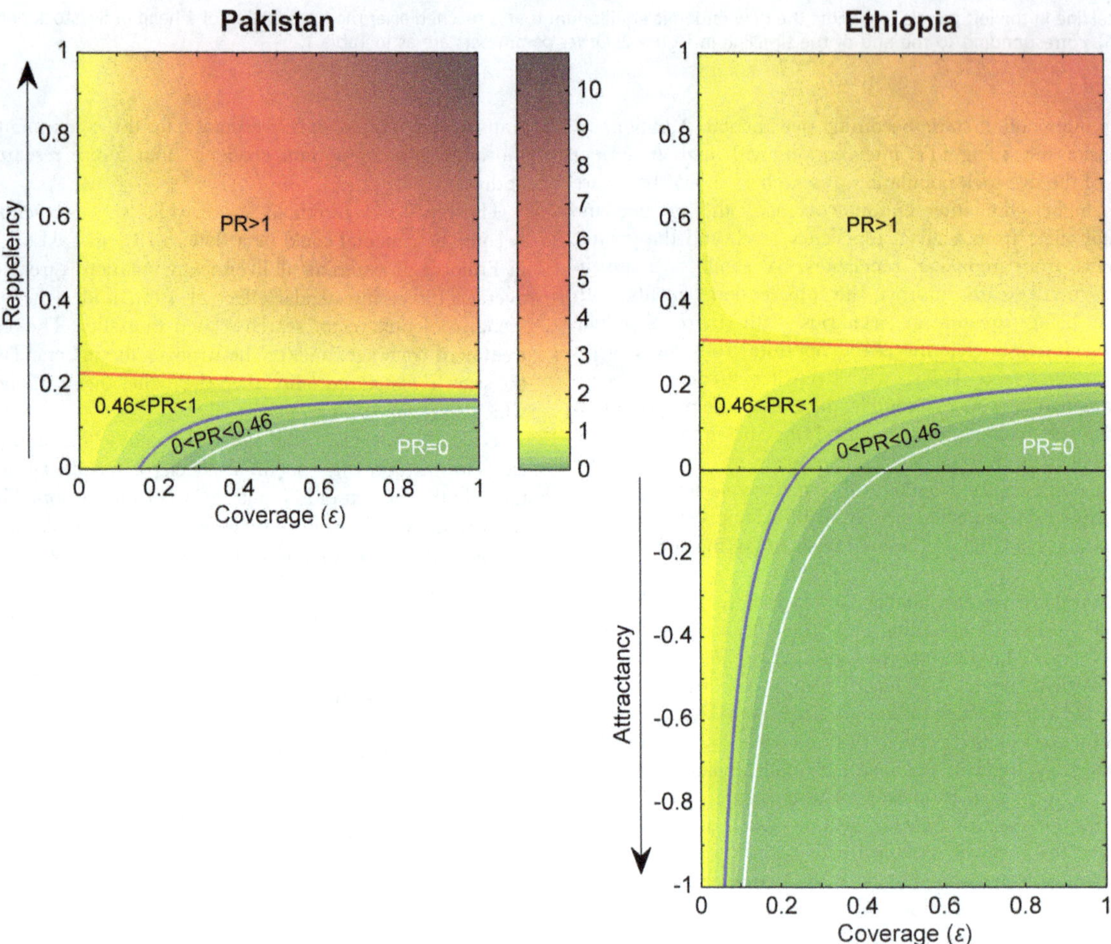

Figure 5. Predicted impact of Insecticide Treatment of Livestock on malaria prevalence – with repellency ($\alpha > 0$) or attractancy ($\alpha < 0$) for $k = 0.1$. This figure shows how the diversionary properties of the insecticide affect the coverage required to achieve a given prevalence ratio (PR: prevalence with ITL / baseline prevalence). Blue line: PR = 0.46 (like the observed in the Pakistan trial); White line: PR = 0; Red line: PR = 1 (above which treating livestock increases malaria prevalence). Along the y axis, α is varying from no diversion ($\alpha = 0$) to maximum repellency ($\alpha = 1$) or maximum attractancy ($\alpha = -1$). The colour bar shows the scale of PR values, from 0 to ≈11 in Pakistan and up to ≈5 in Ethiopia. Other parameters are as in Table 2.

captured by the model, since repellency reduces the availability of treated livestock, increasing the time required to find a bloodmeal host and consequently increasing the vector search-related mortality. The impact of repellency increasing the interval between bloodmeals is something that could be explored by extending the model to explicitly account for that possibility.

We also assume that the probability of vectors being repelled to humans after attempting to bite on livestock, depends only on the proportion of livestock population that is treated with insecticide (coverage,ε), on the repellency probability of the insecticide ($\alpha > 0$), and on the relative number and availability of livestock or human hosts. Additionally, the model assumes that repellency and coverage are independent. In reality, however, the occurrence of a repellent effect can depend on additional factors such as characteristics of the: a) insecticide (chemical compound, formulation and concentration); b) intervention (concentration of the insecticide on the animal's coat, which will eventually decrease with time after application); and c) mosquito vector [73]. Also, the insecticide concentration is likely to be heterogeneous throughout the animal's surface, and the place where the mosquitoes land on the animals can therefore be determinant.

With regards to the mode of action of insecticides applied on livestock depending on the properties of the insecticide itself, some pyrethroids are more toxic to vectors than repellent (e.g. deltamethrin, used in the Pakistan ITL trial), other pyrethroids are more repellent than toxic (e.g. permethrin), and other classes of insecticides (e.g. organophosphates) are just toxic and non-repellent. Yet, even the typical toxic deltamethrin tends to be repellent at low dosages. Namely, as the applied dose of deltamethrin decays over time it goes from being toxic to non-toxic but repellent and then to just repellent.

Due to this, a big concern during the Pakistan ITL trial [41] was that mosquitoes would be repelled onto humans as the dosage of deltamethrin decayed, but it appears malaria was still controlled because the insecticide was reapplied regularly before there was too much decay. This explanation is consistent with the findings from the present work where, on one hand, when accounting for repellency the model results are more compatible with the observed Pakistan trial results, than when assuming that the insecticide had no diversion effect. On the other hand, the predictions suggest that the stronger and/or longer lasting the insecticidal effect, the highest is the repellency threshold above which the intervention is likely to become detrimental. Addition-

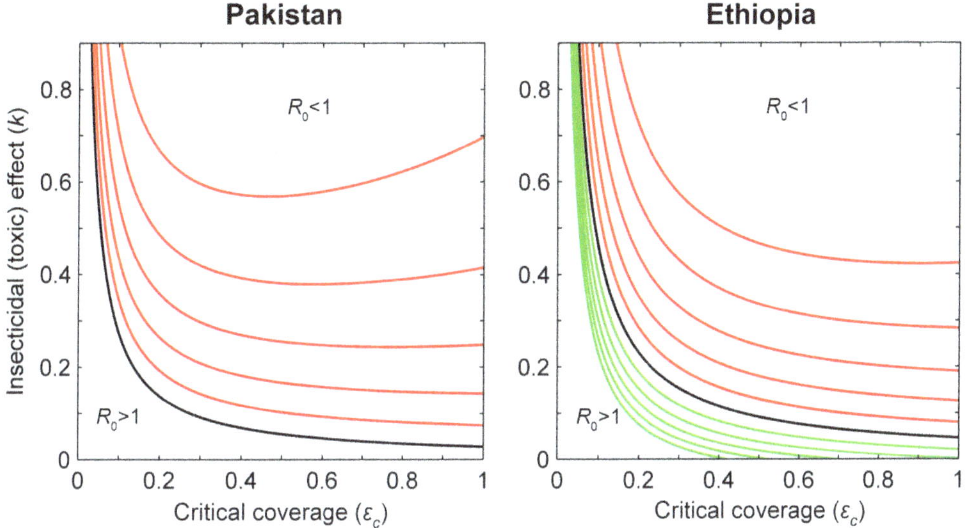

Figure 6. Critical proportion of ITL as a function of the insecticidal (*k*), and diversionnary effect (α). The lines show the combination of values of coverage and insecticidal probability required to achieve $R_0 = 1$, above which R_0 will be decreased below 1, for a given diversion probability (α). Black line: $\alpha = 0$, no repellency or attractancy (is the same as the white line in Figure 4); Red lines: $\alpha > 0$, repellency increasing from 0.1 to 0.5 (top), at intervals of 0.1; Green lines: $\alpha < 0$, attractancy increasing from −0.1 to −0.5 (bottom), at intervals of 0.1. Other parameters are as in baseline simulations (Table 2).

ally, at the high treatment coverage applied in the trial, there is only a small difference between the repellency level with which the observed reduction in prevalence would be achieved, and the repellency threshold. This supports the hypothesis that the intervention effort applied in the Pakistan trial was sufficiently high to make the repellency effects non evident.

Increasing livestock attractiveness to vectors

By increasing the attractiveness of insecticide treated animals to malaria vectors, it could be possible to further enhance the impact of ITL in malaria control in settings with more opportunistic vectors, such as *An. arabiensis* in Ethiopia, as shown in this work. This could eventually enable extending the geographic regions where ITL might reduce malaria burden, to include also areas with more anthropophilic vectors, such as *An. gambiae s.s.*, the most competent malaria vector in sub-Saharan Africa. Given the potential benefits this could bring, it would be worthwhile further exploring this hypothesis in future work.

In practice, however, insecticides tend to be non-attractant (i.e. neutral or repellent). Therefore, to artificially increase livestock attractiveness would require developing an insecticide that has also attractancy properties (in addition to its toxic insecticidal effect), or alternatively, treat livestock with an attractant substance on top of applying a standard insecticide. Although this may sound somewhat speculative, it is not much different from what has been successfully tested in other systems, where synthetic attractants have been applied to baits or traps to increase their attractiveness to tsetse flies [74,75,76], anopheline mosquitoes [58,59], and other insects of medical and veterinary importance [77].

Regarding possible detrimental implications of artificially attracting more mosquitoes into livestock, these are likely to be minimal. Attracting a mosquito to a cow does not necessarily mean the mosquito will succeed in biting/blood feeding as it may be killed or knocked down by exposure to the insecticide before taking up blood, and that is usually the case, namely with pyrethroids. The expected reduction in mosquito survival due to increased exposure to the insecticide toxicity should actually lead to less biting. Therefore, it is unlikely there would be additional disease burden or economic costs, as long as the attractancy would be specific for malaria vectors and would not cause increased number of biting flies or other arthropods that are vectors of pathogens to livestock, and would also not cause a reduction in the animal's blood through excessive biting that could decrease milk or meat yield.

Optimizing insecticide-treated livestock interventions

It is important to highlight that, although we explored the impact that treating livestock with insecticides could have on malaria transmission, this intervention has been traditionally used with a veterinary purpose, to control tsetse flies, ticks and other ectoparasites, and the diseases they transmit to animals, improving livestock health and productivity, such as milk and meat yield. Therefore, when evaluating the cost-effectiveness of the intervention, both the animal health benefits and the public health benefits need to be captured ('One health'). Given the potential double side benefits of veterinary interventions like this, and given the central role of livestock in poor tropical settings, to control human disease and improve livestock health will have disproportionate economic impact that needs to be captured, as accounting for it could promote the wider implementation of the intervention. Namely, if the costs of ITL are allocated to the human health and the animal health sectors in proportion to the benefits, the intervention might be profitable and cost-effective for both sectors. Here lies a challenge to the Public Health community, which will require strengthened collaboration with the Animal Health community.

In addition to the animal health/productivity benefits, ITL uses much less insecticide than traditional malaria control methods, such as indoor spraying of houses with residual insecticide, making ITL very cheap from a human disease control perspective. In the Pakistan trial, sponging livestock with deltamethrin was shown to achieve a reduction in malaria burden similar to indoor residual spraying but with 80% less campaign costs. Furthermore, if accounting for the increase in milk production by the treated cattle, associated with clearance of tick infestations, the economic gain would be enough to cover all insecticide and labor costs [41].

The mathematical model developed here could be used to examine the economic aspects of the 'One Health' approach to disease control, encompassing both human and animal health benefits at a societal level. The model provides a framework for quantifying the benefits of ITL as a reduction in the human health burden (expressed as prevented DALYs, Disability Adjusted Life-Years), associated reduction in health care costs (expressed as $), as well as the improvements in animal health and productivity (expressed as $). The cost-effectiveness of ITL, accounting for both the human and veterinary benefits, could then be compared with other interventions that deliver only human health benefits, such as indoor residual spraying (IRS) and insecticide-treated bednets (ITNs), and the relative attractiveness of ITL across epidemiological settings and animal production systems examined.

The use of any animal-based intervention for malaria control will only be a component of the broader integrated malaria control approach, and will have to be deployed alongside case detection, treatment and prevention. The relative importance of animal-based interventions within the broader approach will vary between settings. Also, the adoption of any recommended intervention is intimately related to the socio-economics of the setting and it is therefore vital to understand the drivers for adoption by the target population.

In Pakistan very high treatment coverage was achieved with a free campaign and the animal owners were enthusiastic because they could see the benefits of tick elimination and improved milk and meat yield [41]. Previously to the campaign the insecticide treatment of livestock for ectoparasites was normally *ad hoc* done by householder according to perceived need, which would lead to only partial coverage at any one time. Therefore, a subsidized campaign approach is recommended, similarly to the externally funded campaigns of IRS.

Although the empirical evidence for Africa is lacking, some inferences can be made from tsetse control work. In particular, the experience from controlling human sleeping sickness in southeast Uganda by targeting the cattle reservoir of the human infective parasite shows that large scale campaigns can also reach very high (>80%) coverage levels with insecticide and trypanocidal treatment. Additionally, reducing the volume of insecticide, and so the price of ITL treatment, through restricted application protocols to target insecticide use to those areas of the cattle where tsetse or anopheline mosquitoes preferentially feed, have the potential to drive routine ITL adoption by small-holder farmers [35,43]. To drive the private uptake of ITL usage, farmers need to see a direct benefit to their animals. Experience from the sleeping sickness work shows that for effective control through ITL it is important that the insecticide products used work against both ticks and the human disease vectors (such as synthetic pyrethroids), as tick control is often the main motivation for farmers to use ITL [34].

ITL is particularly useful for malaria control where vectors, in addition to bloodfeeding on livestock, are (or have became) exophagic (feeding outdoors, therefore escaping to ITNs exposure) and/or exophilic (resting outdoors, and thereby evading IRS).

One cannot rule out that long term and intensive use of ITL may lead to selection for anthropophily, with a consequent shift in preference from animals to humans (assuming that host preference is determined by genetic polymorphisms [78,79,80]). Therefore, changes in the HBI (as a proxy for host preference) should be monitored in regions where repeated campaigns are undertaken [14,41]. Additionally, selection for anthropophily could be countered by combining ITL with indoor strategies to control anthropophilic and endophilic mosquitoes, like ITNs and IRS [19].

At the time of the field studies in the settings to which to which the ITL model was parameterized (Konso region of Ethiopia and NWFP in Pakistan) most people were not using bednets. Future work could expand the present model to investigate the use of livestock-based interventions alongside ITNs or IRS, to provide additional insights to the potential impact that combining these strategies might have on malaria transmission.

A concern inherent to any vector control intervention based on insecticides is the potential development of resistance. Namely, pyrethroid resistance is becoming increasingly wide spread across anopheline mosquitoes [81,82] and several other arthropods that feed on livestock, such as ticks [83,84]. It has been argued that the treatment of livestock with pyrethroids is not likely to induce stronger selection pressure for resistance in malaria vectors than insecticide-treated bednets or indoor residual spraying of houses and cattle sheds, but nevertheless, appropriate monitoring of the vector populations is required if wide scale and long term ITL interventions are implemented [14,41,54].

It has also been recommended that research efforts should target the identification of alternative non-pyrethroid insecticides for livestock treatment [54]. Possible candidates have recently been suggested from the avermectins class of insecticides, which have since long been used in veterinary and human medicine against several helminths and arthropod pests [85] and were latest shown to be also toxic to anopheline mosquitoes. Namely, feeding on bovine blood treated with ivermectin reduced survivorship and fecundity of *An. gambiae s.s.* and *An. arabiensis* [86,87] and may possibly also inhibit the sporogony of *P. falciparum* as it was recently shown in treated humans [88]. Another promising avermectin is the more recent eprinomectin which has similar antihelminthic and ectoparasiticidal action as ivermectin in cattle, but with much less mammary excretion, allowing its use in pregnant and lactating animals, on the contrary of ivermectin [87]. Any of these avermectines could overcome the problems of pyrethroid resistance as well as repellency upon malaria vectors, and could be administered as part of mass livestock vaccination campaigns, simultaneously benefiting animal and human populations. Additionally, while pyrethroids can only be administered topically, both ivermectin and eprinomectine are available topically (as pour-on) and also as injectable formulation (subcutaneous administration), which could surmount the difficulty faced with pyrethroids of achieving high enough concentrations of product throughout the animal's skin. Malaria vectors would however need to bite the animal and take a bloodmeal to be exposed to the insecticide, but every biting mosquito would be exposed and die more promptly, therefore requiring a smaller dose, compared to pyrethroids. Further studies are needed to assess the effects of livestock treated with the recommended dose of ivermectin or eprinomectine upon wild populations of malaria vectors.

Conclusions

A mathematical model was developed to predict the different effects of untreated and insecticide-treated livestock in malaria outcomes in different regions. Similarly to previous work, our model indicates that the zooprophylactic effect of untreated livestock depends on whether 1) the pre-existing malaria vector population had reached its maximum density, 2) livestock abundance and availability to the vector is sufficiently high, and 3) vector mortality related with host-search pre-livestock introduction was sufficiently low. We additional find that, as expected, the insecticide-treatment of livestock is likely to be more beneficial to humans in settings with highly zoophilic malaria vectors as in Pakistan and other areas of South Asia, than in settings with moderately zoophilic vectors, as *An. arabiensis* in sub-Saharan African. Nevertheless, the intervention could also substantially decrease malaria burden in the latter settings, under certain conditions, as illustrated here with the predictions for Ethiopia. Namely, in regions with moderately zoophilic vectors the benefits of the intervention will be maximized if 1) treating most of the livestock population with a product that has a stronger or longer lasting toxic insecticidal effect than what was used in the Pakistan trial, and that has little (ideally null) repellency effect (such as the non-pyrethroids ivermectin or eprinomectin), or 2) if the attractiveness of the treated animals to malaria vectors could be increased.

It is hoped that this work may lead to increasing awareness about the non-linear effects of livestock on malaria transmission, and to the implementation of a community-based trial of insecticide-treated livestock in an African region where *An. arabiensis* predominates, and where this strategy could potentially contribute to the integrated control of human malaria and livestock diseases.

Supporting Information

Text S1 Formulation of livestock effects. S1.1. Livestock effects on Human blood index. S1.2. Livestock effects on vector mortality.

Text S2 Malaria model endemic equilibrium solutions.

Text S3 Model parameterization. S3.1. Untreated livestock model parameterization. S3.2. Insecticide-treated livestock model parameterization for Pakistan and Ethiopia.

Text S4 Sensitivity analyses. S4.1. Sensitivity analysis of the effects of untreated livestock. *Figure S1. Sensitivity analysis of the effects of livestock availability/density vs. vector search-related mortality on several malaria outcomes, at the new endemic equilibrium.* S4.2. Sensitivity analysis of the effects of insecticide-treated livestock. *Figure S2. Sensitivity analysis of the effects of repellency/attractancy vs. insecticidal probability (k) on the prevalence ratio. S4.2.1. Sensitivity analysis of the impact of vector search-related mortality upon the effects of insecticide-treated livestock. Figure S3. Sensitivity analysis of the effects of repellency/attractancy vs. vector search-mortality on the prevalence ratio. Figure S4. Sensitivity analysis of the effects of repellency/attractancy vs. vector search-mortality on the critical proportion of insecticide-treated livestock.*

Acknowledgments

This work is dedicated to Professor Clive R. Davies, who supervised Ana O. Franco's PhD when this work started but sadly passed away in March 2009. We are grateful to Iñaki Tirados for help with the Ethiopian data, Simon Brooker and Steve Torr for useful discussions and comments on an earlier version of this work, and the Collective Dynamics group at the Instituto Gulbenkian de Ciência (Portugal) for helpful suggestions.

Author Contributions

Conceived and designed the experiments: AOF PGC CRD MGMG. Performed the experiments: AOF. Analyzed the data: AOF. Contributed reagents/materials/analysis tools: AOF MR. Wrote the paper: AOF MGMG PGC MR.

References

1. Zinsstag J, Schelling E, Waltner-Toews D, Tanner M (2011) From "one medicine" to "one health" and systemic approaches to health and well-being. Prev Vet Med 101: 148–156.
2. Escalar G (1933) Applicazione sperimentale della zooprofilassi in Ardea. Rivista di Malariologia 12: 373–380.
3. W.H.O. (1982) Manual on environmental management for mosquito control with special emphasis on mosquito vectors. Offset Publication No. 66. Geneva: World Health Organization. 283 p.
4. Hacket LW (1937) Malaria in Europe. Oxford, UK: Oxford University Press.
5. Brumpt E (1944) Revue critique: Zoophylaxie du paludisme. Annales de Parasitologie Humaine et Comparée 20.
6. Service MW (1991) Agricultural development and arthropod-borne diseases: a review. Revista de Saúde Pública 25: 165–178.
7. W.H.O. (1991) Joint WHO/FAO/UNEP/UNCHS Panel of Experts on Environmental Management for Vector Control (PEEM): Report on the Ninth (1989) and Tenth (1990) Meetings. Geneva, Switzerland: World Health Organization. WHO–CWS/91.7 WHO–CWS/91.7. 28 p.
8. Bettini S, Romi R (1998) [Zooprophylaxis: old and new problems]. Parassitologia 40: 423–430.
9. Franco AIO (2010) Effects of livestock management and insecticide treatment on the transmission and control of human malaria. PhD thesis. London School of Hygiene and Tropical Medicine, University of London, United Kingdom.
10. Charlwood JD, Dagoro H, Paru R (1985) Blood-feeding and resting behaviour in the *Anopheles punctulatus* Dönitz complex (Diptera: Culicidae) from coastal Papua New Guinea. Bulletin of Entomological Research 75: 463–475.
11. Burkot TR, Dye C, Graves PM (1989) An analysis of some factors determining the sporozoite rates, human blood indexes, and biting rates of members of the *Anopheles punctulatus* complex in Papua New Guinea. The American Journal of Tropical Medicine and Hygiene 40: 229–234.
12. van der Hoek W, Konradsen F, Dijkstra DS, Amerasinghe PH, Amerasinghe FP (1998) Risk factors for malaria: a microepidemiological study in a village in Sri Lanka. Transactions of the Royal Society of Tropical Medicine and Hygiene 92: 265–269.
13. Bouma M, Rowland M (1995) Failure of passive zooprophylaxis: cattle ownership in Pakistan is associated with a higher prevalence of malaria. Transactions of the Royal Society of Tropical Medicine and Hygiene 89: 351–353.
14. Hewitt S, Kamal M, Muhammad N, Rowland M (1994) An entomological investigation of the likely impact of cattle ownership on malaria in an Afghan refugee camp in the North West Frontier Province of Pakistan. Medical and Veterinary Entomology 8: 160–164.
15. Russel PF (1934) Zoophrophylaxis failure. An experiment in the Philipines. Rivista di Malariologia 13: 610–616.
16. Schultz GW (1989) Animal influence on man-biting rates at a malarious site in Palawan, Philippines. The Southeast Asian Journal of Tropical Medicine and Public Health 20: 49–53.
17. Ghebreyesus TA, Haile M, Witten KH, Getachew A, Yohannes M, et al. (2000) Household risk factors for malaria among children in the Ethiopian highlands. Transactions of the Royal Society of Tropical Medicine and Hygiene 94: 17–21.
18. Seyoum A, Balcha F, Balkew M, Ali A, Gebre-Michael T (2002) Impact of cattle keeping on human biting rate of anopheline mosquitoes and malaria transmission around Ziway, Ethiopia. East African Medical Journal 79: 485–490.
19. Habtewold T (2004) Interaction between *Anopheles*, cattle and human: exploration of the effects of various cattle management practices on the behaviour and control of *Anopheles arabiensis* in Ethiopia. PhD Thesis. Greenwich: University of Greenwich, U.K. 249 p.
20. Subramanian S, Manoharan A, Sahu S, Jambulingam P, Govardhini P, et al. (1991) Living conditions and occurrence of malaria in a rural community. Indian Journal of Malariology 28: 29–37.
21. Service MW (1993) Mosquito ecology. Field sampling methods. London: Chapman & Hall.
22. Gillies MT, De Meillon B (1968) The Anophelinae of Africa south of the Sahara. Publications of the South African Institute for Medical Research, No. 54. South African Institute for Medical Research, Johannesburg.
23. White BN, Magayuka SA, Boreham PFL (1972) Comparative studies on sibling species of the *Anopheles gambiae* Giles complex (Diptera Culicidae) bionomics and vectorial activity of species A and species B at Segera, Tanzania. Bulletin of Entomological Research 62: 295–317.
24. Charlwood JD, Edoh D (1996) Polymerase chain reaction used to describe larval habitat use by *Anopheles gambiae* complex (Diptera: Culicidae) in the environs of Ifakara, Tanzania. Journal of Medical Entomology 33: 202–204.
25. Minakawa N, Mutero CM, Githure JI, Beier JC, Yan G (1999) Spatial distribution and habitat characterization of anopheline mosquito larvae in

Western Kenya. The American Journal of Tropical Medicine and Hygiene 61: 1010–1016.
26. McLaughlin RE, Focks DA (1990) Effects of cattle density on New Jersey light trap mosquito captures in the rice/cattle agroecosystem of southwestern Louisiana. Journal of the American Mosquito Control Association 6: 283–286.
27. Saul A (2003) Zooprophylaxis or zoopotentiation: the outcome of introducing animals on vector transmission is highly dependent on the mosquito mortality while searching. Malaria Journal 2: art. no.32.
28. Habtewold T, Walker AR, Curtis CF, Osir EO, Thapa N (2001) The feeding behaviour and *Plasmodium* infection of *Anopheles* mosquitoes in southern Ethiopia in relation to use of insecticide-treated livestock for malaria control. Transactions of the Royal Society of Tropical Medicine and Hygiene 95: 584–586.
29. Gupta S, Swinton J, Anderson RM (1994) Theoretical studies of the effects of heterogeneity in the parasite population on the transmission dynamics of malaria. Proceedings of the Royal Society of London Series B-Biological Sciences 256: 231–238.
30. Collins WE, Jeffery GM (2003) A retrospective examination of mosquito infection on humans infected with *Plasmodium falciparum*. The American Journal of Tropical Medicine and Hygiene 68: 366–371.
31. USDA (1976)Control of insects affecting livestock. 99 p.
32. Thomson MC (1987) The effect on tsetse flies (*Glossina* spp.) of deltamethrin applied to cattle either as a spray or incorporated into ear-tags. Tropical Pest Management 33: 329–335.
33. Bekele J, Asmare K, Abebe G, Ayelet G, Gelaye E (2010) Evaluation of Deltamethrin applications in the control of tsetse and trypanosomosis in the southern rift valley areas of Ethiopia. Vet Parasitol 168: 177–184.
34. Bardosh K, Waiswa C, Welburn SC (2013) Conflict of interest: use of pyrethroids and amidines against tsetse and ticks in zoonotic sleeping sickness endemic areas of Uganda. Parasit Vectors 6: 204.
35. Torr SJ, Maudlin I, Vale GA (2007) Less is more: restricted application of insecticide to cattle to improve the cost and efficacy of tsetse control. Medical and Veterinary Entomology 21: 53–64.
36. George JE (2000) Present and future technologies for tick control. Ann N Y Acad Sci 916: 583–588.
37. Foil LD, Hogsette JA (1994) Biology and control of tabanids, stable flies and horn flies. Revue Scientifique et Technique (International Office of Epizootics) 13: 1125–1158.
38. Schmidtmann ET, Lloyd JE, Bobian RJ, Kumar R, Waggoner JW, et al. (2001) Suppression of mosquito (Diptera: Culicidae) and black fly (Diptera: Simuliidae) blood feeding from Hereford cattle and ponies treated with permethrin. Journal of Medical Entomology 38: 728–734.
39. Nasci RS, McLaughlin RE, Focks D, Billodeaux JS (1990) Effect of topically treating cattle with permethrin on blood feeding of *Psorophora columbiae* (Diptera: Culicidae) in a southwestern Louisiana rice-pasture ecosystem. Journal of Medical Entomology 27: 1031–1034.
40. Standfast HA, Muller MJ, Wilson DD (1984) Mortality of *Culicoides brevitarsis* (Diptera: Ceratopogonidae) fed on cattle treated with ivermectin. Journal of Economic Entomology 77: 419–421.
41. Rowland M, Durrani N, Kenward M, Mohammed N, Urahman H, et al. (2001) Control of malaria in Pakistan by applying deltamethrin insecticide to cattle: a community-randomised trial. Lancet 357: 1837–1841.
42. Reisen WK, Milby MM (1986) Population dynamics of some Pakistan mosquitoes: changes in adult relative abundance over time and space. Annals of Tropical Medicine and Parasitology 80: 53–68.
43. Habtewold T, Prior A, Torr SJ, Gibson G (2004) Could insecticide-treated cattle reduce Afrotropical malaria transmission? Effects of deltamethrin-treated Zebu on *Anopheles arabiensis* behaviour and survival in Ethiopia. Medical and Veterinary Entomology 18: 408–417.
44. Mahande AM, Mosha FW, Mahande JM, Kweka EJ (2007) Role of cattle treated with deltamethrin in areas with a high population of *Anopheles arabiensis* in Moshi, Northern Tanzania. Malaria Journal 6: 109.
45. Chareonviriyaphap T (2012) Behavioral Responses of Mosquitoes to Insecticides, Insecticides - Pest Engineering, Dr. Farzana Perveen (Ed.). InTech. Available from: http://www.intechopen.com/download/get/type/pdfs/id/28262 (Accessed 1 August 2013).
46. Lines JD, Myamba J, Curtis CF (1987) Experimental hut trials of permethrin-impregnated mosquito nets and eave curtains against malaria vectors in Tanzania. Medical and Veterinary Entomology 1: 37–51.
47. Takken W (2002) Do insecticide-treated bednets have an effect on malaria vectors? Tropical Medicine & International Health 7: 1022–1030.
48. Charlwood JD, Graves PM (1987) The effect of permethrin-impregnated bednets on a population of *Anopheles farauti* in coastal Papua New Guinea. Medical and Veterinary Entomology 1: 319–327.
49. Magesa SM, Wilkes TJ, Mnzava AE, Njunwa KJ, Myamba J, et al. (1991) Trial of pyrethroid impregnated bednets in an area of Tanzania holoendemic for malaria. Part 2. Effects on the malaria vector population. Acta Tropica 49: 97–108.
50. Githeko AK, Adungo NI, Karanja DM, Hawley WA, Vulule JM, et al. (1996) Some observations on the biting behavior of *Anopheles gambiae s.s.*, *Anopheles arabiensis*, and *Anopheles funestus* and their implications for malaria control. Experimental Parasitology 82: 306–315.
51. Bøgh C, Pedersen EM, Mukoko DA, Ouma JH (1998) Permethrin-impregnated bednet effects on resting and feeding behaviour of lymphatic filariasis vector mosquitoes in Kenya. Medical and Veterinary Entomology 12: 52–59.
52. Kolaczinski JH, Reithinger R, Worku DT, Ocheng A, Kasimiro J, et al. (2008) Risk factors of visceral leishmaniasis in East Africa: a case-control study in Pokot territory of Kenya and Uganda. International Journal of Epidemiology 37: 344–352.
53. McLaughlin RE, Focks DA, Dame DA (1989) Residual activity of permethrin on cattle as determined by mosquito bioassays. Journal of the American Mosquito Control Association 5: 60–63.
54. Hewitt S, Rowland M (1999) Control of zoophilic malaria vectors by applying pyrethroid insecticides to cattle. Tropical Medicine & International Health 4: 481–486.
55. Vythilingam I, Ridhawati, Sani RA, Singh KI (1993) Residual activity of cyhalothrin 20% EC on cattle as determined by mosquito bioassays. Southeast Asian J Trop Med Public Health 24: 544–548.
56. Elliot M (1989) The pyrethroids: early discovery, recent advances and the future. Pesticide Science 27: 337–351.
57. W.H.O. (1990) Deltamethrin. Environmental Health Criteria 97. Geneva: World Health Organization.
58. Okumu FO, Killeen GF, Ogoma S, Biswaro L, Smallegange RC, et al. (2010) Development and field evaluation of a synthetic mosquito lure that is more attractive than humans. PLoS One 5: e8951.
59. Jawara M, Awolola TS, Pinder M, Jeffries D, Smallegange RC, et al. (2011) Field testing of different chemical combinations as odour baits for trapping wild mosquitoes in The Gambia. PLoS One 6: e19676.
60. Ross R (1911) The Prevention of Malaria. London: Murray.
61. Macdonald G (1952) The analysis of equilibrium in malaria. Tropical Diseases Bulletin 49: 813–829.
62. Nåsell I (1985) Hybrid Models of Tropical Infections. In: Levin S, editor.Lecture Notes in Biomathematics. New York: Springer-Verlag. pp. 46–50.
63. Sota T, Mogi M (1989) Effectiveness of zooprophylaxis in malaria control: a theoretical inquiry, with a model for mosquito populations with two bloodmeal hosts. Medical and Veterinary Entomology 3: 337–345.
64. Killeen GF, McKenzie FE, Foy BD, Bogh C, Beier JC (2001) The availability of potential hosts as a determinant of feeding behaviours and malaria transmission by African mosquito populations. Transactions of the Royal Society of Tropical Medicine and Hygiene 95: 469–476.
65. Killeen GF, Smith TA (2007) Exploring the contributions of bed nets, cattle, insecticides and excitorepellency to malaria control: a deterministic model of mosquito host-seeking behaviour and mortality. Transactions of the Royal Society of Tropical Medicine and Hygiene 101: 867–880.
66. Kawaguchi I, Sasaki A, Mogi M (2004) Combining zooprophylaxis and insecticide spraying: a malaria- control strategy limiting the development of insecticide resistance in vector mosquitoes. Proceedings of the Royal Society of London Series B-Biological Sciences 271: 301–309.
67. Hurd H (2003) Manipulation of medically important insect vectors by their parasites. Annual Review of Entomology 48: 141–161.
68. Lord CC, Woolhouse MEJ, Heesterbeek JAP (1996) Vector-borne diseases and the basic reproduction number: a case study of African horse sickness. Medical and Veterinary Entomology 10: 19–28.
69. Charlwood JD, Smith T, Kihonda J, Heiz B, Billingsley PF, et al. (1995) Density independent feeding success of malaria vectors (Diptera: Culicidae) in Tanzania. Bulletin of Entomological Research 85: 29–35.
70. Anderson RM, May RM (1991) Infectious Diseases of Humans: Dynamics and Control. Oxford: Oxford University Press.
71. Diekmann O, Heesterbeek JA, Metz JA (1990) On the definition and the computation of the basic reproduction ratio R0 in models for infectious diseases in heterogeneous populations. Journal of Mathematical Biology 28: 365–382.
72. van den Driessche P, Watmough J (2002) Reproduction numbers and sub-threshold endemic equilibria for compartmental models of disease transmission. Mathematical Biosciences 180: 29–48.
73. IVCC. Proceedings of the Innovative Vector Control Consortium (IVCC) - Insect Repellent Workshop; 2007 22–23 January; London, UK.
74. Rayaisse JB, Tirados I, Kaba D, Dewhirst SY, Logan JG, et al. (2010) Prospects for the development of odour baits to control the tsetse flies Glossina tachinoides and G. palpalis s.l. PLoS Negl Trop Dis 4: e632.
75. Vale GA, Lovemore DF, Flint S, Cockbill GF (1988) Odour-baited targets to control tsetse flies, Glossina spp. (Diptera: Glossinidae), in Zimbabwe. Bulletin of Entomological Research 78: 31–49.
76. Vale GA, Hall DR (1985) The role of 1-octen-3-ol, acetone and carbon dioxide in the attraction of tsetse flies, Glossina spp. (Diptera: Glossinidae), to ox odour. Bulletin of Entomological Research 75: 209–218.
77. Chaniotis BN (1983) Improved trapping of phlebotomine sand flies (Diptera: Psychodidae) in light traps supplemented with dry ice in a neotropical rain forest. J Med Entomol 20: 222–223.
78. Coluzzi M, Sabatini A, Petrarca V, Di Deco MA (1979) Chromosomal differentiation and adaptation to human environments in the *Anopheles gambiae* complex. Transactions of the Royal Society of Tropical Medicine and Hygiene 73: 483–497.
79. Donnelly MJ, Townson H (2000) Evidence for extensive genetic differentiation among populations of the malaria vector *Anopheles arabiensis* in Eastern Africa. Insect Molecular Biology 9: 357–367.

80. Petrarca V, Nugud AD, Ahmed MA, Haridi AM, Di Deco MA, et al. (2000) Cytogenetics of the *Anopheles gambiae* complex in Sudan, with special reference to *An. arabiensis*: relationships with East and West African populations. Medical and Veterinary Entomology 14: 149–164.
81. Curtis CF, Miller JE, Hodjati MH, Kolaczinski JH, Kasumba I (1998) Can anything be done to maintain the effectiveness of pyrethroid-impregnated bednets against malaria vectors? Philosophical Transactions of the Royal Society of London Series B, Biological Sciences 353: 1769–1775.
82. Ranson H, N'Guessan R, Lines J, Moiroux N, Nkuni Z, et al. (2011) Pyrethroid resistance in African anopheline mosquitoes: what are the implications for malaria control? Trends Parasitol 27: 91–98.
83. Beugnet F, Chardonnet L (1995) Tick resistance to pyrethroids in New Caledonia. Veterinary Parasitology 56: 325–338.
84. Rodriguez-Vivas RI, Alonso-Díaz MA, Rodríguez-Arevalo F, Fragoso-Sanchez H, Santamaria VM, et al. (2006) Prevalence and potential risk factors for organophosphate and pyrethroid resistance in *Boophilus microplus* ticks on cattle ranches from the State of Yucatan, Mexico. Veterinary Parasitology 136: 335–342.
85. Wilson ML (1993) Avermectins in arthropod vector management - prospects and pitfalls. Parasitology Today 9: 83–87.
86. Fritz ML, Siegert PY, Walker ED, Bayoh MN, Vulule JR, et al. (2009) Toxicity of bloodmeals from ivermectin-treated cattle to *Anopheles gambiae s.l.* Annals of Tropical Medicine and Parasitology 103: 539–547.
87. Fritz ML, Walker ED, Miller JR (2012) Lethal and sublethal effects of avermectin/milbemycin parasiticides on the African malaria vector, Anopheles arabiensis. J Med Entomol 49: 326–331.
88. Kobylinski KC, Foy BD, Richardson JH (2012) Ivermectin inhibits the sporogony of Plasmodium falciparum in Anopheles gambiae. Malar J 11: 381.
89. Warrel DA, Gilles HM (2002) Essential Malariology. London: Hodder Arnold. 348 p.
90. Nedelman J (1985) Some New Thoughts About Some Old Malaria Models - Introductory Review. Mathematical Biosciences 73: 159–182.
91. Molineaux L (1988) The epidemiology of humans malaria as an explanation of its distribution, including some implications for its control. In: Wernsdorfer WH, McGregor SI, editors. Malaria, Principles and Practice of Malariology.London: Churchill Livingstone. pp. 913–998.
92. Mahmood F, Reisen WK (1981) Duration of the gonotrophic cycles of *Anopheles culicifacies* Giles and *An. stephensi* Liston, with observations on reproductive activity and survivorship during winter. Mosquito News 41: 22–30.
93. Krafsur ES (1977) The bionomics and relative prevalence of *Anopheles* species with respect to the transmission of *Plasmodium* to man in western Ethiopia. Journal of Medical Entomology 14: 180–194.
94. Krafsur ES, Armstrong JC (1982) Epidemiology of *Plasmodium malariae* infection in Gambella, Ethiopia. Parassitologia 24: 105–120.
95. Verhage DF, Telgt DS, Bousema JT, Hermsen CC, van Gemert GJ, et al. (2005) Clinical outcome of experimental human malaria induced by *Plasmodium falciparum*-infected mosquitoes. The Netherlands Journal of Medicine 63: 52–58.
96. Rickman LS, Jones TR, Long GW, Paparello S, Schneider I, et al. (1990) *Plasmodium falciparum* -infected *Anopheles stephensi* inconsistently transmit malaria to humans. The American Journal of Tropical Medicine and Hygiene 43: 441–445.
97. Taye A, Hadis M, Adugna N, Tilahun D, Wirtz RA (2006) Biting behavior and *Plasmodium* infection rates of *Anopheles arabiensis* from Sille, Ethiopia. Acta Tropica 97: 50–54.
98. Reisen WK, Boreham PF (1982) Estimates of malaria vectorial capacity for *Anopheles culicifacies* and *Anopheles stephensi* in rural Punjab province Pakistan. Journal of Medical Entomology 19: 98–103.
99. Tirados I, Costantini C, Gibson G, Torr SJ (2006) Blood-feeding behaviour of the malarial mosquito *Anopheles arabiensis*: implications for vector control. Medical and Veterinary Entomology 20: 425–437.

PERMISSIONS

All chapters in this book were first published in PLOS ONE, by The Public Library of Science; hereby published with permission under the Creative Commons Attribution License or equivalent. Every chapter published in this book has been scrutinized by our experts. Their significance has been extensively debated. The topics covered herein carry significant findings which will fuel the growth of the discipline. They may even be implemented as practical applications or may be referred to as a beginning point for another development.

The contributors of this book come from diverse backgrounds, making this book a truly international effort. This book will bring forth new frontiers with its revolutionizing research information and detailed analysis of the nascent developments around the world.

We would like to thank all the contributing authors for lending their expertise to make the book truly unique. They have played a crucial role in the development of this book. Without their invaluable contributions this book wouldn't have been possible. They have made vital efforts to compile up to date information on the varied aspects of this subject to make this book a valuable addition to the collection of many professionals and students.

This book was conceptualized with the vision of imparting up-to-date information and advanced data in this field. To ensure the same, a matchless editorial board was set up. Every individual on the board went through rigorous rounds of assessment to prove their worth. After which they invested a large part of their time researching and compiling the most relevant data for our readers.

The editorial board has been involved in producing this book since its inception. They have spent rigorous hours researching and exploring the diverse topics which have resulted in the successful publishing of this book. They have passed on their knowledge of decades through this book. To expedite this challenging task, the publisher supported the team at every step. A small team of assistant editors was also appointed to further simplify the editing procedure and attain best results for the readers.

Apart from the editorial board, the designing team has also invested a significant amount of their time in understanding the subject and creating the most relevant covers. They scrutinized every image to scout for the most suitable representation of the subject and create an appropriate cover for the book.

The publishing team has been an ardent support to the editorial, designing and production team. Their endless efforts to recruit the best for this project, has resulted in the accomplishment of this book. They are a veteran in the field of academics and their pool of knowledge is as vast as their experience in printing. Their expertise and guidance has proved useful at every step. Their uncompromising quality standards have made this book an exceptional effort. Their encouragement from time to time has been an inspiration for everyone.

The publisher and the editorial board hope that this book will prove to be a valuable piece of knowledge for researchers, students, practitioners and scholars across the globe.

LIST OF CONTRIBUTORS

Rafael A. Molina-López
Centre de Fauna Salvatge de Torreferrussa, Catalan Wildlife-Service, Forestal Catalana, Spain
Departament de Sanitat i Anatomia Animals, Faculty of Veterinary, Universitat Autònoma de Barcelona, Barcelona, Spain

Jordi Casal and Laila Darwich
Departament de Sanitat i Anatomia Animals, Faculty of Veterinary, Universitat Autònoma de Barcelona, Barcelona, Spain
Centre de Recerca en Sanitat Animal, UAB-IRTA, Campus Universitat Autònoma de Barcelona, Barcelona, Spain

Daniela Meloni, Katia Varello, Cristina Casalone,Cristiano Corona, Francesco Ingravalle and Elena Bozzetta
Centro di Referenza Nazionale per le Encefalopatie Animali, Istituto Zooprofilattico Sperimentale del Piemonte, Liguria e Valle d'Aosta, Turin, Italy

Aart Davidse and Jan P. M. Langeveld
Central Veterinary Institute of Wageningen UR, Lelystad, The Netherlands

Anne Balkema-Buschmann and Martin H. Groschup
Friedrich-Loeffler Institut, Federal Research Institute for Animal Health, Insel Riems, Germany

Zunita Zakaria, Latiffah Hassan and Chen Hui Cheng
Faculty of Veterinary Medicine Universiti Putra Malaysia, Serdang, Malaysia

Erkihun Aklilu
Faculty of Veterinary Medicine Universiti Putra Malaysia, Serdang, Malaysia
Faculty of Veterinary Medicine, Universiti Malaysia Kelantan, Pengkalan Chepa, Kota Bharu, Malaysia

Charlotte C. Burn
Veterinary Clinical Sciences, The Royal Veterinary College, North Mymms, Hertfordshire, United Kingdom

Jessica M. Hoffman and Daniel E.L. Promislow
Department of Genetics, University of Georgia, Athens, Georgia, United States of America,

Kate E. Creevy
Department of Small Animal Medicine and Surgery, College of Veterinary Medicine, University of Georgia, Athens, Georgia, United States of America

Jean-Jacques Panthier
CNM Project, Université Paris-Est Créteil, Ecole Nationale Vétérinaire d'Alfort, Maisons-Alfort, France
UMR955 de Génétique Fonctionnelle et Médicale, Institut National de la Recherche
Mouse Functional Genetics URA2578, Centre National de la Recherche Scientifique, Institut Pasteur, Paris, France

Jérôme Mary
CNM Project, Université Paris-Est Créteil, Ecole Nationale Vétérinaire d'Alfort, Maisons-Alfort, France
UMR955 de Génétique Fonctionnelle et Médicale, Institut National de la Recherche Antagene, La Tour de Salvagny, France

Marie Maurer, Laurent Guillaud, Laurent Guillaud, Geneviève Aubin-Houzelstein and Laurent Tiret
CNM Project, Université Paris-Est Créteil, Ecole Nationale Vétérinaire d'Alfort, Maisons-Alfort, France
UMR955 de Génétique Fonctionnelle et Médicale, Institut National de la Recherche Agronomique, Maisons-Alfort, France
Antagene, La Tour de Salvagny, France

Marilyn Fender
CNM Project, Pickett, Wisconsin, United States of America

Thomas Bilzer
Institut für Neuropathologie, Heinrich-Heine-Universität, Düsseldorf, Germany

Natasha Olby
College of Veterinary Medicine, Neurology Faculty, North Carolina State University, Raleigh, North Carolina, United States of America

Jacques Penderis
College of Medical, Veterinary and Life Science, School of Veterinary Medicine, University of Glasgow, Glasgow, United Kingdom

G. Diane Shelton
Department of Pathology, University of California San Diego, La Jolla, California, United States of America

Jean-Laurent Thibaud, Inés Barthélémy and Stéphane Blot
Unité Propre de Recherche de Neurobiologie, Université Paris-Est Créteil, Ecole Nationale Vétérinaire d'Alfort, Maisons-Alfort, France

Christophe Hitte
UMR6290, Centre National de la Recherche Scientifique, Institut de Génétique et Développement de Rennes, Université de Rennes1, Rennes, France

Lena Maria Lorenz
London School of Hygiene and Tropical Medicine, Department of Disease Control, London, United Kingdom

Marta Ferreira Maia
London School of Hygiene and Tropical Medicine, Department of Disease Control, London, United Kingdom
Ifakara Health Institute, Bagamoyo, Pwani Region, United Republic of Tanzania

Ayimbire Abonuusum
Kumasi Centre for Collaborative Research in Tropical Medicine, Kumasi, Ghana

Rolf Garms and Thomas Kruppa
Bernhard-Nocht Institute for Tropical Medicine, Hamburg, Germany

Peter-Henning Clausen and Burkhard Bauer
Free University of Berlin, Faculty of Veterinary Medicine Institute for Parasitology and Tropical Veterinary Medicine, Berlin, Germany

John D. Mitchell and Declan J. McKeever
Royal Veterinary College, Hatfield, Hertfordshire, United Kingdom

Quintin A. McKellar
University of Hertfordshire, Hatfield, Hertfordshire, United Kingdom

Benjamin M. Croak, Mathew S. Crowther and Richard Shine
School of Biological Sciences A08, University of Sydney, Camperdown, New South Wales, Australia

Jonathan K. Webb
School of the Environment, University of Technology Sydney, Broadway, New South Wales, Australia

Kyoung-Min Lee and Kyung-Ha Ahn
Department of Neurology, Seoul National University Hospital, Seoul, Republic of Korea

Johannes Charlier and Jozef Vercruysse
Department of Virology, Parasitology and Immunology, Faculty of Veterinary Medicine, Ghent University, Merelbeke, Belgium

Miel Hostens
Department of Reproduction, Obstetrics and Herd Health, Faculty of Veterinary Medicine, Ghent University, Merelbeke, Belgium

Jos Jacobs
Elanco Animal Health, Vosselaar, Belgium

Bonny Van Ranst
Uniform-Agri BV, Assen, The Netherlands

Luc Duchateau
Department of Physiology and Biometrics, Faculty of Veterinary Medicine, Ghent University, Merelbeke, Belgium

John C. Maerz, Amanda L. Coleman and Susan B. Wilde
D. B. Warnell School of Forestry and Natural Resources, University of Georgia, Athens, Georgia, United States of America

John R. Fischer
Southeastern Cooperative Wildlife Disease Study (SCWDS), Department of Population Health, Wildlife Health Building, College of Veterinary Medicine, University of Georgia, Athens, Georgia, United States of America

Albert D. Mercurio, Sonia M. Hernandez and Michael J. Yabsley
D. B. Warnell School of Forestry and Natural Resources, University of Georgia, Athens, Georgia, United States of America
Southeastern Cooperative Wildlife Disease Study (SCWDS), Department of Population Health, Wildlife Health Building, College of Veterinary Medicine, University of Georgia, Athens, Georgia, United States of America

Angela E. Ellis
The Athens Veterinary Diagnostic Laboratory, College of Veterinary Medicine, University of Georgia, Athens, Georgia, United States of America

Leslie M. Shelnutt
The University of Georgia College of Veterinary Medicine, University of Georgia, Athens, Georgia, United States of America

Helen M. Higgins and Martin J. Green
Population Health and Welfare Group, School of Veterinary Medicine and Science, University of Nottingham, Sutton Bonington, United Kingdom

Eamonn Ferguson
Personality, Social Psychology, and Health Research Group, School of Psychology, University of Nottingham, Nottingham, United Kingdom

Robert F. Smith
Division of Livestock Health and Welfare, School of Veterinary Science, University of Liverpool, Neston, United Kingdom

Liora Benhamou, Maya Bronfeld, Izhar Bar-Gad and Dana Cohen
The Leslie and Susan Gonda Multidisciplinary Brain Research Center, Bar-Ilan University, Ramat-Gan, Israel

Emanuela Dalla Costa, Michela Minero and Elisabetta Canali
Università degli Studi di Milano, Dipartimento di Scienze Veterinarie e Sanità Pubblica, Milan, Italy

Dirk Lebelt and Diana Stucke
Pferdeklinik Havelland / Havelland Equine Hospital, Beetzsee- Brielow, Germany

Matthew C. Leach
Newcastle University, School of Agriculture, Food & Rural Development, Newcastle upon Tyne, United Kingdom

Wendy Prudhomme O'Meara
Department of Medicine, Duke University School of Medicine, Durham, North Carolina, United States of America
Duke Global Health Institute, Durham, North Carolina, United States of America
Department of Epidemiology and Nutrition, Moi University School of Public Health, Eldoret, Kenya
United States Agency for International Development-Academic Model Providing Access to Healthcare Partnership, Eldoret, Kenya

Nathan Smith
Duke Global Health Institute, Durham, North Carolina, United States of America

Samson Ndege
Department of Epidemiology and Nutrition, Moi University School of Public Health, Eldoret, Kenya
United States Agency for International Development-Academic Model Providing Access to Healthcare Partnership, Eldoret, Kenya

Emmanuel Ekal
Ministry of Public Health and Sanitation, Nairobi, Kenya

Donald Cole
Division of Global Health, Dalla Lana School of Public Health, University of Toronto, Toronto, Ontario, Canada

Keren Cox-Witton, Rupert Woods and Victoria Grillo
Australian Wildlife Health Network, Mosman, New South Wales, Australia

Andrea Reiss and Martin Phillips
Zoo and Aquarium Association Australasia, Mosman, New South Wales, Australia

Rupert T. Baker
Healesville Sanctuary, Zoos Victoria, Healesville, Victoria, Australia

David J. Blyde
Sea World, Gold Coast, Queensland, Australia

Wayne Boardman and Ian Smith
Adelaide Zoo, Zoos South Australia, Adelaide, South Australia, Australia

Stephen Cutter and Dion Wedd
Territory Wildlife Park, Berry Springs, Northern Territory, Australia

Claude Lacasse
Australia Zoo Wildlife Hospital, Beerwah, Queensland, Australia

Helen McCracken
Melbourne Zoo, Zoos Victoria, Parkville, Victoria, Australia

Michael Pyne
Currumbin Wildlife Sanctuary, Currumbin, Queensland, Australia

Simone Vitali
Perth Zoo, South Perth, Western Australia, Australia

Larry Vogelnest
Taronga Zoo, Taronga Conservation Society Australia, Mosman, New South Wales, Australia

Chris Bunn and Lyndel Post
Australian Government Department of Agriculture, Canberra, Australian Capital Territory, Australia

Toyotaka Sato, Torahiko Okubo, Masaru Usui and Yutaka Tamura
Laboratory of Food Microbiology and Food Safety, Department of Health and Environmental Sciences, School of Veterinary Medicine, Rakuno Gakuen University, Ebetsu, Japan

Shin-ichi Yokota
Department of Microbiology, Sapporo Medical University School of Medicine, Sapporo, Japan

Satoshi Izumiyama
Nemuro District Agriculture Mutual Aid Association, Nakashibetsu, Japan

Miranda van Rijen
Laboratory for Microbiology and Infection Control, Amphia Hospital, Breda, The Netherlands

Erwin Verkade
Laboratory for Microbiology and Infection Control, Amphia Hospital, Breda, The Netherlands
Laboratory for Medical Microbiology and Immunology, St. Elisabeth Hospital, Tilburg, The Netherlands

Brigitte van Cleef
Laboratory for Microbiology and Infection Control, Amphia Hospital, Breda, The Netherlands
Laboratory for Medical Microbiology and Immunology, St. Elisabeth Hospital, Tilburg, The Netherlands
Centre for Infectious Disease Control Netherlands, National Institute for Public Health and the Environment, Bilthoven, The Netherlands

Jan Kluytmans
Laboratory for Microbiology and Infection Control, Amphia Hospital, Breda, The Netherlands
Laboratory for Medical Microbiology and Immunology, St. Elisabeth Hospital, Tilburg, The Netherlands
Department of Medical Microbiology, VU University medical centre, Amsterdam, The Netherlands

Marjolein Kluytmans-van den Bergh
Amphia Academy Infectious Disease Foundation, Amphia Hospital, Breda, The Netherlands

Birgit van Benthem, Thijs Bosch and Leo Schouls
Centre for Infectious Disease Control Netherlands, National Institute for Public Health and the Environment, Bilthoven, The Netherlands

Maria Chiara Ciuffreda
Department of Cardiothoracic and Vascular Sciences - Coronary Care Unit and Laboratory of Clinical and Experimental Cardiology, Fondazione IRCCS (IRCCS: Institute for Treatment and Research) Policlinico San Matteo, Pavia, Italy
Laboratory of Experimental Cardiology for Cell and Molecular Therapy, Fondazione IRCCS Policlinico San Matteo, Pavia, Italy

Valerio Tolva and Renato Casana
Surgical Department, IRCCS Istituto Auxologico Italiano, Milan, Italy

Massimiliano Gnecchi
Department of Cardiothoracic and Vascular Sciences - Coronary Care Unit and Laboratory of Clinical and Experimental Cardiology, Fondazione IRCCS (IRCCS: Institute for Treatment and Research) Policlinico San Matteo, Pavia, Italy
Laboratory of Experimental Cardiology for Cell and Molecular Therapy, Fondazione IRCCS Policlinico San Matteo, Pavia, Italy
Department of Molecular Medicine, Unit of Cardiology, University of Pavia, Pavia, Italy
Department of Medicine, Cape Town University, Cape Town, South Africa

Emilio Vanoli
Department of Cardiology, IRCCS Multimedica, Sesto San Giovanni, Milan, Italy

Carla Spazzolini
Center for Cardiac Arrhythmias of Genetic Base, IRCCS Istituto Auxologico Italiano, Milan, Italy

John Roughan
Institute of Neuroscience, Comparative Biology Centre, University of Newcastle, Newcastle upon Tyne, United Kingdom

Laura Calvillo
Laboratory of Cardiac Arrhythmias of Genetic Base, IRCCS Istituto Auxologico Italiano, Milan, Italy

Inge Santman-Berends, Gerdien Van Schaik and Maaike Gonggrijp
Department of epidemiology, GD Animal Health, Deventer, The Netherlands

Saskia Luttikholt, René Van den Brom and Piet Vellema
Department of small ruminant health, GD Animal Health, Deventer, The Netherlands

Han Hage
Department of cattle health, GD Animal Health, Deventer, The Netherlands

Manuela da Silva Solcà, Leila Andrade Bastos, Carlos Eduardo Sampaio Guedes, Marcelo Bordoni, Lairton Souza Borja and Washington Luis Conrado dos-Santos
Laboratório de Patologia e Biointervenção, Centro de Pesquisa Gonçalo Moniz–Fundação Oswaldo Cruz, Salvador, Bahia, Brazil

Daniela Farias Larangeira
Laboratório de Patologia e Biointervenção, Centro de Pesquisa Gonçalo Moniz–Fundação Oswaldo Cruz, Salvador, Bahia, Brazil

Escola de Medicina Veterinária, Universidade Federal da Bahia, Salvador, Bahia, Brazil

Pétala Gardênia da Silva Estrela Tuy and Leila Denise Alves Ferreira Amorim
Instituto de Matemática -Departamento de Estatística, Universidade Federal da Bahia, Salvador, Bahia, Brazil

Eliane Gomes Nascimento
Centro de Referência em Doenças Endêmicas Pirajáda Silva (PIEJ), Jequié, Bahia, Brazil

Deborah Bittencourt Mothé Fraga
Laboratório de Patologia e Biointervenção, Centro de Pesquisa Gonçalo Moniz-Fundação Oswaldo Cruz, Salvador, Bahia, Brazil
Escola de Medicina Veterinária, Universidade Federal da Bahia, Salvador, Bahia, Brazil
Instituto Nacional de Ciência e Tecnologia em Doenças Tropicais (INCT - DT), Salvador, Bahia, Brazil

Geraldo Gileno de SáOliveira and Patrícia Sampaio Tavares Veras
Laboratório de Patologia e Biointervenção, Centro de Pesquisa Gonçalo Moniz-Fundação Oswaldo Cruz, Salvador, Bahia, Brazil
Instituto Nacional de Ciência e Tecnologia em Doenças Tropicais (INCT - DT), Salvador, Bahia, Brazil

R. Michele Anholt and John Berezowski
Faculty of Veterinary Medicine, University of Calgary, Calgary, Alberta, Canada
Veterinary Public Health Institute, University of Bern, Bern, Switzerland

Carl S. Ribble and Craig Stephen
Faculty of Veterinary Medicine, University of Calgary, Calgary, Alberta, Canada
Centre for Coastal Health, Nanaimo, British Columbia, Canada

Margaret L. Russell
Community Health Sciences, University of Calgary, Calgary, Alberta, Canada

M. Gabriela M. Gomes
Instituto Gulbenkian de Ciência, Oeiras, Portugal

Ana O. Franco
Instituto Gulbenkian de Ciência, Oeiras, Portugal
Faculty of Infectious and Tropical Diseases, London School of Hygiene and Tropical Medicine, London, United Kingdom

Mark Rowland, Paul G. Coleman and Clive R. Davies
Faculty of Infectious and Tropical Diseases, London School of Hygiene and Tropical Medicine, London, United Kingdom

Index